FIFTH EDITION

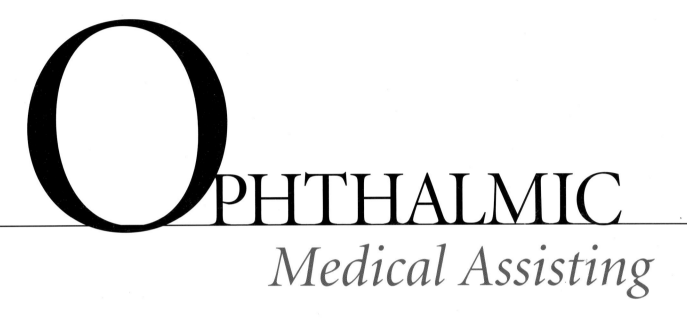

OPHTHALMIC
Medical Assisting

An Independent Study Course

Executive Editors:
Emanuel Newmark, MD, FACS
Mary A. O'Hara, MD, FACS, FAAP

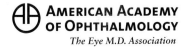

**AMERICAN ACADEMY
OF OPHTHALMOLOGY**
The Eye M.D. Association

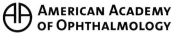
AMERICAN ACADEMY OF OPHTHALMOLOGY
The Eye M.D. Association

655 Beach Street
P.O. Box 7424
San Francisco, CA 94120-7424

Clinical Education Secretaries

Gregory L. Skuta, MD, *Senior Secretary for Clinical Education*
Louis B. Cantor, MD, *Secretary for Ophthalmic Knowledge*

Ophthalmology Liaisons Committee

Carla J. Siegfried, MD, *Chair*
Amy Chomsky, MD
JoAnn A. Giaconi, MD
Miriam T. Schteingart, MD
Samuel Solish, MD
Richard Allen, MD
Martha Schatz, MD
Kyle Arnoldi, CO, COMT
Diana Shamis, CO
Annquinetta F. Dansby-Kelly, RN, CRNO

Academy Staff

Richard A. Zorab, *Vice President, Ophthalmic Knowledge*
Hal Straus, *Director of Publications*
Susan R. Keller, *Acquisitions Editor*
Kimberly A. Torgerson, *Publications Editor*
D. Jean Ray, *Production Manager*
Denise Evenson, *Designer*
Debra Marchi, CCOA, *Administrative Assistant*

Authors/Revisers for This Edition

Emanuel Newmark, MD, FACS (Co-Executive Editor),
  Atlantis, Florida
Mary A. O'Hara, MD, FACS, FAAP (Co-Executive Editor),
  Sacramento, California
Donna M. Applegate, COT, New Albany, Indiana
D. Hunter Cherwek, MD, New York, New York
Neil T. Choplin, MD, San Diego, California
Peter C. Donshik, MD, FACS, Bloomfield, Connecticut
Lee R. Duffner, MD, FACS, Hollywood, Florida
Lindreth G. DuBois, MEd, MMSc, CO, COMT, Atlanta,
  Georgia
William H. Ehlers, MD, Avon, Connecticut
Mitchell J. Goff, MD, Salt Lake City, Utah
David A. Goldman, MD, Palm Beach Gardens, Florida
Damien F. Goldberg, MD, Torrance, California
Karl C. Golnik, MD, Cincinnati, Ohio
Erich P. Horn, MD, MBA, Oakland, California
Heather Machin, RN, Brisbane, Australia
Mark Mattison-Shupnick, ABOM, FNAO, Petaluma,
  California
Helen B. Metzler, COT, CCRP, ABO, Eugene, Oregon
Kenneth B. Mitchell, MD, Morgantown, West Virginia
Martha P. Schatz, MD, San Antonio, Texas
Larry B. Schwab, MD, Morgantown, Virginia
Frank W. Scribbick III, MD, San Antonio, Texas
Diana J. Shamis, MHSE, CO, COMT, Gainesville, Florida
Charles B. Slonim, MD, FACS, Tampa, Florida
Morgan L. Taylor III, CPA, COE, Atlantis, Florida
Sue J. Vicchrilli, COT, OCS, Murray, Utah
Jay S. Wallshein, MD, MBA, Atlantis, Florida

The Academy provides this material for educational purposes only. It is not intended to represent the only or best method or procedure in every case, nor to replace a physician's own judgment, directions, or orders, or give specific advice for case management. Including all indications, contraindications, side effects, and alternative agents for each drug or treatment is beyond the scope of this material. All information and recommendations should be verified, prior to use, with current information included in the manufacturers' package inserts or other independent sources, and considered in light of the patient's condition and history. Reference to certain drugs, instruments, and other products in this publication is made for illustrative purposes only and is not intended to constitute an endorsement of such. Some materials may include information on applications that are not considered community standard, that reflect indications not included in approved FDA labeling, or that are approved for use only in restricted research settings. The FDA has stated that it is the responsibility of the physician to determine the FDA status of each drug or device he or she wishes to use, and to use them with appropriate patient consent in compliance with applicable law. The Academy specifically disclaims any and all liability for injury or other damages of any kind, from negligence or otherwise, for any and all claims that may arise from the use of any recommendations or other information contained herein. The authors listed made a major contribution to this module. Substantive editorial revisions may have been made based on reviewer recommendations.

Financial Disclosures

The authors, reviewers, and consultants disclose the following financial relationships: **Peter C. Donshik, MD, FACS**: (C) Osuka; (S) CIBA Vision, Inspire Pharmaceuticals, Santen, Vistakon, Johnson & Johnson Vision Care. **Lindreth G. DuBois, MEd, MMSc, CO, COMT:** (P) SLACK; (S) National Eye Institute, Pfizer. **David A. Goldman, MD:** (C) Alcon Laboratories, Allergan, Bausch + Lomb Surgical, Lumenis. **Damien F. Goldberg, MD:** (C) Ista Pharmaceuticals, QLT, Santen; (L) Alcon Laboratories, Allergan. **Karl C. Golnik, MD:** (C) Alcon Laboratories. **Helen B. Metzler, COT, CCRP, ABO:** (C) Regneron; (E) Eli Lilly, Genentech, Neurotech, NIH, Novartis Pharmaceuticals, Pfizer. **Charles B. Slonim, MD, FACS:** (C, L) Bausch + Lomb Surgical. **Morgan L. Taylor III, CPA, COE:** (L) Lenstec.

The following contributors state that they have no significant financial interest or other relationship with the manufacturer of any commercial product discussed in the chapters that they contributed to this book or with the manufacturer of any competing commercial product: Donna M. Applegate, COT; Charlene S. Campbell, COMT; D. Hunter Cherwek, MD; Neil T. Choplin, MD; Lee R. Duffner, MD, FACS; William H. Ehlers, MD; JoAnn A. Giaconi, MD; Mitchell J. Goff, MD; Erich P. Horn, MD, MBA; Susan R. Keller; Heather Machin, RN; Kenneth B. Mitchell, MD; Emanuel Newmark, MD, FACS; Mary A. O'Hara, MD, FACS, FAAP; Martha P. Schatz, MD; Frank W. Scribbick III, MD; Diana J. Shamis, MHSE, CO, COMT; Kimberly A. Torgerson; Sue J. Vicchrilli, COT, OCS; Jay S. Wallshein, MD, MBA.

C = Consultant fee, paid advisory boards or fees for attending a meeting
E = Employed by a commercial entity
L = Lecture fees (honoraria), travel fees or reimbursements when speaking at the invitation of a commercial sponsor
S = Grant support for the past year (all sources) and all sources used for this project if this form is an update for a specific talk or manuscript with no time limitation

Library of Congress Cataloging-in-Publication Data

Ophthalmic medical assisting : an independent study course. -- 5th ed. / executive editors, Emanuel Newmark, Mary A. O'Hara.
  p. ; cm.
  Includes bibliographical references and index.
  ISBN 978-1-61525-153-7 (softcover)
  I. Newmark, Emanuel, 1936– II. O'Hara, Mary A., 1953– III. American Academy of Ophthalmology.
  [DNLM: 1. Ophthalmic Assistants--Programmed Instruction. 2. Eye Diseases--Programmed Instruction. 3. Ophthalmology--Programmed Instruction. WW 18.2]

  617.7'0232--dc23

                                                                    2011041159

Printed in the United States of America.
15 14 13 12 11   5 4 3 2 1

CONTENTS

PROCEDURE BOXES

PREFACE

The fifth edition of *Ophthalmic Medical Assisting: An Independent Study Course* boasts a new look and significant enhancements and additions. The editors updated the images to reflect current practice and added several chapters to appeal to a broader, worldwide audience. Unlike the practice of law, which is specific to the locality and country of origin, the practice of ophthalmology is universal and its sophistication dependent only upon the availability of newer diagnostic and treatment technologies. Therefore, we have adopted the fifth edition to include subjects outlined in the 2009 International Joint Commission on Allied Health Personnel in Ophthalmology (JCAHPO) Core Curriculum for Ophthalmic Assistants.

We kept all the fourth edition chapters with appropriate updates where indicated. We added a new chapter on strabismus and motility because it is an area that is often confusing to the novice learner and thus more difficult to master. We trust that you will find this new chapter easy to read and understand. We also added chapters on low vision and community eye health and set off the area of ethics and medical legal issues into a separate chapter in order to consolidate these items in one location. The glossary has been expanded to include new terminology, and the resources were updated to include more recent publications.

As in the previous edition, the fifth edition includes procedure boxes that outline in stepwise fashion the method to perform common clinical tests and other activities. Many of the boxes are enhanced with diagrams to augment the learning process. A list of procedure boxes in the front matter can be referenced for a quick review on "how to do it."

This study book can be utilized in a variety of educational settings; it can be the basis of an entire study course of ophthalmic assisting or a reference to be consulted as necessary. The companion course examination, available as a separate online product, partially fulfills the requirements for applying to take the assistant certifying examination offered by JCAHPO.

Acknowledgments

We thank our predecessors who originally developed this self-study course and all contributors past and present. Special thanks are extended to the Academy Ophthalmology Liaisons Committee, which provided the vision and guidance for this edition and assisted with review.

We are grateful for the work of the Academy staff and the generosity of our ophthalmology colleagues who so ably revised existing chapters and created new chapters. We extend special appreciation to the ophthalmic technicians who revised several chapters and the talented individuals specializing in the area of low vision, opticianry, and international eye care.

The following contributors reviewed the fourth edition for currency and served as peer reviewers for the fifth edition: Kyle Arnoldi, CO, COMT; Amy S. Chomsky, MD; JoAnn A. Giaconi, MD; James W. Gigantelli, MD, FACS; Mary A. O'Hara, MD, FACS, FAAP; Miriam T. Schteingart, MD; Carla J. Siegfried, MD; Samuel P. Solish, MD; and Mary Nehra Waldo, BSN, RN, CRNO. Mary A. O'Hara, MD, FACS, FAAP, contributed the new chapter on ocular motility and contributed to the chapter on low vision. Portions of the low vision chapter were reproduced from *Eye Care in Developing Nations*, fourth edition, by Larry Schwab, MD, with permission from Manson Publishing Ltd, London, UK. D. Hunter Cherwek, MD, Karl C. Golnik, MD, and Heather Machin, RN, developed the new chapter on community health eye care.

Many of the photographs were updated for this edition, thanks to the contributions of the following individuals: Richard Allen, MD; Neal H. Atebara, MD; Charlene S. Campbell, COMT; John J. Cardamone Jr; Brice Critser, CRA; JoAnn A. Giaconi, MD; Mitchell J. Goff, MD; David A. Goldman, MD; Susan Lewandowski, COA; Thomas D. Lindquist, MD, PhD; Mark Mattison-Shupnick, ABOM; William Mathers, MD; Emanuel Newmark, MD, FACS; Tina Newmark, RN, MS; Paris Royo, MD; and Jay S. Wallshein, MD, MBA. In addition, several companies contributed product photographs as examples of different kind of equipment: Accutome, Bausch + Lomb, Enhanced Vision, Haag-Streit USA, Icare Finland Oy, Lumenis Vision, Reichert Technologies, SciCan, The Harloff Company, and Topcon Medical Systems.

Finally, to the students, we congratulate you for choosing to study this critical and rewarding field of ophthalmic medical assisting.

Emanuel Newmark, MD, FACS
Mary A. O'Hara, MD, FACS, FAAP
Executive Editors

INTRODUCTION TO THE COURSE

To the Ophthalmologist

Ophthalmic medical assistants are an important part of the eye care team. They enhance the ophthalmologist's efforts and contribute significantly to the overall quality of patient care. But just as ophthalmic medical assistants do not practice independently, neither do they gain their professional training independently. In this sense, ophthalmologists are an important part of the assistant-training team. They not only instruct but also motivate the assistants they employ.

So even though this book is subtitled *An Independent Study Course*, it has been constructed with special attention to the ophthalmologist's role in the education and professional development of assistants, particularly those just beginning in the profession. To ensure that your assistants' training is as effective as possible, consider scheduling regular meetings to review and discuss the coursework together and present practical instruction that complements the course material presented.

It is important to recognize that the assistant will most effectively learn the practical skills presented in this book when reading of the text is regularly supplemented with hands-on, supervised training. Sponsoring ophthalmologists are encouraged to make such training available to their beginning assistants.

Text Instructional Features

Ophthalmic Medical Assisting: An Independent Study Course helps you direct your assistant's education by providing special instructional exercises and information at the end of each chapter, as described below.

Self-Assessment Test

These exercises can help you gauge your assistant's progress in understanding the basic course content. Encourage your assistant to respond to these study items as each chapter is completed (answers are found at the back of the textbook). Use the exercises as a springboard for discussion with your assistant to clarify some of the more

difficult concepts in ophthalmology and to discuss individual office policy.

Suggested Activities

These activities help your assistant integrate the course content into daily work responsibilities in your office. They suggest practical ways to apply each chapter's information and skills under the supervision of the ophthalmologist or staff member in charge of assistant training. By overseeing these activities, you can ensure that your assistant receives the information and guidance appropriate to practice and policy in your office. You may consider reviewing each chapter and developing additional or alternative activities to assign to your assistant.

Suggested Resources

These are listings of additional topic information available in various formats. You can help your assistant by reviewing these listings and recommending or supplying the resources that you feel are most helpful. You may consider using these suggestions in building a basic office reference library for your current and future ophthalmic medical assisting trainees.

Independent Study Course Examination

Students who work through this course textbook are encouraged to complete the companion course examination, available as a separate online product. Your participation as a sponsoring ophthalmologist, with the educational responsibility that implies, helps ensure that students functionally comprehend the concepts and skills presented in this course and can apply them to their work. The result is a well-trained, motivated, and confident ophthalmic medical assistant who truly contributes to your patients' well-being and to the efficient operation of your practice.

To the Student

Welcome to *Ophthalmic Medical Assisting: An Independent Study Course*. Please read this section before beginning your studies. It contains important information about the components and features of the course, with suggestions for completing the course successfully. Please also share this section and the preceding section, "To the Ophthalmologist," with the ophthalmologist in your office who will be overseeing your participation in this course.

Course Level

Ophthalmic Medical Assisting: An Independent Study Course is a program of self-study for beginners in the field. It assumes that you have at least completed high school, with some courses in basic science and mathematics, though you may have additional formal education beyond high school. The course also assumes that you have had at least 3 months' experience working in an ophthalmology office.

Course Components and Suggested Approaches

The complete course consists of this self-study textbook and the separate online examination, which is described below. You may elect to read the textbook from cover to cover for your own education, or you may turn to selected portions as needed for professional reference on the job. Alternatively, you may choose to test your knowledge by completing the multiple-choice online examination and obtain your examination score. Because of the complexity and diversity of the course content, plan to spend at least 3 months working through the textbook before attempting the course examination. Additional specific information about taking the examination based on this text and submitting it to the Academy appears later in this section and at the start of the online examination itself.

Sponsoring Ophthalmologist

Just as you perform your day-to-day duties on the job under the direction of an ophthalmologist, you will be most successful in this course if a sponsoring ophthalmologist is available to help you direct your studies, understand the material, and apply the course information and skills to your job responsibilities.

Textbook Organization and Features

This textbook presents a blend of fundamental medical and scientific information and basic practical skills often required of beginning ophthalmic medical assistants. Because you must frequently apply basic concepts or information from one chapter to more technically complex material in a succeeding chapter, it is strongly recommended that you read the chapters in order.

To add structure to your independent studies and gain the most from the course, use the following approach and in-text learning aids as described below.

Chapter Introductions

Each chapter begins with an overview of the chapter's content and its relevance to on-the-job ophthalmic medical assisting. The introductions describe the principal topics in the order in which you will encounter them and, as such, help you determine your learning objectives for each chapter.

Procedure Boxes

Numbered, step-by-step instructions for performing 44 basic ophthalmologic tests or procedures appear throughout the book. Share the instructions in these procedure boxes with your ophthalmologist or other trainer, who can assist you in performing a test or procedure for the first time and tell you whether certain procedures are performed differently in your office.

In addition, it is important to obtain hands-on instruction in the procedures you are expected to carry out in your office. Actual supervised training and practice under the guidance of an ophthalmologist or an experienced technician is the most effective way to ensure that you have mastered the practical skills presented in this book.

Self-Assessment Test

Answer the questions and study items at the end of each chapter soon after you read the chapter. You will gain the most by trying to answer the questions based on your recall of information rather than looking up the answers. Then check your responses against the Answers to Self-Assessment Tests grouped by chapter at the end of the book. Where definitions, descriptions, or explanations are called for, your response need not match the printed answer word for word as long as your response indicates that you understand the general concept. It is helpful to have your trainer check your responses to clarify any points you may not have understood. Make note of the questions you missed and reread the relevant portions of the text to make sure you understand the material before proceeding to the next chapter.

Suggested Activities

A list of activities follows the Self-Assessment Test at the end of each chapter. The activities suggest ways for you to apply the chapter's information to the development of your practical skills. They encourage not only independent investigation but also interaction with other staff members, and they frequently involve the guidance of the ophthalmologist or experienced office staff. Be sure the person overseeing your studies is aware of these activities, because many involve the supervised use of office materials and equipment.

Suggested Resources

This last part of each chapter directs you to suggested resources that you might use to further investigate the topics covered in the chapter.

Glossary

A glossary of more than 600 important terms used in the text appears at the end of the book. Pronunciations of scientific and technical terms are provided. Every term included in the glossary is also boldfaced upon its first significant appearance in the book, with its definition immediately following or appearing in nearby text. Occasionally, a term is boldfaced and defined more than once, especially if it has appeared in some chapters earlier.

Independent Study Course Examination

Successful completion of the optional course examination partially fulfills the requirements for applying to take the assistant certifying examination offered by the Joint Commission on Allied Health Personnel in Ophthalmology (JCAHPO). Becoming a certified ophthalmic medical assistant through the JCAHPO process has many professional benefits, which are described in Chapter 1 of this textbook. Contact information for JCAHPO also appears there, if you wish to obtain further information about their certifying examination. Successful completion of the *Ophthalmic Medical Assisting* course examination alone does not constitute professional certification as an ophthalmic medical assistant.

The fifth edition online examination is appropriate for use only with the fifth edition of *Ophthalmic Medical Assisting: An Independent Study Course*. The examinations for the different editions are not interchangeable.

The course examination consists of an online program with 228 multiple-choice questions. Each examination has its own identifying number and is intended for use by one student only. You are allowed to refer to the textbook to complete your examination.

Upon purchasing the online examination, the Academy registers you for the exam and records your identification number when you submit your completed answers. The online program electronically scores your examination right away, and returns the results to you, noting any questions you missed. Those receiving a passing grade receive a confirmation from the Academy verifying successful completion of the course, which serves as your permanent record. If you do not receive a passing grade, you may take the exam one more time (included in the initial purchase cost). The exam may be taken as many times as needed for additional purchase. Detailed information about completing and submitting the examination may be found in the examination booklet itself.

1 INTRODUCTION TO OPHTHALMIC MEDICAL ASSISTING

Welcome to ophthalmic medical assisting. You have chosen to learn more about a fascinating, rewarding, and growing profession. As an important member of the ophthalmic health care team, you will assist in the effort to prevent, detect, diagnose, and manage conditions that can interfere with one of our most precious senses: sight.

As an orientation to your study of ophthalmology and ophthalmic medical assisting, this chapter introduces you to the field of ophthalmology and to the members of the ophthalmic health care team. This chapter also includes important information about professional development and continuing education.

What Is Ophthalmology?

Ophthalmology is a specialized branch of medicine. This medical and surgical specialty is concerned with the eye and its surrounding structures, the eye's proper function, eye diseases and disorders, and all aspects of vision. Ophthalmology is one of the oldest specialties in medicine, dating back to the middle of the nineteenth century, when the ophthalmoscope was invented. The ophthalmoscope is an instrument used to examine the retina and optic nerve, which are structures in the back of the eye (Figure 1.1). This instrument provided the first opportunity for physicians to see blood vessels inside an organ without surgery. In addition, ophthalmology was the first medical specialty to develop a certification process.

The American Board of Ophthalmology administers a testing procedure to assure that every board-certified ophthalmologist has met an appropriate level of competence in the field. Most specialties of medicine now have a similar certifying process. Since 1992, recertification in ophthalmology has been required every 10 years.

Ophthalmology is an ever-changing specialty with amazing developments in the last 40 years. The ability to prevent and manage previously blinding eye

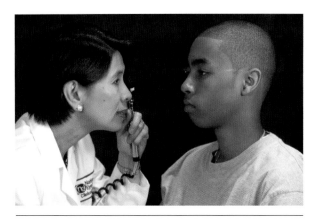

Figure 1.1   The ophthalmologist uses a direct ophthalmoscope to examine the structures in the back of the eye. *(Image courtesy of National Eye Institute, National Institutes of Health.)*

diseases has improved markedly, thanks to new technology and medications. One major medical advance of the last few decades is laser surgery for diabetic eye disease. Laser surgery dramatically reduces the complications that can lead to blindness in individuals with diabetes. Laser surgery and most types of minor eye surgery have been moved out of the hospital operating room and into the office setting (Figure 1.2).

Visual rehabilitation with intraocular lens implantation during cataract surgery can restore vision to countless patients who in past decades would have had to wear thick eyeglasses or contact lenses to achieve good vision. New kinds of intraocular lenses have been developed, which can reduce or eliminate the need for eyeglasses. Cataract surgery is now an outpatient procedure, requiring only a few hours' stay for most patients, rather than a several day stay in the hospital as in the past. Retinal

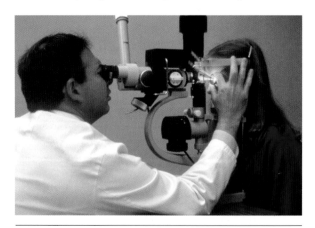

Figure 1.2   Today many laser and minor eye surgeries take place in the office setting, rather than in the hospital operating room.

detachment, a condition in which the light-sensitive tissue at the back of the eye becomes detached from the underlying layer, resulting in loss of peripheral vision or blindness, is now largely repairable through surgery. The most aggressive type of macular degeneration, a disease primarily affecting elderly patients, now has effective treatments, which can stabilize or even reverse central vision loss. Glaucoma, a disease associated with increased pressure inside the eye, is largely controllable. Contact lens technology has improved, and millions of people wear lenses comfortably to improve vision during all kinds of activities.

Who Provides Eye Care?

Internationally, various medical and nonmedical personnel participate in eye care. The multiplicity of participants may produce some confusion as to who specifically has what responsibilities for a patient's eye health and vision. The ophthalmic assistant should have a clear understanding about these individual health professionals and the role they play in eye health care.

Ophthalmologist

The **ophthalmologist** (sometimes referred to as an *eye physician and surgeon* or a *medical eye specialist*) is a medical doctor (MD, Doctor of Medicine degree, or DO, Doctor of Osteopathy degree) specializing in the prevention, diagnosis, and medical as well as surgical treatment of vision problems and eye diseases. An ophthalmologist typically completes a bachelor's degree to satisfy requirements for scientific training, 4 years of medical school, 1 year of postgraduate clinical experience, and at least 3 years of specialized ophthalmologic training (called a *residency* in ophthalmology). Ophthalmologists may also complete a fellowship (another 1 or 2 years of training) after residency in preparation for practice in a subspecialty area of ophthalmology (eg, retinal specialist).

An ophthalmologist's training prepares him or her to deal with a variety of problems, including correction of refractive errors with eyeglasses or contact lenses; repair of a lacerated or drooping eyelid; treatment of dry, crossed, or lazy eyes; or other eye disorders such as glaucoma, cataract, retinal detachment, diabetic retinopathy, or visual problems from brain tumors. Ophthalmologists not only diagnose and treat eye diseases but also strive to preserve vision through educating the public and patients about the best way to care for their eyes.

Although the majority of ophthalmologists are capable of treating the entire spectrum of eye conditions, some concentrate on conditions related to only one area of the eye. These ophthalmologists are called *subspecialists*. Ophthalmic subspecialists may focus their care on patients who have problems requiring orbital and plastic surgery (oculoplastics), corneal and external eye disease, or eye disorders such as glaucoma, retinal problems, or nerve problems (neuro-ophthalmology). *Pediatric ophthalmologists* are physicians who specialize in treating eye and vision difficulties primarily in children.

Optometrist

The **optometrist** is an independent practitioner who completes a 4-year postgraduate, doctoral-level course in optometry after typically obtaining a bachelor's degree. This training prepares optometrists to prescribe eyeglasses and contact lenses as well as to detect eye disease. In some states, optometrists are permitted to diagnose and medically treat some eye diseases. Doctors of optometry do not attend medical school and do not train to perform ophthalmic surgery, unlike ophthalmologists, who have a full medical education, followed by extensive clinical and surgical training in ophthalmology, with thousands of hours devoted to the care and treatment of sick patients.

Optician

The **optician** is an independent professional usually State licensed to make (dispense) eyeglasses and contact lenses according to prescriptions supplied by an ophthalmologist or optometrist. This professional is sometimes referred to as a *dispensing optician* or an *ophthalmic dispenser*. An optician can obtain his or her training through several models. Some enroll in an online independent study course, followed by a 6-month practicum. Others obtain a 2- to 4-year on-the-job apprenticeship program supervised by a licensed optician, optometrist, or ophthalmologist. Lastly, formal training is offered at some community colleges, leading to a 2-year associate's degree or a 1-year certificate.

Registered Nurse

A **registered nurse** completes a 2- to 4-year education program before taking an examination to be licensed as a professional registered nurse (RN). Ophthalmic RNs have additional experience, education, and training in caring for patients with problems related to the eye.

Ophthalmic RNs often provide direct care, perform ophthalmic diagnostic testing, plan and provide patient education, help patients find and use needed services, assist the ophthalmologist in surgery, or serve as directors of ophthalmic surgery or clinical services. RNs who have at least 2 years of experience in ophthalmic nursing and who pass a comprehensive written examination may use the credential *certified registered nurse in ophthalmology* (CRNO). Nurse practitioners or clinical nurse specialists are registered nurses with an advanced degree. They provide more complex ophthalmic nursing care such as taking preoperative histories, performing physical examinations, or assessing and treating patients at home and in various other clinical settings.

Orthoptist

The **orthoptist** is a specialized member of the ophthalmic medical personnel team. The orthoptist completes an undergraduate degree and then 2 years of postgraduate training before passing a national certifying examination. The orthoptist's areas of expertise include testing visual function, particularly in infants and children, evaluating eye muscle disorders, and evaluating impairments in binocular vision such as double vision. The orthoptist assists in diagnosis, management, and nonsurgical treatment of eye muscle imbalance and related visual impairments. Orthoptists work with and under the direction of ophthalmologists.

Ocularist

The **ocularist**, another specialized member of the ophthalmic team, fabricates and fits patients with prostheses (artificial eyes or shells), which replace a surgically removed eye or cover an unsightly eye. According to the American Society of Ocularists (ASO), typically a person learns how to make artificial eyes through an apprenticeship with an approved ocularist (a Board Approved Diplomate Ocularist). The ASO apprentice program requires the apprentice to spend 5 years (10,000 hours) in practical training and study all aspects of ocular prosthetics. Upon successful completion of all requirements, the ASO awards the title Diplomate of the American Society of Ocularists.

Ophthalmic Photographer

The **ophthalmic photographer** photographs the eye structures for diagnosis and documentation. Many ophthalmic medical assistants do photographic work in an ophthalmologist's office. However, to become a *certified* ophthalmic photographer, a person must undergo special training and also pass a competency examination.

Ophthalmic Medical Assistant

The term **ophthalmic medical assistant** is often used to describe any individual who helps the ophthalmologist with diagnostic and treatment-oriented procedures. Individuals, organizations, or publications may also refer to those who assist the ophthalmologist as *technical personnel*, *allied health personnel*, *technicians*, or *ophthalmic medical personnel*. For the sake of simplicity, this text uses the terms *ophthalmic medical assistant*, *ophthalmic assistant*, and *assistant* interchangeably to refer to individuals at the entry level of experience. As of January 2009, the ophthalmic allied health profession was approved as a separate occupational listing of "Ophthalmic Medical Technician" by the United States Bureau of Labor Statistics Standard Occupational Classification (SOC). The SOC listing recognizes ophthalmic personnel at all levels of certification offered by the Joint Commission on Allied Health Personnel in Ophthalmology (JCAHPO).

The ophthalmic medical assistant helps the ophthalmologist in a variety of diagnostic and administrative tasks. By assisting with tasks that do not require the ophthalmologist's specific expertise, a skilled ophthalmic medical assistant enables the ophthalmologist to spend quality time with the patient, completing only those diagnostic and treatment functions that the ophthalmologist must personally perform. This also allows the ophthalmologist to see and treat more patients. The ophthalmic medical assistant can, in effect, multiply the ophthalmologist's efforts.

The ophthalmologist may ask the ophthalmic medical assistant to perform the following tasks:

- Schedule and greet patients.
- Help patients to understand and adhere to physician-prescribed treatments.
- Perform certain tests and use ophthalmic instruments that provide diagnostic information.
- Assist with office surgical procedures.
- Administer topical medications or diagnostic drugs prescribed by the ophthalmologist for testing or treatment.

These tasks and others vary from office to office, depending on the individual ophthalmologist's needs and policies. Even so, ophthalmic medical assistants should always treat patients in a helpful, friendly manner. Certainly, ophthalmic medical assistants need not be either servile or overly familiar, but they should express an honest concern and respect for the individual patient through their facial expressions, voice, and behavior. A caring attitude, coupled with skill in your job and a professional manner and appearance, will allow you to make a significant contribution to the patient's overall well-being and total visual health. (See Chapter 20 for more information about medical ethics and how they affect you.)

What Is Certification?

JCAHPO is an organization established in 1969 to promote the education and utilization of allied health personnel in ophthalmology. Although JCAHPO employs the term *ophthalmic medical personnel* to denote all individuals who assist the ophthalmologist, the organization also recognizes that ophthalmic medical personnel do not all have the same degree of skill and education. A central part of JCAHPO's mission is the commitment to administer a certification process to acknowledge these differences. JCAHPO recognizes 3 core levels of certified ophthalmic medical personnel: *Certified Ophthalmic Assistant* (COA), *Certified Ophthalmic Technician* (COT), and *Certified Ophthalmic Medical Technologist* (COMT). JCAHPO also offers 3 additional specialty certifications: Certified Diagnostic Ophthalmic Sonographer (CDOS), Registered Ophthalmic Ultrasound Biometrist (ROUB), and Ophthalmic Surgical Assisting (OSA). Regardless of the level of credential or specialty, JCAHPO certification attests to the skills and knowledge of individuals at each of these levels after they meet certain educational and experiential prerequisites and pass a certification examination. This credential provides evidence to employers and patients that the certified individual has achieved a certain level of competence. The JCAHPO credential is similar to the certification received by physicians or nurses who have met the requirements of their respective certification processes.

The ophthalmic medical assistant grows professionally in stages by using a combination of reading, continuing education courses, formal instruction, and clinical experience.

Each successive core level of ophthalmic medical assisting requires more knowledge, skill, and experience, and individuals can make the transition from ophthalmic assistant to technician in a modular fashion. Although some individuals advance directly to one of the upper levels of certification through formal schooling, the certification process also allows an individual to achieve the first level of certification without formal schooling by completing an independent study course such as this one and working for a certain length of time under the supervision of an ophthalmologist. The certification procedure also permits individuals to advance to the next level of certification through a combination of continuing education and clinical experience, or by completing a formal training program. The CDOS, ROUB, and the OSA certifications, in addition to the 3 core levels, reflect specialization among ophthalmic medical personnel.

Although certification as an ophthalmic medical assistant is not necessary for the successful performance of the tasks required by this position and, to date, certification has not been required by any state law, JCAHPO certification can be an important part of a career in ophthalmic assisting. When you apply for an ophthalmic assisting position, certification assures potential employers that you have certain skills and knowledge. In addition, certification shows pride in your work and a professional attitude toward what you do.

You can obtain information about certification directly from JCAHPO:

Joint Commission on Allied Health Personnel in
    Ophthalmology
2025 Woodlane Drive
St Paul, MN 55125-2998
Telephone: 800-284-3937
E-mail: jcahpo@jcahpo.org
Internet: www.jcahpo.org

Professional Development

Membership in a professional organization is another important part of professional development. The Association of Technical Personnel in Ophthalmology (ATPO) is the professional organization for ophthalmic medical personnel. Although ATPO has a strategic alliance with JCAHPO to help them provide member services, increase efficiency, and contain costs, JCAHPO is not the membership organization for ophthalmic medical personnel. Certified individuals cannot "belong" to JCAHPO, but they achieve and maintain certification through

JCAHPO's certification and recertification processes. However, both certified and noncertified ophthalmic medical personnel *can* belong to ATPO. Joining ATPO helps strengthen this membership organization, allowing ATPO to effectively represent the interests of ophthalmic medical personnel and advance the profession. ATPO also provides numerous professional benefits relating to continuing education resources for ophthalmic medical personnel.

You can contact ATPO directly to find out more about member benefits:

Association of Technical Personnel in
    Ophthalmology
2025 Woodlane Drive
St Paul, MN 55125-2998
Telephone: 800-482-4858
E-mail: ATPOmembership@atpo.com
Internet: www.atpo.org

Ophthalmic medical personnel may also join other ophthalmic organizations such as the Ophthalmic Photographers Society (OPS) or the American Society of Ophthalmic Registered Nurses (ASORN) for continuing education opportunities or other activities.

JCAHPO certification not only implies a specific level of skill and knowledge but also, along with membership in ATPO or other ophthalmic organizations, signifies that the individual is interested in ongoing professional development and lifelong learning. This means a commitment to keeping your skills up to date and developing new ones through the process of continuing education.

Continuing education is obtained through courses, reading, and other educational activities. Courses are available through formal ophthalmic medical assistant training programs, hospitals, and colleges as well as through annual and regional continuing education programs. ATPO, OPS, ASORN, JCAHPO, and other ophthalmic organizations offer courses in conjunction with the annual meeting of the American Academy of Ophthalmology. The Academy is the membership organization representing the majority of ophthalmologists in the United States and Canada. Courses offered by the Academy and other organizations that meet at the same time may be useful for ophthalmic medical personnel.

Individuals wishing to obtain continuing education to maintain certification or advance to a higher level of certification must be sure that the continuing education activity is approved by JCAHPO. Many ophthalmic organizations apply for JCAHPO approval of their continuing education offerings. JCAHPO lists these courses on their website and in the JCAHPO/ATPO newsletter. You can receive this newsletter simply by asking to have your name added to the mailing list.

Many organizations publish newsletters or journals that list or provide continuing education opportunities that may be of interest to you. See Table 1.1 for additional information. The organizations most likely to be initially helpful for a newcomer to ophthalmic assisting are ATPO and JCAHPO. Both organizations offer continuing education opportunities year round at select regional and annual meetings, as well as through online resources such as webinars and the E-Learning website www. actioned.org.

Table 1.1 Selected Resources for Professional Development of Ophthalmic Personnel

ACTIONed: www.actioned.org

American Academy of Ophthalmology: www.aao.org

American Orthoptic Council: www.orthoptics.org

American Society of Ocularists: www.ocularist.org

American Society of Ophthalmic Registered Nurses: www.asorn.org

Association of Technical Personnel in Ophthalmology: www. atpo.org

Canadian Society of Ophthalmic Medical Personnel: www.eyesite.ca

Contact Lens Association of Ophthalmologists: www.clao.org

Contact Lens Society of America: www.clsa.info

Joint Commission on Allied Health Personnel in Ophthalmology: www.jcahpo.org

My Eye Career for Ophthalmic Medical Technicians: www.myeyecareer.org

Ophthalmic Photographers Society: www.opsnet.org

Opticians Association of America: www.oaa.org

SELF-ASSESSMENT TEST

1. Match the types of ophthalmic health professionals with their duties.

   _____ ocularist

   _____ ophthalmologist

   _____ optometrist

   _____ orthoptist

   _____ ophthalmic medical assistant

   _____ optician

   a. measures and fits patients with artificial eyes

   b. helps with diagnosis, management, and nonsurgical treatment of eye muscle imbalance

   c. dispenses eyeglasses and contact lenses from prescriptions supplied by others

   d. prescribes and/or fits eyeglasses and contact lenses and screens for eye diseases as a nonphysician professional

   e. prevents, diagnoses, and medically and surgically treats problems of the eye as a medical doctor

   f. helps the doctor in a variety of clinical and administrative tasks

2. List the 3 levels of certified ophthalmic assisting in order of level of training and experience.

3. Ophthalmic medical assistants may be required to do all tasks except which of the following?

   a. Perform diagnostic tests.

   b. Assist with office surgical procedures.

   c. Administer certain medications to patients.

   d. Diagnose patients' eye conditions.

   e. Schedule and greet patients.

4. Which of the following is a specialty certification offered by JCAHPO?

    a. SOC

    b. OSA

    c. ATPO

    d. COT

5. Ophthalmologists who confine their practice to diagnosing and treating a defined area of the eye or disease are called

    a. retinologists

    b. subspecialists

    c. oculist

    d. specialists

SUGGESTED ACTIVITIES

1. Contact the Association of Technical Personnel in Ophthalmology (ATPO) and the Joint Commission on Allied Health Personnel in Ophthalmology (JCAHPO) to request membership and certification information as well as other information on ophthalmic assisting as a career. The site, www.myeyecareer.com, is a resource developed by JCAHPO and offers additional information about a career in eye care.

2. Discuss with the doctor in your office what tasks you might be called upon to perform.

3. Meet with an experienced assistant in one or more ophthalmology offices to discuss the career path for the ophthalmic medical assistant.

4. Find out, from other assistants, whether there is a local group of ophthalmic medical assistants in your area that you could join. Such groups offer support through study and continuing education opportunities.

5. Ask the doctor in your office if you may observe a variety of patient visits to gain first-hand knowledge about the tasks of an ophthalmic medical assistant.

6. Interview the ophthalmic medical assistants in your office or in another ophthalmology practice and ask them to describe their daily routine, what they like best about their position, and what they like least about their duties.

7. Determine in what ways you can add to your basic and continuing education. For example, research what DVDs, audiotapes, books, and courses are available to you. Good resources to start with include the JCAHPO/ATPO newsletter *Viewpoints*, the ATPO website at www.atpo.org, the JCAHPO website and online bookstore at www.jcahpo.org, the E-Learning website at www.actioned.org, and the American Academy of Ophthalmology's annual product catalog.

SUGGESTED RESOURCES

Cassin B. *Fundamentals for Ophthalmic Technical Personnel.* Philadelphia: Saunders; 1995.

Cassin B, Rubin ML, eds. *Dictionary of Eye Terminology.* 5th ed. Gainesville, FL: Triad; 2006.

DuBois LG. Instrument maintenance. In: *Fundamentals of Ophthalmic Medical Assisting.* DVD. San Francisco: American Academy of Ophthalmology; 2009.

Introducing Ophthalmology: A Primer for Office Staff. 2nd ed. San Francisco: American Academy of Ophthalmology; 2002.

Ledford JK. *Handbook of Clinical Ophthalmology for Eyecare Professionals.* Thorofare, NJ: Slack; 2000.

Ledford JK., Hoffman J. *Quick Reference Dictionary of Eyecare Terminology.* 5th ed. Thorofare, NJ: Slack; 2008.

Riordan-Eva P, Whitcher JP, eds. *Vaughn & Asbury's General Ophthalmology.* 17th ed. New York: McGraw-Hill; 2008.

Stein HA, Stein RM. *The Ophthalmic Assistant: A Text for Allied and Associated Ophthalmic Personnel.* 8th ed. St Louis: Mosby; 2006.

2 ANATOMY AND PHYSIOLOGY OF THE EYE

The ability to see is produced by the actions of various parts of the eye, nerve cells, and the brain. These structures take form beginning in the second week of pregnancy. Problems during early pregnancy can cause congenital defects that can interfere with the development of vision. Structures surrounding the eye, such as the lids and lashes, protect and assist this organ in its visual function. If any component of the visual system fails to operate properly, sight may be impaired. The ophthalmic medical assistant plays an important role in helping the ophthalmologist detect, treat, and prevent disorders that may affect vision. To provide such help, the assistant must be able to describe and recognize the parts of the visual system and understand how they function. The assistant should be acquainted with the normal appearance of these structures and with deviations from normal.

This chapter introduces you to the eye as the primary organ of vision and to its surrounding structures. The chapter considers in detail the anatomy (structure) and physiology (function and operation) of the various parts of the visual system and discusses the relationship of the eye to the brain in the visual process. This chapter also introduces you to a set of diseases and disorders affecting the part of the eye under discussion. Chapter 3 discusses these conditions in depth.

The Eye as an Optical System

When a person looks at an object, that object reflects light rays to the eye. As the rays pass through the optical system of the **globe**, or **eyeball**, they are bent to produce an upside-down image of the object at the back of the inner eyeball. Here the image is converted to electric impulses that are carried to the brain, where the image is translated so that the object is perceived in its upright position.

The first part of the eye's optical system is the clear, round membrane at the front of the globe, called the **cornea**. This transparent membrane begins the process of focusing light the eye receives. Behind the cornea is a colored circle of tissue called the **iris**. The iris controls the amount of light entering the eye by enlarging or reducing the size of the opening in its center, called the **pupil**.

Immediately behind the iris is the **crystalline lens** (or, more simply, the **lens**), the second part of the optical focusing system of the eye. The large space behind the crystalline lens is filled with a clear, jelly-like substance called the **vitreous**, or vitreous body. Because the vitreous is optically transparent, light rays focused by the cornea and lens can pass through it unaffected to produce an image on the inner back surface of the eye, the **retina**. The light-sensitive cells of the retina convert the image to electric impulses that are carried to the brain by the **optic nerve**. The electric impulses are integrated in the brain's visual cortex to produce the sensation of sight. Figure 2.1 shows the principal structures involved in the eye as an optical system.

The Globe

The range of front-to-back or **axial length** of the normal eye is between 23 and 25 millimeters (mm) in length. The width is labeled at 24 mm. The central thickness of the cornea (known as **CCT**) is 545 micrometers (μm) or just over 0.5 mm. This can be measured either optically or

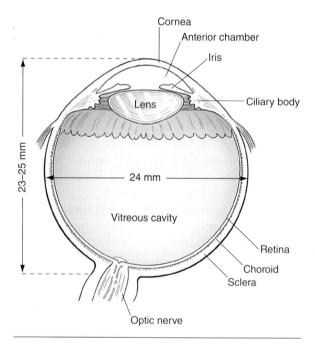

Figure 2.1 The eye as an optical system. *(Reprinted, with permission, from Chalam KV, Basic and Clinical Science Course, Section 2, Fundamentals and Principles of Ophthalmology, San Francisco: American Academy of Ophthalmology, 2011–2012.)*

with ultrasound with a test called **pachymetry**. The cornea is thinnest centrally and is thicker in the periphery to approximately 1000 μm or 1 mm. Corneal pachymetry is an important test to be performed in the evaluation of glaucoma. The average horizontal diameter of the cornea is 11.5 mm. The average **refracting power** of the cornea is 42 **diopters** and the average refracting power of the crystalline lens is 18 diopters. The total refracting power of the normal eye is therefore around 60 diopters.

The parts of the eye and their anatomy and physiology are considered in greater detail later in this chapter, following a discussion of the tissues that surround the eye.

The Adnexa

The tissues and structures surrounding the eye are called the **adnexa**. They include the orbit, the extraocular muscles, the eyelids, and the tear-producing and tear-draining lacrimal apparatus. These structures serve to protect and support the globe.

Orbit

The **orbit** is the pear-shaped bony cavity in the skull comprising 7 bones that house the globe, the extraocular muscles, the blood vessels, and the nerves, all of which are cushioned by layers of fat. The globe is situated within the bony orbit in such a way that it is protected from major injury by a rim of bone (Figure 2.2).

The bony orbit is surrounded by air-filled chambers called the sinuses. Nasal allergies or infections can spread to the sinuses and patients with sinus disease can complain of pain around the eye. Rarely, infections or cancers can spread to the orbit from the sinuses.

A fracture in the floor of the orbit that results from blunt-force trauma is termed a **blowout fracture**. Evaluation of the orbit is performed with conventional x-ray, computed tomography (CT) scanning, magnetic resonance imaging (MRI), and ultrasonography.

Extraocular Muscles

The muscles that control movement of the globe are called **extraocular muscles** to distinguish them from muscles inside the eyeball. The 6 extraocular muscles are named by their positions or attachments in relation to the globe. These attachments also determine the direction of movement of the eyeball when the muscles contract:

- The **medial rectus muscle** rotates the eye inward toward the nose, a movement called *adduction*.

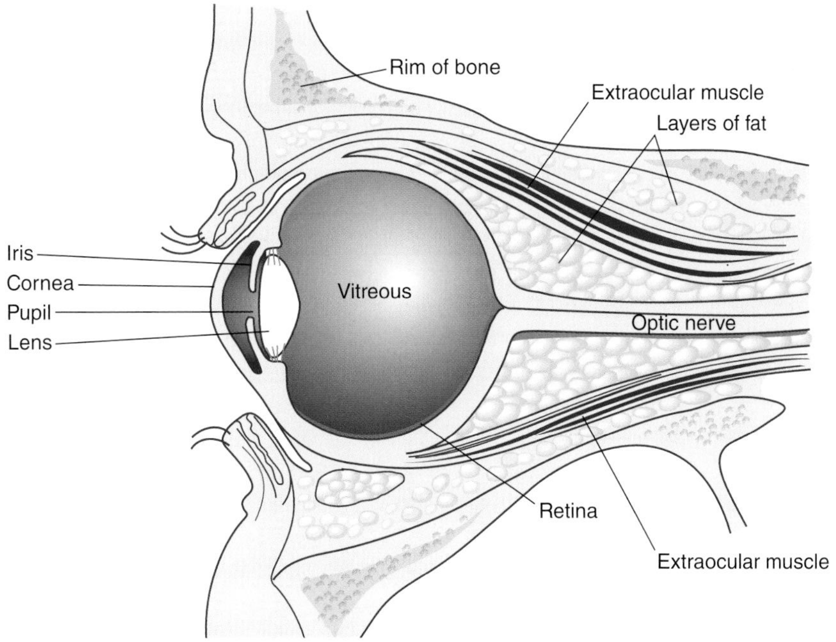

Figure 2.2 The orbit.

- The **lateral rectus muscle** rotates the eye outward toward the temple, a movement called *abduction*.

- The **superior oblique muscle** primarily causes a torsional movement and twists the eye down and inward, a movement called *incyclotorsion*.

- The **inferior oblique muscle** primarily causes a torsional movement and twists the eye up and outward, a movement called *excyclotorsion*.

- The **superior rectus muscle** is the primary muscle responsible for turning the eye upward. Secondarily incyclotorsion.

- The **inferior rectus muscle** is the primary muscle responsible for turning the eye downward. Secondarily excyclotorsion.

(See Figure 9.1 for anatomy of the extraocular muscles and Figure 9.2 for illustration of movements of the eye.)

Movement of the eye in most directions usually requires the coordinated contraction and relaxation of two or more muscles. For example, when a person looks directly upward, the superior rectus muscle acts together with the inferior oblique muscle to raise the eye, while the inferior rectus muscle and superior oblique muscle relax. When a person looks toward their nose, the medial rectus muscle contracts while the lateral rectus muscle relaxes.

In addition to the coordinated action of muscles in one eye, proper vision requires coordination of the contraction of muscles in the two eyes. The extraocular muscles must rotate each globe so that both eyes are directed toward the same target; that is, both eyes must be in visual alignment. Movement of the two eyes in visual alignment generally requires the coordinated action of different muscles for the left and right eyes. When a person looks to the right, the medial rectus muscle of the left eye contracts; at the same time so does the lateral rectus muscle of the right eye. During this maneuver, the right medial rectus muscle and the left lateral rectus muscle both relax. Conversely, when a person looks to the left, the lateral rectus muscle of the left eye contracts in coordination with the medial rectus muscle of the right eye and the opposites relax.

The eyes are kept in visual alignment by the coordinated contraction and relaxation of the 6 pairs of external ocular muscles. When the eyes are directed toward a single target and are perfectly aligned, **binocular vision** results. The brain blends the separate images received by the two eyes so that the person perceives a single view, a process called **fusion**.

Weakness, paralysis, or other restriction of an extraocular muscle in one eye may prevent coordinated movement of that eye in relation to the other. If the extraocular muscles do not work in a coordinated manner, the eyes become misaligned and vision may be disturbed, a condition called **strabismus**. If the misalignment is significant, the brain may be unable to fuse the two images. The result in adults and older children is double vision. In infants and young children the result is suppression of vision in one eye. For a complete discussion of suppression and double vision (diplopia) as well as a condition called amblyopia ("lazy eye"), refer to Chapter 9.

Eyelids and Conjunctiva

The **eyelids** are the complex movable cover of the outer portion of the eyeball. They consist of an upper and lower component of skin, tarsus, delicate muscles, eyelashes, glands, and conjunctiva. All of these components are discussed in detail below. They help protect the eye from injury, exclude light, and aid in the lubrication of the ocular surface. A film of tears is normally present on the outer surface of the eye, and the blinking action of the upper lid spreads this tear film evenly over the ocular surface to provide a clear layer that does not interfere with vision.

The almond-shaped opening between the upper and lower lids is called the **palpebral fissure**. The point where the lids meet on the nasal (inner) side of the palpebral fissure is called the **medial canthus**. The temporal (outer) junction of the lids is called the **lateral canthus**.

The margin, or edge, of the eyelid contains several structures. On the **anterior** (front) edge are rows of hair follicles for the eyelashes. The eyelashes, technically known as **cilia**, help protect the surface of the eye by sweeping away airborne dust particles and other foreign matter when the eyelids blink.

The eyelashes normally curl upward on the upper lid and downward on the lower eyelid. Occasionally, an eyelash may grow in the wrong direction and rub against the surface of the eye, irritating the cornea. This eyelid abnormality is called **trichiasis**. Under other conditions, a lash follicle may become inflamed and produce

a reddened, sore lump near the outer edge of the lid, known as a **stye** or **external hordeolum**.

On the **posterior** (back) margin of the eyelid (the edge closest to the globe) is a row of tiny holes, the openings of oil-secreting glands that are hidden in the tissue of the eyelids. These glands are called the **meibomian glands**. The oil they secrete becomes part of the tear film that lubricates the outer surface of the eyeball. Figure 2.3 depicts the external eyelids and associated structures.

As with the lash follicles, a meibomian gland may become inflamed and infected, in this case producing a swelling on the inner eyelid called an **internal hordeolum**. Over time, this inflammation may produce a lump called a **chalazion** on the outer lid. Yet another lid condition is **blepharitis**, a common inflammation that produces reddened and crusted lid margins.

The eyelids themselves are composed of 3 layers: an outer layer of skin, a middle layer of fibrous tissue and muscle, and an inner layer of tissue called the conjunctiva. Within the middle layer of the upper and lower eyelids is a dense, plate-like framework, the **tarsus** or **tarsal plate**, which gives the eyelids their firmness and shape. Also located in the middle layer is the **orbicularis oculi**, a circular muscle that closes the eye when it contracts, as in winking. A second muscle, the **levator palpebrae superioris**, is attached to the upper tarsal plate. When it contracts, it raises the upper lid.

Sometimes the levator muscle loses its ability to lift the eyelid to its full extent, the upper lid droops and cannot lift fully. This condition is called **ptosis**. Malformation of the eyelid tissues or damage to them may cause the lower lid margin to fall or pull away from the eye, a condition called **ectropion**. Conversely, the upper or lower lid margins may be turned inward, a condition

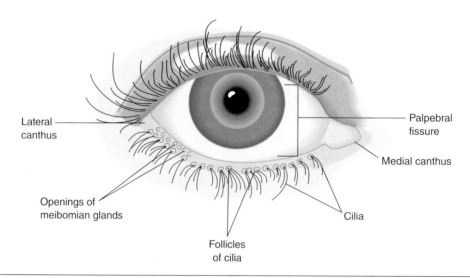

Figure 2.3 The external eyelids.

called **entropion**. Either condition produces continuous irritation and possible damage to the cornea.

The third layer of the eyelids, the **conjunctiva**, is a thin, translucent mucous membrane that lines the inner surface of the lids and the outer front surface of the eyeball, except for the cornea. The portion of this tissue lining the eyelids is called the **palpebral conjunctiva**; the section covering the outer eyeball is called the **bulbar conjunctiva**. The area where the palpebral and bulbar portions of the conjunctiva meet beneath the upper and lower lids is actually a loose pocket of conjunctival tissue, called the **fornix** or **cul-de-sac**. Figure 2.4 shows the eyelid and the conjunctiva.

The slippery nature of the conjunctival tissue helps the eyelids slide easily against the outer surface of the eyeball. Coursing through the conjunctiva is an elaborate network of fine blood vessels that help nourish the underlying tissue of the eyelids and the surface of the eyeball.

Irritation, allergy, or infection may cause the small conjunctival blood vessels to swell, making the conjunctiva appear red, a condition called **conjunctivitis**. Infectious conjunctivitis is commonly called "pink eye." Occasionally, one of the conjunctival blood vessels may rupture, allowing blood to flow under the tissue. These **subconjunctival hemorrhages** may occur after violent coughing or often without explanation. They usually resolve in a few weeks without treatment and are not a threat to the health of the eye. However, recurring subconjunctival hemorrhages could indicate a systemic medical problem, a condition affecting the body as a whole.

Lacrimal Apparatus

The **lacrimal apparatus** (Figure 2.5) consists of the orbital structures that produce tears and the ducts that drain the excess fluid from the front of the eyes into the nose. A small amount of tears is produced continuously during the waking hours, not just when the eye is irritated or when a person cries. The tears become part of a 3-layered coating called the **tear film** that covers the front surface of the globe. This film helps provide ocular comfort and clear vision, and gives moisture and nourishment to the eye.

The outer layer of the tear film is formed from the oily substance secreted by the meibomian glands of the eyelid. This layer helps prevent evaporation of moisture from the middle layer. The middle aqueous layer supplies moisture, oxygen, and nutrients to nourish the cornea. This layer is produced by the **lacrimal gland**, located in the lateral part of the upper lid (the side away from the nose) just under the upper orbital rim. Other smaller, accessory lacrimal glands are distributed throughout the upper fornix. The innermost layer of the tear film is composed of a **mucinous** (sticky) fluid produced by specific

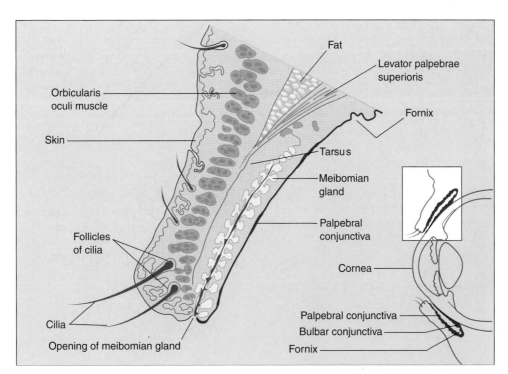

Figure 2.4   Cross section of the eyelid.

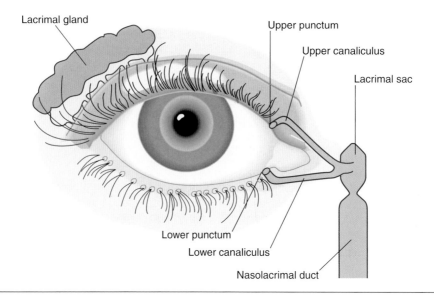

Figure 2.5 The lacrimal apparatus.

cells in the conjunctiva called **goblet cells**. This layer promotes an even spread of the tear film over the cornea.

Dry eyes are a common complaint, especially among elderly people.

Patients with dry eyes complain of irritation and a feeling of grittiness, described medically as a **foreign-body sensation**. The tests used to detect dry eyes include the **Schirmer tear test** and **phenol red thread test**. These tests are discussed in Chapter 8.

The tear film is evenly spread over the surface of the eye when the lids close during a blink. The excess tears then form a "tear lake" along the lower lid margin before passing through tiny openings, the **upper punctum** and **lower punctum**. These puncta (plural of **punctum**) are located on the upper and lower eyelid margins near the nose.

The puncta are entrances to tubes called the **upper canaliculus** and **lower canaliculus**. These canaliculi (plural of canaliculus) join together and connect with the **lacrimal sac**. Tears entering the puncta pass through the canaliculi and into the lacrimal sac. The lacrimal sac empties by means of the **nasolacrimal duct** into the nasal cavity, where the tears become part of the fluid that moistens the mucous membrane of the nose. Passage of excess tears through this system is the reason you have to blow your nose after crying and the reason patients have a "funny taste" in their mouth after using eyedrops.

Inflammation of the lacrimal sac is called **dacryocystitis**. This relatively common condition usually occurs as a result of obstruction of the nasolacrimal duct. Such obstruction results in chronic tearing. If the blockage is severe, surgery may be required.

The Eye

The globe is an almost perfect sphere that houses the optical structures directly involved in the visual process. The globe is often divided anatomically into two parts. The front of the eye, or **anterior segment**, includes the structures between the front surface of the cornea and the vitreous. The remainder of the eyeball, the **posterior segment**, is composed of the vitreous and the retina.

Cornea and Sclera

The outermost, front part of the globe is the **cornea**, which appears as a bulge. The cornea is a thin, tough, crystal-clear membrane, often referred to as the "window of the eye." Transparency of the cornea results from its highly ordered cell structure and from its lack of blood vessels, a characteristic that distinguishes it from other tissues. The cornea receives its nourishment from the tear film that covers it and from a specialized fluid called *aqueous humor* that flows beneath it.

The curvature of the cornea and its transparency permit it to perform its principal function, which is to focus light rays reflected to the eye. The cornea contributes about two-thirds of the focusing power of the eye. The tear film aids in this process by providing a smooth surface over the cornea.

The cornea is made up of 5 layers (Figure 2.6), listed from the outside surface in:

- corneal epithelium
- Bowman's membrane
- corneal stroma
- Descemet's membrane
- corneal endothelium

The nerves that supply the cornea lie immediately beneath the **corneal epithelium**, the cornea's first line of defense against infection and injury. **Bowman's membrane** acts as an anchor for the epithelial layer. The **corneal stroma** is the main body of the cornea. Laser or other corneal refractive surgeries involve the epithelium and stromal layers. The stroma and **Descemet's membrane** contribute rigidity to the cornea. The cells of the **corneal endothelium** serve as pumps to maintain a proper fluid balance within the cornea. When the corneal epithelium is injured, a **corneal abrasion**, or scratch, results. Even a small scratch can be very uncomfortable because of the nerves beneath the epithelial layer. These injuries are very common, but they heal rapidly if they do not become infected. A **corneal ulcer** may result if an injury to the corneal epithelium becomes infected. When inflammation spreads and clouds the normally transparent cornea, loss of vision can result.

The white tissue surrounding the cornea is a continuation of the fibrous outer layer that forms the main structural component of the globe, protecting the intraocular contents. This tissue is called the **sclera**. The exposed part of the sclera is covered with the thin, translucent bulbar conjunctiva. What appears as the "white of the eye," therefore, is actually two layers of tissue: the sclera and the almost invisible conjunctiva that covers it. The junction between the sclera and the cornea is called the **limbus**. The limbus is also the point where the bulbar conjunctiva terminates, since it does not cover the cornea.

Anterior Chamber

Between the cornea and the iris is a small compartment, called the **anterior chamber**, filled with a clear, transparent fluid called **aqueous humor**. The aqueous humor is produced by secretory tissue located behind the iris. As the fluid is produced, it flows across the back of the iris, through the pupil, and into the anterior chamber.

The aqueous fluid leaves the eye at the junction of the cornea and the iris, called the **anterior chamber angle**, or **filtration angle**. From there it passes through the trabecular meshwork, a spongy structure that filters the aqueous fluid and controls its rate of flow out of the eye. After passing through the trabecular meshwork, aqueous humor drains through a conduit in the sclera called the **canal of Schlemm**, then through collector channels called **aqueous veins** and lastly into the venous vessels on the conjunctiva to return to the general circulation. The balance between the outflow and the production of aqueous fluid maintains the intraocular pressure and is extremely important to the proper function of the eye. Figure 2.7 depicts the anterior chamber angle and the direction of aqueous flow.

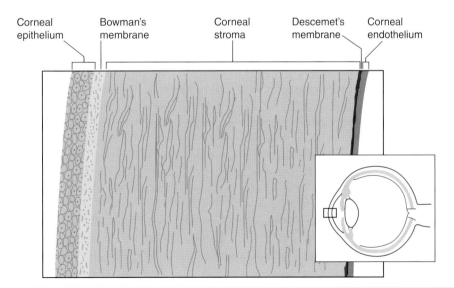

Corneal epithelium　Bowman's membrane　Corneal stroma　Descemet's membrane　Corneal endothelium

Figure 2.6 The 5 layers of the cornea.

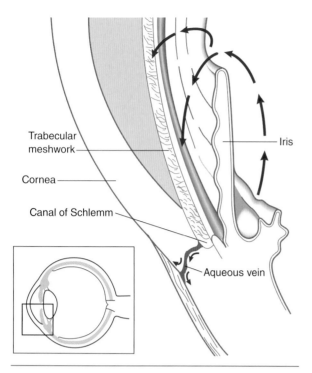

Figure 2.7 The anterior chamber angle and the flow of aqueous fluid.

If drainage of aqueous fluid is impaired, pressure inside the eye rises, increasing the risk for glaucoma. Increased pressure in the eye can damage the optic nerve, leading to visual field loss and eventually blindness if not appropriately treated.

Uvea: Iris, Ciliary Body, Choroid

The **uvea**, or **uveal tract**, is the main vascular compartment of the eye. It consists of 3 parts: iris, ciliary body, and choroid. The uveal tract is responsible for providing most of the blood supply and much of the nourishment to the eye.

The **iris** is a colored diaphragm of tissue that is stretched across the rear of the anterior chamber behind the cornea. By varying the size of the pupil, the circular opening in its center, the iris controls the amount of light entering the inner part of the eye. Fibers of the **dilator muscle** stretching from the pupil to the boundaries of the iris contract to widen (dilate) the pupil in reduced light conditions. The **sphincter muscle** that encircles the pupil contracts to make the pupil smaller in response to bright light. The pupil itself appears black because the interior of the eye is dark.

The iris varies in color from one individual to another and may also change color in the same person with age. In newborn infants, the iris often appears blue due to an absence of pigment in the transparent tissue. As the eye develops, the more permanent iris color becomes apparent.

The space between the back of the iris and the front of the vitreous is called the **posterior chamber**. This space is filled, like the anterior chamber, with aqueous fluid.

The **ciliary body** is a band-like structure made of muscle and secretory tissue that extends from the edge of the iris and encircles the inside of the sclera toward the front of the eye. The inner surface of the ciliary body is arranged in folds, rows, or ridges called **ciliary processes**. These structures secrete the aqueous humor that fills the anterior and posterior chambers. The muscle fibers in the ciliary body form the **ciliary muscle**. The ciliary body supports another structure in the eye, the crystalline lens, by means of connecting fibers.

The third part of the uveal tract, the **choroid**, is a continuation of the ciliary body in the form of a layer of tissue that lies between the sclera and the retina, the innermost surface of the posterior segment of the eyeball. The choroid is made up largely of blood vessels, which supply nourishing blood to the outer layers of the retina. Figure 2.8 shows the structures of the uveal tract.

Crystalline Lens

The transparent structure located immediately behind the iris, suspended in the posterior chamber, is the crystalline lens. The lens is suspended by transparent fibers called **zonules** that radiate from the lens and attach to the ciliary body. The lens itself consists of an outer clear, elastic capsule filled with a clear inner "core" called the nucleus that is surrounded by **cortex** (a clear, paste-like protein).

The lens completes the process of focusing light rays reflected to the eye, a process begun by the cornea. While the cornea is the primary refractive structure, the lens is responsible for approximately one-third of the total refractive power of the eye. The overall refractive power of the eye is approximately 60 diopters, 40 of which are attributed to the cornea and 20 to the crystalline lens. In contrast to the cornea, the curvature of the lens can change in order to focus images of objects that are closer to the eye. This action, called **accommodation**, occurs with the help of muscles of the ciliary body. When the ciliary muscle contracts, the zonules relax, permitting the lens to become rounder and increasing its focusing power.

Elasticity of the crystalline lens decreases as part of the normal aging process. By the age of 45, a significant amount of the lens' ability to increase its curvature is lost and the individual is no longer able to focus on very near objects, a condition called **presbyopia**. For this reason, many people over the age of 45 wear reading glasses. Also with aging, proteins of the lens deteriorate, leading to **opacification** (clouding) of the lens called a **cataract**. When the cloudiness progresses to the point that it

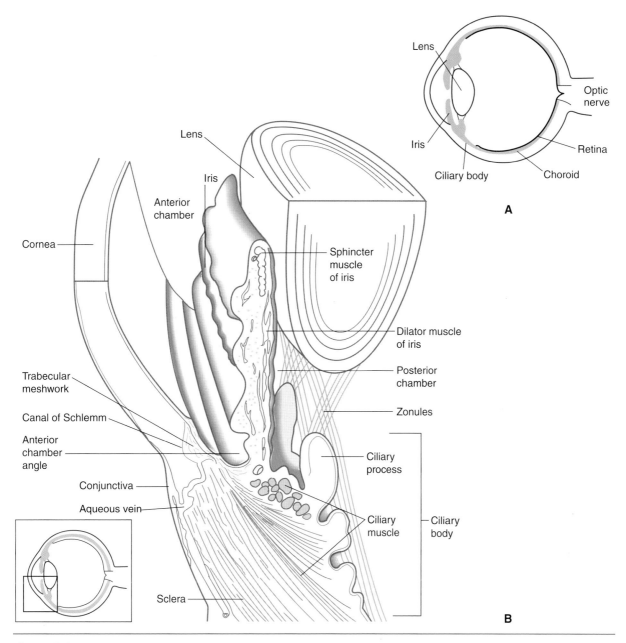

Figure 2.8 The uveal tract. **A.** The iris, ciliary body, and choroid in relation to other structures of the eye. **B.** Details of the uveal structure.

interferes with the patient's daily routine or totally blocks vision, the cataract can be surgically removed. An appropriate refractive lens (spectacles, contact lenses, or intraocular lenses) is used to replace the lost optical power of the cloudy lens.

Vitreous

The vitreous is a clear, jelly-like substance that fills the intraocular cavity behind the lens. This substance acts as a shock absorber and maintains the spherical shape of the globe. Normally, the vitreous is optically transparent, so that light rays bent by the cornea and the lens can pass unimpeded to focus an image on the retina.

The vitreous may liquefy as part of the normal aging process, occasionally producing small clumps or strands of concentrated gel floating in the now-fluid vitreous. These particles, called **floaters**, cast shadows on the retina and appear to the patient as moving spots. Although annoying, they rarely require treatment. However, in some cases floaters can be indicative of more serious diseases of the eye.

Retina

The retina is a transparent layer of tissue that forms the innermost lining of the globe. The layer consists mainly of nerve cells and is actually an extension of the brain. The posterior two-thirds of the retina is called the "visual portion" because it is the surface on which images are focused by the cornea and lens.

The retina is composed of an inner layer of nerve cells and an outer **pigment epithelium** that lies against the choroid. The base of the nerve cell layer contains two types of **photoreceptor** (light-sensitive) cells, the **rods** and the **cones**, each with a different function in the visual process. The rods are largely responsible for vision in reduced light ("night vision") and for peripheral (side) vision. The cones provide sharp central vision and the perception of color.

The retina is nourished by blood vessels on its surface and by the vessels in the choroid underneath. The central retinal artery enters and the central retinal vein exits at a location in the retina known as the **optic disc**, or **optic nerve head**. Close to the center of the retina is a specialized area known as the **macula**. The center of the macula is called the **fovea** (Figure 2.9). Because most of the cone cells are concentrated in the macula, proper function of this area is crucial to the finely detailed central vision needed for reading and other detailed visual tasks.

Injury to the macula or degeneration of this part of the retina, due to factors that are mostly age-related, reduces visual acuity (sharpness) of the central vision. In extreme cases, the eye may be left with only peripheral vision. If other areas of the retina are damaged, blind spots will occur in corresponding parts of the visual field.

When light stimulates the rods and the cones in the retinal photoreceptor layer, electric (nerve) impulses are generated in these cells and relayed to **bipolar cells**, which lie above the rods and cones. The nerve impulses then pass to **ganglion cells** at the top, or innermost surface, of the retina. The ganglion cells possess long, fiber-like **axons**, which course over the surface of the retina and converge at the optic disc, at the back of the eye. The axons from the ganglion cells form the **optic nerve**. The optic nerve thus resembles a cable of uninterrupted axon strands or nerve fibers, each carrying a visual message, as the nerve exits the globe. Because no rods or cones are present at the optic disc, this small area is sightless and is called the **physiologic blind spot** in the field of vision. Figure 2.10 illustrates the structures at the junction of the retina and the optic disc.

The optic disc has a small central depression called the *cup*. The comparison of the size of the central cup to the size of the optic nerve is called the *cup/disc ratio*. This is expressed as either a percentage (as "30% cup") or a decimal fraction (as "0.3 cup"). An enlarging cup can be a sign of glaucoma. The tissue surrounding the cup is called the **rim** (Figure 2.11). Thinning of the rim may accompany enlargement of the cup in patients with glaucoma. A pale appearance to the cup and rim is called **optic atrophy** and may be a sign of serious neurologic diseases.

The fibers in the optic nerve travel onward to relay stations in the **central nervous system** to bring visual information to the brain. A disease like glaucoma can

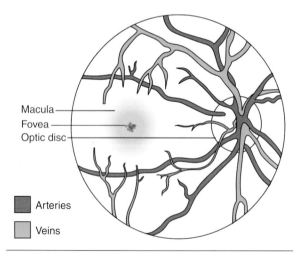

Figure 2.9 The macular area and the optic disc with the retinal blood supply.

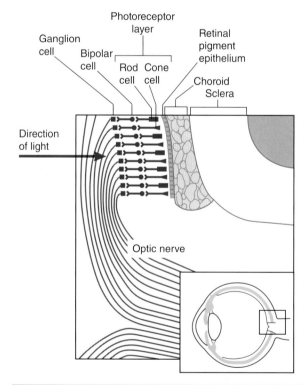

Figure 2.10 The retina at its junction with the optic disc.

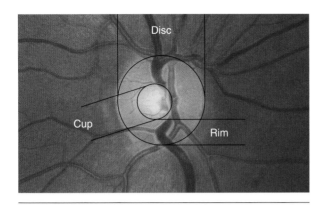

Figure 2.11 Photograph of a normal optic disc with the cup and rim areas noted. *(Image courtesy of Charlene S. Campbell, COMT.)*

destroy ganglion cells and their axons reducing the **nerve fiber layer** of the retina which can be measured clinically.

Visual Pathway

The route taken by light-generated nerve impulses after they leave the eye is called the **visual pathway** or **retrobulbar visual pathway**. The initial portion of this pathway consists of the optic nerve from each eye. The two optic nerves merge at a point behind the eyes in the brain called the **optic chiasm**. Here axon fibers from the nasal retina of each eye cross to the opposite side of the chiasm, while axons from the temporal retina of each eye continue on their respective sides of the chiasm. The realigned axons emerge from the chiasm as the left and right **optic tracts** and end in the left and right **lateral geniculate bodies**. At these midbrain "way stations," the axons of the optic tracts **synapse** (connect) to nerve cells called **optic radiations**, which travel to the right and left halves of the **visual cortex** at the back of the brain. Figure 2.12 depicts the visual pathway and its principal structures.

The purpose of the apparently complex crossing of nerve fibers from the nasal retina of the two eyes becomes clear in the context of the visual messages they carry. The image received by the nasal retina of the left eye is essentially the same as the image focused on the temporal retina of the right eye. Conversely, the image on the nasal retina of the right eye is closely similar to the image on the temporal retina of the left eye. Although the left and right optic tracts emerge from the chiasm with nerve fibers from *both* eyes, the visual message each optic tract carries is of an image from one direction, or field of vision.

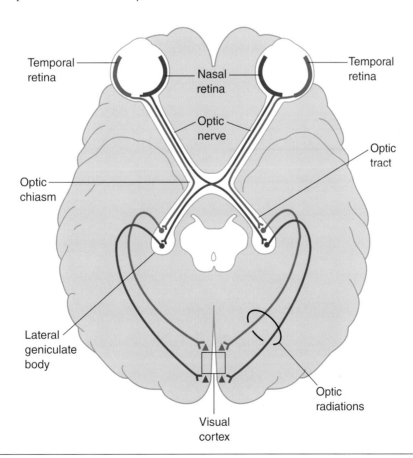

Figure 2.12 The visual pathway.

The visual messages transmitted in the form of nerve impulses from the two eyes are integrated in the visual cortex of the brain to create the sensation of sight. The object originally viewed by both eyes is perceived as a single image, seen upright and from the correct perspective.

Disorders affecting different parts of the visual pathway produce characteristic changes in the field of vision. The nature of visual field disturbances, therefore, can help in determining which part of the visual pathway is affected. Your ophthalmologist may order specialized visual field testing to detect or monitor these changes.

SELF-ASSESSMENT TEST

1. Briefly describe how the eye converts light rays to a perceived image, naming the principal structures involved in the process.

2. Name the 4 primary structures included in the adnexa.

3. Describe the structure and function of the orbit.

4. Match the 6 extraocular muscles with their functions.

    _____ medial rectus   a. outward rotation

    _____ lateral rectus   b. upward rotation

    _____ superior rectus   c. downward rotation

    _____ inferior rectus   d. inward rotation

    _____ superior oblique   e. excyclotorsion, up and outward

    _____ inferior oblique   f. incyclotorsion, down and inward

5. What are the 3 functions of the eyelids?

6. Name the 3 layers of the eyelid.

7. What are the 2 principal functions of the lacrimal apparatus?

8. Give 2 reasons why tears are important to the functioning of the eye.

9. What is the relationship between the lacrimal gland, lacrimal sac, and nasolacrimal duct?

10. Name the 3 layers of tear film and their functions.

11. On the cutaway view of the eye, identify the following structures: cornea, sclera, lens, vitreous, retina, cilia, conjunctiva.

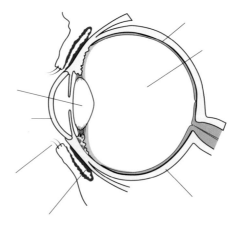

12. What is the principal function of the cornea?

13. Match the 5 layers of the corneal tissue with their functions. (Two of the layers perform the same function.)

____ endothelium   a. serves as first line of defense against infection and injury

____ epithelium   b. contributes rigidity

____ Bowman's membrane   c. acts as anchor for epithelium

____ Descemet's membrane   d. maintains proper fluid balance

____ stroma

14. What is the main function of the sclera?

15. Why is a balance between the inflow and outflow of aqueous humor important?

16. Describe the course of aqueous humor into and out of the eye, naming the principal ocular structures involved.

17. Name the 3 main structures that make up the uveal tract.

18. Describe how the pupil dilates and contracts, naming the muscles involved.

19. What is the function of the ciliary processes?

20. What is the main function of the choroid?

21. Which structure besides the cornea provides the eye's focusing power?

22. What is the physiologic process and purpose of accommodation?

23. The lens is attached to the ciliary body by transparent fibers called _____.

24. What is the main function of the vitreous?

25. The retina includes a photoreceptor layer containing 2 types of cells: _____ and _____.

26. How are the functions of these 2 types of retinal photoreceptor cells different?

27. Briefly describe how the retina works to produce sight.

28. The macula contains most of the _____ cells.

29. Describe the route of nerve impulses through the retrobulbar visual pathway.

SUGGESTED ACTIVITIES

1. Obtain a commercial model eye. Under supervision of your ophthalmologist or other trainer, disassemble it and reassemble it, naming the various structures as you do so.

2. Cover the labels on a poster of the anatomy of the eye with a sheet of paper or strips of masking tape and write in the labels. Then compare your labels with those on the poster to see how accurate you were.

SUGGESTED RESOURCES

Cassin B, ed. *Fundamentals for Ophthalmic Technical Personnel*. Philadelphia: Saunders; 1995.

Cassin B, Rubin ML, eds. *Dictionary of Eye Terminology*. 5th ed. Gainesville, FL: Triad; 2006.

Goldberg S, Trattler W. *Ophthalmology Made Ridiculously Simple*. 4th ed. Miami: MedMaster; 2008.

Marieb E. *Human Anatomy and Physiology*. 6th ed. San Francisco: Benjamin Cummings; 2003.

Stein HA, Stein RM. *The Ophthalmic Assistant: A Text for Allied and Associated Ophthalmic Personnel*. 8th ed. St Louis: Mosby; 2006.

3 DISEASES AND DISORDERS OF THE EYE

Various disorders may interfere with the normal function of the eye and ocular adnexa and thereby affect sight. To help the ophthalmologist correct or prevent damage to the visual system, the ophthalmic medical assistant must be able to recognize common eye problems and understand how and why they developed. It is also important for the assistant to know the medical terms used to describe these disorders and the disease mechanisms that produced them. In addition, the assistant should have a general knowledge of the kind of treatment needed to manage or correct the problem.

This chapter introduces you to the general concepts of disease and to the processes by which diseases evolve. The specific disorders that may occur in various parts of the eye and ocular adnexa are discussed in detail. You will learn the causes of these disorders, their effects on vision, and the procedures used to treat them. Such information will help you to understand and perform diagnostic tests and other responsibilities of ophthalmic medical assisting.

Mechanisms of Disease and Injury

The term **disease** means a specific process in which **pathologic** (abnormal) changes result in malfunction of a particular part or system of the body. A variety of biologic or other mechanisms can cause disease. However, because none of the body's parts or systems exists in isolation, pathologic changes in one part of the body frequently affect the operation of another part. Thus, the process that is the **etiology** (cause) of one disease may itself be a disease process or the result of another disease. The term *cell injury* is associated with disease because the processes that produce disease change, damage, and destroy **cells**, the microscopic units that compose a tissue (cornea, iris, and retina). The mechanisms of disease and injury can be divided into 10 general types: infectious, inflammatory, allergic, ischemic, metabolic, congenital, developmental, degenerative, neoplastic, and traumatic.

Infectious Process

Humans share this planet with many kinds of animals and plants, including unnumbered varieties of very small organisms visible only with a microscope. These **microorganisms** are present in the air we breathe, in the food we eat, and on the objects we touch. They are even present inside our bodies. In many cases, we live in harmony with these bacteria, fungi, and **viruses** and even benefit from some of them. For example, bacteria present in the intestine feed on waste matter and produce a vitamin that promotes blood clotting. However, penetration of some microorganisms through the body's natural defenses and into the tissues can have very damaging results. Invasion and multiplication of these harmful microorganisms, called **infection**, can injure cells by competing for nutrients and producing toxic substances or simply by interfering with the cells' normal activities and reproduction.

Bacterial and fungal infections frequently begin in the tissues immediately surrounding the microorganism's point of entry. Such infections are described as local. If they are unchecked, the infections may spread to surrounding tissues and become diffuse. In some cases, infections can get into the bloodstream and cause trouble at sites quite remote from the point of entry.

Inflammatory Process

The body generally reacts to infection first by a local protective tissue response called **inflammation**. Specialized cells move to the affected area and act to destroy the injurious agent, while other cells release fluids to dilute any toxic substances produced by the infectious agent. Still other cells then proceed to wall off both the offender and the damaged tissue. Inflammation generally produces pain, heat, redness, and swelling in the region affected. Although inflammation develops in response to infection, it may also occur following any injury or damage to tissue. Inflammation is often the body's response to foreign substances, such as bacteria or chemicals. The body releases its army of scavenger cells to try to neutralize the invading organism or substance. The medical term for inflammation of a tissue or organ is obtained by adding the suffix "itis" to the name of the tissue or organ. Thus, inflammation of the iris is known as iritis, inflammation of the retina, retinitis, and so forth.

Inflammation that flares up quickly and remains for only a short period is called **acute** inflammation. If the condition persists for a long period, it is called **chronic** inflammation. The terms *acute* and *chronic* are also applied to infection and other disease processes, depending on whether they are brief or persistent. Although the purpose of inflammation starts out as protective, the changes it produces can result in a loss of function of the tissue or organ involved. Inflammation thus can itself act as a disease process.

Allergic Process

The body's initial inflammatory response to infection is generally followed by a wider and more complex **immune reaction**. Part of this response is the development of **antibodies** to proteins present in the specific infecting microorganism. If a person is later re-exposed to the same invader, the antibodies will serve to neutralize the microorganism and may prevent recurrence of the infection. Even if reinfection is prevented, however, inflammation may still occur.

Many people have an overactive immune system that produces antibodies not only to infecting microorganisms, but to foods they eat, to plant pollens in the air they breathe, and to medications they take. Re-exposure to these substances causes these people to have **allergic reactions**. Generally, the reactions are no more serious than a runny nose, watery eyes, and an occasional skin reaction, but in some people they produce difficulties in breathing, such as asthma, or even death. Allergy, therefore, is an important disease mechanism. As with microbial infection, allergic reactions may be accompanied by inflammation.

Ischemic Process

Ischemia is the term given to a severe reduction in the blood supply to any part of the body. The cells of most body structures depend on the blood carried by nearby vessels for nutrients and oxygen and as a means to remove waste products. Interruption of the blood flow to a particular body part can occur if the vessels become **occluded** (blocked)—for example, by a blood clot—or if the vessels break as the result of injury or high blood pressure. Even a relatively short period of ischemia and the resulting **hypoxia** (loss of oxygen) can lead to damage or death of the cells the vessels serve.

Metabolic Process

Metabolism refers to the combination of all the physical and chemical processes by which the body converts food into the building blocks of the body's tissues and into the energy the body uses. An extraordinary number of individual processes are involved to build and repair the machine that is the body and to keep it running. In addition to food and water, the metabolic processes require various substances and agents to assist the chemical reactions. Examples include minerals, vitamins, agents called **enzymes**, which accelerate the processes, and **hormones**, which regulate the process.

Most of the enzymes and hormones needed are produced by special tissues or organs in the normal individual. In some people, a defect may cause an enzyme or hormone production to increase, decrease, or stop altogether. This change in production can cause a series of problems in bodily function, leading to damage or change in organs, including the eye. Examples of overproduction of a hormone include increased thyroid hormone in the disease **hyperthyroidism** and increased cortisol levels in **Cushing disease**. A familiar example of decreased hormone production is the disease **diabetes mellitus**. People with this condition are unable to produce enough of the hormone **insulin** required for the metabolism of sugar. Sugar then accumulates in the blood and spills over into the urine, upsetting many organ systems and damaging tissue, including the eye.

Congenital Process

Various disease processes develop in the child or adult because of an outside influence, such as infection or injury, or for no known reason. In some individuals, these processes or their effects may be present from the time of birth; that is, they are **congenital**. Congenital disease, as well as congenital malformations or malfunctions of the eye and other body structures, may be **genetic** (inherited), or they may be acquired during development of the fetus or during delivery.

Developmental Process

Development of the body tissues and structures begins at conception and continues throughout gestation. Growth and development continue after birth and through puberty until a person reaches adulthood. In some fetuses, babies, and young people, one or another organ, body structure, or body system may not develop properly or at all, due to genetic factors, infection, trauma, or unknown causes. Faulty development of these structures or systems results in their inability to function properly.

Degenerative Process

Automobile parts tend to wear out with age. This is also the case with parts of the eye and other organs of the body. Gradual deterioration in the structure or function of body tissues is called **degenerative** disease, a process often occurring with advanced age. Age is not the only cause, however; genetic factors may be responsible for degenerative pathology in young people and even children, as well as in the elderly. Injury, infection, and inflammation may also lead to degenerative disease.

Neoplastic Process

A **neoplasm** is a new growth of different or abnormal tissue, such as a tumor or a wart. The growth may be **benign**—that is, not dangerous to the well-being of the individual—or it may be **malignant** (cancerous). The cells in malignant tissue are abnormal and multiply at an extraordinary rate. These cells may also **metastasize**—spread to other parts of the body—and begin to produce new tumors, eventually overwhelming the normal function of the body structures and draining them of their food and oxygen. While generally more inconvenient than dangerous, benign neoplasms can cause problems by physically interfering with the operation of neighboring structures.

Traumatic Process

Trauma is a sudden wound or injury to the eye or other part of the body from an external source. The injury may be a cut or a blow or a fragment of wood or metal penetrating the eye. These are examples of physical or mechanical trauma, but the body is vulnerable to other kinds of assault. **Toxins** (poisons) may be a serious cause of trauma, whether they are received by mouth, contact with the skin, inhalation, or from a snake or insect bite. **Thermal trauma** is the term for burns or freezing of tissues. **Chemical trauma** is a major concern of the ophthalmologist because of the serious and rapid damage caused by such chemicals as acid or alkali entering the eye. By its nature, the traumatic disease process often requires emergency care and treatment.

Signs, Symptoms, and Syndromes

All of the disease processes described can affect the vision of individuals and prompt them to seek the help of an ophthalmologist. The changes in vision they experience and the pain or other effects they feel are called **symptoms**. Abnormal changes observed by the physician on examination of the patient are called **signs**. Some signs and symptoms may be the same in a particular condition. However, distinction between the terms is useful because symptoms tend to be more subjective or personal, while signs are usually objective. **Syndrome** is the term given to a set of signs or symptoms that is characteristic of a specific condition or disease.

Both signs and symptoms are important

in the diagnosis of disease.

Abnormalities of the Adnexa

Many disease processes can affect the ocular adnexa. Infections and inflammation of the orbit, eyelids, and lacrimal system are among conditions commonly seen in the ophthalmology office. Disorders of the extraocular muscles that affect functional vision are often seen in pediatric ophthalmology practices.

Orbit

Because the orbit is made of solid bone and is open only at the front, any increase in volume of the orbital contents will push the eyeball forward—a condition called **proptosis** or **exophthalmos** (Figure 3.1). Exophthalmos often occurs in **Graves disease**, a condition of unknown origin that involves the thyroid gland situated anteriorly in the throat and causes the soft tissues surrounding the eyeball to swell. Studies to determine thyroid function are performed on patients with exophthalmos.

Unilateral proptosis (only one eye bulging) may indicate an orbital tumor. A decrease in vision or abnormal results of imaging of the orbit is further evidence of a tumor. **Hemorrhage** (accumulation of blood from a broken vessel) or **edema** (swelling from large amounts of fluid) that results from inflammation or infection in the orbit may also result in proptosis. The blood or fluid may spontaneously resorb.

Diffuse infection of tissues in the orbit is called **orbital cellulitis**. This condition may also produce grossly swollen eyelids and red eyes, sometimes without proptosis.

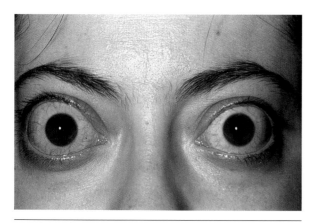

Figure 3.1 Proptosis (exophthalmos).

Symptoms of orbital cellulitis include decreased vision and ocular pain that is made worse with eye movement. Because of its nearness to the brain, orbital cellulitis can be a life-threatening disease. Treatment often includes antibiotics taken by mouth or by injection, and hospitalization may be necessary.

Trauma to the eye or orbit with a blunt object, like a ball or a fist, can break the bony orbital floor or walls and push the eyeball and orbital contents into the **sinuses** (bony air caverns of the skull). This **blowout fracture** (orbital floor) may require surgery to reconstruct the orbit and to release the orbital tissue trapped in the fracture. The eyeball may also be injured and need repair.

Extraocular Muscles

When the extraocular muscles are not functioning properly or are not in good balance, the eyes can go out of alignment, a condition called **strabismus**. In strabismus, the fovea of one eye may not be directed at the same object as the fovea of the other eye. As a result, the patient may complain of **diplopia** (double vision).

Strabismus comes in a number of different forms, depending on where in the motility system the problem lies. In the most common form of strabismus, the cause is thought to be due to an imbalance of muscle tone mediated by an abnormal brain signal. The muscle with more tone will tend to pull the eye out of alignment with the other eye. Congenital strabismus is usually of this type. Strabismus can also be caused by other processes as well. If the nerve controlling a particular muscle is damaged, such as in trauma or stroke, misalignment of the eyes will occur in the direction of gaze controlled by that muscle. This is called *paralytic strabismus*. Strabismus may also occur when a muscle loses elasticity from scarring, trauma, or inflammation, as in Graves disease. This is called restrictive strabismus.

Strabismus can be classified by the direction of the misalignment. Outward deviation of the eye is called an **exo deviation** and inward deviation of the eye is called an **eso deviation**. It can further be named depending on whether the deviation is continually manifest or visible in which case it is called a **tropia** (Figure 3.2). By contrast, some people's brains are able to overcome the misalignment tendency and control it. This type of deviation can only be elicited by covering one eye, so that the brain's ability to fuse the images is blocked. This is called a **phoria**. For example, someone whose eye is obviously turned out has an exotropia and someone whose eye turns out intermittently but is straight most of the time might be said to have an exophoria.

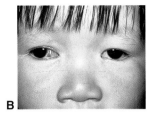

Figure 3.2 Strabismus. **A.** Esotropia. Right eye is turned inward (light reflex is at the temporal corneal margin). **B.** Exotropia. Right eye is turned outward (light reflex is at the nasal corneal margin).

Treatment of congenital strabismus generally consists of prescription glasses, patching, penalization of the dominant eye with drops or surgically altering the muscles to straighten the eyes. This is usually done at an early age because delays can risk a permanent loss of binocular vision and **stereopsis** (3-dimensional visual perception). To prevent the confusion produced by the diplopia of misaligned eyes, the brain of a child tends to ignore the image of the deviating eye—a condition known as **suppression**. This is generally the case in children under 6 years of age because of their greater neural adaptability. If a child has suppressed the vision from one eye over a period of time, the unconscious habit continues even after surgery has produced normal alignment of the eyes. This suppressed deviating eye can also develop amblyopia (decreased vision). This condition can often be corrected by retraining the nonworking amblyopic eye if started in childhood. This is accomplished by placing a patch over the dominant eye or using drops to make it blur, forcing the amblyopic eye to work. Once the amblyopia has been persistent past the age of 7, it is often permanent. The exact age when amblyopia is no longer treatable may extend beyond age 7 and is still being established. Nevertheless, it is important to diagnose and treat amblyopia and strabismus as soon as possible to maximize treatment options.

Nystagmus is a condition in which the eyes shift involuntary in a rhythmic beating motion. Usually, the eye is driven off its intended gaze position with a sudden jerk back to the original position. Occasionally, the direction is vertical, circular, oblique, or rotary, but a side-to-side movement is most common. The presence of nystagmus indicates there is a problem with the brain and not with the extraocular muscles. Nystagmus may be self-limiting but typically not treatable. Occasionally, under certain circumstances, it can be improved with surgery.

Eyelids

Bacterial infection of a gland surrounding an eyelash follicle produces a localized **abscess** known as a **stye** or **external hordeolum** (Figure 3.3A). Treatment consists of hot moist packs and antibiotic drops. Occasionally, the abscess must be **incised** (lanced) and drained. Infection of a meibomian gland results in an abscess on the inside of the eyelid called an **internal hordeolum** (Figure 3.3B). Inflammation accompanies these infections and, in the case of the meibomian gland, may remain long after recovery from infection in the form of a nontender **granulomatous** (solid) lump called a **chalazion** (Figure 3.3C). The lump may eventually be absorbed without treatment or it can be removed surgically.

Blepharitis is a common, low-grade, chronic infection with inflammation of the lid margins, generally produced by bacteria (Figure 3.3D). The lid margins appear slightly red with crusts along the lash line. Treatment includes careful eyelid cleaning and topical antibiotic–corticosteroid treatment, with oral antibiotics needed in special situations, and often for many weeks. The condition is recurrent and predisposes the eyelid to styes and chalazia.

Several disease processes can alter the normal position of the eyelids and thus directly or indirectly affect vision. **Ptosis** is an abnormality in which the upper eyelid droops, due to muscle or nerve damage or to mechanical causes (Figure 3.3E). Congenital ptosis may be caused by partial paralysis of the **oculomotor nerve**, which activates the levator palpebrae muscle. Treatment is surgical. Acquired ptosis is caused by any disease process affecting the nerve supply to the upper levator palpebrae muscle or by degenerative changes in one levator palpebrae tendon. Examples include injuries, diabetes, myasthenia gravis, or tumors that press on the nerve. Treatment of acquired ptosis is directed against the primary disease, but surgical correction of the ptosis may be required.

Ectropion is a turning of the lid margin outward and away from the eyeball (Figure 3.3F). Excessive drying of the cornea could result in exposure keratopathy, causing irritation and tearing. The condition is generally caused by age-related degenerative changes or by scarring. Treatment is surgical and directed to the specific cause.

In **entropion** (Figure 3.3G), the eyelid margins are turned inward, causing **trichiasis**, in which the eyelashes rub against the eyeball and produce tearing, discomfort, and possible scratching of the cornea. The condition may be caused by excessive action of the orbicularis oculi muscle or by scarring and is treated surgically.

Lagophthalmos is a condition in which the globe is not completely covered when the eyelids are closed. It may be caused by facial-nerve paralysis, trauma, or an enlarged or a protruding eye. Treatment is directed to the primary disease.

Benign tumors are very common on the skin surface of the eyelids. Surgical removal may be necessary,

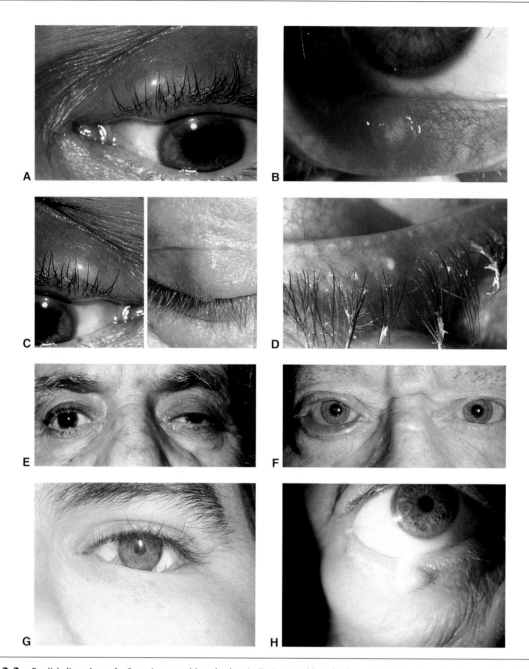

Figure 3.3 Eyelid disorders. **A.** Stye (external hordeolum). **B.** Internal hordeolum. **C.** Chalazion. **D.** Blepharitis. **E.** Ptosis. Left upper eyelid droops. **F.** Ectropion. Right lower eyelid is turned outward. **G.** Entropion. Lower left eyelid is turned inward. **H.** Basal cell carcinoma.

especially if vision is disturbed. **Basal cell carcinoma** is the most common malignant lid tumor (Figure 3.3H). The tumor has a characteristic appearance of a pit surrounded by raised "pearly" edges. Surgical removal is curative if it is performed early.

Lacrimal Apparatus

The tear-producing lacrimal gland is generally free of disease, although tear production may decline with age. **Dacryocystitis** (inflammation of the lacrimal sac) in the

drainage portion of the lacrimal system occurs occasionally (Figure 3.4). Dacryocystitis is usually caused by blockage of the nasolacrimal duct. Major signs and symptoms include tearing with pain, swelling, and tenderness. In infants under 1 year of age, the condition generally results from a congenitally narrow nasolacrimal duct. The duct often widens spontaneously by 1 year of life, but it may be probed open if the narrowing persists. Dacryocystitis occurs in adults as a result of chronic lacrimal system obstruction because of inflammation, facial injury, or tumor. Antibiotics are helpful if

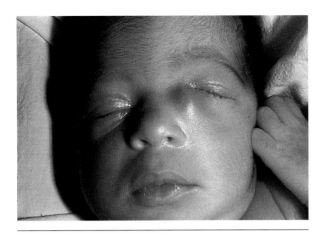

Figure 3.4 Dacryocystitis.

a bacterial infection is present. Surgery may be required if an infection is recurrent.

Keratoconjunctivitis sicca (dry eye syndrome) is a common complaint in the general population, particularly among elderly people and individuals with certain autoimmune diseases. Patients with dry eye syndrome complain of irritation and a foreign-body sensation. This condition is caused by a decrease in the middle aqueous layer. Rapid tear breakup time causes dry spots in the tear film over the cornea, and some patients experience blurred vision. Present treatment is the use of artificial tears in the form of eyedrops. In more severe cases, closure of the lacrimal puncta and the use of cyclosporine ophthalmic emulsion eyedrops may be indicated.

Abnormalities of the Eye

Although the eye is a small organ, its complexity makes it susceptible to a variety of disease processes. Whether they result from infection, inflammation, trauma, systemic disease, or other disease processes, many eye disorders have the capacity to threaten vision. Fortunately, many diseases that may have led to blindness in the past are capable of being treated successfully today. (See Chapter 21.)

Conjunctiva

The conjunctiva that lines the inner surface of the eyelids folds on itself to cover the outer surface of the globe except for the cornea, as already described. Diseases that affect the palpebral conjunctiva almost always involve the bulbar portion of this tissue as well. The bulbar conjunctiva is the eye's first line of defense after the eyelids. As such, it is exposed to dust, pollens, and other foreign matter. **Conjunctivitis** (inflammation of the conjunctiva) is a very common disease, often due to infection with bacteria or viruses, or to allergy. Inflammation causes the small blood vessels in the palpebral and bulbar conjunctiva to dilate (or "become injected" in clinical terminology), so that the conjunctiva appears bright pink in color (Figure 3.5A).

Bacterial conjunctivitis ("pink eye") is recognized by a **mucopurulent** discharge, that is, a thick fluid containing mucus and pus—products of the mucous membranes, dead cells, bacteria, and the white blood cells of the immune system. Recovery generally occurs within 2 weeks without treatment, but antibiotic drops and ointment in the eye can speed the process.

Viral conjunctivitis produces a watery discharge and changes in the follicles of the palpebral conjunctiva. The everted eyelid conjunctival surface appears to be covered with hundreds of tiny bumps. Some individuals develop corneal involvement with severe photophobia (light sensitivity). The infection generally runs its course in 1 to 3 weeks. Some forms of viral conjunctivitis require treatment, although the treatment is often nonspecific, providing only symptomatic relief. Strict adherence to the OSHA universal precautions (Chapter 7) helps prevent spread of the conjunctivitis to office staff and other patients.

Allergic or vernal (springtime) conjunctivitis causes tearing and itching. Redness and swelling are also present. **Topical** (surface) application of a mast cell stabilizer/antihistamine eyedrop usually controls the condition.

Ophthalmia neonatorum is conjunctivitis occurring in the first 30 days of life, the newborn period. The disease may be produced by various bacteria or viruses to which the infant is exposed during passage through an infected birth canal. Silver nitrate solution, sometimes administered to newborns to prevent eye infection, may itself produce conjunctivitis. Laboratory studies are required to determine the specific cause or responsible microorganism and to select treatment. The disease is rare in modern medical practice.

Occasionally, one of the tiny blood vessels that course through the conjunctiva may rupture, allowing blood to flow under the tissue. These **subconjunctival hemorrhages** (Figure 3.5B) occur after violent sneezing or coughing, rubbing of the eyes, or often without explanation. These hemorrhages usually have no symptoms, but the appearance of a bright-red flat area on the conjunctiva may alarm a patient. The condition resolves in a few weeks, and no treatment is required.

A **pinguecula** is a small, benign, yellow-white mass of degenerated tissue of the bulbar conjunctiva (Figure 3.5C). The mass may be located on either side of, but not on, the cornea and may be present in both eyes.

Pingueculae do not threaten vision but can cause minor eye irritation. A **pterygium** is a wedge-shaped growth of the bulbar conjunctiva, probably the result of chronic sun exposure (Figure 3.5D). Unlike a pinguecula, the abnormal tissue gradually grows onto the cornea and may cause irritation, chronic redness, foreign-body sensation, blurred vision, and sensitivity to light. The growth can be surgically removed but may recur. Both pingueculae and pterygia are probably caused by chronic ultraviolet light damage to the conjunctival surface.

Nevi (freckles) are very common tumors involving the bulbar conjunctiva. They appear as yellowish pink or brown areas on the conjunctiva. Nevi are considered benign, but a small percentage becomes malignant. Rarely do they require surgical removal.

Cornea and Sclera

Inflammation of the cornea is referred to as **keratitis**. The cornea may lose its luster and even its transparency. Trauma to the cornea may produce **abrasion** (scratch) and **laceration** (tear) of the protective epithelial layer. The doctor can observe these **lesions** (breaks in the tissue) by staining the epithelium with special dyes. If the lesions do not become infected and the cause of the inflammation is removed, the corneal epithelium will regenerate and heal itself without treatment. On the other hand, bacterial or fungal infection of the lesions can produce a **corneal ulcer**. The corneal epithelium becomes eroded, and the cornea loses its transparency and develops a gray-white opacity that can obscure vision. With an infected cornea, pus often accumulates in the anterior chamber, a condition called **hypopyon** (Figure 3.6). The bulbar conjunctiva appears quite red. Symptoms include

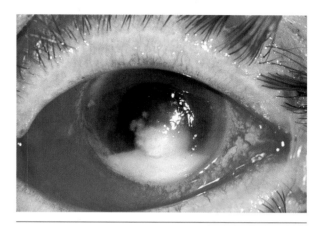

Figure 3.6 Hypopyon with corneal ulcer. Note pus layer in anterior chamber obscuring iris structure.

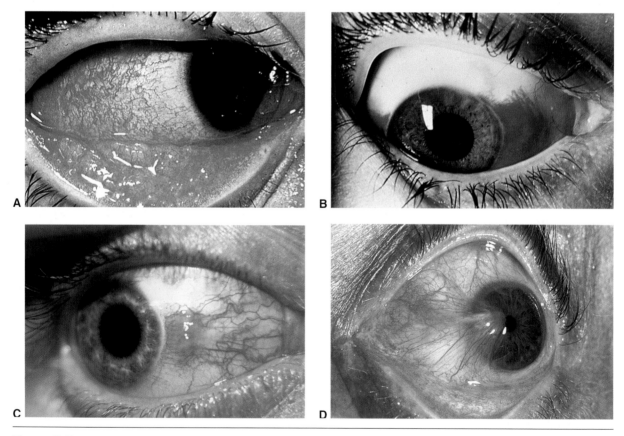

Figure 3.5 Conjunctival disorders. **A.** Conjunctivitis. **B.** Subconjunctival hemorrhage. **C.** Pinguecula. **D.** Pterygium.

moderate to severe pain, sensitivity to light, and excessive flow of tears. Laboratory studies are necessary to determine the specific causative microorganism. Treatment includes antibiotics administered topically (by drops), subconjunctivally, and systemically (by mouth and/or injection). Most ulcers respond to treatment but usually leave a scar on the cornea and possibly decreased vision.

Herpes simplex virus, the virus that produces cold sores, can also lead to keratitis and corneal ulcer. An ocular herpes simplex infection produces symptoms similar to but less severe than those associated with bacterial or fungal ulcers. The doctor may observe a corneal opacity and, through the use of a fluorescent dye, a **dendritic** (branch-shaped) figure can be seen on the corneal surface (Figure 3.7). Treatment starts with antiviral medication applied to the eye and may also be given orally. If unsuccessful, simple scraping of the corneal epithelium often helps heal the ulcer. Herpes simplex ulcers tend to recur. Repeated attacks can lead to severe corneal scarring or thinning, which in turn may require a corneal transplant.

Arcus senilis is a common degenerative change of the cornea usually affecting persons over the age of 50. The outer edge of the cornea gradually becomes opaque, generally in both eyes. Vision is unaffected, and there are no other symptoms. No treatment is needed.

Keratoconus is a degenerative corneal disease of genetic origin. The cornea thins and assumes the shape of a cone, seriously affecting vision. Mild or moderate cones permit treatment with contact lenses, but more severe cones require corneal transplant surgery to restore useful vision.

Inflammation of the sclera, known as **scleritis**, may occur in patients with autoimmune diseases (eg, rheumatoid arthritis). **Episcleritis**, inflammation of the layer overlying the sclera, may result from allergy, although the exact cause is uncertain. It is less painful than scleritis.

Anterior Chamber

Infection or inflammation within the eye may cause a pool of pus (**hypopyon**) to layer at the bottom of the anterior chamber. Blood may also pool in the anterior chamber (**hyphema**) as the result of trauma or certain diseases (Figure 3.8). Treatment is generally directed to the primary disease.

Malformation and malfunction of structures within the anterior chamber angle are responsible for a very common and potentially blinding condition called **glaucoma**. Glaucoma exists when the **intraocular pressure** is too high for continued normal function of the eye. An abnormally high pressure eventually can damage the optic nerve, causing an irreversible loss of visual field and ultimately loss of visual acuity. As explained in Chapter 2, the intraocular pressure is maintained by a balance between the steady secretion of aqueous humor from the ciliary body behind the iris and the steady outflow of the fluid through the trabecular meshwork in the anterior chamber angle. If drainage of aqueous humor out of the eye is hindered, the intraocular pressure rises and over time damages ocular tissue. Such interference with drainage of the aqueous humor and the resulting damage may have multiple causes.

If glaucoma is detected early and intraocular pressure is reduced to normal or tolerable levels by medication or laser or incisional surgery, the progression to blindness can be retarded or halted completely. The diagnosis of glaucoma depends on the measurement of the intraocular pressure, the patient's **visual field** (ie, the height and breadth of space seen by the eye when it looks straight ahead), the corneal thickness, and examination of the optic nerve head. Measuring intraocular pressure by itself is not enough to assure the absence of glaucoma. Intraocular pressure can vary throughout the day and might be normal in a patient with early glaucoma at the time of the examination.

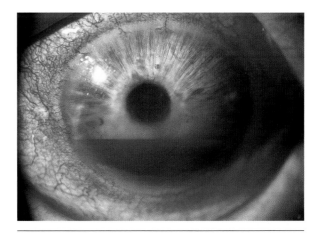

Figure 3.8 Hyphema. Note blood layer in anterior chamber obscuring iris structure.

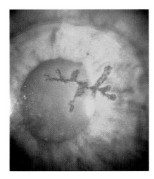

Figure 3.7 Dendritic appearance of a corneal ulcer caused by herpes simplex virus.

Many forms of glaucoma have no symptoms, even while they gradually cause irreversible destruction of vision.

Scientific studies show that central corneal thickness is a risk factor for glaucoma. A thicker cornea results in higher measured intraocular pressure, and a reduced-thickness cornea results in a lower measurement. Therefore, assessment of corneal thickness with a **pachymeter** is important in patients at risk of developing glaucoma and in previously diagnosed glaucoma patients. Reduced corneal thickness increases the risk of developing glaucoma.

Several devices are available to map or image the optic nerve and retina. The *Heidelberg retinal tomograph* (HRT), *GDxVCC nerve fiber analyzer*, and *optical coherence tomographs* are the most common instruments used. (See Chapter 10.) These imagers are a useful adjunct in detecting early changes of glaucomatous damage.

TYPES OF GLAUCOMA Four main types of glaucoma have been identified, primarily on the basis of etiology: primary open-angle glaucoma (or chronic open-angle glaucoma); primary angle-closure glaucoma (or primary closed-angle glaucoma); secondary glaucoma (open and closed); and congenital (developmental) glaucoma.

Primary open-angle glaucoma accounts for 60% to 90% of all adult glaucomas. In this form of glaucoma, the anterior chamber angle appears in its normal open position. Resistance to aqueous drainage occurs in the outflow channels between the trabecular meshwork and the episcleral blood vessels of the body's circulation (Figure 3.9). The intraocular pressure usually rises slowly over a long period of time, even years. Most patients are without symptoms, although some may complain of mild discomfort in the eyes, tearing, and halos around lights. Loss of vision starts at the periphery (outer edges) of the visual field and often is not noticed by the patient until it has nearly reached the center. By this time, the optic nerve has lost most of its function permanently.

Detection of open-angle glaucoma depends heavily on intraocular pressure measurements, visual field studies, and examination of the optic nerve head. Treatment of this type of glaucoma consists mainly of medication to lower intraocular pressure. If medication fails to control the pressure, laser or incisional surgery may be used to reduce aqueous production or to provide new channels for aqueous outflow.

Primary angle-closure glaucoma results from a structural abnormality of the eye. It generally occurs in people over age 60 and accounts for about 10% of all glaucomas. In a small percentage of people, the distance between the iris and cornea is shorter than normal. As these people age, the natural increase in the size of the lens, located immediately behind the iris, blocks the flow of aqueous humor through the pupil, gradually bowing the iris forward until its outer edge blocks the aqueous outflow channels in the anterior chamber angle (Figure 3.10). Intraocular pressure rises rapidly the moment the blockage occurs, producing a sudden glaucoma. Patients report severe eye pain and redness, blurred vision, rainbow-colored halos around lights, headache, and sometimes nausea and vomiting. An angle-closure attack requires emergency treatment with pressure-reducing medication, usually followed by laser surgery (iridotomy) to open the anterior chamber angle.

Various ocular and other diseases can reduce drainage, causing the intraocular pressure to rise. These

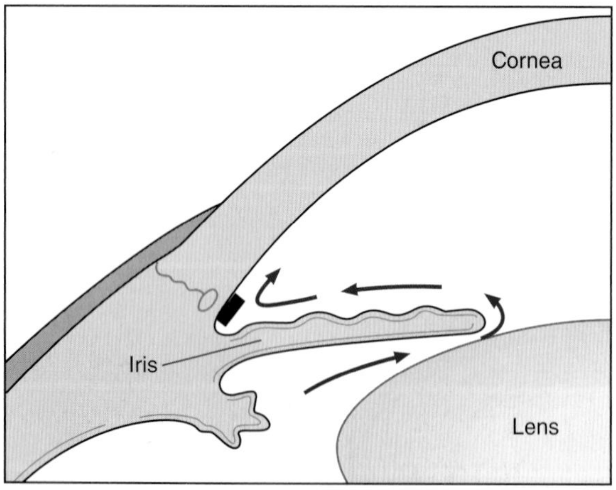

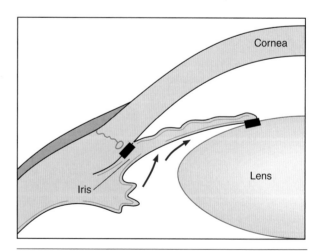

Figure 3.9 Primary open-angle glaucoma. Black rectangle shows area of open angle.

Figure 3.10 Primary angle-closure glaucoma. Black rectangles show areas of blockage.

disease processes include inflammation, tumors, blood vessel blockage, eye trauma, proliferative diabetic retinopathy, and certain medications taken for other disease conditions. The resulting glaucoma is called **secondary glaucoma** because it occurs secondary to another disease or cause. Treatment is directed both at the primary disease condition and at reduction of intraocular pressure with medications.

Congenital glaucoma is a rare disease in infants due to a malformation of the anterior chamber angle. These patients often have other ocular deformities. Treatment is primarily surgical.

Uveal Tract

The iris, ciliary body, and choroid together form the uvea or uveal tract. Inflammation, infection, and tumors that affect one part of the uveal tract often eventually involve the other parts. **Iritis** (inflammation of the iris) causes pain, photophobia, and blurred vision. This condition must be differentiated from glaucoma because treatment includes use of medications to dilate the pupil, agents that could be dangerous in glaucoma. Topical steroids are also used in iritis, and these medications may also be harmful in glaucoma by increasing the intraocular pressure. The progression of iritis may itself produce secondary glaucoma.

Local and systemic diseases, particularly diabetes, may cause **neovascularization** (the abnormal growth of new blood vessels) on the surface of the iris. The iris may develop a reddish color. This condition, called **rubeosis iridis**, may cause bleeding into the anterior chamber or may obstruct the anterior chamber angle, causing secondary angle-closure glaucoma. Treatment is directed to the primary disease and to the conditions produced by the rubeosis. For example, panretinal laser photocoagulation is used to treat rubeosis caused by a central retinal vein occlusion. Tumors, cysts, nodules, and nevi may also develop on the iris. If they produce symptoms, surgical removal may be necessary.

Dysfunction of the muscles within the iris, usually due to a fault in the nerves that supply them, may cause the pupils to be of unequal size, a condition called **anisocoria**. The iris muscle or nerve injury or damage of the visual pathway in the brain may prevent the pupils from dilating or contracting normally in response to light. Treatment, if indicated, generally consists of surgical repair of the iris damage or is directed to the primary disease causing the faulty nerve function.

Crystalline Lens

The inner core of the lens begins to harden soon after birth, and elasticity of the structure decreases gradually as part of the normal aging process. Sometime between about age 40 and age 45, the ability of the lens to accommodate for near vision has deteriorated to the point that many people require reading glasses. This condition is called **presbyopia**.

Another effect of aging is the natural deterioration of the proteins of the lens with a progressive loss of transparency. Such opacification of the lens is called a **cataract** (Figure 3.11). When the cloudiness is sufficient to interfere with the patient's daily routine or totally blocks vision, the cataract can be surgically removed. Absence of the crystalline lens, usually because of cataract extraction, is called **aphakia**. The lost optical power of the lens must be replaced by a contact lens, intraocular lens, or eyeglasses for more normal vision (**aphakic correction**). Correction with an intraocular lens is called **pseudophakia**. Today, intraocular lens implantation is the most common method of replacing the lost optical power after cataract removal.

Cataracts can also result from injury or disease, or may be congenital. Congenital cataracts may be genetic in origin or secondary to maternal infections. Cataracts of genetic origin may also develop in children or adults. Treatment consists of surgical removal of the cataract in the visually impaired. Milder cataracts may only need an optical correction.

Vitreous

Protein condensations in the vitreous or separation of the vitreous gel from the retina (posterior vitreous detachment) may occur as part of the normal aging process. The particles and vitreous collagen fibers, called **floaters**, are seen by the patient as spots or cobwebs. No treatment is required, and floaters are of no concern unless they suddenly increase in number. In that event, they may indicate a retinal detachment.

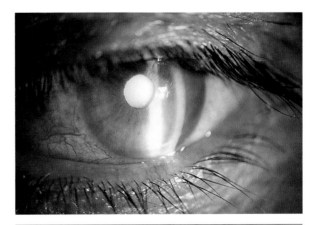

Figure 3.11 Mature cataract. Note the white appearance in the pupillary opening.

Infection of the vitreous and adjacent tissues by bacteria accidentally introduced through injury or surgery is an emergency situation. This condition, called **endophthalmitis**, can destroy an eye within days. Treatment consists of massive doses of antibiotics given locally and systemically. Surgical removal of the infected vitreous may also be required.

Abnormal retinal vessels may produce a hemorrhage into the vitreous that interferes with vision. The blood is usually absorbed over time without treatment. If blood persists, the vitreous can be removed surgically (**posterior vitrectomy**).

Retina

Retinal detachment (separation of the sensory layers of the retina from the underlying pigment layer) is a vision-threatening emergency requiring surgical repair. Three major mechanisms for retinal detachment exist: rhegmatogenous, exudative, or tractional. In the **rhegmatogenous retinal detachment**, liquid vitreous enters the subretinal space through a retinal tear or hole. The condition may occur as the result of trauma, preexisting weaknesses of the retina, or from posterior vitreous detachment. The patient notices stars or flashes of light at one corner of the eye, followed several hours later by a sensation of a curtain moving across the eye and a painless loss of vision. Treatment consists of sealing the tear by **cryopexy** (freezing by surgical means), **photocoagulation** ("welding" with light from a laser), **pneumatoretinopexy** (injection of gas into the eye), **scleral buckle** (placing a block of silicone or other material on the eye to indent the wall), **posterior vitrectomy**, or some combination of these.

An **exudative retinal detachment** results from fluid collecting in the subretinal space as a result of abnormalities of the underlying retinal pigment epithelium, choroid, or sclera.

Long-standing and poorly controlled diabetes mellitus produces a progression of pathologic changes in the retina called **diabetic retinopathy**. Abnormalities of the capillaries may leak exudates and blood into the retina. In some cases, the development of new vessels and fibrous tissue may follow. A **tractional retinal detachment** can result from pulling on the retina by the fibrous growth. This progressive form of change is called **proliferative diabetic retinopathy** and can often be prevented or delayed by tight glycemic control and laser surgery of the retina.

Acquired immunodeficiency syndrome (**AIDS**) results from infection with the **human immunodeficiency virus** (**HIV**). AIDS patients have a deficient immune system and, as a result, are susceptible to a variety of bacterial, viral, fungal, and parasitic infections of various tissues including the retina. Treatment consists of intraocular and systemic antibiotics or antivirals selected on the basis of the infecting microorganism.

Age-related macular degeneration (**AMD**), as its name describes, is a degenerative disease affecting older people. Two forms of AMD exist, dry and wet. The dry form is characterized by **drusen** (yellow-white deposits in the retinal pigment epithelium) and **atrophic** (loss of tissue) spots. The wet form is characterized by leaking and bleeding from fragile new blood vessel growth (**neovascular net**) underlying the macula. The wet form can cause rapid loss of central vision. The wet form of AMD can be treated by **laser photocoagulation** surgery, **photodynamic therapy** (**PDT**), intravitreal injections of corticosteroids and/or **antivascular endothelial growth factor** (**anti-VEGF**). Nutritional supplements may slow the intermediate and advanced stages of the dry form of AMD.

Retinitis pigmentosa is a hereditary, progressive retinal degeneration that affects both eyes, usually in children. It begins with loss of vision in dim light, followed by loss of peripheral vision, progressing after years to blindness. There is some evidence that nutritional supplements may retard the progression of the disease.

Vascular occlusions (blockage of the blood vessels that serve the retina) result in **hypoxia** (lack of oxygen) and death of the retinal tissue. These obstructions of the retinal artery or vein more commonly affect older people with hypertension or diabetes. (Also see "Cerebral Vascular Accident" in Chapter 4.) There is no treatment, and blindness frequently results, except in cases of occlusions further down the macular tree (a branch vein) with secondary macular edema, which may be improved with laser surgery.

Optic Nerve

Disease processes affecting the function of the optic nerve are called *optic neuropathies*. They can be temporary or permanent and have various causes.

Chronic increased intraocular pressure may produce destruction of the nerve fibers in the optic disc and retina (glaucoma).

Increased pressure within the skull (**intracranial**) can produce **papilledema**, swelling of the optic disc with engorged blood vessels due to optic nerve compression. In the early stages of the process the normal physiologic blind spot is enlarged on visual field testing, but the rest of the vision is normal. If the pressure on the optic nerve is not normalized, permanent severe vision loss can occur over time. Treatment is directed to the primary cause of the increased intracranial pressure.

Optic neuritis (inflammation of the optic nerve) can produce sudden, but reversible, loss of sight. This inflammation may be due to infections or immune reactions. Some patients may show signs of multiple sclerosis and may warrant neurological imaging. Treatment may consist of large doses of corticosteroids or antibiotics.

Occlusion of the blood supply to the optic nerve can cause sudden severe vision loss and is called **anterior ischemic optic neuropathy**. No treatment exists.

Visual Pathway

Damage of nerve fibers in the retrobulbar (behind the eye) visual pathway may occur as the result of pressure due to a tumor in the surrounding tissues, stroke (ischemia or hemorrhage within the brain), or trauma. Inflammation or disease may also affect the function of the nerve cells. The location of the damage in the retrobulbar visual pathway causes characteristic changes in the visual field. Treatment is directed to the cause of the neural damage. Pathologic conditions of the visual pathway and changes in the field of vision are discussed in detail in Chapter 11.

SELF-ASSESSMENT TEST

1. Name the 10 general types of disease/injury processes.

2. Distinguish between a sign, symptom, and syndrome.

3. When the orbital volume increases, the resulting protrusion of the eyeball is called _____ or _____.

4. What alterations in the appearance of the eye may be caused by orbital cellulitis?

5. Define *strabismus* and state 3 possible causes.

6. Match the names of the conditions with their descriptions.

   ____ external hordeolum

   ____ chalazion

   ____ blepharitis

   ____ ectropion

   ____ internal hordeolum

   ____ trichiasis

   ____ ptosis

   ____ entropion

   ____ lagophthalmos

   a. abscess caused by infection of a gland surrounding a lash follicle

   b. abscess caused by infection of meibomian gland

   c. nontender solid lump under lid

   d. red and encrusted lid margins

   e. inward turning of lid margin

   f. globe not completely covered when lids are closed

   g. outward turning of lid margin

   h. eyelash(es) rubbing against the eyeball usually causing irritation

   i. droopy upper lid

7. Define *keratoconjunctivitis sicca* and name the usual treatment.

8. Name the condition resulting from inflammation of the lacrimal sac.

9. Distinguish between the signs and symptoms of bacterial, viral, and allergic conjunctivitis.

10. Describe a subconjunctival hemorrhage and its probable cause.

11. Distinguish between a pinguecula and a pterygium with respect to appearance and symptoms.

12. Name the symptoms and treatment of a bacterial or fungal corneal ulcer.

13. Describe how a corneal ulcer caused by the herpes simplex virus differs from a bacterial or fungal corneal ulcer.

14. Describe the condition known as *keratoconus*.

15. Describe what happens when drainage of aqueous humor is hindered, and name the resulting pathologic condition.

16. Match the 4 main types of glaucoma with their descriptions.

_____ primary open-angle

_____ primary angle-closure

_____ secondary

_____ congenital

a. malformation of anterior chamber angle along with other ocular deformities

b. reduced aqueous drainage resulting from another disease

c. reduced aqueous drainage in outflow channels between trabecular meshwork and blood vessels

d. blocked drainage because the iris is bowed forward due to a swollen lens

17. Please circle all that apply to aid in establishing the diagnosis of glaucoma.

a. family history

b. vision

c. intraocular pressure

d. gonioscopy

e. visual field

f. corneal thickness

g. optic nerve examination

18. What principal change occurs in a lens affected by a cataract?

19. Name 4 possible causes of cataracts.

20. What are floaters?

21. What is the name of an infection of the vitreous and adjacent tissues?

22. What is a retinal detachment?

23. What symptoms do patients experience with a retinal detachment?

24. How is eye function altered as a result of age-related macular degeneration?

25. What is papilledema?

26. Name 4 possible causes of damage to the nerve cells of the visual pathway.

SUGGESTED ACTIVITIES

1. Ask your ophthalmologist to allow you to observe patients who have any of the diseases or disorders described in this chapter. Note any variations in the signs described, and ask the physician to explain the apparent differences. It is important to remember that an individual rarely shows all the possible signs or symptoms of a condition.

2. Select one structure of the adnexa or the eye and list as many disorders and diseases as you can, including their possible causes, signs, symptoms, and treatments.

SUGGESTED RESOURCES

Cassin B. *Fundamentals for Ophthalmic Technical Personnel.* Philadelphia: Saunders; 1995: 397–432.

Goldberg S, Trattler W. *Ophthalmology Made Ridiculously Simple.* 4th ed. Miami: MedMaster; 2008.

Harper RA, ed. *Basic Ophthalmology.* 9th ed. San Francisco: American Academy of Ophthalmology; 2010.

Stein HA, Stein RM. *The Ophthalmic Assistant: A Text for Allied and Associated Ophthalmic Personnel.* 8th ed. St Louis: Mosby; 2006.

4

SYSTEMIC DISEASES AND OCULAR MANIFESTATIONS

Diseases that affect one or more of the major systems of the body are called *systemic diseases*. Examples of systemic diseases are diabetes mellitus, which affects the body's endocrine and cardiovascular systems; hypertension, which affects the cardiovascular system; and cancer, which can affect various organs and body systems. Systemic diseases often produce distinctive changes in the eye's external and internal structures. Because the eye is so readily accessible to inspection, information from an examination of the eye can help physicians detect the presence of systemic disease. Alternatively, patients known to have systemic diseases may develop ocular problems that require attention from an ophthalmologist.

This chapter reviews some of the common systemic diseases that manifest ocular pathologic changes. Knowledge of these ocular changes helps the ophthalmic medical assistant to understand these patients' problems and assist with their care.

Major body systems include the cardiovascular, respiratory, endocrine, and nervous systems. In the **cardiovascular system**, the heart pumps blood, and the veins and arteries deliver the blood to and from the heart throughout the body. The structures in the **respiratory system** (nasal passages, trachea, bronchi, and lungs) are involved in the exchange of oxygen for carbon dioxide in the blood. Oxygen is an essential ingredient for many bodily functions. Carbon dioxide is a waste product of metabolism. Multiple glands in the **endocrine system** produce **hormones** that regulate functions such as sugar metabolism (insulin), growth and body metabolism (thyroid hormone), and sexual development and function (estrogen and testosterone). The **nervous system** (brain, spinal cord, and peripheral nerves) functions as the wiring system of the body. Messages are sent to create certain actions, and messages are received so further actions can be taken. The eyes function as an important receptor in this system.

Five main categories of disease types provide a framework for approaching ocular manifestations of systemic disease: inflammatory and autoimmune, metabolic, vascular (including ischemic), infectious, and malignant.

Inflammatory and Autoimmune Diseases

Numerous diseases may be characterized as inflammatory, autoimmune, or both. Only the conditions that result in significant ocular involvement are discussed here.

Myasthenia Gravis

Myasthenia gravis is a chronic autoimmune condition that interferes with proper nerve transmission in the skeletal muscles, causing selective muscle weakness. This weakness is caused by a deficiency in a chemical (called a *neurotransmitter*) that is released from the nerve ending and is supposed to stimulate a receptor on the associated muscle causing the muscle to contract. The disease can occur at any age. The ocular manifestations of myasthenia gravis include **ptosis** (Figure 4.1) and **diplopia**. Patients

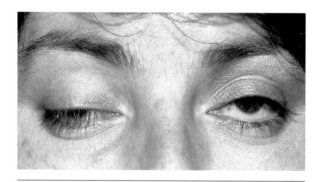

Figure 4.1 Ptosis in a patient with myasthenia gravis. The right upper eyelid has a greater degree of ptosis than the left.

may also complain of limited eye movements. Muscle stimulants and other systemic medications may help.

Rheumatoid Arthritis

Rheumatoid arthritis is a chronic disease of unknown origin that causes pain, stiffness, inflammation, swelling, and sometimes destruction of the joints. Dry eyes are common in patients with rheumatoid arthritis. Other ocular manifestations include uveitis (inflammation of the uveal tract), scleritis (inflammation of the sclera), episcleritis (inflammation of the superficial tissue overlying the sclera), and corneal ulcers (Figure 4.2). Treatments vary according to the specific problem: artificial tears, lubricating ointments, cyclosporine-A, topical steroids, moisture chambers (eg, goggles), and punctal occlusion for dry eye; topical and systemic corticosteroids and other potent anti-inflammatory drugs for uveitis and scleritis; and scleral or corneal patch grafts for perforations. Treatment for the more severe systemic manifestations of rheumatoid arthritis requires corticosteroids or even stronger medications that suppress the immune system.

Sarcoidosis

Sarcoidosis causes inflammation and microscopic nodules called granulomas that affect almost all systems of the body. The most common ocular manifestation of sarcoidosis is uveitis (inflammation of the uveal tract), which can cause cellular deposits on the cornea (Figure 4.3) inflammatory cells in the anterior chamber (iritis) or vitreous (vitritis) and scarring of the pupil (synechiae). In some patients, sarcoidosis affects the choroidal and the retinal vessels, as well as the optic nerve and lacrimal gland. Ocular problems related to sarcoidosis are treated with topical or systemic corticosteroids.

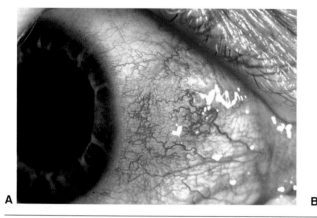
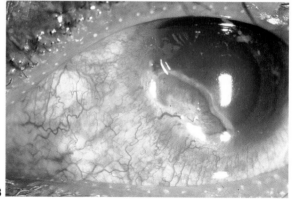

Figure 4.2 Ocular manifestations of rheumatoid arthritis. **A.** Scleritis. **B.** Corneal ulcer.

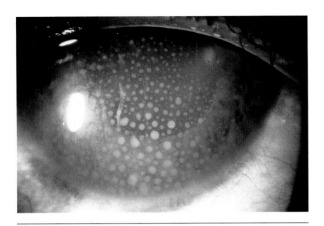

Figure 4.3 Cellular deposits on the cornea resulting from uveitis caused by sarcoidosis.

Sjögren Syndrome

Sjögren syndrome is a combination of dry eyes and dry mouth in the patient. This disorder can appear without known cause or it may be associated with other inflammatory or immunologic diseases such as rheumatoid arthritis. The dry eyes of Sjögren syndrome result in the corneal condition **keratoconjunctivitis sicca**. Symptoms include photophobia and a sensation of burning, grittiness, or foreign body sensation. The ophthalmologist often treats the ocular symptoms of Sjögren syndrome with artificial tears and/or lubricating ointment applied at bedtime. Topical anti-inflammatories (eg, corticosteroids, immunomodulators such as cyclosporine-A) are often required to reduce the ocular immunologic response. Closure of the lacrimal puncta is sometimes necessary to prevent the tears from escaping the ocular surface.

Systemic Lupus Erythematosus

Systemic lupus erythematosus (SLE) can affect many body systems and organs, including the skin, blood vessels, lungs, and kidneys. The disease primarily afflicts women, and the cause is unknown. Dry eyes, scleritis, and corneal ulcers may result from SLE. However, the most common eye conditions produced by SLE are those affecting the vessels of the retina (retinal vasculitis) and the optic nerve itself (Figure 4.4). Corticosteroids, administered either topically or systemically, are frequently the treatment of choice.

Thyroid Disorders

The thyroid gland, a part of the endocrine system, helps regulate the body's metabolism. The many types of thyroid dysfunction, sometimes manifested as

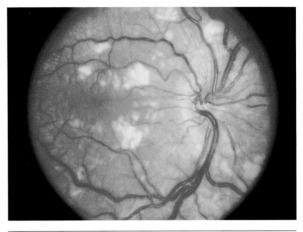

Figure 4.4 The retinopathy seen in the fundus of a patient with SLE; the characteristic yellowish white patches are known as cotton-wool spots.

inflammatory disorders, can cause a wide variety of eye problems known collectively as *thyroid ophthalmopathy* (Figure 4.5A). This group of conditions produces various degrees of swelling of the eyelids and orbital tissues, specifically the extraocular muscles. As an autoimmune disease, the body's immune system attacks the thyroid gland, which creates the thyroid dysfunction. Unfortunately, the receptors of the cells of the extraocular muscles are almost identical to the appearance of the thyroid cell receptors and, therefore, the immune system also attacks the extraocular muscles when it attacks the thyroid gland. The results of such extraocular muscle swelling include **proptosis**, also referred to as *exophthalmos*, and associated problems with lid and ocular muscle movement. Severe exophthalmos causes **exposure keratopathy** (Figure 4.5B), which exposes the delicate ocular surface and is associated with drying of the conjunctiva and corneal surface, and can lead to loss of vision from corneal scarring or perforation. Swelling in the orbit can lead to compression of the optic nerve and, if left untreated, can also result in visual loss.

Treatment for the thyroid condition itself sometimes relieves the eye problems, but thyroid ophthalmopathy may persist or even progress despite restoration of normal thyroid function. Therapy specifically for the eye conditions ranges from the use of artificial tears for corneal surface problems to orbital decompression surgery for severe exophthalmos and compressive optic neuropathy.

Multiple Sclerosis

Multiple sclerosis (MS) is a chronic disease of the nervous system affecting the white matter of the spinal cord and brain. Optic nerve inflammation (optic neuritis)

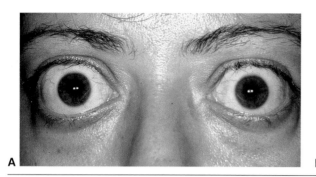 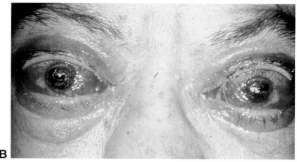

Figure 4.5 Thyroid ophthalmopathy. **A.** Retracted lids and proptosis. **B.** Corneal damage (exposure keratopathy).

resulting from MS is frequent in young adults. A positive diagnosis is difficult to establish but may involve examination of spinal fluid, magnetic resonance imaging (MRI) scans, and assessment of the patient's long-term pattern of symptoms.

Metabolic Disorders

Of all the metabolic diseases, diabetes is the one that carries the greatest risk of blindness.

Diabetes Mellitus

According to the American Diabetes Association, diabetes mellitus afflicts more than 25 million people in the United States. Unfortunately, nearly one-third are unaware that they have the disease. Diabetes affects a variety of organs and organ systems, from the peripheral nerves to the kidneys. The effects of diabetes on the vascular system can cause progressive stages of damage including leakage of fluid from blood vessels and oozing of protein substances into the retina (*nonproliferative diabetic retinopathy*).

Diabetics can also develop a state of very poor retinal circulation (nonperfusion) or ischemia and ultimately neovascularization (uncontrolled growth of new blood vessels over the surface of the retina). This proliferation of blood vessels can lead to blindness due to vitreous hemorrhage or tractional retinal detachment. This condition is known as *proliferative diabetic retinopathy* (Figure 4.6). In addition, diabetic patients can accumulate fluid in the macula that can significantly decrease vision. The occurrence of blindness among people with diabetes is 25 times that of the general population. Blood sugar and blood pressure control is critical in decreasing the risk of development and progression of diabetic retinopathy especially with early stages of diabetic retinopathy. Therefore, ophthalmologists strongly encourage diabetics to maintain a glycosylated hemoglobin (HbA_{1c}) level less than 7% (a blood test that assesses the quality

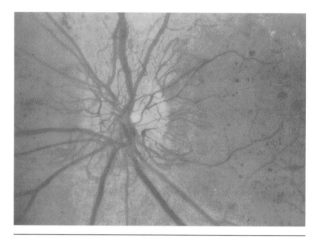

Figure 4.6 Fundus of a patient with diabetic retinopathy; new vessels are growing on the optic disc.

of long-term blood sugar control) and a blood pressure level less than 140/85.

Diabetic retinopathy can severely damage retinal structures before patients notice any loss of vision. For this reason, diabetic patients require routine ophthalmological examinations to detect possible retinopathy and follow its progression at intervals determined by the extent of the retinopathy. Laser surgery has been found to be effective in preventing blindness from diabetic retinopathy. Traditional surgical treatment may be required to remove a vitreous hemorrhage or repair retinal detachments that may complicate proliferative diabetic retinopathy. Injecting the eye's vitreous humor with a corticosteroid (eg, triamcinolone acetonide) and, more recently, an antivascular endothelial growth factor (anti-VEGF), has been shown to improve diabetic macular edema.

Vascular Diseases

Problems with the blood vessels—the circulatory system—can lead to a host of diseases that affect the eye or the visual system.

Cerebral Vascular Accident

Stroke and cerebral hemorrhage (bleeding within the brain) are the principal types of cerebral vascular accident (CVA). A CVA is an example of an interaction between the nervous system and the vascular system. A variety of systemic conditions that affect the heart and circulatory system can impair or block blood vessels and lead to a loss of blood flow to the brain, called a *stroke*. Without blood and the oxygen it carries, the brain's tissues quickly die. Unless the blood supply is restored rapidly, damage becomes irreversible. When a stroke occurs in a part of the brain involved with vision (visual pathways or visual cortex), a visual field defect can result.

A primary cause of eye problems associated with interrupted blood flow is an embolus (plural: emboli), a plaque of cholesterol, a clot of blood cells, or calcium, that plugs tiny vessels of the retina and/or the optic nerve and blocks blood circulation for a finite period (Figure 4.7). These obstructions can produce a sudden loss of vision, often in just one eye, and may be transient. Such incidents of temporary visual loss may be the first indication that a patient has a circulatory problem requiring medical attention. These emboli typically originate from the carotid vessels or the heart. Sometimes the embolus causes a prolonged blockage of the retinal artery, producing permanent visual loss called a *retinal artery occlusion*. The position of the embolus within the retinal vascular tree determines the name of the condition. For example, an embolus in the central retinal artery is called a **central retinal artery occlusion** (**CRAO**). If the obstruction occurs farther down the vascular tree, it is referred to as a **branch retinal artery occlusion** (**BRAO**).

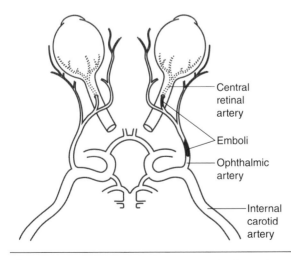

Figure 4.7 Emboli that can cause a cerebral vascular accident may also become lodged in arteries leading to the eye and cause temporary or permanent visual loss.

Giant Cell Arteritis

Giant cell arteritis, also known as **temporal arteritis**, affects the circulation of blood in the medium-sized arteries and is, therefore, considered a vascular disease. However, giant cell arteritis can also be classified as an inflammatory or immunologic disorder. It primarily afflicts people over the age of 60. The effects of giant cell arteritis on certain cranial arteries, including those supplying the eye, lead to a number of potential systemic and eye problems. The optic nerve may become severely damaged from a reduced blood supply, causing visual loss (ischemic optic neuropathy). Loss of vision can also result when the central retinal artery becomes occluded. Eye muscle imbalance may also occur.

Ocular signs and symptoms often serve as the first indication to the doctor that the patient has giant cell arteritis. Urgent blood testing and/or biopsy (surgery to remove and test suspect tissue) of the temporal artery may be required, as well as prompt drug therapy (eg, corticosteroids) to prevent blindness or death. Treatment of the systemic condition, which may include corticosteroids, can also be effective for the ocular conditions.

Migraine

Migraine usually produces intense headache and possibly nausea, often preceded by scintillations—visual sensations of flashing or whirling lights. Ophthalmic migraine produces only the scintillations and, in some patients, pupillary dilation and temporary partial or complete loss of vision. Although not completely understood, the causes of migraine are thought to involve a problem with the circulatory system of the brain or, in the case of ocular migraine, the occipital cortex, the part of the brain associated with vision. Migraine also may stem from a treatable vascular disease. Specific systemic drugs may be used to help relieve symptoms and prevent their frequent recurrence.

Hypertension

Systemic hypertension (high blood pressure) impairs blood circulation. In the eye, this circulatory impairment may produce problems in the vessels supplying the retina, choroid, and optic nerve. Hypertension can lead to small hemorrhages and other characteristic changes in the retina and its vessels even without creating noticeable visual problems (Figure 4.8). An ophthalmologist's retina (fundus) examination, therefore, is often important in detecting and diagnosing the presence of hypertensive retinopathy and following its course. Various methods

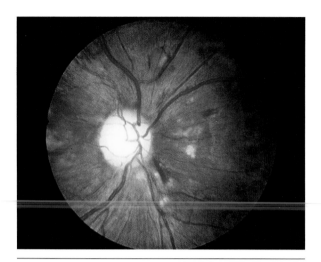

Figure 4.8 Characteristic retinal changes due to hypertension include flame-shaped hemorrhages and whitish cotton-wool patches.

of controlling systemic blood pressure, ranging from dietary to drug treatments, can help overcome many of the eye problems associated with systemic hypertension.

Infectious Diseases

Infectious diseases are of special concern because they can produce irreversible ocular damage in a relatively short period. These diseases are acquired and transmitted by various methods. Several infectious conditions have important ophthalmologic implications.

Acquired Immunodeficiency Syndrome

Acquired immunodeficiency syndrome (AIDS) is an infection caused by the human immunodeficiency virus (HIV). The presence of HIV affects the ability of the body's immune system to combat many different kinds of additional infections. The disease may be present in a variety of forms. Some patients harbor HIV for many years with no extreme effects on their immune systems, while the immune systems of others with HIV are compromised within a year or two of infection. AIDS was once untreatable and invariably fatal. More people with HIV are now able to live symptom free because of the advent of a number of antiretroviral drugs such as reverse transcriptase inhibitors, protease inhibitors, fusion inhibitors, and integrase inhibitors. These drugs have significantly prolonged the longevity of the AIDS patient.

HIV can be sexually transmitted but also can be acquired through blood transfusions or direct or indirect contact with blood or body fluids from individuals infected with HIV. A fetus can contract HIV during gestation from an HIV-infected mother.

Eye problems frequently occur in patients with AIDS. These problems are associated with opportunistic infections, which are infections that are able to proliferate in an immune-deficient patient. Retinal infections are common, particularly cytomegalovirus (CMV) retinitis (Figure 4.9), especially in those individuals who are severely immune-compromised with CD4 counts less than 50 (a total cell count of a subtype of white blood cell called helper T lymphocytes). A normal CD count is 1000 cells per cubic milliliter of blood (range 500 to 1500). A noninfectious HIV retinopathy that resembles diabetic retinopathy may also be present. Kaposi sarcoma is a vascular growth of malignant cells on the lid and conjunctiva. Another viral eye infection that may afflict AIDS patients is herpes zoster. Herpes zoster ophthalmicus is a painful infection that affects both the eyelids and the eye. It can affect virtually all layers of the eye from the cornea to the retina.

Chlamydial Infections

A bacterium called **chlamydiae** is responsible for this group of infections. One form of chlamydia, which affects the urologic, reproductive, and sex organs, is transmitted sexually. This type of chlamydia occurs commonly among sexually active young people. Genital infections can be transmitted to the eye, causing chlamydial, or inclusion, conjunctivitis (see Figure 7.2B).

Symptoms of chlamydial conjunctivitis include eye redness and discharge. Diagnosis of this type of conjunctivitis

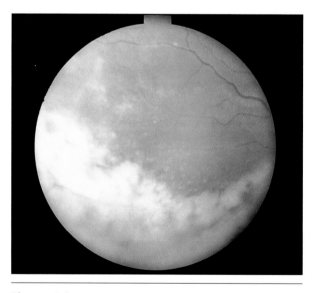

Figure 4.9 Yellowish lower area of the retina infected with cytomegalovirus in a patient with AIDS is easily distinguished from upper, uninfected area.

is usually made through special microbiologic testing. Proper diagnosis is important not only to select the correct treatment, but also to treat the sexual partners of the infected patient and to prevent further spread of the primary disease. Treatment for this condition usually includes use of systemic, and possibly topical, antibiotic drugs.

Herpes Infections

The viruses **varicella-zoster** and **herpes simplex** can infect numerous body systems, creating a variety of effects in each. The varicella-zoster virus, which causes chicken pox, can affect the peripheral nervous system. When it does, it causes a condition called *shingles*— painful nerve inflammation with swelling and skin eruptions. When it involves the eye, herpes zoster ophthalmicus can cause uveitis, corneal inflammation, and other intraocular conditions. It is sometimes complicated by opportunistic bacterial eye infection, producing reddened eyes and swollen lids (Figure 4.10). The retina and other parts of the eye may also become infected. Treatment for the eye condition usually consists of topical corticosteroids, cycloplegic drops, and/or systemic antiviral medications.

Herpes simplex virus type 1 causes fever blisters, while type 2 produces genital infections. Known as *ocular herpes simplex* when it occurs in the eye, type 1 infection can lead to blepharitis, conjunctivitis, keratitis, and other, more severe corneal conditions. Retinal infection, though rare, may also occur. Treatment for ocular herpes simplex may involve oral systemic antiviral drugs as well as topical antiviral agents, depending on the area and severity of infection.

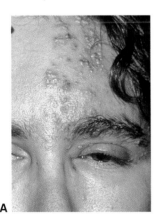 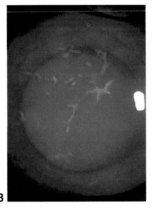

Figure 4.10 Herpes zoster ophthalmicus. **A.** Skin eruptions near the eye and swollen lids. **B.** Diseased cornea stained with diagnostic fluorescein shows the characteristic branchlike (dendritic) pattern of herpetic keratitis.

Histoplasmosis

Histoplasmosis is a systemic fungal infection contracted by inhaling dust from soil containing spores of the fungus. It is particularly common in the Mississippi and Ohio River Valleys and the river valleys of South America, Asia, and Africa. Histoplasmosis principally affects the pulmonary system, causing flu-like symptoms, but can infect a number of other body systems as well. The exact effect of histoplasmosis on the eye is controversial. Eye conditions related to contact with the fungus, referred to as **ocular histoplasmosis**, involve choroidal and retinal scarring and subretinal hemorrhages from choroidal neovascularization.

Syphilis

Syphilis is a highly contagious sexually transmitted disease caused by the bacterium *Treponema pallidum*. Syphilis can mimic almost any other inflammatory infectious disease. Adults may become infected through sexual activity, and newborns can contract the disease, in the birthing process, from an infected mother. Uveitis is the principal ocular condition associated with syphilis, but defects in pupillary function, retinal vasculitis, and optic neuropathy may also occur. Syphilis is treated with penicillin; untreated syphilis can result in blindness.

Toxoplasmosis

Toxoplasmosis is an infection caused by a protozoan, *Toxoplasma gondii*, which may be passed from mother to fetus (congenital toxoplasmosis). It also can be contracted from contact with animal feces (acquired toxoplasmosis), such as when changing cat litter or with ingestion of contaminated undercooked meat. The congenital form of this disease severely affects the central nervous system of the fetus or newborn (often resulting in death), while the acquired form may cause only mild fever, swollen glands, and general illness. Ocular toxoplasmosis occurs as an active retinochoroiditis or inactive retinochoroidal scar associated with uveitis and vitritis (inflammation of the vitreous). This infection may also occur in association with AIDS.

Neoplastic Diseases

Systemic malignancies such as cancer or leukemia can produce ocular manifestations that may require therapy to prevent visual loss.

Metastatic Carcinoma

Metastatic carcinoma is the term used to describe cancer that produces tumors (growths that can be malignant and potentially lethal) in more than one part of the body. The originating tumor is called the primary tumor while the same type of tumor found in other parts of the body is called the metastatic tumor. Tumors in the eye often develop as a result of tumors that have originated elsewhere in the body, notably from cancer in the breast or lungs (Figure 4.11). Such metastatic (secondary) carcinomas can lead to loss of vision through invasion by the tumor cells into the choroid, a primary site for metastatic cancer. *Metastases* may also appear in the orbit. Some of these tumors may respond to treatment with radiation or chemotherapy.

Blood Dyscrasias

Blood dyscrasias are defined as any abnormal or pathologic condition of the blood. An example of a serious blood dyscrasia is leukemia, a well-known type of cancer. This disorder can adversely affect the optic nerve, retinal blood vessels, and other portions of the retina (Figure 4.12). Because changes in retinal appearance may be present before visual symptoms develop, patients known to have blood dyscrasias often require regular ophthalmologic examinations.

Cerebral Neoplasms

Brain tumors may cause increased intracranial pressure and headaches. Visual field defects and pupillary abnormalities may be the first signs of a brain tumor. Swelling of the optic nerve head, or papilledema, may be detected on funduscopy. Computed tomography (CT) and MRI scans help confirm the diagnosis.

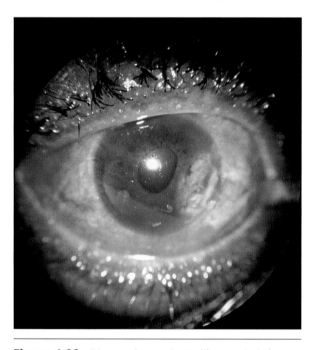

Figure 4.11   Iris mass in a patient with metastatic lung carcinoma.

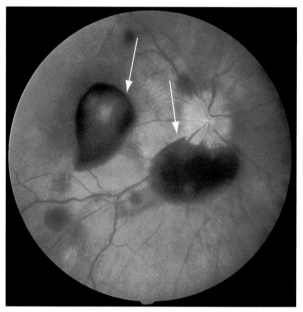

Figure 4.12   Fundus of a patient with leukemia, displaying preretinal (arrows) and retinal hemorrhages.

SELF-ASSESSMENT TEST

1. Name some of the main hormones produced by the endocrine glands.

2. What are the 5 categories of systemic disease that have ocular manifestations?

3. What are the symptoms of keratoconjunctivitis sicca?

4. Outline the effects of diabetes on the retinal vascular system.

5. Diabetics should be encouraged to maintain glycosylated hemoglobin and blood pressure at what level?

6. What is the primary cause of eye problems associated with interrupted ocular blood flow?

7. Name 2 opportunistic infections seen in the eyes of AIDS patients.

8. Metastatic eye tumors commonly originate from which 2 organs?

9. What 2 eye findings are usually the first signs of a brain tumor?

10. A diagnosis of multiple sclerosis, although difficult to establish, is based on what diagnostic tests?

SUGGESTED ACTIVITIES

1. Outline the complications of HIV infection and how they relate to the eye.

2. Present a 5-minute talk on "shingles involving the face" to the office staff.

3. Ask your ophthalmologist or senior technician if you could shadow them when they are examining diabetic patients.

4. Interview a patient with chronic disease about how it impacts his or her life.

SUGGESTED READING

Beers MH, ed. *The Merck Manual of Medical Information: Home Edition*. 2nd ed. Whitehouse Station, NJ: Merck Publishing Group; 2003.

Harper RA, ed. *Basic Ophthalmology*. 9th ed. San Francisco: American Academy of Ophthalmology; 2010: 165–182.

Fraunfelder FT, Roy FH, eds. *Current Ocular Therapy 5*. Philadelphia: Saunders; 2000.

Morgan RA. *How Systemic Diseases Affect the Visual System* [audio lecture, product 04-07]. St Paul, MN: Joint Commission on Allied Health Personnel in Ophthalmology.

Stenson SM, Friedberg DN, eds. *AIDS and the Eye*. New Orleans: Contact Lens Association of Ophthalmologists; 1995.

Wright KW, ed. *Textbook of Ophthalmology*. Baltimore: Lippincott Williams & Wilkins; 1997.

5 OPTICS AND REFRACTIVE STATES OF THE EYE

As the primary organ of vision, the eye operates much like a camera. Light rays reflected from objects pass through the optical system of the eye, cornea, and lens and are focused to form images of the objects on the light-sensitive retina. Various diseases of the eye and the visual pathway can interfere with vision or even totally destroy sight. However, nonpathologic imperfections in the optical system of an essentially healthy eye may also produce less than satisfactory vision. In this case, the "camera" isn't broken; it just produces pictures that are out of focus or distorted. Such nonpathologic imperfections in the eye's optical system, known as refractive errors, can be corrected by the use of supplementary lenses in the form of eyeglasses or contact lenses, by refractive corneal surgery, or by implantation of an intraocular lens.

Ophthalmic medical assistants usually participate in the measurement of refractive errors that may be present. Such assistance requires a basic knowledge of optics—the science that studies the properties and behavior of light—especially as it pertains to lenses used to correct refractive errors. In addition to discussing optics, lenses, and the nature of refractive errors, this chapter also discusses the basic principles and elements of the procedures used to discover, measure, and correct refractive errors. It also includes instructions for performing and recording the results of two important related tests: lensometry and keratometry.

Principles of Optics

Optics is the branch of physical science that deals with the properties of light and vision. To simplify the study of this complex subject, the science of optics has been divided into different areas. The two principal areas that most concern ophthalmology are **physical optics**, which describes the *nature of light in terms of its wave properties*, and **geometric optics**, which *deals with the transmission of light as rays* and is concerned with the effect of lenses on light and the production of images.

What is commonly referred to as light is the very small *visible* portion of a wide spectrum of **electromagnetic radiation** (Figure 5.1). The spectrum ranges from invisible cosmic, gamma, and x-rays, through visible light waves, to invisible radio and television signals. All of these forms of energy travel through space and various substances as waves, each wave having a crest and a trough just as ocean waves do.

Violet light has the shortest wavelength; red, the longest.

One way of differentiating the types of electromagnetic energy is by wavelength—the distance between crests of the wave. X-rays, for example, have a wavelength of about one billionth of a centimeter, while, at the opposite end of the spectrum, radio waves have a wavelength that is measured in kilometers. The wavelengths of light visible to the human eye lie roughly in the middle of the spectrum of electromagnetic radiation, ranging from about 400 to 750 *billionths* of a meter (nanometers). These wavelengths comprise light with the colors red, orange, yellow, green, blue, indigo, and violet (easily remembered by the mnemonic *ROY G BIV*).

As with all forms of energy in the electromagnetic spectrum, light can travel through certain substances but may be blocked by others. Substances that completely block light are called **opaque**; those that transmit light but significantly interfere with its passage are referred to as **translucent**; substances that permit the passage of light without significant disruption are referred to as **transparent**. It is the behavior of light rays as they pass through transparent objects that most affects the correction of refractive errors.

Refraction

Light rays are **refracted** (bent) when they pass at an angle from one transparent medium, such as air, into another transparent medium, such as water, glass, or plastic, and are refracted once again when they exit the second medium. A simple illustration of refraction can be obtained by poking a straw into a glass of water (Figure 5.2). If you look at the straw from directly above, you will see it continue straight into the water; if you look at it from an angle, the straw appears to bend at the point where it enters the water. This phenomenon is due to the differences in the speed at which light travels through various substances.

Light travels through a vacuum at a speed of 300,000 kilometers per second (about 186,000 miles per second). On passage through other transparent media or substances, light slows down somewhat, depending on the **optical density** (compactness) of the particular substance. The ratio of the speed of light in a vacuum to its speed in a specific substance is called the **refractive index** of that substance:

$$\text{refractive index} = \frac{\text{speed of light in a vacuum}}{\begin{array}{c}\text{speed of light in a}\\\text{specific substance}\end{array}}$$

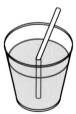

Figure 5.2 Refraction. Viewed at an angle, a straw appears to bend when it enters the water in a glass.

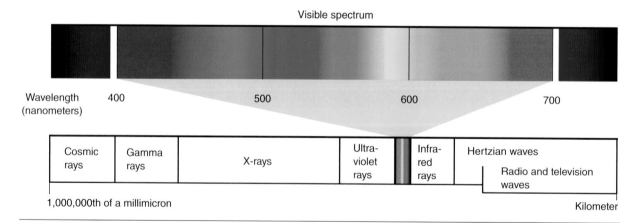

Figure 5.1 The spectrum of electromagnetic radiation. Note the narrow band of visible light.

The more optically dense the substance, the slower the speed of light and the higher the refractive index. Refractive indices of some common substances are presented in Table 5.1. Because the speed of light in air is close to that in a vacuum, the refractive index of air is 1.00. The refractive indices of other, denser substances are all greater than 1.00. The refractive index of transparent substances such as glass or plastic (that is, the extent to which these substances bend light) is a useful property considered in the manufacture of lenses. The principal refractive properties of lenses relate to the surface curvatures and the index of refraction.

Refractive Properties of Curved Lenses

Lenses are transparent optical devices shaped in ways that can alter normal vision (such as with microscopes and telescopes) and improve poor vision (such as with eyeglasses and contact lenses). An understanding of how curved lenses are formed and how they refract light to achieve various optical effects may be gained by considering the refractive properties of prisms.

A **prism** is a triangular piece of glass or plastic with **plane** (flat) sides, an **apex** (top), and a **base** (bottom). When a light ray passes through a prism, the emerging light ray bends in a direction toward the base of the prism (Figure 5.3A). If two identical prisms are placed together base to base, light rays passing through the glass or plastic will be refracted to **converge** (come together) at some point on the other side of the prisms (Figure 5.3B). If, on the other hand, two prisms are placed together apex to apex, the light rays will **diverge** (spread apart) on the other side of the prisms (Figure 5.3C).

Smoothing the sharp angles of adjacent prisms into curves where they meet yields the two basic forms of lenses. The first type is called a **convex lens** (Figure 5.4A). This lens is a piece of glass or plastic in which one or both surfaces are curved outward. In the second type, the **concave lens** (Figure 5.4B), one or both surfaces

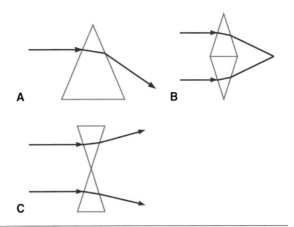

Figure 5.3 Passage of light through prisms. **A.** Prism deviates light toward its base. **B.** Light rays passing through two prisms placed base to base converge. **C.** Light rays passing through two prisms placed apex to apex diverge.

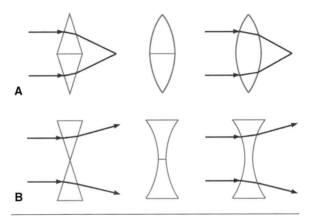

Figure 5.4 A pair of prisms smoothed to form (**A**) a convex lens and (**B**) a concave lens, and the subsequent matching refractive characteristics of the lenses.

are curved inward. These simple forms retain the same light-converging or light-diverging properties of the pair of prisms from which they are derived.

Convergence, Divergence, and Focal Point

The effects of lenses on light are generally considered in terms of straight light rays that emanate or are reflected from a distant object. These rays are said to be **parallel** to one another; that is, they travel side by side in the same direction.

A light ray that is perpendicular to a lens and strikes the center of a lens of any shape passes undeviated through the lens material, regardless of the lens' index of refraction. However, the light velocity alters depending on the density of the lens material. This pathway is known as the **principal axis** of the lens, and the light

Table 5.1 Index of Refraction for Substances of Interest in Ophthalmology

Substance	Index
Air	1.00
Water	1.33
Aqueous humor	1.34
Cornea	1.38
Crystalline lens	1.39
CR 39 plastic eyeglass lenses	1.49
Crown glass eyeglass lenses	1.52

ray is called the **axial** or **principal ray**. Parallel light rays from a distant source that enter the lens at any point other than the center are called **paraxial rays**.

With convex lenses, the paraxial rays from a distant source are refracted by the lens material and converge at a point somewhere along the principal axis behind the lens, that is, on the side of the lens opposite from the object (Figure 5.5). This point is known as the **focal point** of the lens. If you placed a piece of paper or a screen at the exact focal point, you would see a clear, real image of the object from which the light rays originally emanated, although the image would be inverted (upside down) and reversed (Figure 5.6). Convex lenses are called **positive** or **plus lenses**.

With concave lenses, the paraxial rays from a distant source are refracted by the lens material and diverge as they emerge from the lens (Figure 5.7). As a result, they cannot be focused behind the lens, and they produce no real image. However, if the direction of the diverging light rays is extended backward in a drawing, an imaginary or "virtual" focal point can be found in front of the lens where the lines meet the principal axis, that

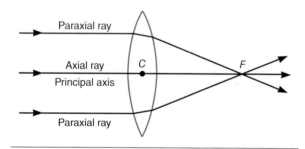

Figure 5.5 Passage of light rays through a convex (converging) lens. C = center of lens. F = focal point on principal axis behind lens.

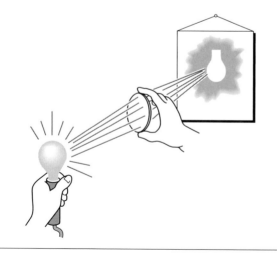

Figure 5.6 A real, inverted image of the light source is seen when a screen is placed at the focal point of the convex lens.

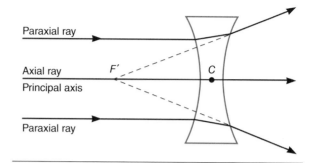

Figure 5.7 Passage of light rays through a concave (diverging) lens. C = center of lens. F′ = virtual focal point on principal axis in front of lens.

is, on the same side of the lens as the object. A **virtual image** of the light source can be seen at this point, but it cannot be focused on a screen. Concave lenses are called **negative** or **minus lenses**.

Lens Power and Focal Length

The **vergence power**, or simply **power**, of a lens is a measure of its ability to converge or diverge light rays. This ability depends on the refractive index of the lens material and on the shape of the lens. Steeply curved convex lenses of a given material produce greater convergence than do less curved convex lenses of the same substance and thus are more powerful. Similarly, concave lenses with greater curvature cause more divergence than do concave lenses with less curvature and thus are more powerful. The greater the convergence or divergence of light rays by a lens, the closer to the lens the focal point will be. (Figure 5.8). In other words, the distance between the focal point and the lens, the **focal length**, is related *inversely* to the power of the lens (that is, the stronger the lens, the shorter its focal length). Lens power is considered in terms of focal length, as follows: the power of a lens is equal to the *reciprocal* of the focal length measured in meters and is expressed in units called **diopters**:

$$D = 1/F$$

where D = lens power in diopters and F = focal length in meters. For example, a convex lens with a focal length of 2 meters has a power of 1/2, or 0.50 D; a convex lens with a focal length of 0.25 meter has a power of 1/0.25, or 4.00 D.

As described earlier, concave (minus) lenses cause light rays from a distant source to diverge, producing a virtual image in front of the lens. For this reason, the power of a minus lens is expressed in negative diopters. For example, a concave lens with a focal length of 2 meters has a power of –1/2, or –0.50 D; a concave lens with a focal length of –0.25 meter has a power of –1/0.25,

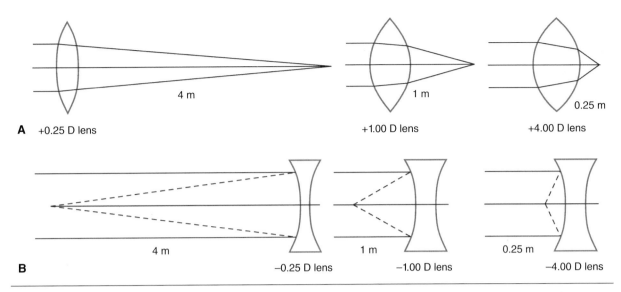

Figure 5.8 The relationship of lens power to focal length. **A.** Three examples of plus, or convex (converging), lenses. **B.** Three examples of minus, or concave (diverging), lenses.

or –4.00 D. Understanding the basis and methods of expressing lens power is important in measuring and correcting refractive errors of the eye.

Refractive States of the Eye

The principles of optics and the properties of lenses discussed above apply equally to the optical system of the human eye. The eye is a plus-power system consisting of the convex cornea and crystalline lens, which refract light rays reflected from objects and focus them to produce real images on the retina. The overall converging power of the eye is approximately 60 D, about 40 of which are attributed to the cornea and about 20 to the crystalline lens. Because the normal lens can change its curvature and thus its power, it allows for the fine adjustment of focus. This capability, called **accommodation**, is important because, although the screen (retina) on which images are focused is fixed in its distance from the refractive elements of the eye, the objects on which gaze is directed are not.

The term **refractive state** refers to the relative ability of the refractive components of the eye (the cornea and lens) to bring objects into focus on the retina. The two principal refractive states are **emmetropia**, where parallel light rays are focused perfectly on the retina, and **ametropia**, where light rays are not perfectly focused on the retina due to various **refractive errors**. A condition associated with diminished accommodation is **presbyopia**, which primarily affects near vision and is a normal condition of aging.

Emmetropia

In the normal eye, light rays from a distant object are focused sharply on the retina by the relaxed lens without the need of any accommodative effort. This condition is called *emmetropia* (Figure 5.9). Light rays emanating from a near object are divergent and, therefore, an emmetropic eye has to accommodate to see the object clearly. In contrast, a myopic eye sees a near object clearly without corrective lenses or accommodation. Accommodation adds plus power to the eye. A hyperopic eye accommodates to see clearly for both distance and near.

Ametropia

When the relaxed, or nonaccommodating, eye is unable to bring light rays from a distant object into focus, the condition is called *ametropia*. Three basic conditions may produce this refractive error: myopia; hyperopia, or hypermetropia; and astigmatism.

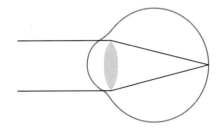

Figure 5.9 The emmetropic eye: parallel rays of light focus sharply on the retina.

MYOPIA   Also known as nearsightedness, **myopia** is a condition in which the cornea and lens of the nonaccommodating eye have too much plus power for the length of the eye. As a result, images of distant objects are focused in front of the retina and thus appear blurred (Figure 5.10). Near vision in people with myopia is almost always good. Because of the greater relative plus power of their optical system, myopic individuals not wearing corrective lenses require less accommodation for near vision than do people with normal eyes.

HYPEROPIA   Also known as farsightedness, hyperopia is a condition in which the cornea and lens have too little plus power for the length of the nonaccommodating eye. As a result, light rays from a distant object come to a focus at a point theoretically behind the retina and the image appears blurred (Figure 5.11). For many individuals, accommodation by the lens, which adds plus power to the eye's optical system, can supply the needed additional converging power and bring the distant light rays into focus on the retina. Healthy children have an ample reserve of accommodation and, if hyperopic, can unconsciously accommodate for both distant and near objects. As accommodative ability gradually declines with maturity, these hyperopic individuals will notice a loss of clarity in near and distance vision.

Almost all infants are hyperopic at birth, but generally the eye lengthens and approaches "normal" size as the infant matures. Hyperopia may occur if the eye does not

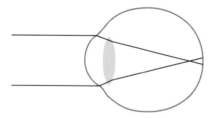

Figure 5.10   The myopic eye: parallel rays of light are brought to a focus in front of the retina.

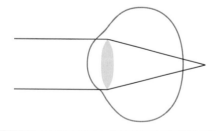

Figure 5.11   The hyperopic eye: parallel rays of light would come to a focus behind the retina in the unaccommodated eye.

reach a "normal" size or if the entire optical power is too weak for whatever its length.

ASTIGMATISM   The cornea of the normal eye and of most myopic and hyperopic individuals has a uniform curvature, with resulting equal refracting power over its entire surface; this is the **spherical cornea**. In some individuals, however, the curvature of cornea is not uniform—the toric cornea—and curvatures are greater in one meridian than another, much like a football. The result is different levels of myopia or hyperopia in different optical planes. Light rays refracted by the **toric cornea** are not brought to a single point focus; retinal images from objects both distant and near are blurred and may appear broadened or elongated. This refractive error is called **astigmatism**.

The **principal meridians**—the meridians of maximum and minimum corneal curvature—are at right angles to each other in astigmatism and are usually (but not necessarily) vertical and horizontal. In **regular astigmatism**, which is the more common form, the shape of the corneal surface would resemble the surface of a football standing on one end or on its side or, less often, tipped to one side. In **irregular astigmatism**, which is less common, the corneal "football" would have an irregular or bumpy shape. Various types of regular astigmatism have been identified on the basis of the refractive power and position of the focal points of the principal meridians (Figure 5.12).

PRESBYOPIA   **Presbyopia** is a progressive loss of the accommodative ability of the crystalline lens due to the natural processes of aging. To understand presbyopia, consider the mechanism of accommodation (Figure 5.13). An emmetropic eye can focus light rays from distant objects on the retina without the aid of accommodation. However, light rays from near objects (those closer than 20 feet, or 6 meters, which is the generally accepted minimum distance for testing far visual acuity) would normally focus behind the retina unless accommodation—an increase in the curvature and thus the plus power of the crystalline lens—occurred. This accommodative mechanism is particularly strong in children but gradually diminishes with age as the lens loses its elasticity. The normal hardening of the lens begins at birth but generally does not cause a problem until about the age of 40 or 45. When the loss of accommodation interferes with, or prevents, clear near vision, the result is presbyopia.

Presbyopia may occur in the presence of emmetropia, myopia, and hyperopia, as well as astigmatism. Its onset results in increasing difficulty with near visual work, such

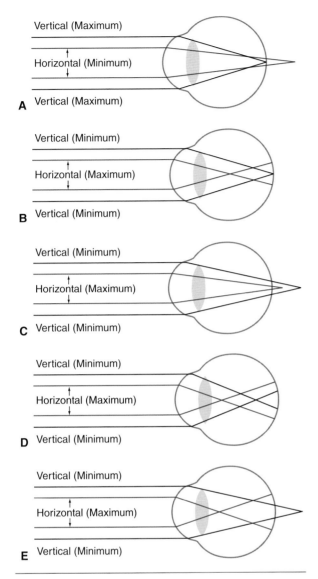

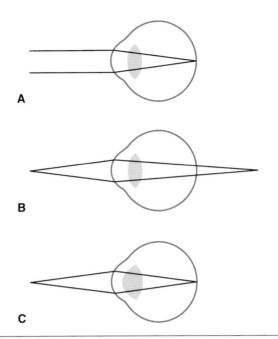

Figure 5.13 Accommodation in the emmetropic eye. **A.** No accommodation is necessary to focus light rays from a distant object. **B.** Rays from a near object are focused behind the retina, unless (**C**) accommodation is brought into play.

Types and Uses of Corrective Lenses

The principal refractive errors of the eye can be corrected by the use of ophthalmic lenses in the form of eyeglasses or contact lenses, refractive surgery, or surgical implantation of an artificial lens (intraocular lens implants). For a more detailed discussion of contact lenses and refractive surgery, refer to Chapters 14 and 18.

Lenses used to correct refractive errors are generally made of glass or plastic and, like all lenses, refract light rays as described earlier in this chapter. In various forms, corrective lenses can supply needed additional convergence of light rays (as in hyperopia), compensate for excess convergence of light rays (as in myopia), correct refractive errors that are not uniform in all meridians of the eye (as in astigmatism), and provide near vision that has been reduced due to presbyopia.

Table 5.2 lists the principal ophthalmic lens types, shapes, and corrective uses. The basic types of ophthalmic lenses used to test for and correct refractive errors are spheres, cylinders, and a combination of both (spherocylinders). Although they are not lenses in the traditional sense, prisms are sometimes categorized as such because they are incorporated into eyeglasses to correct extraocular muscle imbalance. Ophthalmic medical assistants require an understanding of the specific properties and

Figure 5.12 Classes of regular astigmatism. **A.** Simple hyperopic astigmatism: one meridian focuses light on the retina, the other theoretically behind the retina. **B.** Simple myopic astigmatism: one meridian focuses light in front of the retina, the other on the retina. **C.** Compound hyperopic astigmatism: both meridians focus light theoretically behind the retina. **D.** Compound myopic astigmatism: both meridians focus light in front of the retina. **E.** Mixed astigmatism: one meridian focuses light in front of the retina, the other behind the retina.

as reading small print (especially in dim light), sewing, and the like. However, this effect and the age at which a myopic or hyperopic individual might first perceive this difficulty can vary according to the type and extent of the refractive error and whether an individual wears corrective lenses or contact lenses. Presbyopia does not develop at the same rate in individuals, and its onset may manifest clinically at any time during the fourth or fifth decade of life.

Table 5.2 Properties and Uses of Ophthalmic Corrective Lenses

Lens Type	Lens Shape and Power	Corrective Use
Sphere	Convex (+)	Hyperopia
	Concave (−)	Myopia
Cylinder	Spherocylindrical (+ or −)	Astigmatism
Prism	Plane, with at least 2 nonparallel surfaces	Double vision

uses of these lenses in order to take measurements used in arriving at a patient's eyeglass or contact lens prescription and to measure the optical characteristics of existing corrective lenses.

Spheres

A lens that has the same curvature over its entire surface and, thus, the same refractive power in all directions, or meridians, is referred to as a **spherical lens** or **sphere**. These terms were adopted because the lens may be thought of as having been cut from a sphere of glass or plastic. Because of its uniform curvature and refractive ability, a spherical lens is able to focus light rays at a single point (Figure 5.14).

> Spherical lenses may be convex or concave and of any dioptric power.

Spherical plus-power (convex) lenses are used to provide clear near and distance vision for hyperopic

individuals. Plus-power spherical lenses also provide near vision to emmetropic individuals with presbyopia; corrective eyeglasses for this purpose are sometimes referred to as reading glasses, since wearers use them only for reading and other near work. Spherical minus-power (concave) lenses are used to provide distance vision for those with myopia. Because near vision is often good with myopia, myopic individuals who develop presbyopia may need only remove their glasses to read and do close work.

For some patients, segmented 2- or 3-part eyeglass lenses—**bifocals** and **trifocals**—may be prescribed (Figure 5.15). In these eyeglasses, commonly referred to as **multifocal lenses**, the uppermost portion carries the minus or plus sphere correction (and cylinder if needed) for distance vision, while the power of the lowermost segment is for near vision (14 to 16 inches). The lower segment is always plus power added to the distance correction. The difference between the power of the upper segment and that of the lower segment is called the **add**. In the case of myopia, the adjustment is a less negative (or more positive) correction, while a hyperopic individual receives plus power in addition to that required for distance vision. The middle segment in trifocals corrects vision for an intermediate distance (2 to 4 feet). (See Chapter 12 for a discussion

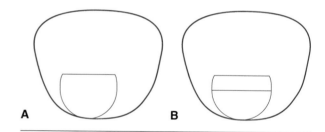

Figure 5.15 Flat top multifocal lenses. **A.** Bifocal. **B.** Trifocal.

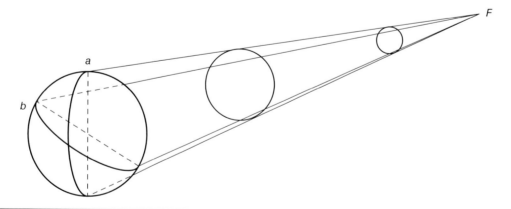

Figure 5.14 Refraction by a spherical lens (in this case, a planoconvex sphere). Because its radii of curvature (*a*, *b*) are equal, a sphere brings light rays to a single point focus (*F*).

about the types and specific uses of these and other multifocal lenses.)

Cylinders

Cylindrical lenses, or **cylinders**, differ from spheres in that they have curvature, and thus refractive power, in only one meridian. They may be convex or concave and of any dioptric power. The meridian perpendicular to (90° from) the meridian with curvature is called the **axis** of the cylinder (Figure 5.16). By convention, the orientation (position in space) of the cylinder is indicated by the axis, which ranges from 0° (horizontal) through 90° (vertical), to 180° (same as 0°). In contrast to a spherical lens, a cylinder focuses light rays to a focal line rather than to a point (Figure 5.17).

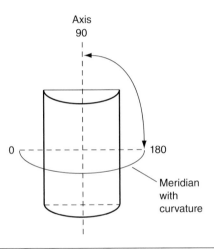

Figure 5.16 The axis of a cylinder is located 90° from its meridian with curvature.

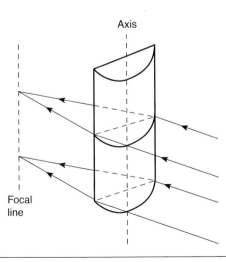

Figure 5.17 Refraction by a cylinder. Because a cylinder has refracting power in only one meridian (perpendicular to its axis), it focuses light to a focal line.

Pure cylindrical lenses are used in ophthalmology mostly for testing purposes. Theoretically, a pure cylindrical lens—one that possesses power in only one meridian—might be used to correct astigmatism. However, most astigmatic individuals are hyperopic or myopic as well and require correction in more than one meridian. To provide the correction they need, a lens formed from the combination of cylinder and sphere (spherocylinder) is generally required.

Spherocylinders

A **spherocylinder**, as its name suggests, is a combination of a sphere and a cylinder. It is sometimes also called a **toric lens**.

If a spherical lens may be imagined as cut from an object shaped like a basketball, a spherocylindrical lens can be thought of as cut from an object shaped like a football. Unlike the spherical "basketball," which has the same curvature over its entire surface, the spherocylindrical "football" has different curvatures varying continuously between a meridian of maximum curvature to a meridian 90° away of minimum curvature (Figure 5.18).

Because the perpendicular radii of its curvature are not equal, a spherocylinder does not focus light to a single focal point, as does a sphere. Rather, it refracts light along each of its two meridians to two different focal lines (Figure 5.19). The clearest image is formed at a point between these two focal lines, which is given the geometric term *circle of least confusion*. The ability of a spherocylindrical lens to refract light along each of

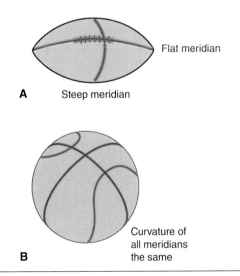

Figure 5.18 Examples of spherocylinders. **A.** A toric (spherocylindrical) football has different curvatures in each of 2 principal meridians. **B.** A spherical basketball possesses the same curvature over its entire surface.

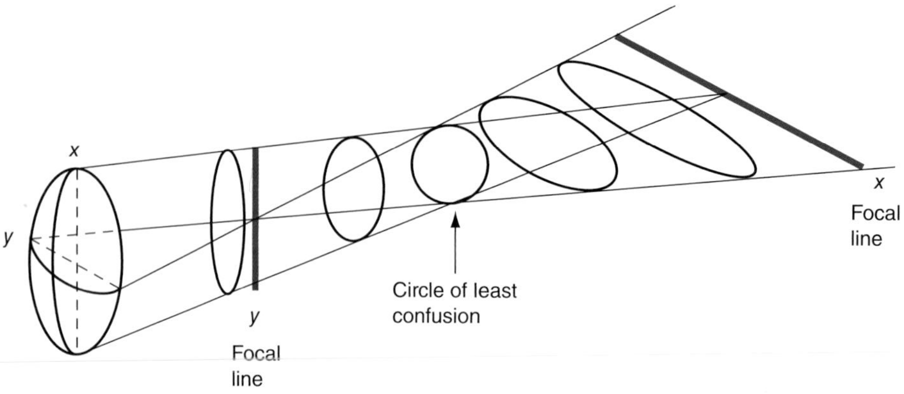

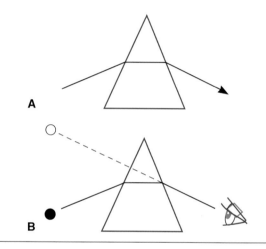

Figure 5.19 Refraction by a spherocylinder. Because its perpendicular radii of curvature (*x*, *y*) are not equal, a spherocylinder does not focus light to a point, but to 2 lines (*y* focal line, *x* focal line) in different places. The clearest image is formed at the circle of least confusion.

two meridians makes it ideal to correct myopia or hyperopia that is combined with astigmatism. The spherocylinder can supply varying amounts of plus and/or minus correction to each of the two principal meridians of the astigmatic eye.

Two properties of a spherocylinder must be recorded in order to prescribe the appropriate correcting lens for an astigmatic individual or to measure a patient's existing corrective lens: (1) the amount (in dioptric power) and the type of correction (plus or minus) in each of the two principal meridians; and (2) the position of the astigmatic axis. The latter must be known because although the meridians are usually perpendicular to each other, they may not be oriented in a strictly vertical (90°) and horizontal (180°) position. The technique of measuring these properties of spherocylindrical lenses, as well as specific properties of other types of lenses, is called **lensometry**.

Prisms

Because of its shape, a prism deviates (refracts) light rays toward its base. This effect causes objects viewed through prisms to appear displaced toward the prism apex (Figure 5.20). Depending on the refractive power and orientation of a prism, an object can be seen to appear in various locations other than its actual position. Because of this unique refracting property, prisms are employed in a number of ophthalmic instruments. Prisms are used to measure extraocular muscle imbalances, and they can be incorporated into eyeglass lenses to correct **diplopia** (double vision).

The refractive power of a prism depends on its refractive index and the size of its apex angle. This power is measured in terms of the prism's ability to deviate a ray of light and is expressed in prism diopters, notated with

Figure 5.20 Prisms. **A.** Because of its shape, a prism refracts light rays toward its base. **B.** If an object is viewed through a prism, the object appears displaced toward the prism apex.

the Δ symbol. (Figure 5.21). A prism measuring 1 prism diopter (1Δ) deviates parallel rays of light 1 centimeter at a distance of 100 centimeters (1 meter) from the prism. A prism that deviates rays 1 centimeter at a distance of 2 meters measures 0.5Δ; a prism that deviates rays 1 centimeter from a distance of one-half meter (0.5 m) measures 2Δ. Knowledge of this measurement convention is important in understanding the power and orientation of a prism needed to test for visual misalignments and correct double vision.

Components of Refraction

In eye care, the term *refraction* is used to describe the process of measuring a patient's refractive error and determining the optical correction needed to focus light

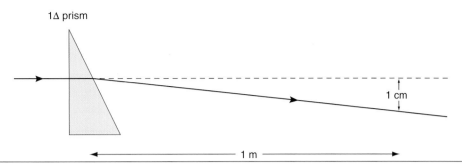

1Δ prism

1 cm

1 m

Figure 5.21 Prism refractive power. A prism measuring 1Δ deflects a light ray 1 centimeter at a distance of 1 meter.

rays from distant objects onto the retina and provide the patient with clear vision.

The process of refraction comprises two main components: refractometry, a multifaceted measurement of refractive errors with a variety of specific instruments and techniques, and clinical judgment, which is required to prescribe appropriate optical correction. Ophthalmic medical assistants are often responsible for many of the measurements involved in refractometry; the ophthalmologist provides the clinical judgment needed to verify the refractometric results, assess related needs of the patient, and prescribe appropriate correction. Because considerable skill and experience are required to perform the complex steps of refractometry well, this section provides only general descriptions and principles of these processes.

Refractometry may be divided into 3 steps: retinoscopy, refinement, and binocular balancing. These steps may be performed manually with a variety of instruments and materials or partly with automated refractors. The automated units can be moderately accurate and very efficient, but their utility will depend on their ability to produce the specific kinds of information the ophthalmologist needs to determine the appropriate correction. Performance of manual refractometry is an important skill for ophthalmic medical assistants. Even in practices where automated refractors are used, knowledge of the principles and methods of manual refractometry is required to use the equipment properly.

Whether manual or automatic, refractometry may be performed either with or without the use of cycloplegic drops, solutions of drugs that temporarily paralyze the ciliary muscle and thus block accommodation. Known as **cycloplegic refraction**, this method is useful in measuring refractive errors in patients under 20 years of age, whose powerful accommodative ability may contribute to false measurements and lead to inadequate correction of their refractive problem. When performed without cycloplegic drugs, as is the case with most adult patients,

the method of measurement is referred to as a **manifest refraction**.

The ophthalmologist usually determines whether manifest or cycloplegic refractometry is more appropriate for a given patient. Specific information about the uses, actions, and administration of cycloplegic drops appears in Chapter 6.

Retinoscopy

Retinoscopy is the initial step in refractometry. It is used to determine the approximate nature and extent of a refractive error and to estimate the type and power of the lens needed to correct that error. Retinoscopy is sometimes referred to as **objective refractometry** because it requires no participation or response from the patient. For some patients, such as children, individuals with developmental disabilities, and others unable to communicate well, retinoscopy is the only way to determine the refractive error.

In performing retinoscopy, the examiner uses a **retinoscope**, an instrument consisting of a light source and a viewing component (Figure 5.22). A mirror in the retinoscope directs an adjustable beam of light at the patient's eye, while the examiner observes the eye through the viewer. Two basic types of retinoscopes are available: one produces a spot of light; the other, a streak. The discussion here is limited to the more commonly used streak retinoscope.

One eye is examined at a time in retinoscopy. If the patient's accommodation has not been blocked by cycloplegic drops, the patient is asked or otherwise guided to **fixate** (gaze steadily at) a distant object. An alternate technique to neutralize the accommodative effort by the patient is to temporarily "fog" the patient's fellow eye with a plus lens. The examiner projects the streak of light from the retinoscope directly into the patient's eye. The light beam passes through the optical system of the eye and is reflected back by the patient's retina, appearing as a "retinoscopic reflex" in the patient's pupil.

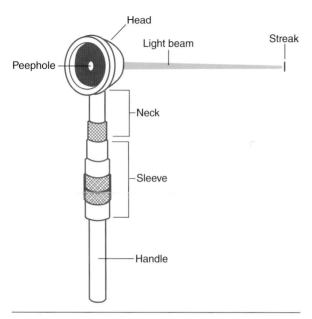

Figure 5.22 A retinoscope.

The examiner, who sees the reflex as a red-orange glowing line (Figure 5.23A), watches its movement while sweeping the light across the pupil. As the light sweeps across the pupil, the different types of refractive errors of the eye produce characteristic movements of the reflex.

The direction in which these reflexes move is affected by the retinoscopic lighting effect chosen by the

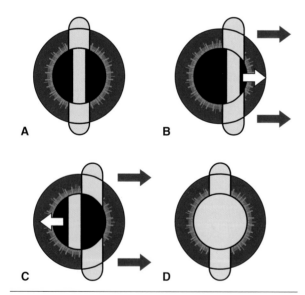

Figure 5.23 Reflexes produced by the streak retinoscope. **A.** Normal. **B.** "With" motion: the reflex moves in the same direction as the streak of light, indicating a hyperopic eye. **C.** "Against" motion: the reflex moves in the direction opposite to that of the streak, indicating a myopic eye. **D.** Neutralization point: there is no apparent movement of the reflex, and the pupil is filled with a red glow.

examiner. Retinoscopes allow the user to change lighting effects by raising or lowering a sleeve on the instrument handle. The **plano** (flat) **mirror effect** produces slightly divergent rays. The **concave mirror effect** produces convergent rays. The most commonly used retinoscopes require the sleeve to be raised to achieve the plano mirror effect and lowered to achieve the concave mirror effect. These positions are referred to as "sleeve up" and "sleeve down" respectively. To determine the plano mirror position, shine the streak against the palm of your hand in both the sleeve-up and sleeve-down positions. The streak will appear thickest when in the plano mirror position.

When the plano mirror effect of the retinoscope (usually "sleeve up") is being used, the hyperopic eye usually causes the retinoscopic reflex to move in the same direction as the streak of light. This movement is termed "**with motion**" (Figure 5.23B). The myopic eye usually causes the reflex to move in the opposite direction from the streak, termed "**against motion**" (Figure 5.23C). An astigmatic eye causes different types or degrees of movement in the two principal meridians; astigmatic retinoscopic reflexes vary greatly and can be difficult to interpret, and further discussion of them is beyond the scope of this text.

As might be imagined, with and against motions are reversed if the examiner uses the concave mirror effect. However, for the purposes of this text, the succeeding discussions will assume that the plano mirror effect is in use.

The examiner can affect movement of the retinal reflex by placing corrective lenses between the patient's eye and the retinoscope. The objective is to find the lens power that will "neutralize" the reflex and fill the pupil with light (Figure 5.23D). The lens that achieves this **neutralization point** is the approximate correction for the patient's refractive error. Such a lens will neutralize the reflex regardless of the retinoscope's movement or the mirror effect used. If the eye has an astigmatic error, neutralization will have to be done for both the maximum and the minimum meridians. The axis of the neutralizing spherocylinder must be identified and specified for the refraction to be complete.

During retinoscopy and neutralization, the examiner selects various lenses to introduce before the patient's eye by means of a **trial lens set** (Figure 5.24A) and **trial frame** (Figure 5.24B) or with a **refractor**, also called a **Phoroptor** (Reichert Technologies, Depew, New York), which stores a range of trial lenses that can be dialed into position (Figure 5.25). When "with" motion is observed (hyperopia), plus lenses are added sequentially until sufficient power is present to achieve the neutralization

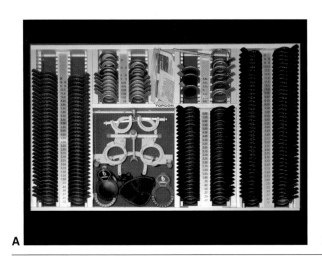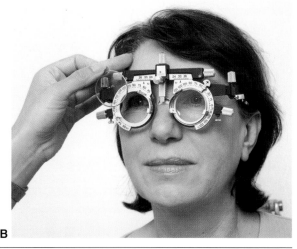

A   **B**

Figure 5.24 Trial lens and frame. **A.** A trial lens set consists of a variety of concave and convex lenses. **B.** A trial frame allows manual insertion of multiple lenses selected from a trial set. *(Part A Image courtesy of Brice Critser, CRA, Department of Ophthalmology and Visual Sciences, University of Iowa, Part B reprinted, with permission, from Wilson FM II, Blomquist PH,* Practical Ophthalmology, *6th ed, San Francisco: American Academy of Ophthalmology, 2009.)*

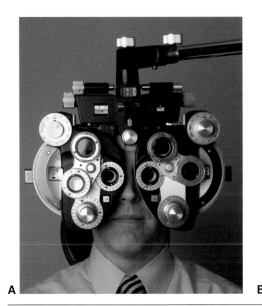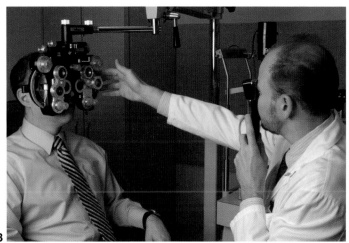

A   **B**

Figure 5.25 A phoropter (**A**) stores trial lenses that (**B**) can be dialed into position. *(Image courtesy of Brice Critser, CRA, Department of Ophthalmology and Visual Sciences, University of Iowa.)*

point. When "against" motion occurs (myopia), minus lenses are added until the neutralization point is reached.

Because the examiner must be much closer to the patient than 20 feet (optical infinity) to perform retinoscopy and neutralization, an additional adjustment to the dioptric power of the neutralizing lens must be made to correct for the distance between the examiner and the patient (the "working distance"). The amount of adjustment needed can be easily calculated using a variation of the formula D = 1/F previously discussed: D = 1/working distance in meters. As an example, if the working distance is 50 cm, then D = 1/0.5 m = 2 D. This working-distance

lens power is algebraically subtracted from the retinoscopy lens power that created neutralization in order to yield the patient's refractive error.

See Procedure 5.1 for guidelines about retinoscopy using the plus cylinder convention.

Refinement

The second step in refractometry is **refinement**. Also performed on one eye at a time, refinement consists of a group of procedures that provides a very precise measurement of refractive error and appropriate lens correction.

Procedure 5.1 Performing Retinoscopy Using the Plus Cylinder Convention

1. Have the patient fixate on the chart with a "fogged" fellow eye.

2. Start with too much minus on the test eye because conversion of "with" motion to "against" motion is easier to observe.

3. Add plus power until the first meridian is neutralized.

4. Using the Phoroptor, add plus cylinder in the axis perpendicular (90° away) to the previously neutralized axis until the second meridian is neutralized.

5. Subtract the working distance.

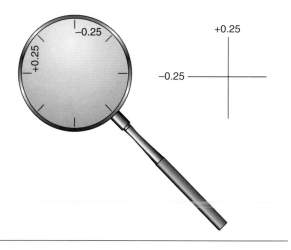

Figure 5.26 The cross cylinder, used to refine the selection of corrective cylindrical lenses for astigmatism. *(Reprinted, with permission, from Wilson FM II, Blomquist PH, Practical Ophthalmology, 6th ed, San Francisco: American Academy of Ophthalmology; 2009.)*

It serves to refine (confirm) the information produced by retinoscopy. Refinement is sometimes referred to as **subjective refractometry** because it requires patient participation and reaction ("I can see better with this lens than with that one"). Because of its subjective nature, refinement is not possible with infants, some toddlers, and other patients who are unable to communicate adequately.

In the first step of the process, the patient views letters of various sizes on a special visual acuity chart placed at a distance of 20 feet from the patient. (This is usually the standard eye chart of letters or numbers that is familiar to many people through school or driver's license screening procedures.) The examiner leads the patient by presenting a choice of lenses in the refractor or trial frame while asking a series of questions about the relative clarity of the images seen on the chart. The patient's responses guide the examiner to selecting the most appropriate lens to correct the refractive error in each of the patient's eyes.

The **cross cylinder** is a common refinement instrument used to confirm first the axis and then the power of a correcting cylindrical lens for astigmatism. The cross cylinder is a special lens consisting of two cylinders of equal power, one minus and one plus, with their axes set at right angles to each other (Figure 5.26). The technique, which requires choices and responses by the patient, is extremely accurate.

Binocular Balancing

Performed on both eyes at once, **balancing** (sometimes called **binocular balancing**) helps ensure that the optical correction determined by refractometry for distance vision does not include an uneven overcorrection or undercorrection for the two eyes. Such an anomaly can result from errors introduced by the patient's natural accommodation. Obviously, then, this procedure is unnecessary in patients who have undergone cycloplegic refraction or in patients whose accommodation is minimal or absent (patients over 60 years of age or those who have had cataracts removed). However, balancing procedures provide an additional check of the monocular refraction despite small inequalities of visual acuity.

One technique used for balancing involves "fogging" the end-point refractive correction in both eyes with plus spheres. The rotary prisms or the 6 D base-up prism on the Phoroptor are used to separate the images seen by the right and left eyes. This allows the patient to compare the clarity of the two images. If the original refraction was correctly balanced, the fogged images will look equally blurred. If one image appears clearer, the refraction may be unbalanced, and the refractometrist must consider making adjustments accordingly. Detailed instruction in balancing techniques can be found in many of the "Suggested Resources" listed at the end of this chapter.

Interpretation of Prescriptions

The outcome of refraction is an optical prescription—a written description of the optical requirements for correcting the patient's refractive error. The optical correction exactly counteracts the error of the eye; ie, an eye with 2 D of too much plus power (myopia) is corrected with a –2 D lens. The ophthalmologist uses the information gathered during refractometry—power of sphere, and power and axis of cylinder for each eye if cylinder is required—together with other patient considerations only a doctor can evaluate to supply a prescription for corrective lenses. Ophthalmic medical assistants must understand the format used for writing eyeglass lens prescriptions to record accurately the results of refractometry and to interpret refractive data on patient medical charts and forms.

The prescription for spectacle lenses follows a standard format. The power of the sphere (abbreviated *sph*) is recorded first with its sign (+ = plus, or convex sphere; – = minus, or concave sphere), followed by the power of the cylinder with its sign and axis if a cylinder is required. The axis is designated by ×, followed by a number of degrees. A prescription is recorded for each eye, using the abbreviations **OD** (*oculus dexter*) for the right and **OS** (*oculus sinister*) for the left eye.

A typical prescription for a patient with simple hyperopia might be:

OD +2.00 sph

OS +2.25 sph

For simple myopia, the prescription might be:

OD –2.50 sph

OS –2.25 sph

No cylinder is required in the two examples above. A prescription for corrective spherocylindrical lenses might read:

OD plano $\bigcirc$ +0.75 × 90°

OS plano $\bigcirc$ +0.50 × 90°

In this example, plano means "no sphere power"; $\bigcirc$ is the symbol for "combined with"; +0.75 and +0.50 indicate the sign and power of the cylinders; and 90° indicates their axes. For myopia combined with astigmatism, the prescription might look like the following:

OD –75 $\bigcirc$ +0.50 × 150°

OS –100 $\bigcirc$ +0.50 × 120°

In writing prescriptions, some people omit the $\bigcirc$ sign and the degree designation. Thus, the previous example might be recorded as:

OD –75 +0.50 × 150

OS –100 +0.50 × 120

For bifocal prescriptions, the word *add,* a plus sign, and the power of the added sphere in the bifocal segment used to correct the presbyopia are appended to the distance correction. A typical bifocal prescription for one eye might read:

–2.50 $\bigcirc$ +1.00 × 90° add +2.00

For a trifocal, a typical prescription for one eye would show first the near add, followed by the intermediate correction:

–2.50 $\bigcirc$ +1.00 × 90° add +2.50 int +1.25

Transposition of Prescriptions

The majority of ophthalmology offices today require refractive measurements and prescriptions involving spherocylindrical lenses to be written in plus-cylinder form, as expressed in the earlier examples, but some prefer to express them in minus-cylinder form. Optometrists and opticians generally use the minus-cylinder form. Conversion from one form of expression to the other, known as **transposition**, may be required to accommodate office preference or to read prescriptions from another office. Ophthalmic medical assistants may encounter the need for transposition in performing lensometry (discussed later in this chapter).

Transposition is nothing more than a simple mathematic manipulation of a lens prescription.

Prescription transposition steps follow:

1. Add algebraically the cylindrical power to the spherical power.

2. Reverse the sign of the cylinder, from plus to minus or vice versa as appropriate.

3. Add or subtract 90° to make the new axis 180° or less.

Here are two examples of plus-cylinder expressions with their minus-cylinder forms:

$$+3.00 +2.00 × 90 = +5.00 -2.00 × 180$$
$$-4.00 +3.00 × 45 = -1.00 -3.00 × 135$$

Automated Refractors

Automated refractors exist for both objective and subjective refractometry, eliminating the need to use a Phoroptor or trial frame and lenses. The automated objective refractors use infrared light to provide information similar to that derived by manual retinoscopy. Automated subjective refractors rely totally on patient responses, the same as manual refractometry performed with Phoroptors or trial lenses and frames. Combination objective/subjective refractors allow the operator to use patient responses to check visual acuity before and after the measurement as well as to refine sphere, cylinder, and axis after the objective measurement has been made. In general, automated refractors of all types are expensive, which might be a drawback in some practices. General advantages and disadvantages of the differing types are described in the sections that follow.

Objective Refractors

Automated objective refractors are simple to operate. Minimal storage and use space is required—a consideration in small offices. However, refractometric results may be variable and are not accurate enough to allow prescription without refinement. Furthermore, accurate results may not be possible in patients with certain diseases or disorders, such as immature cataracts, or certain physiologic characteristics, such as small pupils.

Subjective Refractors

Some subjective automated refractors allow testing of both distance and near vision and permit overrefraction of a patient's present eyeglasses. Some models feature an automated sequence of refracting steps, and others allow two different refractions to be compared with the push of a button. However, despite many automated features, a subjective refractor still requires a skilled, well-trained operator.

Objective/Subjective Refractors

With objective and subjective capability in the same instrument, a combination automated refractor may save space in the office, because it eliminates the need for the traditional 20-foot testing distance required by manual refinement. Figure 5.27 shows a typical combination refractor. As with purely subjective refractors, though, combination units require operator skill and knowledge for accurate refinement.

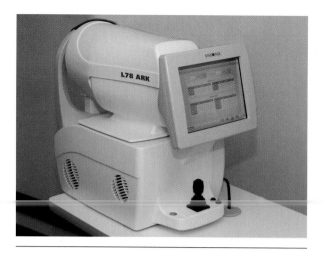

Figure 5.27 An automated refractor. *(Image courtesy of Brice Critser, CRA, Department of Ophthalmology and Visual Sciences, University of Iowa.)*

Lensometry

Lensometry is a procedure used to measure the prescription of a patient's existing eyeglass lenses or the power of contact lenses. This technique is often called *neutralization*, but should not be confused with neutralization as the word applies to retinoscopy. Lensometry is performed (usually by the ophthalmic medical assistant) with a specialized instrument known as a **lensmeter** or **vertometer**.

Lensometry measures 4 principal properties of lenses: spherical and cylindrical power in diopters; axes, if the lenses have a cylinder component; presence and direction of a prism incorporated into the lenses; and optical centers. Lensometry performed on a patient's eyeglasses before refraction can provide a starting point for the current refraction. This information is also useful in revealing changes in refractive error. Lensometry also serves to confirm that a patient's new glasses have been made in accordance with the doctor's prescription.

Types of Lensmeters

Instruments used to perform lensometry may be either manual or automated. Figure 5.28A shows a manual lensmeter (sometimes spelled *lensometer*) with the significant parts labeled; Figure 5.28B shows a lensmeter in use. To use manual instruments well, the operator needs a thorough understanding of not only lensometry itself, but also the principles of ophthalmic corrective lenses.

Automated lensmeters (Figure 5.29) measure an eyeglass lens prescription "at the push of a button." Little understanding of lensometry principles is necessary to operate the instrument. Automated lensometry can be

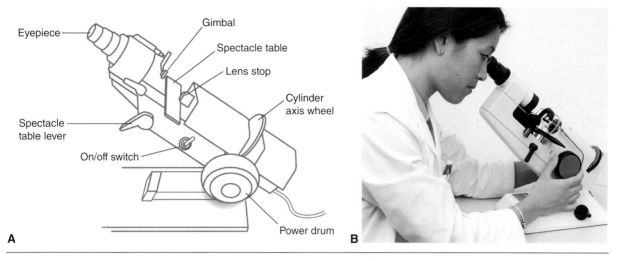

Figure 5.28 A manual lensmeter. **A.** Schematic of a manual lensmeter. **B.** Lensmeter in use. *(Part B reprinted, with permission, from Wilson FM II, Blomquist PH,* Practical Ophthalmology, *6th ed, San Francisco: American Academy of Ophthalmology; 2009.)*

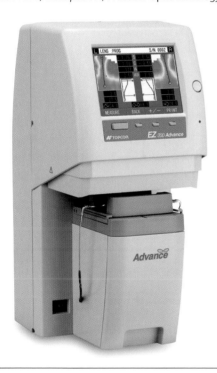

Figure 5.29 An automated lensmeter. *(Image courtesy of Topcon Medical Systems, a subsidiary of Topcon Corporation.)*

faster than manual methods, but speed depends on the operator. If the lens being measured is not properly centered in the lensmeter, an inaccurate reading may result. In addition, these instruments are more expensive than manual ones. Because not all ophthalmology offices have automated equipment and because a manual lensmeter reading may be more accurate than an improperly obtained automated lensmeter reading, ophthalmic medical assistants should develop basic skills in manual lensometry.

Elements of Lensometry

The first steps in performing lensometry on lenses of all types are (1) focusing the instrument eyepiece; (2) positioning the eyeglass lens to be measured on the spectacle table (or frame-support platform) of the lensmeter; (3) measuring the sphere power and, if present, cylinder power and axis, either in plus-cylinder or in minus-cylinder form; and (4) marking the optical center (optional).

Lensometry always begins with focusing the eyepiece, followed by positioning the lenses. For multifocal lenses, the distance portion is positioned and measured first. Sphere and cylinder power may be measured and expressed in either plus- or minus-cylinder form, but because the preference for either method may vary from office to office, ophthalmic medical assistants should be able to obtain these measurements in lensometry in both formats. Procedure 5.2 describes the steps for performing lensometry on single-vision lenses and the distance portion of multifocal lenses.

Incorrect eyepiece focusing can lead to errors in measuring sphere power, so proper focus should be verified each time the instrument is used. To avoid errors in measuring the cylinder axis, one must ensure that the bottom of the eyeglasses is set firmly on the spectacle table.

Lensometry Technique for Multifocal Lenses

After measuring the sphere, cylinder, and axis for the distance portion of a multifocal lens, one then obtains a reading for the bifocal or trifocal adds. The procedure for measuring bifocal or trifocal segments by lensometry is the same, as described in Procedure 5.3.

Procedure 5.2 Performing Basic Lensometry

Focusing the Eyepiece

The focus of the lensmeter eyepiece must be verified each time the instrument is used, to avoid erroneous readings.

1. With no lens or a plano lens in place in the lensmeter, look through the eyepiece of the instrument. Turn the power drum until the mires (the perpendicular crossed lines), viewed through the eyepiece, are grossly out of focus.

2. Turn the eyepiece in the plus direction, normally counterclockwise. This will fog (blur) the target seen through the eyepiece.

3. Slowly turn the eyepiece in the opposite direction until the target is clear, then stop turning. This procedure focuses the eyepiece.

4. Turn the power drum to focus the mires. The mires should focus at a power-drum reading of zero, which is plano. If the mires do not focus at plano, repeat the procedure from step 1.

Positioning the Eyeglasses

1. Place the eyeglasses on the movable spectacle table with the earpieces facing away from you. You are now prepared to read the back surface of the lenses, normally the appropriate surface from which to measure.

2. While looking through the lensmeter eyepiece, align the eyeglass lens so that the mires cross in the center of the target. You are then looking through the optical center of the lens. It is usually appropriate to measure the right lens first, followed by the left lens.

Measuring Sphere and Cylinder Power

The plus-cylinder technique employs the following steps:

1. Turn the power drum to read high minus (about −10.00).

2. Bring the closely spaced mires, often called *single lines*, into sharp focus by rotating the power drum counterclockwise while at the same time rotating the cylinder axis wheel to straighten the single lines where they cross the widely spaced perpendicular set of mires, often called *triple lines*.

3. If the single lines and triple lines come into focus at the same time, the lens is a sphere (Figure A). If only the single lines focus, you have identified the sphere portion of a spherocylinder. In either case, record the power-drum reading at this point as the power of the sphere.

4. If cylinder power is present, after noting the power-drum reading for the sphere, measure cylinder power by moving the power drum farther counterclockwise or rotating the drum toward you (less minus or more plus), bringing the triple lines into sharp focus (Figure B).

5. Calculate the difference between the first power-drum reading for the focused single lines and the second power-drum reading for the focused triple lines, and record this figure as the plus-cylinder power of the lens.

6. Read the axis of the cylinder off the cylinder axis wheel.

Example (plus cylinder):

single line focused at −2.50

triple lines focused at −1.00

cylinder power = +1.50

4. If cylinder power is present, move the power drum farther clockwise or rotate the drum away from you (more minus or less plus), bringing the triple lines into sharp focus.

5. Calculate the difference between the single-line reading on the power drum and the triple-line reading on the power drum, and record this figure as the minus-cylinder power.

6. Read the axis of the cylinder off the cylinder axis wheel.

The minus-cylinder technique employs the following steps:

1. Turn the power drum to read high plus (about +10.00).

2. Bring the single lines into sharp focus by rotating the power drum clockwise while simultaneously rotating the cylinder axis wheel to straighten the single lines where they cross the perpendicular set of triple lines.

3. If the single lines and the triple lines come into focus at the same time, the lens is a sphere. Record the power-drum reading at this point as the sphere power.

(continued)

Procedure 5.2 (Continued)

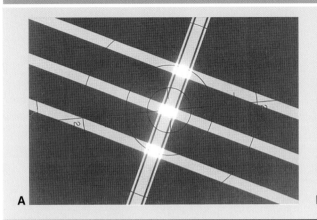

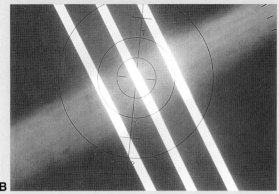

A

B

Procedure 5.3 Measuring Multifocal Power

Measuring Bifocal Power

1. After measuring the sphere and cylinder distance portion of bifocal eyeglass lenses, center the bifocal add at the bottom of the lens in the lensmeter gimbal (the ring-like frame) and refocus on the triple lines (if working in plus-cylinder technique) or the single lines (if working in minus-cylinder technique).

2. The add, or bifocal reading, is the difference between the distance reading of the triple-line focus (in plus-cylinder technique) or the single-line focus (in minus-cylinder technique) and the new triple- or single-line focus. Always read from the same type of line (single or triple) in the distance part and the bifocal part. If the bifocal lens has a high power, turn the glasses around and place the front surface of the eyeglass lens against the lens stop to read the bifocal power.

3. If the distance portion of the eyeglass lens is found to be a sphere, measure the sphere power of the bifocal segment. Record as the add the algebraic difference between the distance and bifocal sphere power readings (the distance subtracted from the bifocal). For example, if the sphere power in the distance segment is –1.00 and the sphere power in the near segment is +1.00, the bifocal add is +1.00 – (–1.00) = +2.00. The add is always written as a positive number.

Measuring Trifocal Power

To measure the trifocal segment directly, follow the same procedure as for the bifocal segment, reading the distance segment first, the intermediate segment second, and the near segment last.

Remember that the absolute power of the bifocal segment is always more positive (or less negative) than the sphere power in the upper portion of an eyeglass lens. The add is the total difference in dioptric power between the upper segment and the lower segment. For example, if the distance portion is +1.00 sph and the bifocal measures +3.00 sph, the bifocal add is +2.00. Similarly, if the distance portion is –1.00 sph and the bifocal measures +1.00, the bifocal add is +2.00.

PROGRESSIVE ADDITION (PROGRESSIVE ADD) MULTIFOCAL LENSES These lenses differ from traditional bifocal or trifocal eyeglasses in that no discrete, visible line divides the distance and reading portions of the lenses (Figure 5.30). Optical compromises required by the manufacturing processes used to eliminate the discrete lines on the lens often produce unwanted cylinder power, distortion, or blurred transition zones between the distance and near segments, which poses difficulties in performing lensometry. When looking at progressive add eyeglasses through the lensmeter, take care to select the area with the least distortion in both the distance and the reading portions of the lenses before taking a reading. Be sure to read the add as close to the bottom of the lens as possible. Once the proper areas are found, the lensometry technique is the same as for conventional multifocals. For specific information about the characteristics and uses of progressive add multifocal lenses, refer to Chapter 12.

Lensometry Technique for Prisms

Lensometry measures not only the power of a prism but also the orientation of the prism's base. The prism orientation may horizontal as base in (toward the nose) and base out (toward the temple), or vertical as in base up,

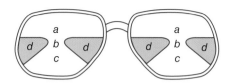

Figure 5.30 Progressive add bifocals. A transition zone (*b*) lies between the distance (*a*) and the near (*c*) portions. That zone, as well as other areas of the lens (*d*), contain optical compromises that may make lensometry readings difficult to obtain.

or base down or a combination of vertical and horizontal prism. Procedure 5.4 describes the steps for obtaining these measurements.

Placement of Optical Centers

For ideal visual correction, the optical center of eyeglass lenses must be placed directly in front of the patient's pupils. The lensmeter may be used to verify the position of the optical center of a lens. Refer to Chapter 12 for details about the purpose of measuring optical centers of lenses and the lensometry technique for doing so.

Keratometry

Keratometry is the measurement of a patient's corneal curvature. Keratometry is performed with a device called a **keratometer** or an **ophthalmometer**. As such, it provides an objective, quantitative measurement of corneal astigmatism, measuring the corneal front surface meridians of maximum and minimum curvature as well as designating the angular direction of these two meridians. Keratometry is also helpful in determining the appropriate fit of contact lenses and is an essential measurement before refractive surgery. Figure 5.31 illustrates the components of a typical manual keratometer. Procedure 5.5 describes the steps for obtaining measurements with this instrument. Various types of automated keratometers, sometimes combined with automated refractors, are in use in many ophthalmology offices.

Procedure 5.4 Measuring Prism Power and Orientation

In general, the existence of prescribed prism power in an eyeglass lens is revealed if the lensmeter mires are not centered in the central portion of the lensmeter target, provided that the lens is being measured at the place on the lens that rests in front of the patient's pupil. Once you have determined the presence of a prism, measure prism power and determine orientation as follows:

1. Count the number of black concentric circles from the central cross of the lensmeter target to the center of the vertical and/or horizontal crossed mires (see the figure). Each circle represents 1 prism diopter.

2. Record the direction of the thick portion (base) of the prism by determining the direction of the displacement of the mires. For example, if the mires are displaced upward, the prism base is base up; downward displacement indicates base down; displacement toward the nose, base in; and displacement toward the temple, base out.

3. Prism-compensating devices are incorporated into some lensmeters. Such devices permit the

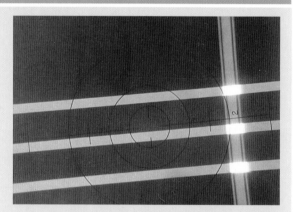

measurement of prism without using the concentric circles. To avoid recording prism power that is not actually present when using these devices, be sure that the prism-compensating device is set to zero. Auxiliary prisms are available for use with some lensometers to assist in measuring glasses with prism power greater than the number of concentric circles.

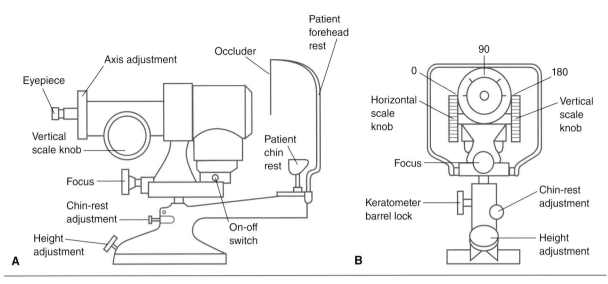

Figure 5.31 A typical manual keratometer. **A.** Side view. **B.** Rear view (examiner's perspective).

Procedure 5.5 Performing Keratometry

1. Looking through the eyepiece of the keratometer, use the eyepiece to focus the reticule (cross hair) in the same way as for the lensmeter.

2. Adjust the height of the keratometer table or platform so that the patient can comfortably put the chin and forehead on the appropriate rests.

3. Instruct the patient to place the forehead and chin firmly against the rests. Use the occluder attached to the keratometer to cover the eye not being measured.

4. Use the instrument's chin-rest adjustment knob to position the keratometer to the patient's eye roughly in line with the keratometer barrel. Then use the height-adjustment knob of the keratometer to position the light reflections at the level of the cornea. Swivel the instrument horizontally to align with the patient's eye. These actions should both make the patient comfortable at the instrument and bring the light reflections from the keratometer into the patient's cornea.

5. Ask the patient to look into the barrel of the instrument for a reflection of the eye or at a fixation light if one is used.

6. Look through the eyepiece and use the focus knob to focus on the general area of the eye.

7. Lock the keratometer barrel when you see 3 circles through the eyepiece, which represent reflections from the patient's eye.

Steps 1 through 7 may need to be repeated during the remainder of the procedure to readjust the instrument.

8. Further align the keratometer with the eye by raising or lowering the keratometer by means of the height-adjustment knob and horizontal-swiveling capability until the reticule is in the center of the bottom-right circle (Figure A).

9. To obtain proper focus, rotate the focus knob until the bottom-right circles converge to form a fused image (Figure B).

10. Finding the axis is critical when taking an exact measurement. To locate the proper axis, look at the aiming marks (mires) and rotate the keratometer until the pluses between the two bottom circles line up as shown in Figure C.

11. With the horizontal scale knob on the left, the pluses between the circles can be moved and aligned (Figure D). Some keratometers have different mires. Check with your doctor or read the instruction manual that came with the keratometer.

12. With the vertical scale knob on the right, the minuses between the circles can be moved until they align (Figure E).

13. Often it is not possible to obtain good readings in the vertical meridian using the minuses for alignment. In this case, the keratometer should be rotated 90°, and the pluses aligned using the horizontal scale knob, as described in step 11.

(continued)

Procedure 5.5 (Continued)

A proper measurement can be obtained when the following conditions are met simultaneously:

- The reticule is in the center of the bottom-right circle.

- The keratometer is focused with fusion of the bottom-right circles.

- The pluses between the circles are in the same plane and are fused.

- The minuses between the circles are in the same plane and are fused.

You may need to readjust one or all of the control knobs until every element of proper measurement is obtained. In addition, it is critical that the eyepiece be properly focused at the start of the procedure.

Recording Keratometry Measurements

Figure F illustrates a possible measurement of an astigmatic cornea. This information can be recorded in one of three ways:

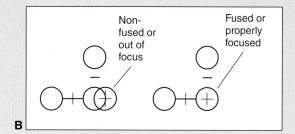

1. $\mathsf{K}\ \dfrac{42.25 \times 135}{46.50 \times 45}$

2. K R 42.25 × 135 / 46.50 × 45
   L

3. 46.5/A.M. 42.25 × 135 (A.M. = axis meridian)

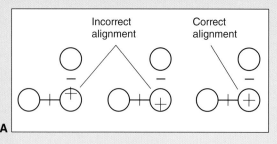

A

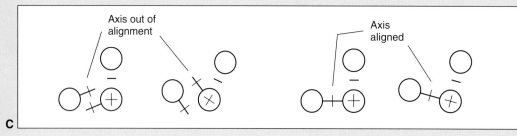

C

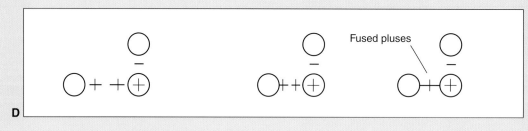

D

(continued)

Procedure 5.5 (Continued)

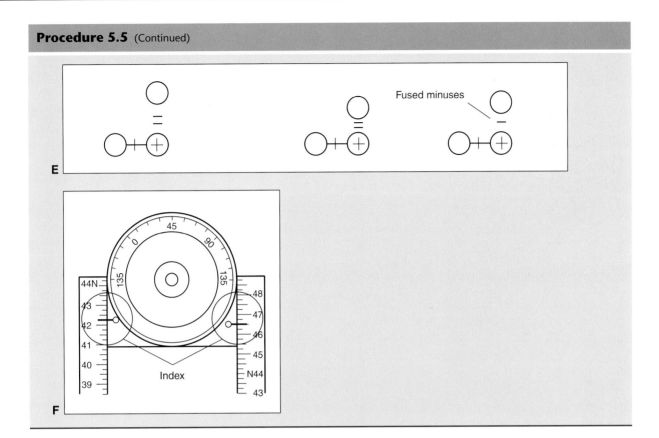

E

F

SELF-ASSESSMENT TEST

1. Define the following terms: *refractive index, focal point, focal length,* and *diopter.*

2. Name the principal refractive properties of a convex lens and a concave lens.

3. Distinguish between *emmetropia* and *ametropia.*

4. Define and describe the physiologic characteristics of myopia, hyperopia, and astigmatism.

5. Define *presbyopia.*

6. Name at least 3 methods of correcting refractive errors of the eye.

7. Define and state the purpose of an *add* in multifocal lenses.

8. Define a *spherocylinder.*

9. State the principal refractive characteristic of a prism.

10. State the purpose of incorporating a prism into a corrective lens.

11. The refractive power of a prism is measured in units called _____.

12. A 0.5Δ prism deviates parallel rays of light 1 cm at a distance of _____ m from the prism.

13. Name the kind of ophthalmic lens used to correct the following refractive errors: myopia, hyperopia, and astigmatism.

14. Define *refraction* as the term is used in eye care.

15. Name the 2 main components of refraction.

16. Name the 3 separate steps of refractometry.

17. Distinguish between *cycloplegic refraction* and *manifest refraction.*

18. Define and distinguish between *objective refractometry* and *subjective refractometry.*

19. Name 4 instruments or devices that may be used during refraction.

20. Define *with motion* and *against motion.*

21. Name the 3 components of the lens prescription shown below:

    +2.75   −1.50   × 135
      a.   b.   c.

22. Transpose the following lens prescription:

    +4.25   +1.50   × 135

23. Define *lensometry.*

24. List the 4 properties of lenses that can be measured by a lensometer.

25. Name the type of lens identified by lensometry when the single and triple perpendicular lines come into focus simultaneously.

26. The lensmeter power-drum reading on the distance portion of a multifocal lens measures −1.50 sph. The power-drum reading for the bifocal is +0.25. What is the bifocal add?

27. Define *keratometry.*

28. List the 4 conditions that must be met simultaneously to obtain a proper measurement with a keratometer.

SUGGESTED ACTIVITIES

1. Ask a senior technician or an ophthalmologist in your office if you can observe while he or she performs retinoscopy, lensometry, and keratometry. At a convenient time, ask him or her to demonstrate the equipment used in these procedures and allow you to try the procedures.

2. Ask an optician's office staff if you can have damaged or unwanted eyeglass lenses in various styles (single-vision, bifocals, and trifocals). With a permanent marker, label each lens in a corner with a different identifying letter or number. Ask your senior technician to read each lens by lensometry and note the identifying letter or number and the lensometry reading for each on a sheet of paper. Then practice your lensometry technique by reading each lens yourself. Compare your readings with those of the technician, and discuss the reasons for any discrepancies.

3. Check the tables of contents and indexes of books included in the "Suggested Resources" list and read the pertinent chapters or sections for more information on subjects covered in this chapter.

4. Ask the ophthalmologist in your office to consider obtaining the *Retinoscopy and Subjective Refraction* DVD listed in the "Suggested Resources" section. Three areas are covered: retinoscopy: minus cylinder technique; retinoscopy: plus cylinder technique; and subjective refraction: cross-cylinder technique.

SUGGESTED RESOURCES

Abrams D. *Duke-Elder's Practice of Refraction.* 10th ed. Edinburgh: Churchill Livingston; 1993.

Azar DT. *Refractive Surgery.* 2nd ed. St Louis: Elsevier-Mosby; 2007: 89–145.

Cassin B. Section II: optics. In: *Fundamentals for Ophthalmic Technical Personnel.* Philadelphia: Saunders; 1995.

Corboy JM. *The Retinoscopy Book: An Introductory Manual for Eye Care Professionals.* 5th ed. Thorofare, NJ: Slack; 2003.

DuBois LG. Neutralization of spectacles. In: *Fundamentals of Ophthalmic Medical Assisting.* DVD. San Francisco: American Academy of Ophthalmology; 2009.

Guyton DL. *Retinscopy and Subjective Refraction.* DVD. San Francisco: American Academy of Ophthalmology; 1986. Reviewed for currency: 2007.

Keeney AH, Hagman RE, Fratello CJ, et al. *The Dictionary of Ophthalmic Optics.* Boston: Butterworth-Heinemann; 1995.

Milder B, Rubin ML. *The Fine Art of Prescribing Glasses Without Making a Spectacle of Yourself.* 3rd ed. Gainesville, FL: Triad; 2004.

Rubin ML. *Optics for Clinicians.* 25th anniversary ed. Gainesville, FL: Triad; 1993.

Stein HA, Stein RM. *The Ophthalmic Assistant: A Text for Allied and Associated Ophthalmic Personnel.* 8th ed. St Louis: Mosby; 2006.

6

BASICS OF OPHTHALMIC PHARMACOLOGY

Pharmacology is the term given to the study of the medicinal use and actions of drugs. Also called *medications*, drugs play an important role in most medical practices. In the ophthalmology office, medications are used chiefly to diagnose and treat diseases and to test for normal eye functions. As part of their duties, beginning ophthalmic medical assistants may call in the doctor's prescription for a specific medication to the pharmacy and may record drug information on the patient's history chart. As they become more familiar with medications used to treat eye disorders, assistants may administer certain kinds of drugs on instruction of the doctor. The experienced assistant, especially one who assists in surgical procedures, may need to set out certain types of medications for the doctor to use during certain procedures. To carry out these responsibilities, assistants should have a basic understanding of drug actions, patient reactions to these agents, and the general types and uses of pharmaceuticals in the ophthalmology practice. In addition, assistants must know how and when to administer medications. Any assistant who administers drugs should also be able to recognize the symptoms of allergic reactions, as well as when such reactions require treatment and how to summon help.

This chapter provides an overview of drug delivery systems and describes the procedures for administering eyedrops and ointments to patients. The chapter also discusses the types, actions, and functions of medications commonly used in the ophthalmology office, with an emphasis on their side effects and allergic reactions and, most important, the first aid procedures required for adverse drug reactions. Throughout the chapter, brand names of drugs are mentioned (in parentheses following the generic names) only for the purpose of familiarizing technicians with some of the names they may encounter in office practice or clinic.

Delivery Systems of Drugs

Patients may receive ophthalmic drugs by 3 principal methods: (1) **topical systems**, whereby drugs are applied directly to the surface of the eye or surrounding skin; (2) **injections**, whereby drugs are injected with a hypodermic needle into or around the eye or into another part of the body; and (3) **oral systems**, whereby drugs are taken by mouth.

Drug delivery has advanced over the years, and other systems of drug delivery have been introduced with specific emphasis on controlled release of drugs to specific areas of the eye. Sustained release, through the use of **implantable intraocular drug delivery devices**, has allowed drug delivery without the need for multiple injections. Development is also underway to introduce delivery systems of drugs that involve transscleral technology. This system of drug delivery diffuses medication through the sclera and into the eye. Also in the future, the use of nanoparticle technology may replace eyedrops and intravitreal injections.

Topical Systems

Topical drugs include liquid drops in the form of solutions, suspensions, and ointments for use on the surface of the eye or eyelids. Topical drug application is the major route of administration of drugs in the practice of ophthalmology. These agents work well in a variety of tests and treatments involving external and anterior eye structures. Ophthalmic medical assistants often apply topical drugs to patients who are undergoing eye tests. To enhance the absorption of the drops into the ocular tissues and allow less to drain into the nose and down the throat, instruct patients to close their eyes for 2 minutes after applying the drops. This maneuver is especially helpful in limiting the amount of medication that could have systemic side effects.

The Academy has endorsed the uniform use of a color-coding system for the caps and labels of topical ocular medications. (See Table 6.1 and "Suggested Resources.")

The color-coding system is in constant transition and many manufacturers of generic drugs are not always adhering to the prescribed color codes. Assistants must be aware that they cannot fully rely on the colors.

SOLUTIONS A drug in **solution** is completely dissolved in an inert liquid called the **vehicle**, such as sterile salt water. Because the normal eye is **hydrophobic** (resists water), a topical solution may also contain a chemical to overcome this natural resistance. The solution may also include a preservative ingredient to prevent bacteria or other organisms from growing during storage. Occasionally, the preservative agent can irritate the eyes of some patients, causing redness, tearing, or pain.

Solutions are used frequently in ophthalmologic practice because they are easy to apply as drops and do not interfere with vision, except, of course, for drugs that may alter vision as part of their desired action, such as medications used to dilate pupils. Adverse reactions can occur when using solutions. If a reaction does occur, use artificial tears or eye irrigation solution to wash out the eye. If the patient is at home he or she should be instructed to use fresh running tap water (if artificial tears are not available). The eyes must be washed out thoroughly and then the patient should see the ophthalmologist. A prominent disadvantage of solutions is that the drops do not remain in contact with the surface of the eye for long; like tears, the medicinal drops drain through the lacrimal system into the nose and throat. Because solutions drain out of the eye, more frequent application may be

Table 6.1 Examples of Color Codes for Caps and Labels of Ocular Medications

Class	Color	Pantone Number
Anti-infectives	Tan	467
Anti-inflammatories/steroids	Pink	197
Mydriatics and cycloplegics	Red	1797
Nonsteroidal anti-inflammatories	Gray	4
Miotics	Dark green	348
Beta-blockers	Yellow	Yellow C
Beta-blocker combinations	Dark Blue	281
Adrenergic agonists	Purple	2583

required if they are used as a treatment. Solutions also may cause effects in other parts of the body.

SUSPENSIONS   A **suspension** is a liquid vehicle in which particles of the drug are "suspended." Like solutions, suspensions may contain a preservative ingredient to inhibit the growth of bacteria and other unwanted organisms during storage. Suspensions are also easy to apply as drops and do not interfere with vision unless that is the desired action of the drug. Disadvantages of suspensions are that, like solutions, they do not remain in contact with the eye surface for long and that particles may settle out in the container during storage. If the active drug falls to the bottom of the bottle, it will not be delivered in an adequate amount unless the user shakes the container vigorously before each application. The ophthalmic medical assistant should check each container of medication before use in case it requires this procedure. (Some labels specify "Shake well before using.")

OINTMENTS AND GELS   In the form of an **ointment** or **gel**, the drug is dissolved or suspended in an oily or greasy vehicle. The chief advantage of an ointment or gel is that the drug remains in contact with the eye or lid longer than when in liquid solution or in liquid suspension. The greasy character makes the drug less likely to wash away with tears—a useful property in patients with excessive tearing or in crying children. However, ointments and gels may blur vision due to their inherent greasiness (although this effect can be rendered irrelevant by application at bedtime), and they can be difficult to apply correctly.

Injections

With **injections**, the drug in solution is introduced into a part of the body by a needle. In ophthalmology, drug injections primarily serve as a means of applying treatment, but they can also be used in some testing or diagnostic procedures. Injections into other parts of the body are usually given by a registered nurse or medical doctor. In preparation for an eye injection by the ophthalmologist, an anesthetic drop is given to deaden the surface by placing it into the inferior cul-de-sac and a broad spectrum microbicide (kills germs) is applied to the eyelids and site of injection.

Four types of injections are available in the practice of ophthalmology: into the eye (such as intravitreal, Figure 6.1) or around the eye (periocular, retrobulbar, or subconjunctival); into a vein (intravenous); into a muscle (intramuscular); and under the skin (subcutaneous).

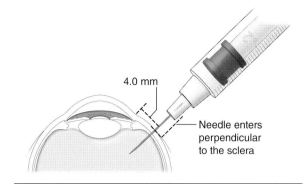

Figure 6.1   Intravitreal injection. *(Reprinted, with permission, from Dunn JP, et al, Basic Techniques of Ophthalmic Surgery, San Francisco: American Academy of Ophthalmology, 2009. Illustration by Mark M. Miller.)*

The intravenous, intramuscular, and subcutaneous injections are classified as **systemic drug delivery** because the active drug travels through the body's circulatory system before actually reaching the eye. Intravitreal injections have been associated with intraocular complications and therefore the patients, after the injection, should be instructed to immediately report symptoms such as pain, redness, or loss of vision or visual field.

Intravitreal medications are injected into the eyeball typically in order to reduce swelling and inflammation inside the eye. A good example of an intravitreal medication is a corticosteroid, triamcinolone (Trivaris, Triesence). This drug has been proven to help treat eye conditions like cystoid macular edema, diabetic macular edema, and some cases of wet macular degeneration, among others.

The most common intravitreal injections for wet macular degeneration are pegaptanib (Macugen), ranibizumab (Lucentis), and bevacizumab (Avastin). These agents work on a certain chemical substance created by the body to stimulate growth of new blood vessels. This chemical is called **vascular endothelial growth factor** (VEGF: pronounced "veg-F"). Medications in this category are anti-VEGF agents.

Oral Systems

Drugs taken orally (by mouth) include tablets, capsules, and liquids. Oral drug intake belongs to the systemic drug delivery category because, as with certain types of injections, the active agent must travel through one or more other body systems before reaching the eye. The practice of ophthalmology uses few oral drugs. However, for patients with certain conditions, such as glaucoma, infections, and allergic reactions, oral drugs fill an important medical need.

Implants

Intravitreal implants are intended to provide sustained drug delivery to the posterior segment of the eye. Although they are surgically inserted, it is important that ophthalmic assistants be aware of this drug delivery system. Retisert is an intravitreal implant that releases 3 to 4 µg of fluocinolone acetonide (a corticosteroid) per day for about 30 months. Figure 6.2 shows the Retisert implant inside the eye. The therapeutic benefit of implants is a constant release of medication and eliminates the doctor's concern of whether the patient is administering their medication as instructed. Ozurdex is a sustained-release intravitreal implant of dexamethasone (a corticosteroid) and is approved for macular edema associated with branch and central vein occlusions.

Improving Compliance

In order to improve patient adherence with taking their medication and improve absorption, several recommendations for patients have been suggested:

- Take drops with other routine tasks such as teeth brushing.

- Take multiple drops at least 5 minutes apart to avoid washing out or diluting each medication but close enough in timing to prevent missing the sequence of multiple drops.

- Set alarms on a watch or cell phone as reminders to take the medication.

- Prepare a daily log or schedule and mark off each drop after use.

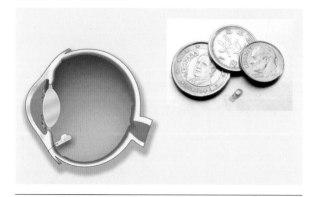

Figure 6.2 An intravitreal implant provides sustained drug delivery to the posterior segment of the eye. *(Images courtesy of Bausch & Lomb.)*

Administration of Topical Eyedrops and Ointments

Most topical ophthalmic drugs are available as a solution, a suspension, or an ointment. The ophthalmic medical assistant commonly aids the ophthalmologist by instilling eyedrops or applying ointments to patients in the office. Refer to Procedure 6.1 for step-by-step instructions.

Purposes and Actions of Drugs

Ophthalmic drugs may be used as a part of a test to diagnose eye disorders, as a principal treatment of eye conditions, or as an adjunct to surgical eye treatment. In addition to their desired action for each use, drugs of all kinds have certain side effects, some of which can be harmful. Because ophthalmic medical assistants often apply topical drugs or assist in ordering or setting up medications for the doctor to administer, they need to be familiar with the most common types of drugs used in ophthalmic practice and their general uses and actions.

Diagnostic Medications

Medications used to diagnose eye conditions include mydriatics, cycloplegics, dyes, and anesthetics. Most of these are available as topical solutions, and some are prepared as ointments. Some of these drugs also produce effects that make them additionally useful in treating certain eye disorders.

MYDRIATICS The act of dilating the pupil is called **mydriasis**. Thus, mydriatic drugs cause the pupil to dilate, usually by stimulating the iris dilator muscle. Mydriatic drops are used mainly to facilitate the examination of the lens and fundus. During this examination, the more fully dilated pupil allows a greater area of the lens and fundus to be visualized. A large pupil is essential to aid in the diagnosis and treatment of eye diseases.

Occasionally mydriatics may be used to improve the vision of patients with cataracts or other media opacities, but they are usually used to diagnose eye conditions. Dilating drops are also used during the treatment of some conditions such as amblyopia and inflammation.

Side effects associated with mydriatics include stinging on administration, headache, increased blood pressure, and photophobia. Because these agents open the pupil,

Procedure 6.1 Administering Eyedrops and Ointments

Preliminaries

1. Have the patient sit or lie down.

2. Wash your hands thoroughly.

3. Check the physician's instructions—what medication and which eye?

4. Select the correct medication and strength and also check the expiration date. Always read the label. Many ophthalmic medication bottles look alike.

5. If the medication to be used is a suspension, shake the container well to ensure the drug is distributed consistently throughout the liquid.

6. To maintain sterility of the bottle contents, do not allow the inside edge of the bottle cap to contact any surface or object other than the bottle. Avoid touching the bottle tip to the lids, lashes, or surface of the eye.

Instilling Eyedrops

Improperly instilled eyedrops do not reach the eye. The following technique helps ensure optimal drug delivery.

1. Have the patient recline or tilt the head far back. If a patient has difficulty bending the neck back, have him recline in the exam chair.

2. Ask the patient to look up, with both eyes open.

3. Use the little finger or ring finger of the hand holding the bottle to gently pull down the skin over the cheekbone, pulling the lower lid down and out. This motion exposes the conjunctival cul-de-sac, creating a cup to catch the drops.

4. Squeeze the bottle gently to expel a drop of medication. Try to direct the drop toward the cul-de-sac, not toward the sensitive surface of the cornea (Figure A).

5. Instruct the patient to close both eyes gently for 2 minutes or apply light pressure at the inner corner of the eyelids for 60 seconds (Figure B).

These actions help prevent systemic absorption by reducing the amount of the drug that drains into the lacrimal system, to the nose, and eventually down the throat. Alternately and equally as effective, a patient can be instructed to keep his eyelids gently closed for 2 minutes to decrease systemic absorption. These maneuvers also increase the time available for absorption of the drug and thereby improve its effectiveness.

6. Wipe any excess drops from the patient's lids with a clean tissue.

7. Record the following information in the patient's chart:

   a. Medication name and strength

   b. Time administered

   c. Which eye received the medication

Applying Ointments

Perform steps 1 through 6 of "Preliminaries" earlier in this box. Then continue with steps 1 through 5 below.

1. If the tube of ointment has been opened prior to this use, express one-half inch of ointment onto a fresh cotton ball, gauze, or tissue and discard it.

2. Squeezing the tube lightly and with even pressure, apply the ointment along the conjunctival surface of the lower lid, moving from the inner to the outer canthus (Figure C). Usually one-half inch of ointment is enough. Avoid touching the tip of the tube to the eye, eyelashes, or skin to prevent contamination of the tube. With a twisting motion, detach the ointment from the tip of the tube.

3. Instruct the patient to close the eyes gently.

4. Wipe any excess ointment from the skin with a fresh cotton ball, gauze, or tissue; then discard it properly.

5. Record the application of ointment in the patient's chart, as described in step 7 above.

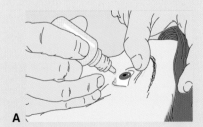
A

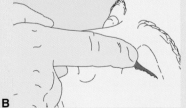
B

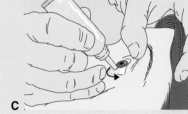
C

mydriatics may precipitate an attack of angle-closure glaucoma in patients with a narrow anterior chamber angle. The ophthalmologist or ophthalmic assistant should check the patient's anterior chamber angle depth (described in Chapter 8) before using a mydriatic drug. A commonly used mydriatic is phenylephrine, in strengths of 2.5% and 10% (Neo-Synephrine, Mydfrin).

REVERSAL DROPS The pupillary dilation produced by mydriatic drops can be reversed by instilling dapiprazole 0.5% at the end of the eye examination. These drops do not reverse the dilation produced by strong cycloplegic drops such as cyclopentolate. Dapiprazole ophthalmic is no longer available in the United States. Most patients experience transient stinging and redness of their eyes after receiving dapiprazole.

CYCLOPLEGICS **Cycloplegia** is the term applied to the ability of a drug to temporarily paralyze the ciliary muscle. Cycloplegic drugs also temporarily paralyze the iris sphincter muscle, causing passive dilation of the pupil by preventing constriction. By their paralyzing action on the ciliary muscle these agents limit or prevent accommodation, which controls the ability of the crystalline lens to expand and contract for near and far vision. Cycloplegic agents differ from mydriatics in that cycloplegics both dilate the pupil and paralyze accommodation, whereas mydriatics only dilate the pupil.

The principal uses of cycloplegics include the following:

- performing a refraction that requires an absence of accommodation

- conducting a fundus examination

- treating uveitis (inflammation of the uveal tract)

- treating postoperative intraocular inflammation

Cycloplegic refraction is especially important in children, who have a strong accommodation mechanism that can interfere with an accurate determination of the refractive state of the eye unless cycloplegic drops are utilized.

All cycloplegic drugs may sting slightly when administered to the eye. Another important reaction to cycloplegic medication is blurred vision or difficulty seeing at near due to paralysis of accommodation. This altered vision may last from a few hours to days, depending on the type and strength of the drug used. Other major side effects associated with cycloplegics include sensitivity to light, dry mouth, fever, rapid pulse, hallucinations, disorientation, bizarre behavior, and angle-closure glaucoma in patients with a narrow anterior chamber angle.

Cycloplegic drugs may be categorized by the duration of their action. It is recommended to separate the drops in duration of action to avoid confusion with long-acting cycloplegics (eg, cyclopentolate) with the shorter-acting drops (eg, tropicamide). It is important that assistants do not use cyclopentolate drops in a patient who needs a much shorter-acting drug like tropicamide. Atropine should never be used for routine dilation unless the doctor specifically orders its use in advance or it is noted in a specific office protocol (eg, accommodative esotropia).

Shorter-acting compounds are chosen for refraction and retinal examinations because their side effects of blurred vision and paralyzed accommodation decrease soon after application. The most common short-acting cycloplegic compound used in ophthalmology is tropicamide 0.5% and 1.0% (Mydriacyl). A slightly longer-acting drop is cyclopentolate 0.5%, 1.0%, and 2.0% (Cyclogyl).

In children, cyclopentolate is used to obtain a more accurate, objective measurement of the eye's refractive error because of their strong power of accommodation. Cyclopentolate 2% is to be avoided in children to reduce side effects.

Longer-acting compounds are used for refraction and the treatment of uveitis. Examples include homatropine 2.0% and 5.0%; atropine 0.5% and 1.0%; and scopolamine 0.25% (Hyoscine). Because the bottles of cycloplegic agents look alike (that is, most have red tops), it is crucial that the assistant check the label of the bottle before using, to be sure the correct agent will be instilled.

DYES These substances temporarily stain cells or systems within the eye to outline or highlight defects in their structure or function. Ophthalmologists employ topical dyes in clinical practice chiefly to evaluate the ocular surface. Topical dyes also are used in applanation tonometry and contact lens fitting. Dyes administered by injection may be used to evaluate retinal conditions.

The common dyes used in ophthalmology are **fluorescein**, which has fluorescent properties, **rose bengal** (a red dye), and **lissamine green**. They are available for topical use as solutions or in paper strips impregnated with the dye, and available under numerous brand names (Figure 6.3). Fluorescein additionally is available as a

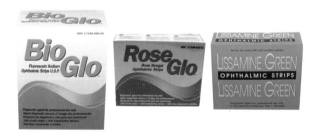

Figure 6.3 Dye strips. *(Images courtesy of Accutome, Inc.)*

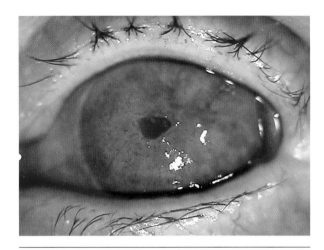

Figure 6.4 Neurotrophic corneal ulcer with rose bengal stain. *(Reprinted, with permission, from Schultze RL, et al,* Focal Points: Neurotrophic Keratitis, *San Francisco: American Academy of Ophthalmology, 2003.)*

solution for injection. Rose bengal stains and highlights degenerating corneal and conjunctival cells (Figure 6.4), and so is used mainly to test for and diagnose dry eye conditions. Fluorescein similarly stains cells, but has other, more complex uses such as identifying dendrites (herpes) in the eye.

For topical testing and diagnostic use, the examiner applies fluorescein drops or a fluorescein-impregnated strip to the eye and exposes the eye to a special cobalt-blue light. Under this lighting condition, the dye fluoresces a bright yellow-green color. In the normal eye, only the tear layer fluoresces, a characteristic that makes the dye useful for applanation tonometry and contact lens fitting. In an abnormal eye, fluorescein can highlight defects in the tear film. It also stains defective or absent corneal epithelium, allowing the doctor to observe and identify corneal abrasions and infections. In addition, aqueous humor leaks from the anterior chamber of the eye can be visualized.

When administered intravenously by a doctor, nurse, or phlebotomy technician, fluorescein courses through the bloodstream to reach the eye.

When the fundus receives the fluorescein dye and is exposed to cobalt-blue light, the dye highlights retinal structures, especially blood vessels. The doctor may use a camera, a slit lamp, or an ophthalmoscope to observe highlighted defects in the retinal vessels. Fluorescein angiography, a diagnostic photographic procedure described

in Chapter 10 utilizes an intravenous injection of fluorescein. Used in this way, fluorescein injection is an important adjunct to diagnosing conditions affecting the retinal vessels, such as diabetic retinopathy. Fluorescein given by injection may cause some patients to experience nausea or, rarely, an allergic reaction. Ophthalmic dyes when applied topically rarely cause allergic reactions. Although it is not used as frequently, indocyanine green (ICG) dye is injected intravenously for ICG angiography.

ANESTHETICS An **anesthetic drop** numbs the surface of the eye, which results in loss of feeling of the tissue. An injection of anesthetic causes paralysis of the affected muscles and deadening of the nerves, which also results in loss of feeling of the surrounding tissue. Anesthetics used in ophthalmology are either a topical solution or injected. These drugs commonly affect only the eye receiving the medication. Most ophthalmic anesthetics act within a minute or so and have an effect lasting from 10 to 20 minutes for topical anesthetics and hours for some injected types. Duration of action depends on the type of topical anesthetic used and amount being applied. Anesthetics can cause irreversible corneal damage and even complete destruction of the cornea if used in excess.

Topical anesthetics are most often used to prevent discomfort during diagnostic procedures such as tonometry, gonioscopy, ultrasonography, and other examinations that involve touching the surface of the eye. These agents are also used in cataract surgery and other therapeutic procedures, such as removal of foreign bodies from the eye and sutures from the cornea. On rare occasions, a topical anesthetic may be used to alleviate pain for the few minutes required to diagnose or treat a painful condition. Injectable anesthetics are used to perform minor and major eyelid surgery and major intraocular and periocular surgery. Although these ophthalmic anesthetics are injected, they still produce only local anesthetic effects; nevertheless, systemic toxicity can occur.

Anesthetics can produce an allergic reaction in a sensitive individual. Topical anesthetics become toxic to the cornea if in contact with the eye for long periods or if used often. They delay the resurfacing of the cornea by the corneal epithelium, which inhibits healing, and they can disrupt the normal stromal architecture, which can cause permanent clouding of the cornea. For these reasons, anesthetics are *not* used as a treatment except to alleviate pain for a few minutes until definitive therapy can be started.

The ophthalmic medical assistant should caution the patient receiving an ophthalmic anesthetic not to rub the eyes, because the numbed eye could be easily scratched without the patient being aware of it until the anesthesia wears off. Never give a patient a topical anesthetic for home use or use one yourself, as a significant toxic corneal reaction could result.

The following topical ophthalmic anesthetics are commonly used:

- cocaine 1% to 4%

- proparacaine 0.5% (Ophthaine, Ophthetic, Alcaine)

- tetracaine 0.5%, 1%, 2% (Pontocaine)

- lidocaine topical 3.5% (Xylocaine)

- benoxinate plus fluorescein (Fluress)

- proparacaine plus fluorescein (Fluoracaine)

Commonly used injectable anesthetics include lidocaine 1% and 2%; mepivacaine 1% and 2%; and bupivacaine 0.25% to 0.75%.

Therapeutic Medications

Medications used to treat certain eye conditions have very specific actions for each individual disorder. Such therapeutic medications are generally prescribed by the doctor for patients to administer themselves. Occasionally, ophthalmic medical assistants may be asked by the physician to either administer such medications to patients or teach patients how to administer the medication to themselves. This class of medications includes miotics and other glaucoma treatments, antimicrobials, antiallergic and anti-inflammatory agents, decongestants, lubricants, and immunomodulators.

Miotics

Miotics cause the iris sphincter muscle to contract, producing miosis (pupillary constriction), which leads to a reduction in the light entering the eye. One effect of a small pupil is to increase the patient's depth of field, which may improve vision in a patient with an uncorrected or poorly corrected refractive error. Miotic agents also cause contraction of the ciliary body muscle, which results in increased accommodation and opening of the trabecular drainage system, allowing an increase in aqueous outflow.

Miotics are less commonly used to treat open-angle glaucoma than in the past, and they are frequently used to break attacks of angle-closure glaucoma. Some accommodative strabismus problems in children can respond to miotic treatment. Miotics may also be used inside the eye during intraocular surgery. Preoperatively miotics are used prior to laser iridotomy, penetrating keratoplasty, and other intraocular surgeries benefiting from a small pupil.

Miotics are available for topical application in the form of solutions and gels. The major side effects of this class of pharmaceuticals include brow ache, myopia, tearing, cataract, and retinal detachment. With the most potent agents, sweating, salivation, abdominal cramps, and diarrhea can occur. The principal miotic agents used in ophthalmology today are pilocarpine (Isopto Carpine) 0.5%, 1%, 2%, 3%, 4%, and 6%; carbachol (Isopto Carbachol) 1.5% and 3%; and echothiophate (Phospholine Iodide) 0.125% (only available one bottle at a time directly from Wyeth Pharmaceuticals, a division of Pfizer).

Glaucoma Medications

Many types of medications exist to treat glaucoma, all of which aim to reduce intraocular pressure, although by diverse mechanisms of action. There is no cure for glaucoma; however, it can be controlled. Some glaucoma agents open the outflow pathways of aqueous fluid in the eye, others decrease the production of the aqueous humor, and still others work through a combination of effects. Side effects of glaucoma medications vary with the type and action of the specific drug. These effects can range from an allergic reaction to blurred vision, increased or decreased blood pressure, and emotional or psychological effects. The major glaucoma medications can be subdivided into 8 categories based on their chemistry or the body system they affect.

BETA-ADRENERGIC BLOCKERS Used in a variety of glaucoma eyedrops, beta-blockers were at one time the drugs of first choice in treating glaucoma. These drugs work by decreasing fluid (aqueous) production in the eye and are often prescribed as an adjunct to or in combination with prostaglandins.

These eyedrops have the potential to reduce the heart rate and may cause adverse side effects in individuals with certain heart problems. Also the use of these agents should be avoided in patients with obstructive lung disease (eg, emphysema). The commercially available drops include the following:

- timolol (Timoptic, Betimol)

- betaxolol (Betoptic)

- levobunolol (Betagan)

- metipranolol (Optipranolol)

- carteolol (Ocupress)

ADRENERGIC-STIMULATING AGENT Now infrequently used in the United States. an adrenergic-stimulating agent works mostly by increasing aqueous outflow. At one time epinephrine was available for use in this category, but now only one agent, dipivefrin, (Propine), is prescribed.

ORAL AND TOPICAL CARBONIC ANHYDRASE INHIBITORS   These agents decrease the formation and secretion of aqueous humor, thereby lowering intraocular pressure. Topical agents include brinzolamide (Azopt) and dorzolamide (Trusopt). Oral agents include acetazolamide (Diamox) and methazolamide (Neptazane). The oral form can cause undesirable side effects that include tingling sensation in hands and feet, loss of appetite, metallic taste and kidney stones.

ALPHA₂ SELECTIVE AGONISTS   These drugs work by decreasing the rate of aqueous humor production and can be used alone or in combination with other anti-glaucoma eyedrops. Common side effects associated with this classification of eyedrop include itching, red or bloodshot eyes (ocular injection), upper lid elevation, and mildly dilated pupils. The FDA-approved drugs in this class include apraclonidine 1.0% and 0.5% (Iopidine) and brimonidine 0.2%, 0.15% and 0.1% (Alphagan and Alphagan P).

PROSTAGLANDINS   A single evening dose is very effective in reducing intraocular pressure. Ocular side effects include stimulation of eyelash growth, hyperemia (redness), increased pigmentation of the iris and eyelid skin. The agents presently available include bimatoprost (Lumigan), latanoprost (Xalatan), and travoprost (Travatan).

HYPEROSMOTICS   These agents decrease intraocular pressure by drawing fluid out of the aqueous and vitreous humors. The mechanism of action is by osmosis (the creation of a fluid force across a permeable membrane): in this case the fluid content of the eye and the bloodstream. An oral formulation of glycerin (**Osmoglyn**) and an injectable formulation of mannitol (**Osmitrol**) are employed in acute cases of high intraocular pressure (acute angle-closure glaucoma) and during intraocular surgery to create a rapid lowering of intraocular pressure producing a "soft eye."

COMBINATION AGENTS   Study results show that half of individuals with glaucoma require more than one type of medication to control the intraocular pressure. For this reason, a few ophthalmic pharmaceutical companies have produced "combination" eyedrops that include two anti-glaucoma medicines in a single drop.

For convenience, your eye doctor might prescribe combined medications. Typically, these combined medications have an additive effect of reducing intraocular pressure. Examples of medications of this type include dorzolamide/timolol (Cosopt), brimonidine/timolol (Combigan), and travoprost/timolol (DuoTrav).

ANTIMICROBIALS   Antimicrobials comprise a large variety of agents, including **antibiotics** for bacterial infections, **antivirals** for viral infections, and **antifungals** for fungal infections. The ophthalmologist has a great many choices among each type of antimicrobial medication for treatment of a specific eye condition. The side effects of antimicrobial products are numerous and complex and often influence the doctor's selection of a specific drug. Adverse reactions to antimicrobials include hypersensitivity to the particular drug and when taken orally, digestive system upset, and toxicity to other body systems. First and foremost, however, the doctor chooses an antimicrobial drug based on its ability to counter the specific microbial organism. The ophthalmic medical assistant should become familiar with this broad category of drugs over time by asking questions and reading the package insert that accompanies every drug.

Antibiotics kill or inhibit the growth of bacteria. For ophthalmic use, these drugs exist as topical drops or ointments to treat superficial infections such as blepharitis, bacterial conjunctivitis, and corneal ulcers. The most common use for antibiotics is before and after surgery as a preventative measure. However, data is sparse proving that antibiotics before and after cataract surgery is helpful in preventing postoperative infections.

Antibiotic solutions can be injected around the eye to treat more severe infections of bacterial corneal ulcers or endophthalmitis. In addition, "fortified" antibiotic drops may be used after mixing by a nurse or pharmacist. When taken orally or injected systemically, antibiotics serve to treat more serious ophthalmic conditions such as severe endophthalmitis, orbital infections (including orbital cellulitis), and acute dacryocystitis.

Antibiotics in common use in ophthalmology exist in a myriad of formulations and scores of brand names. An individual antibiotic can be used alone or with one or more other antibiotics. The following are the most common antibiotics an ophthalmic medical assistant would encounter in daily practice:

- bacitracin ointment, generic
- tobramycin drops and ointment (Tobrex, AKTob)
- erythromycin ointment (generic)
- azithromycin (AzaSite)
- gentamicin drops and ointment (Genoptic, Gentacidin)
- sulfonamide drops and ointment (Bleph-10, Sulf-10)

Examples of the fluoroquinolone group include the following:

- ciprofloxacin drops and ointment (Ciloxan)
- ofloxacin (Ocuflox)
- levofloxacin (Quixin, Iquix)
- gatifloxacin (Zymar, Zymaxid)
- moxifloxacin (Vigamox)
- besifloxacin (Besivance)

With the ever-increasing number of new antibiotics available, the ophthalmologist has the option of using combination drugs for treating ocular diseases, and the ophthalmic medical assistant should become familiar with these. These combinations include those composed of different types of antibiotics and those composed of mixtures of antibiotics and corticosteroid preparations. The following are some of the combination drugs often used in ophthalmology:

- neomycin-polymyxin B-bacitracin (Neosporin), ointment
- neomycin-polymyxin B-gramicidin (Neosporin), solution
- trimethoprim-polymyxin B (Polytrim)
- polymyxin B-bacitracin (Polysporin)
- terramycin-polymyxin B, generic
- neomycin-polymyxin B-dexamethasone (Maxitrol)
- tobramycin-dexamethasone (TobraDex)
- gentamicin-prednisolone (Pred G)
- sulfacetamide-prednisolone (Blephamide, Vasocidin)
- neomycin-bacitracin-polymyxin B-hydrocortisone (Cortisporin)
- neomycin-polymyxin B-prednisolone (PolyPred)
- tobramycin-loteprednol etabonate (Zylet)

ANTIVIRAL AGENTS **Antivirals** inhibit the ability of the virus to reproduce. Antiviral drugs are used to treat the more serious virus-caused ophthalmic conditions such as the herpes simplex and herpes zoster infections. Some of the antiviral drugs and how they are administered in ophthalmology include the following:

- trifluridine (Viroptic), topical
- ganciclovir (Zirgan gel), topical
- ganciclovir (Cytovene), intravenous
- ganciclovir (Vitrasert), intravitreal
- acyclovir (Zovirax), oral and intravenous
- foscarnet (Foscavir), intravenous
- valacyclovir hydrochloride (Valtrex), oral
- famciclovir (Famvir), oral
- valganciclovir (Valcyte), oral
- cidofovir (Vistide), intravenous

ANTIFUNGAL AGENTS **Antifungals** kill fungi and are therefore used to treat a variety of external ocular fungal infections, such as fungal blepharitis, keratitis, and conjunctivitis, and some internal fungal conditions as well. Fortunately, fungal infections of the eye are uncommon. Some of these agents can be toxic to the cornea and are therefore used when the diagnosis is definitive or highly suspicious of fungal disease. Some antifungals and how they are administered in ophthalmologic practice include the following:

- natamycin (Natacyn), topical
- amphotericin B (Fungizone), topical, subcutaneous, intravenous, and intravitreal
- ketoconazole (Nizoral), oral
- voriconazole (Vfend), topical, oral, and intravenous
- fluconazole (Diflucan), oral and intravenous

ANTIALLERGIC AND ANTI-INFLAMMATORY AGENTS **Corticosteroids** (**steroids**) are the chief drugs used to treat allergic reactions and inflammations. Corticosteroids, also called simply steroids, are hormones derived from the body's adrenal gland or made synthetically. Most corticosteroids are modifications of the hormone cortisone. In the treatment of eye disorders, these hormonal agents act by reducing inflammation and can dramatically decrease swelling, redness, and scarring. Most corticosteroids are applied topically in drop or ointment form to treat conditions involving the eyelid or the anterior segment of the eye. Systemic steroid drugs taken orally are used as therapy for disorders of the posterior segment as well as for acute or severe allergic reactions around the eye or elsewhere in the body.

Corticosteroids must be used and administered carefully because of their potentially harmful side effects. The ophthalmic medical assistant should check the patient's medical record for diseases such as hypertension, peptic ulcer, diabetes, and tuberculosis, all of which could worsen through the use of systemic corticosteroids.

These diseases, if present, should be flagged for the attention of the doctor. Side effects of steroid use from topical application can occur also, although most of these happen only after weeks to months of treatment. These side effects include glaucoma, bacterial or viral infection, overgrowth of fungi, slower healing, and cataract.

Steroids are sometimes injected behind, around, and in the eye to treat severe inflammation. Side effects are similar to those from topical use. If taken orally for a long period of time, corticosteroids can retard wound healing, cause swelling of the face and eyelids, promote cataract and glaucoma, lower a patient's resistance to infection, and increase blood sugar and blood pressure. Topical steroids commonly used in ophthalmology include the following:

- hydrocortisone acetate skin cream and ointment 1.0%, generic
- dexamethasone phosphate 0.1% (Maxidex)
- prednisolone acetate 0.12% and 1.0% (Pred Mild, Pred Forte, Omnipred)
- prednisolone sodium phosphate 1% (Inflamase Forte, Prednisol)
- fluorometholone 0.1% and 0.25% (FML, Fluor-OP, FML Forte)
- fluorometholone ophthalmic ointment (FML S.O.P.)
- fluorometholone acetate 0.1% (Flarex)
- rimexolone 1.0% (Vexol)
- loteprednol etabonate 0.2% and 0.5% (Alrex, Lotemax)
- difluprednate 0.05% (Durezol)

Commonly used systemic corticosteroids and their tablet doses include the following:

- hydrocortisone 10 mg (Hydrocortone)
- prednisone 5 mg (Deltasone)
- prednisolone 5 mg, generic
- methylprednisolone 4 mg (Medrol)
- triamcinolone 4 mg (Kenalog)
- dexamethasone 0.75 mg (Decadron)

Because of significant side effects of topical corticosteroids, **nonsteroidal antiinflammatory drugs (NSAIDs)** have been introduced. These medications may be used in the treatment of ocular inflammatory processes and ocular allergies. Commonly used topical ocular NSAIDs include the following:

- flurbiprofen (Ocufen)
- diclofenac (Voltaren)
- ketorolac tromethamine (Acular)
- bromfenac (Xibrom, Bromday)
- nepafanac (Nevanac)

Ocular decongestants act by constricting the superficial blood vessels in the conjunctiva. Ophthalmologists may prescribe decongestants as a cosmetic aid to reduce the eye redness caused by smoke or smog or to soothe eyes fatigued from driving, reading, or close work. Although this effect is soothing and cosmetic, it does nothing to alleviate the cause of the redness. Side effects related to decongestants include allergy, angle-closure glaucoma (rarely), and rebound, which means the superficial blood vessels become even more congested than before the drug was taken. Most decongestants used to treat ophthalmologic conditions are available without a doctor's prescription (also known as over-the-counter products). Some combination products are discussed under the allergy section below. The following brand name drops contains a single active ingredient:

- Visine
- Visine Advanced Relief
- Visine L.R.
- AK-Nefrin
- Murine Tears Plus
- Clear Eyes
- All Clear AR
- All Clear
- AK-Con
- Albalon

Agents for relief of seasonal allergic conjunctivitis are effective in reducing the itching, tearing, conjunctival injection, mucous secretion, and corneal complications of seasonal or vernal allergic conjunctivitis. Available products are an antihistamine (AH), mast cell inhibitor (MCI) or combination. Some brand name agents and their working action include the following:

- cromolyn (Crolom), MCI
- azelastine (Optivar), MCI/AH
- lodoxamide (Alomide), MCI

- nedocromil (Alocril), MCI

- epinastine (Elestat), MCI/AH

- olopatadine (Patanol, Pataday), MCI/AH

- ketotifen (Zaditor, Alaway), MCI/AH

- pemirolast (Alamast), MCI

- bepotastine besilate (Bepreve), MCI/AH

- alcaftadine (Lastacaft) MCI/AH

- emedastine difumarate (Emadine), AH

Sometimes a topical NSAID is useful to treat allergic conjunctivitis and ketorolac (Acular) may be prescribed. Patients can purchase several over-the-counter (OTC) products to treat their allergic eye symptoms. Vasocon-A, NaphconA, Visine A and Opcon A are common brand name products that contain an antihistamine and decongestant. In more acute allergic conditions, topical corticosteroids may be prescribed.

LUBRICANTS Lubricants help the patient to maintain an appropriate tear film balance or to keep the external eye moist. When used in the ointment form they have a more prolonged contact time to protect the eye from dryness. The ophthalmologist prescribes these medications to treat or relieve dry eye conditions, such as keratoconjunctivitis sicca and other tear-deficiency conditions. Side effects of lubricants are allergy to or irritation from the preservative in these agents. Some of the newer lubricant products are preservative-free (PF) and thus can be used more frequently than those with preservatives. The lack of preservatives also makes them less likely to cause side effects. The lubricants used to treat dry eye ophthalmic conditions are mostly bought over the counter. They consist of gel type substances with chemical names found under ingredients including carboxymethylcellulose, glycerin, propylene glycol, methylcellulose, polyvinyl alcohol, hydroxypropyl methylcellulose (hypromellose), povidone, sodium hyaluronate, white petrolatum, and mineral oil. Some common brand names of artificial tear products include the following:

- Clear Eyes CLR

- TheraTears

- Advanced Eye Relief Dry Eye Environment Lubricant Eye Drops, Advanced Eye Relief Dry Eye Rejuvenation Lubricant Eye Drops

- Refresh Tears, Refresh Plus PF, Refresh Liquigel, Refresh Celluvisc PF

- Hypo Tears

- Tears Naturale Forte, Tears Naturale Free, Tears Renewed

- Murocel

- GenTeal Mild

- GenTeal Moderate, GenTeal Gel

- Bion Tears

- Systane, Systane Ultra, Systane Balance

- Akwa Tears

- Visine Tears, Visine Pure Tears PF, Visine Tears Long Lasting Dry Eye Relief

- Murine Tears

- Soothe Lubricant Eye Drops

- Optive, Optive Sensitive PF

- Fresh Kote

Some common brand names of lubricating **ointment** products include the following:

- GenTeal PM

- Tear Naturale PM

- AKWA Tears

- Lacri-Lube SOP

- Hypotears Ointment Tears Renewed

- Refresh PM

- Tears Renewed, Tears Again Eye

A biodegradable insert (a dried miniature hydroxypropyl cellulose rod) is available under the brand name of Lacrisert to be placed in the cul-de-sac of the eyelid to melt slowly for lubrication.

IMMUNOMODULATORS In this class of medications, cyclosporine (Restasis) is a topical emulsion available for treatment of tear deficiency associated with the autoimmune or inflammatory conditions in the eyelids.

OTHER PHARMACEUTICALS Many other kinds of pharmaceutical products are used as treatment of eye-related conditions and for test procedures. Ophthalmic irrigating solutions comprise a group of sterile solutions of saline and other chemicals intended for flushing the eye or for use during surgical procedures. Osmotics are chemical agents in solution form that, when applied to the eye, employ the process of osmosis to reduce corneal edema by drawing fluid out through the corneal epithelium. Examples of drugs that produce effects used in specialized ophthalmic testing procedures include solutions for diagnosing pupillary dysfunction and gels that permit ultrasonic evaluation of the orbit. The ophthalmic assistant should become familiar with these agents by continued reading of the large variety of ophthalmic publications and by experience with the actual ophthalmic drugs used in the office or clinic.

Interpretation of a Prescription

The ophthalmic medical assistant should know how to read the doctor's prescription. Figure 6.5 illustrates a sample prescription. On a pad printed with the doctor's name, the doctor may include the following information on the medical prescription:

- the patient's name and address, and the date of the prescription

- the name of the drug and its concentration or dose (strength)

- the total amount of the drug to be dispensed to the patient (the dispense quantity)

- the directions to the pharmacist as to what to type on the label of the drug, usually written beside the abbreviation "Sig" (for the Latin word signa, meaning mark)

- the signature of the doctor

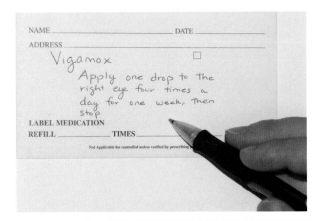

Figure 6.5 Partial view of sample prescription. The preprinted form would have at the top the doctor's name, address, telephone number and a place for the date. The bottom shows instructions for labeling and the number of refills allowed. A blank space at the bottom for the doctor's signature and at the top for the patient's name is not shown in this figure. (*Image courtesy of Jay S. Wallshein, MD.*)

Previously, abbreviations shown in Table 6.2 were used to write directions; however, today these are not used as often (if at all). Most directions are now written literally, as in the following examples: "One drop 8 times a day right eye." "Apply small amount of ointment before bedtime in both eyes." "Take 1 capsule every 12 hours for 2 weeks then stop." "Apply 2 drops to right eye every 4 hours while awake for 10 days then stop." This change away from Latin abbreviations is due to preprinted prescriptions and electronic prescribing and is aimed toward reducing medical errors. Sometimes there is an indication to the pharmacist that the prescription can be refilled; for example, "Repeat X2."

Table 6.2 Abbreviations and Symbols Used in Prescriptions

Abbreviation or Symbol	Meaning
ac	(*ante cibum*) before meals
bid	(*bis in die*) twice a day
dispi	dispense
g	gram
gtt	(*gutta, guttae*) drop, drops
h	(*hora*) hour
hs	(*hora somni*) at bedtime
ml	milliliters
mg	milligram
non rep	(*non repetatur*) do not repeat or refill
OD	(*oculus dexter*) right eye
OS	(*oculus sinister*) left eye
OU	(*oculi uterque*) both eyes, considered separately
pc	(*post cibum*) after meals
po	(*per os*) by mouth; orally
prn	(*pro re nata*) as needed
qd	(*quaque die*) every day (avoid; use qd)
qh	(*quaque hora*) every hour
qid	(*quater in die*) 4 times a day
ql	(*quantum libet*) as much as desired
q4h	(*quaque quarta hora*) every 4 hours
Rx	(*recipe*) prescription
S or Sig	(*signa*) label
Sol or Soln	solution
Susp	suspension
tid	(*ter in die*) 3 times a day
tsp	teaspoon
ung	(*unguentum*) ointment

Frequently, an indication to the pharmacist is made to place the name of the medication on the label or a stop date on the use of the drug may be part of the directions. Glaucoma drugs usually are continued indefinitely but the number of refills may be limited by a state's pharmacy regulations.

Sometimes the doctor's state medical license number and Drug Enforcement Administration (DEA) number is printed, especially if the prescription is for a controlled substance such as a narcotic. Prescriptions for controlled drugs cannot be phoned into the pharmacy by the ophthalmic medical assistant. Additionally, special care should be taken in the office to keep blank prescription pads in a safe place where they cannot be taken or used by unauthorized individuals.

First Aid for Acute Drug Reactions

Ophthalmic medical assistants should become familiar with the office emergency first aid procedure before assisting in the use of or administering ophthalmic medications. You should ask your doctor or a senior technician for any written procedures or guidelines to deal with such an event.

The ophthalmic medical assistant should be prepared to give general first aid if a patient suffers an acute drug reaction immediately or within a few minutes of receiving an ophthalmic drug. Acute drug reactions include fainting; tremors or convulsions, in which the patient shakes or writhes because the drug has overstimulated the central nervous system; and respiratory emergency, in which the patient complains of difficulty in breathing. Procedures for dealing with a patient who feels faint are given in a box in Chapter 15. Instructions for handling tremors or convulsions and respiratory difficulty appear in Procedure 6.2.

Acute allergic reaction, one of the most serious drug reactions, requires immediate attention.

Patients with acute allergic reactions to drugs develop an itching skin rash, difficulty in breathing, or a rapid, weak pulse right after receiving the drug. Because prompt medical treatment is needed, the only action for the ophthalmic medical assistant to take in this situation is to call for the ophthalmologist immediately. The doctor may need to give the patient an antihistamine, adrenaline or corticosteroid by injection, and administer oxygen. In severe cases of swelling in the patient's larynx, a tracheotomy (surgical cutting of the windpipe) may need to be performed.

The ophthalmic medical assistant should know where the following first aid materials are kept and how to make them immediately available to the doctor for an acute allergic reaction:

- oxygen

- diphenhydramine (Benadryl), oral

- epinephrine, injectable

- diazepam (Valium), oral

- cortisone, intravenous

- smelling salts or spirits of ammonia

- syringes and needles

The assistant should also know where to find materials for flushing an eye and the appropriate procedures for ocular and systemic emergencies in the office. (See Chapter 15.)

Procedure 6.2 Giving First Aid

Tremors or Convulsions

1. Call for the ophthalmologist at once.

2. If the patient has tremors, make sure she is seated so that she won't fall and hurt herself. If the patient is having convulsions, help her lie on the floor, cushioning her head. Never insert anything into the mouth.

3. Loosen any tight clothing.

Respiratory Emergency

1. Call for the ophthalmologist if a patient complains of breathing difficulty.

2. If the patient stops breathing altogether, call for the ophthalmologist and initiate cardiopulmonary resuscitation (CPR).

SELF-ASSESSMENT TEST

1. List the 3 principal delivery systems for ophthalmic medications.

2. Name the 3 principal forms of topical ophthalmic medications.

3. Name 3 possible types of eye irritations caused by preservatives used in eyedrops.

4. What is the major advantage of drugs dissolved or suspended in ointments or gels over eyedrops?

5. Which eye care professionals usually inject ophthalmic drugs?

6. Place the following steps for instilling eyedrops or applying ointments in the proper order.

    a. Check the doctor's instructions.

    b. Expose the lower conjunctival cul-de-sac.

    c. Wash your hands thoroughly.

    d. Instruct the patient to open the eyes and look up.

    e. Gently close the eyelids for 2 minutes.

7. Which of the following actions is most important in ensuring adequate drug delivery of an ophthalmic suspension?

    a. Wash your hands thoroughly.

    b. Shake the bottle to distribute the drug thoroughly.

    c. Gently wipe the tip of the applicator with a sterile cotton ball.

    d. Press the patient's lacrimal sac.

    e. Express a small amount onto a cotton ball.

8. Drugs that paralyze the iris sphincter muscle and dilate the pupil are called which of the following?

    a. anesthetics

    b. short-acting agents

    c. corticosteroids

    d. cycloplegics

    e. miotics

9. Mydriatic agents are used for what purpose?

    a. to dilate the pupil

    b. to paralyze the iris sphincter muscle

    c. to treat inflammation of the eyelids

    d. to treat accommodation problems

    e. to treat infections

10. Fluorescein and rose bengal aid in which of the following?

   a. deadening nerves

   b. diagnosing certain corneal problems

   c. treating viral infections

   d. inhibiting bacterial growth

   e. treating angle-closure glaucoma

11. Which 3 kinds of organisms that cause infection do antimicrobials inhibit or kill?

   a. fungi, cysts, and bacteria

   b. bacteria, hormones, and viruses

   c. bacteria, viruses, and osmotics

   d. bacteria, viruses, and fungi

   e. bacteria, microorganisms, and fungi

12. If the doctor's prescription indicates to "apply eyedrops tid," what would you advise the patient that this means?

   a. Use the drops in the morning.

   b. Use the drops once a day.

   c. Use the drops 3 times a day.

   d. Use the entire prescription of drops before discarding the bottle.

   e. Use the drops as needed.

13. Within a few minutes of applying anesthetic eyedrops, the patient complains of itching around the eye and difficulty breathing. What would be your best first action to take?

   a. Loosen the patient's collar.

   b. Suspect an allergic reaction and call for the doctor immediately.

   c. Apply corticosteroid drops.

   d. Begin cardiopulmonary resuscitation (CPR).

   e. Have the patient lie down.

14. Which of the following best defines fluoroquinolone?

   a. an antibiotic used to treat bacterial infections

   b. an antifungal agent used to treat mycotic keratitis

   c. a sunscreen used for ultraviolet (UV) light protection

   d. a medication used to treat migraine headaches

   e. a corticosteroid agent used to treat inflammation

SUGGESTED ACTIVITIES

1. Discuss the use and dispensing of ophthalmic drugs with your ophthalmologist. Be thoroughly familiar with any guidelines or procedures for administering medication to patients.

2. Ask your ophthalmologist or a senior technician if you may observe the treatment or testing of patients that requires the instillation of eyedrops or ointments. Take notes and ask questions in a later discussion.

3. With your ophthalmologist or a senior technician supervising, practice instilling eyedrops and applying ointments on coworkers who have agreed to participate. Be sure to ask the doctor to choose a medication that is safe to use for this practice exercise.

4. Review with your ophthalmologist the procedure for the treatment of acute drug reactions. Ask the doctor to outline all the possibilities of what could go wrong and what would be your best immediate response to help the patient.

5. Collect the printed package inserts of the most common medications used in your doctor's practice. Read them thoroughly, paying special attention to the section on side effects or adverse reactions, and discuss any questions you may have with your ophthalmologist or a senior technician.

SUGGESTED RESOURCES

American Academy of Ophthalmology. *Color Codes for Topical Ocular Medications*. Policy Statement. San Francisco: American Academy of Ophthalmology; 2010. www.aao.org/about/policy. Accessed August 15, 2011.

Cassin B, ed. *Fundamentals for Ophthalmic Technical Personnel*. Philadelphia: Saunders; 1995: chap 4.

DuBois LG. Patient services, installation of medications. In: *Fundamentals of Ophthalmic Medical Assisting*. DVD. San Francisco: American Academy of Ophthalmology; 2009.

Harper RA, ed. *Basic Ophthalmology*. 9th ed. San Francisco: American Academy of Ophthalmology; 2010.

PDR Network. *PDR for Ophthalmic Medicines (Physicians' Desk Reference for Ophthalmic Medicines)*. Montvale NJ: PDR Network; updated annually.

Stein HA, Stein RM. *The Ophthalmic Assistant: A Text for Allied and Associated Ophthalmic Personnel*. 8th ed. St Louis: Mosby; 2006.

7 MICROORGANISMS AND INFECTION CONTROL

Microorganisms, or microbes, are organisms so small they are visible only with the aid of a microscope. Humans exist harmoniously with many microorganisms, but some can cause disease, including eye disease. Ocular infections often start when harmful microorganisms contact and enter the ocular tissues, either through trauma (including contact lens wear) or by means of contaminated (microbe-carrying) instruments, hands, solutions, or medications. Infection is the invasion and multiplication of harmful microbes within the body tissues.

An important responsibility of the ophthalmic medical assistant is to prevent the transmission of disease-causing microorganisms from one patient to another or to office personnel. This responsibility is part of a program of sanitation and microbial control (antisepsis) in the office referred to as standard precautions. The purpose of standard precautions is to reduce the opportunity for harmful microbes to flourish and threaten patients and medical personnel, who may be exposed to possibly infectious materials.

This chapter describes the kinds of microbes that can cause eye disease, and their means of transmission and routes of infection. Most important, it covers the techniques that are used to control the spread of microorganisms, such as standard, universal, and isolation precautions; disinfection; and sterilization.

Types of Microorganisms

Although microorganisms exist in numerous forms, the following groups are most commonly associated with eye disease:

- bacteria (singular: bacterium), including gram-negative and gram-positive types and mycobacteria

- viruses (singular: virus), including herpes simplex virus, herpes zoster virus, and human immunodeficiency virus

- fungi (singular: fungus), including yeasts

- protozoa (singular: protozoan), including amoebas

Scientists usually classify microorganisms according to their size, structure, method of reproduction, or response to laboratory procedures such as *staining* (dyeing with special procedures and coloring agents such as Gram stain). Like all organisms, microorganisms are given names that reflect their classification, with first a *genus* and then a *species* name. The genus name is sometimes abbreviated after the first usage. For example, a common intestinal bacterium with which you may be familiar is named *Escherichia coli* and abbreviated *E coli*.

Bacteria

Bacteria are simple, single-celled microorganisms that reproduce by splitting in two. Although they are widely dispersed in nature, some bacteria cannot live very long when exposed to sunlight and air. Others are relatively resistant, or fastidious, and can survive for hours or days on dust particles in the air or on the surface of objects. Still other bacteria produce spores, a hardy, thick-skinned form that allows them to survive for months and even years until they encounter conditions suitable for growth.

The majority of bacterial infections can be successfully treated with antibiotics.

Bacteria (and certain other microbes) can be classified by their reaction when exposed to dyes in a procedure called **Gram staining**. Knowing an organism's Gram-staining characteristics is useful in predicting the severity and course of an infection and determining which antibiotic(s) to select in treating that infection. In the Gram-staining procedure, a glass microscope slide that has been smeared with a microbial specimen is covered with a dye or dyes, which stain the normally colorless microorganisms. Bacteria that stain purple or blue are referred to as *gram positive*; those that stain pink are referred to as *gram negative* (Figure 7.1). This differentiation allows the clinician to choose a more specific antibiotic based on predicted susceptibility. Generally, gram-negative infections are more problematic, with the exception of methicillin-resistant *Staphylococcus aureus* (MRSA), which is resistant to most antibiotics. So that you may familiarize yourself with the names of bacteria that you may see on patient charts and other medical documents, Table 7.1 lists types of bacteria most commonly associated with ocular infections and their Gram-stain characteristics.

For example, the gram-positive bacterium *Staphylococcus aureus* is a frequent cause of blepharitis, conjunctivitis, and infectious keratitis (stromal infiltrates and epithelial ulceration). Similarly, other *Staphylococcus*

Table 7.1 Bacteria Commonly Recovered from Ocular Infections

Gram Positive (G+)	Gram Negative (G–)
Actinomyces species	*Haemophilus influenzae*
Bacillus cereus	*Moraxella catarrhalis*
Corynebacterium species	*Moraxella lacunata*
Propionibacterium acnes	*Neisseria gonorrhoeae*
Staphylococcus aureus	*Proteus mirabilis*
Staphylococcus epidermidis	*Pseudomonas aeruginosa*
Streptococcus pneumoniae	*Serratia marcescens*
Streptococcus pyogenes	*Streptococcus viridans* group

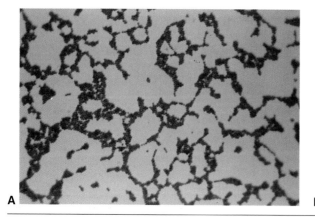
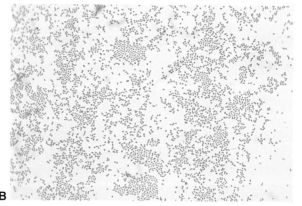

Figure 7.1 Photomicrographs of Gram-stained bacteria. **A.** Gram-positive *Staphylococcus aureus*. **B.** Gram-negative *Neisseria gonorrhoeae*.

species, many of which are considered normal inhabitants on the surface of our bodies and hair, are responsible for infections of the conjunctiva, cornea, lacrimal apparatus, and intraocular fluids.

As a group, gram negative–associated infections are more serious in their natural course. Infections caused by gram-negative organisms (ie, *Pseudomonas aeruginosa*) are often associated with contact lens overwear. Permanent visual impairment may occur within 48 hours even if these infections are diagnosed properly and treated aggressively. Pseudomonas is a common contaminant in eyedrops, cosmetics, and hot tubs. The gram-negative bacterium *Neisseria gonorrhoeae* transmitted through sexual contact or congenital exposure in an infected birth canal can also cause a hyperacute conjunctivitis; this is usually a serious infection (Figure 7.2A) because the bacteria can enter into the eye, invading through an otherwise intact barrier structure.

Mycobacteria, a unique organism capable of intracellular growth, was formerly in our differential diagnosis of infections following LASIK surgery; however, this condition was discovered to be caused by unsterile solutions and this problem has been almost completely eradicated. It is considered an "opportunistic" infection, one that occurs only when exposed to the right environment, and although it rarely occurs, it can be very difficult to combat. The mycobacteria family includes both the tuberculosis and nontuberculosis groups.

Chlamydia trachomatis is responsible for a myriad of ocular infections. These include neonatal conjunctivitis (a conjunctivitis contracted by newborns from an infected birth canal; Figure 7.2B), inclusion conjunctivitis (a common cause of follicular conjunctivitis in sexually active adults), and trachoma, a chronic, severe, scar-producing conjunctivitis. This is why all newborn infants in the United States are given erythromycin ophthalmic ointment at birth, and notably there was a nationwide shortage of this medicine in 2009. In the United States, trachoma is rare and mostly restricted to the southwestern region, especially on Indian reservations, due to contaminated water supplies. Trachoma remains the leading cause of preventable blindness in the Middle East, North Africa, and Southeast Asia. It is also transmitted via a contaminated water supply.

Another group of bacteria that cause syphilis (*Treponema pallidum*) and Lyme disease (*Borrelia burgdorferi*) can less commonly lead to ocular disorders. Infections with these organisms tend to be chronic, cause progressive damage, and involve the nervous system.

Viruses

Among the smallest microorganisms, viruses do not have a cellular structure and so can multiply only within living cells. Because of their unique makeup, viruses are not given genus and species names, but are instead often named for the diseases they cause or the organisms they infect. Many viral infections are self-limited (that is, the disease they cause runs a definite, limited course, like the common cold), and treatment for these is mainly to alleviate symptoms, not to eradicate the organism or cure the infection. Systemic and topical antiviral drugs can effectively control a limited range of viral infections, but they may also be toxic (have "poisonous" side effects) with prolonged use.

Viral infections cannot be controlled with antibiotics.

Members of the **herpesvirus** family include herpes simplex virus type 1 (HSV-1), herpes simplex virus type 2

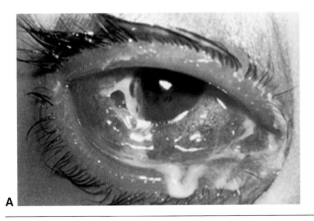
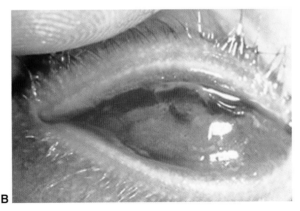

Figure 7.2 Bacterial conjunctivitis. **A.** Hyperacute conjunctivitis due to invasion by *Neisseria gonorrhoeae*. **B.** Neonatal chlamydial conjunctivitis.

(HSV-2), varicella-zoster virus (VZV), cytomegalovirus (CMV), and Epstein-Barr virus (EBV). Once infected or exposed to these viruses, the individual will carry them for life, though there may never be a clinical disease. These viruses are involved in more than 500,000 cases of ocular disease each year, including blepharoconjunctivitis, keratitis, uveitis, retinitis, and conjunctivitis. **Herpes simplex virus type 1**, which causes commonly seen "fever blisters" on the lips and mouth, is responsible for most of the lesions of the cornea and eyelids (Figure 7.3). **Herpes simplex virus type 2** (HSV-2) more commonly infects the genital region and is transmitted by sexual contact. Newborns exposed to HSV-2 during passage through an infected birth canal are at high risk for ocular infection. HSV-2 has become a more common cause of ocular infection over the last several years.

HSV ocular infections can be recurrent. Some authors report upwards of 25% of all initial HSV infections will come back in any of several forms. A conjunctival or epithelial dendrite form may appear. These are "true" recurrent infections. An ulcerative or stromal/endothelial/uveitis form may also present. These are inflammatory, autoimmune-based recurrences, not "true" infections. Antiviral medications are most effective in treating a "true" HSV-related infection, whether it is the primary (first) infection or a recurrent infection. For inflammatory recurrences, the pivotal treatment is the frequent topical use of strong corticosteroids along with topical antiviral drops. In addition, oral antiviral medications are often used in this setting (ie, acyclovir or famciclovir). Despite effective treatments, HSV continues to be one of the leading causes of infectious corneal blindness in the United States and other developed countries due to its high rate of recurrence and its ability to "masquerade" as another condition, making the diagnosis of recurrent episodes more difficult.

Varicella-zoster virus (VZV) produces the common childhood disease chicken pox. Recovery from chicken pox usually leaves the person immune to recurrence, but VZV may reactivate in certain individuals, especially those with an immunocompromised state like acquired immunodeficiency syndrome (AIDS) or cancer, producing a painful skin condition called *zoster* or *shingles*. During these outbreaks or often independent from them, the eye can also become involved, resulting in a painful, severe, and sometimes blinding disease called *herpes zoster ophthalmicus*.

Oral antiviral drugs and topical anti-inflammatory (steroid) medications are used to minimize inflammation of the eye and orbit and to limit subsequent visually compromising scar formation. Patients may be treated for weeks to months while the inflammatory reaction to this infection slowly subsides. Patients may also develop cranial nerve palsies, which might require steroids and antiviral medications for weeks or months while waiting for the inflammation to resolve.

CMV retinitis, an ocular infection due to *cytomegalovirus*, is commonly seen in patients infected with the **human immunodeficiency virus** (HIV), which causes AIDS, and in other immunocompromised patients. However, with the advent of highly active antiretroviral therapy (HAART), this is now an unusual clinical manifestation of this disease. Along with a low white blood cell count, this infection is often the first indication that a patient who has been HIV-positive has made the transition to AIDS.

HIV, which is a type of virus called a *retrovirus*, is indirectly responsible not only for CMV retinitis but also for several other serious infections of the eye. Ocular involvement occurs in 50% to 75% or more of HIV-infected patients. HIV has been isolated from tears as well as from conjunctival and corneal tissue. HIV may

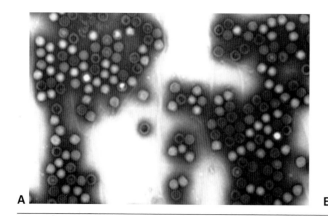
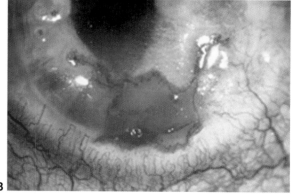

Figure 7.3 Herpes simplex virus type 1 and one result of its infection of the eye. **A.** Photomicrograph of HSV-1. **B.** Corneal ulcer resulting from HSV-1 infection. The ulcer has been stained pink with rose bengal dye. *(Part A courtesy of John J. Cardamone Jr/Biological Photo Service.)*

also be isolated from the contact lenses of infected patients. However, the U.S. government agency called the Centers for Disease Control and Prevention (CDC) says that the virus is not in sufficient quantity in these fluids to be considered an infection risk. The route by which HIV reaches the ocular surface tissues and tears remains uncertain.

Infections from the adenovirus family are responsible for two distinct and common ophthalmic syndromes: epidemic keratoconjunctivitis (EKC) and pharyngoconjunctival fever (PCF), also known as "pink eye."

EKC is a highly contagious disease that is spread by direct contact with contaminated medical personnel or instruments or by indirect contact with exposed surfaces in the exam room, in the waiting area or reception/check-out area, or in the patient's home or work place. Outbreaks are known to occur in ophthalmic offices and clinics, school locker rooms, and college dormitories. EKC infections may lead to development of inflammatory corneal infiltrates that can leave visually significant scars. Although there is no current antiviral treatment, topical steroids are often initiated to both relieve the significant discomfort and, when infiltrates are present, to limit the potential for scarring.

The PCF form of adenoviral conjunctivitis is also contagious, yet it is a milder form that can occur associated with or following a respiratory infection. Ophthalmic personnel who acquire these infections should not be allowed direct patient contact until the infection clears.

Fungi

Fungi are multicellular microorganisms with a more complex structure than that of bacteria. Fungi can be divided into two groups: **yeasts**, which produce creamy or pasty colonies; and **molds**, which produce woolly, fluffy, or powdery growth (Figure 7.4). The fuzzy growth seen on old bread is an example of a fungal mold colony.

Ocular fungal infections, especially those involving the cornea, usually are the result of direct trauma, usually from some type of vegetable matter, such as a scratch from a tree twig, that introduces plant material or soil into the eye. Intraocular fungal infections can result as an extension of keratitis, from another infected source within the body, or from contaminated instruments or solutions. Fungal infections are more common in immunocompromised patients. Fungal infections are more commonly seen in warmer, moister climates such as those seen in the Southeastern United States. A common source of fungal eye infections is the *Candida albicans* species of yeast. The fungus called *Histoplasma capsulatum* causes ocular histoplasmosis, an intraocular (inside

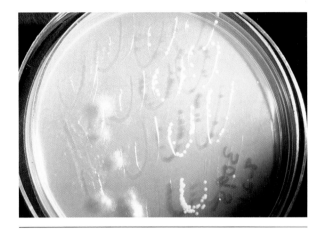

Figure 7.4 Fungi obtained from the cornea of a patient and grown in a laboratory. The left two rows of fluffy streaks are a mold; the right two rows of creamy streaks are a yeast.

the eye) infection. Although both topical and systemic antifungal medications are available to treat fungal infections, the course of treatment is often quite extended and more difficult as compared to bacterial infections.

Protozoa

Protozoa such as *Acanthamoeba* are relatively large and complex single-celled microorganisms found in numerous places all around us, including fresh water, salt water, soil, plants, insects, and animals, even humans. For example, *Acanthamoeba* species flourish in soil, freshwater lakes, hot tubs, swimming pools, and homemade contact lens salt solutions (Figure 7.5). This organism can cause an extremely painful infection of the cornea, and so contact lens wearers must be instructed in special precautions about the care, storage and use of their lenses. (See Chapter 14.)

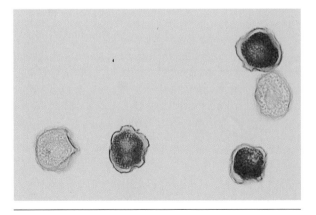

Figure 7.5 Photomicrograph of *Acanthamoeba*, the protozoan that causes *Acanthamoeba* keratitis. *(Image courtesy of William Mathers, MD, University of Iowa.)*

This same type of corneal infection has also been associated with trauma that involves soil or water contaminated with these organisms. The treatment of *Acanthamoeba* is difficult and prolonged. It requires specially formulated medications, some of which are not available in the United States.

In the eye, infection with the protozoan *Toxoplasma gondii*, called **toxoplasmosis**, causes inflammation of uveal and retinal structures. Toxoplasmosis is now one of the most common infections seen in patients with AIDS. It was previously believed to be a congenital infection; however, now it is most often acquired be ingesting undercooked meat products. Oral antibiotics and, occasionally, steroids are used to treat toxoplasmosis.

The risk for any contact lens–associated infection greatly increases if the person sleeps in his or her contact lenses, and this practice should always be discouraged.

Prions

Prions are unique transmissible proteins that represent a threat to humans and can be transmitted in a number of ways. Mad cow disease (bovine spongiform encephalopathy), one of the best known of the prion diseases, may be transmitted to humans who eat tainted meat. Kuru, or laughing sickness, was present in the 1950s in New Guinea in a population of people who engaged in ritualistic cannibalism after death, and many women and children contracted this prion because the men ate the more choice meat and the women and children were left with the organs and brains. Prions may be present in our bodies for years before causing pathology and are difficult to detect. Transplanted tissue (ie, corneas) may carry the prions, infecting the recipient and possibly causing an encephalopathy that is a variant form of Creutzfeldt-Jakob disease. Resistant to common forms of sterilization, this condition can be very frustrating to prevent and treat.

Concern regarding prions extends beyond corneal transplantation. Botulinum toxin and human fibrin tissue adhesive (Tisseel) both contain human serum albumin and have a theoretical risk of prion transmission. The American Red Cross has stopped accepting blood donations from individuals with a history of corneal transplantation.

Transmission of Infectious Diseases

To produce infection, a microorganism must be living, viable, and able to produce offspring and it must gain access to or cross the protective barriers of the invaded organism. Then it must overcome that organism's natural defense mechanisms and find conditions suitable for growth and reproduction.

Although the external ocular structures, conjunctiva, and cornea are constantly challenged by harmful or potentially harmful microbes, infection rarely results. This is due in part to the eye's natural protective barriers and defense mechanisms. Protective barriers and mechanisms that help the eye resist infection include intact skin; eyelids and lashes and an intact blink mechanism; tears, which contain antibacterial substances; and the mucous layer of the conjunctiva and cornea, which repels or traps and expels invading organisms. As long as the outer epithelial and stromal layers of the conjunctiva and cornea remain unbroken, they also form a barrier against most microbial invaders. However, infection can result when the protective layers are broken, such as by trauma, surgery, or debilitating illness, or by seemingly less obvious routes, including contact lens wear or even moderate dry eye conditions.

Disease-causing microorganisms are transmitted from a **reservoir** (the animate or inanimate object that provides a microorganism the means for survival and opportunity for transmission) to a **host** (the animal or plant that provides a microorganism with nutrients and the other conditions that are necessary for survival and reproduction). The principal means of infectious transmission are as follows:

- airborne droplets and particles containing infectious microbes

- direct contact with a contaminated person

- indirect contact with a contaminated person or inanimate object

- common-vehicle transmission, in which microbes are transmitted from a common, inanimate source such as a contaminated food or water supply to infect several people

- vector-borne transmission, which occurs through insects such as mosquitoes and flies (vectors)

Airborne Droplets and Particles

A person infected with certain disease-causing microbes who coughs or sneezes produces a cloud of water droplets containing millions of infectious organisms. When a susceptible individual inhales these airborne droplets, the microbes are brought directly to cells of the upper respiratory tract and can produce infection in the new host. The varicella-zoster virus that causes chicken pox and the bacterium that causes tuberculosis (*Mycobacterium tuberculosis*) can be spread in this way. The excimer laser creates a microscopic plume of organic material, some of which may be biologically active and could theoretically transmit infection.

These could include the hepatitis C and HIV viruses. There is no doubt that many people with hepatitis C and HIV are getting LASIK surgery, sometimes unbeknownst to the patient and the staff. Having these viruses is not a contraindication for surgery; however, procedures for such patients should be done at the end of the day and the suite thoroughly cleaned afterward. As with all cases, the surgical team should wear surgical masks during the excimer procedure.

Direct-Contact Transmission

Direct-contact transmission is the direct transfer of an infectious agent from person to person through close physical contact. The fingers are an especially effective means of direct-contact transmission. Physicians or assistants who touch the infected eye of a patient or an infected lesion (such as a cold sore) on a patient or themselves can carry infectious microbes on their fingers for minutes, hours, or even longer, depending on the organism. Examining the eyes of another patient without first washing the hands provides the opportunity to transfer the infectious microbes from the fingers to the new patient. The use of waterless antibacterial gels has become commonplace in many medical offices, especially after the H1N1 ("swine flu") influenza virus pandemic in 2009, but it is important to realize that these are ineffective against viruses. Many offices employ the use of cotton-tipped applicators in order to avoid direct contact with a patient's eye or periocular skin.

Indirect-Contact Transmission

Indirect-contact transmission involves the transfer of microbes from one host to another via an inanimate object. For example, a tissue or handkerchief used by a person with acute conjunctivitis may carry a high concentration of the offending virus, as do objects handled by the infected person shortly after using the handkerchief. Touching these contaminated objects or surfaces, possibly for an extended period, can expose individuals to the virus if they then bring their own hands to their face or eyes.

An important means of indirect-contact transmission the ophthalmic medical assistant may encounter is contaminated medical instruments, examination equipment, and materials. Door knobs, faucet handles, exam chairs, desk tops, and even paper products (ie, books, magazines, sign-in sheets, and pens) are also potential sources for microbial transmission by indirect contact. Some medical offices will have a designated "dirty room" to examine patients with suspected ocular infections, and this helps in decreasing the spread of microorganisms. These rooms are disinfected after each patient encounter. In addition, any patient testing that requires direct contact like applanation tonometry should be deferred unless medically necessary. In the home setting, towels, sheets, pillowcases, eating utensils, drinking glasses, tabletops, and just about any surface if it has been exposed to infectious organisms may also be potential sources for indirect transmission. Indirect-contact transmission can also occur when the skin or eye is penetrated by wood or metal fragments, such as twigs, nails, and knives, which can be contaminated with disease-causing bacteria or fungi. In addition, contaminated eyedrops and other solutions may transmit infection by indirect contact. The tips of open eyedrop containers should never touch the patient, and should be dated when opened and replaced periodically, even if not empty.

Infectious microbes can reside for minutes, hours, or longer on instruments, needles, other sharp implements, swabs, and other reusable or disposable materials that have contacted an infected patient's blood or body fluid. Special care must be taken to decontaminate instruments as well as to clean or dispose of materials in such a way that those who next contact them will not be exposed to infectious or potentially infectious microbes.

Common-Vehicle Transmission

Common-vehicle transmission involves the transfer of infectious microbes from one reservoir to many people. For example, disease-causing organisms can contaminate and multiply in ocular medications, such as eyedrops, that have been improperly stored or handled or have been opened and used for too long a period. Each patient who then has the contaminated eyedrops instilled is exposed and may become infected. Serious ocular infections can result from the administration of contaminated medications, and special precautions for handling medications are strictly required in medical offices, clinics, and hospitals. (See Procedure 6.1 for information about administering eyedrops and "Aseptic Technique: Handling Sterile Medical Equipment" in this chapter.)

Vector-Borne Transmission

In biology, a vector is an organism that transmits a pathogen to a host. Diseases caused through **vector-borne**

transmission are unlikely to be encountered in most ophthalmology offices and clinics in the United States. In the developing world, trachoma and onchocerciasis are examples of diseases transmitted through flies. (See Chapter 21 for a broader discussion of major causes of reversible irreversible blindness around the world.)

Trachoma is the result of eye infection by *Chlamydia trachomatis*, a microorganism that spreads through eye discharge from infected individuals and through transmission by eye-seeking flies. Years of repeat infection lead to eyelid scarring (entropion), eyelash abnormalities (trichiasis), corneal scarring, and loss of vision. Trachoma continues to be common in many of the poorest and most remote rural areas of Africa, Asia, Central and South America, Australia and the Middle East. Medical treatment consists of antibiotics (oral azithromycin or tetracycline ointment) and surgery to repair entropion. Facial cleanliness and improved water supply have been shown to reduce the risk of infection. Recent data from Vietnam shows that trachoma can be nearly eliminated as a community health problem. In 1960, 80% of Vietnamese people suffered from the disease and 30% became blind from it. The country's Trachoma Control Program was launched in 2000 through 53 districts where the disease was prevalent. Today, cases of active trachoma have dropped to less than 1% of the population.

Onchocerciasis (river blindness) is a parasitic disease caused by the worm *Onchocerca volvulus*. It is transmitted through the bites of infected blackflies, which carry immature larval forms of the parasite microfilariae from human to human. In the human body, the larvae form nodules in the subcutaneous tissue, where they mature to adult worms. These worms can move through the body, and may find their way into ocular tissues except the lens. Inflammation results and visual loss can be due to corneal scarring (keratitis), retinal lesions and optic nerve disease. In a number of countries, onchocerciasis has been controlled through spraying of blackfly breeding sites with insecticide. In addition, a drug is available that kills the microfilariae, alleviating symptoms and reducing transmission.

Infection Control Precautions

Ophthalmic medical assistants, as well as ophthalmologists, work in close proximity to patients, some of whom have ocular infections or are carrying disease-causing microorganisms. Many patients have lowered resistance to infection because of systemic disease, use of certain medications, or age. All medical professionals, including ophthalmic medical assistants, must take the necessary steps to prevent transmission of infectious microbes to the patient, between patients, and to those who may later come in contact with materials contaminated by infectious material from patients. Assistants also have the obligation to protect themselves from infection. A well-designed and scrupulously followed program of microbial control in the medical office can greatly reduce the risk of transmitting infectious organisms between patients and to or from health care workers.

The Centers for Disease Control and Prevention (CDC) has developed specific procedures designed to help health care workers prevent transmission of pathogens and protect themselves and patients from various infections. These procedures are of two types, universal precautions and body substance isolation precautions.

Universal precautions, designed to reduce the risk of transmission of diseases carried in the blood, were initially a response to the AIDS epidemic. Universal precautions require medical workers to assume that all human blood and body fluids containing visible blood may be infectious, potentially harboring HIV, hepatitis B virus (HBV), and other bloodborne *pathogens* (disease-causing microorganisms). Such precautions include hand washing (before and after patient contact) and the use of appropriate barriers (gloves, masks, goggles, etc) to prevent direct contact with potentially infected body fluids. Also, particular sterilization and disinfection measures and infectious waste disposal procedures are to be followed. See Procedure 7.1 for a complete list of these precautions.

The separate standard for body substance isolation precautions, also referred to as *transmission-based precautions*, is more commonly used in hospitals. It is further restrictive and is designed to reduce the risk of disease transmission by body fluids other than blood and moist areas such as mucous membranes. These include droplet precautions for influenza, airborne isolation for pulmonary tuberculosis, or contact isolation for MRSA, a pathogen that is common in clinic and hospital settings. The possibility of a MRSA infection should be suspected in any patient that works in these environments.

The Occupational Safety and Health Administration (OSHA) of the U.S. Department of Labor has created a regulation based on universal precautions to help prevent the transmission of potentially life-threatening microbes and diseases to and from workers who come into contact with blood or blood-contaminated fluids. This regulation, called "Occupational Exposure to Bloodborne Pathogens," applies to all medical offices in the U.S. that have at least one worker whose duties may expose him or her to blood or other potentially infectious materials. Ophthalmic medical assistants should consult the

Procedure 7.1 Following Universal Precautions

The best way to reduce occupational risk of "bloodborne" infection is to follow universal precautions based on the concept that every patient should be treated with the same level of precautionary and preventative measures to ensure the safety of everyone involved, including health care personnel. The following list of universal precautions is extracted from the OSHA regulation "Occupational Exposure to Bloodborne Pathogens." Please refer to this publication for complete instructions and precautionary guidelines. Ophthalmic medical personnel should regularly review all universal precautions presented there, ensure that they understand them completely, and adhere to them at all times.

1. Wash hands before and after patient contact, and immediately if hands become contaminated with blood or other body fluids.

2. Wear gloves whenever there is a possibility of contact with body fluids.

3. Wear masks whenever there is a possibility of contact with body fluids via airborne route.

4. Wear gowns if exposed skin or clothing is likely to be soiled.

5. During resuscitation procedures, ensure that pocket masks or mechanical ventilation devices are readily available for use.

6. Clean spills of blood or blood-containing body fluids using a solution of household bleach (sodium hypochlorite) and water in a 1:100 solution for smooth surfaces and a 1:10 solution for porous surfaces.

7. Health care professionals who have open lesions, dermatitis, or other skin irritations should not participate in direct patient care activities or handle contaminated equipment.

8. Contaminated needles should never be bent, clipped, or recapped. Immediately after use, contaminated sharp objects should be discarded into a puncture-resistant "sharps container" designed for this purpose.

9. Contaminated equipment that is reusable should be cleaned of visible organic material, placed in an impervious container, and returned to central hospital supply or some other designated place for decontamination and reprocessing.

10. Instruments and other reusable equipment used in performing invasive procedures should be disinfected and sterilized as follows:

   • Equipment and devices that enter the patient's vascular system or other normally sterile areas of the body should be sterilized before being used for each patient.

   • Equipment and devices that touch intact mucous membranes but do not penetrate the patient's body surfaces should be sterilized when possible, or undergo high-level disinfection if they cannot be sterilized, before being used for each patient.

   • Equipment and devices that do not touch the patient or that only touch intact skin need only be cleaned with a detergent or as indicated by the manufacturer.

11. Body fluids to which universal precautions always apply are as follows: blood, serum/plasma, semen, vaginal secretions, cerebrospinal fluid, vitreous fluid, synovial fluid, pleural fluid, pericardial fluid, peritoneal fluid, amniotic fluid, and wound exudates.

12. Body fluids to which universal precautions apply only when blood is visible in them are as follows: sweat, tears, sputum, saliva, nasal secretions, feces, urine, vomitus, and breast milk.

physician in their office for detailed information about this standard. For more information on how universal precautions apply specifically to ophthalmology patients and staff, refer to *Minimizing Transmission of Bloodborne Pathogens and Surface Infectious Agents in Ophthalmic Offices and Operating Rooms*, published by the American Academy of Ophthalmology. (See "Suggested Resources" in this chapter.)

The term **standard precautions** designates the range of procedures used to prevent the transmission of infectious microbes between patients and personnel in the medical office. Standard precautions combine the earlier universal and body substance isolation precautions and are the precautions commonly followed today in the health care setting. However, only universal precautions ("Occupational Exposure to Bloodborne Pathogens") are mandated by OSHA. (Refer to this publication or the website www.cdc.gov for complete instructions and precautionary guidelines.) Standard precautions apply to blood, all body fluids, mucous membranes, and nonintact skin.

Procedure 7.2 reviews 6 basic activities that make up standard precautions. However, it is not possible in a physician's office to work with patients in a totally

Procedure 7.2 Basic Standard Precautions

1. Wash hands between contacts with patients.

2. Wear disposable gloves to avoid contact with body fluids or contaminated objects.

3. Use special receptacles ("sharps containers") for disposal of contaminated needles, blades, and other sharp objects.

4. Properly dispose of, disinfect, or sterilize contaminated objects between uses with patients.

5. Wear a fluid-impermeable gown and mask when splashing of bloody or contaminated body fluids is possible.

6. Dispose of eye patches, gauze, and the like that are saturated with blood (blood that can be wrung or squeezed out) in a special red impermeable isolation bag.

Procedure 7.3 Washing the Hands Effectively

1. Turn on the faucets and adjust the water to the warmest comfortable temperature.

2. Wet your hands, wrists, and about 4 inches of your forearms.

3. Apply antiseptic soap from a dispenser and wash your hands with circular strokes for at least 15 seconds.

4. Rinse your hands and forearms.

5. Hold dry paper towels to close the faucets, and discard them when finished.

6. Dry your hands with clean paper towels.

microbe-free environment, nor is it necessary to do so. The following sections discuss specific procedures based on standard precautions to help prevent the spread of infectious microbes. The procedures described here are recommendations and should be confirmed with the physician in charge to ensure that they conform with infection-control practices in your office.

Hand Washing

Hand washing is one of the most important, yet one of the simplest, of the standard precautions. Simply washing with soap and warm water is an effective technique for removing infectious microorganisms from the fingers and hands. Again, washing with soap and water is effective against most bacteria and viruses, but the hand gels are generally only directed toward bacteria. Hand washing does not remove all organisms, but it substantially reduces the risk of transmitting disease-causing microbes. The hands should be washed immediately before and immediately after contact with each patient, and after any procedure or patient contact that might recontaminate the hands. Keeping fingernails short makes it easier to properly wash the hands.

Procedure 7.3 describes the technique suitable for general purpose and patient testing in the office. Often overlooked is the importance of turning off the faucet with clean, dry paper towels. If hands-on assistance in surgical procedures is involved, a lengthier "scrub" is required, as described in Chapter 17.

Use of Personal Protective Equipment

Personal protective equipment such as gloves, masks, and gowns minimizes contact between health care workers and patients, and so minimizes the chances of infection. Wear disposable gloves to avoid contact with body fluids, mucous membranes, or objects contaminated with blood or body fluids. The gloves should be discarded after use with each patient, and hands should be washed before and after wearing gloves.

Health care workers should wear masks or eye protection whenever there is a possibility of contact with body fluids (including if within 16 inches of an operating excimer laser). Gowns should be worn if soiling of exposed skin or clothing is likely. During resuscitation procedures, pocket masks or mechanical ventilation devices should be used.

Cleaning, Disinfection, and Sterilization

Prior to disinfection and sterilization, all equipment should be thoroughly cleaned to remove all organic material. **Disinfection** is the process of inactivating or eliminating most disease-causing microorganisms. Exposure to boiling water for 20 minutes destroys many microorganisms and is a satisfactory method of disinfecting some surgical instruments. However, boiling has disadvantages in that it dulls sharp points and cutting edges and can cause the instruments to rust.

Complex instruments and items made of plastic or certain other substances that can be damaged or destroyed by moist or dry heat can be disinfected by use of a **germicide**, a chemical that kills germs. This germicidal, or chemical, disinfection consists of soaking the item in a solution of the chemical or swabbing those parts that come in contact with the patient's tissues (for example, the prism of the tonometer used to measure intraocular pressure. Chapter 22 presents instructions on cleaning tonometers).

Germicides may be used for high-level chemical disinfection of reusable, heat-sensitive medical devices. Chemical germicides (sterilants) include hydrogen peroxide solution and a number of commercial preparations containing hypochlorite (bleach), such as Presept and Milton; phenolics, such as Stercol and Hycolin; aldehydes, such as formaldehyde and glutaraldehyde; alcohols; and other chemicals.

The problem with germicides is that few, if any, are effective against spores, and they may leave toxic residues. Nonetheless, for certain purposes (such as cleaning the tonometer) they are very useful. Consult manufacturers' recommendations for specifics regarding disinfection of ophthalmic equipment.

Sterilization is the killing of all living microorganisms. Different sterilization methods may be selected, depending on the object or substance to be sterilized. If the sterilized item is to contact sensitive tissues such as those of the eye, the sterilization method chosen must allow no residue of the sterilizing agent or remnants of any organic material to remain that might irritate or damage the tissues. Commonly used methods of sterilization include moist heat, dry heat, and ethylene oxide gas. Plasma sterilization is a newer alternative method.

MOIST HEAT An **autoclave** is a metal chamber that is equipped to use steam under high pressure to destroy microorganisms (Figure 7.6). In principle, it operates much like a kitchen pressure cooker; the increased pressure permits steam to reach temperatures of at least 250° F

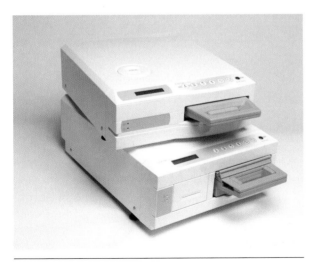

Figure 7.6 Example of an autoclave, used to sterilize materials with moist heat. *(Image courtesy of SciCan, Inc.)*

for 30 minutes or 272° for 15 minutes (the temperatures and times usually required for sterilization). This higher pressure and temperature method is known as "flash" sterilization, and should only be used when there is not enough time for a full sterilization. The time and temperature used for autoclaving can be varied, depending on the kinds and amounts of materials to be sterilized.

Autoclaving is commonly used to sterilize glass and stainless steel objects, some solutions, and materials such as towels and sponges. Items other than solutions are wrapped in paper and tied or taped closed. After sterilization, they are permitted to dry in the autoclave and stored. If the paper cover is unopened and environmental conditions are stable, the items will remain sterile for several months or longer.

DRY HEAT Sterilization using dry heat is an alternative method for autoclaving instrumentation between uses. Although this type of sterilization causes more rapid "aging" of the instruments, it removes a possible source for a form of corneal inflammation, diffuse lamellar keratitis, following LASIK. Formerly, the most common method to sterilize LASIK instruments was the use of steam from distilled water. This water would collect in a drain pan that was difficult to empty completely, and if the water was not drained, the dead infiltrates would collect in the water and be introduced to the next batch of items being sterilized in the steam. For this reason, many LASIK surgeons have switched to dry heat sterilization and the incidence of diffuse lamellar keratitis has decreased dramatically.

ETHYLENE OXIDE GAS This gas effectively sterilizes instruments and various materials with little damaging effect on the articles themselves. It is often used for items made of plastic, rubber, and other substances that would be destroyed by heat or exposure to chemical agents. The disadvantages of ethylene oxide sterilization are that it is slow and costly and the gas is highly flammable and toxic. Still, it is widely used commercially for the production of sterile disposable (single-use) articles such as hypodermic syringes and needles, scalpels and blades, rubber gloves, bandages, sutures, and plastic equipment.

PLASMA STERILIZATION This method is fast evolving into a promising alternative to standard sterilizing techniques. It employs a low temperature hydrogen peroxide gas plasma. The process is usually performed at room temperature and hence poses no dangers associated with high temperatures (unlike autoclaves). It does not involve any chemicals and hence is nontoxic (unlike ethyl alcohol). Time of treatment is fast, on the order of 1 minute or less. The plasma method is versatile and can sterilize almost any material and any shape with nooks and crannies.

Aseptic Technique: Handling Sterile Medical Equipment

After an instrument or container has been sterilized, it is sterile, and that sterility needs to be maintained until it is used. Even when the hands and fingers are properly washed and gloved, they may still contaminate a sterile instrument, bottle, or other item; this contamination is a transmission risk, especially if it occurs at the *functional surface* of the article. The assistant and physician must therefore use **aseptic technique** to protect an article's sterility before and during its intended use. (See Chapter 17 for a discussion of aseptic technique in minor surgical assisting.) In practice, this means handling the item only on a part that will not come in contact with the patient or with other sterile materials.

Proper aseptic technique requires that instruments that have been disinfected or sterilized be picked up by their handles or a nonfunctional part or by using sterile gloves. With sterile gauze pads, adhesive bandages, and similar materials, avoid touching the portions that will contact the wound they are intended to cover.

Relatively inexpensive items such as eyedroppers, rubber gloves, hypodermic syringes, and scalpels are available in single-use, disposable form. These articles are individually paper-wrapped and are sterile. When an item is to be used, carefully open the wrapper and grasp the article by a part that will not be in contact with the patient or with other sterile materials. Disposable eyedroppers, gloves, syringes, and several other items are intended to be used once and discarded. They should never be stored and reused. Once used, they must be considered not only nonsterile, but contaminated.

Occasionally, when handling a sterile article, you may accidentally touch the sterile functional surface. If this occurs or if you are in doubt whether the sterility of the article has been compromised, take it out of action and discard or resterilize the item as appropriate. The cost of the disposable item or of resterilization is less than the damage that can result from contamination.

The rules for handling sterile items apply equally to containers of eyedrops, other liquids, and ointments. Remove the cap without allowing your fingers to touch the lip or tip of the bottle or the inner surface of the lid. Finger contact compromises the sterility of the fluid in the container. Similarly, when instilling topical drops or applying topical ointments, never allow the tip of an eyedropper, dropper bottle, or ointment tube to contact the patient's lashes, lids, or eye. If this occurs, consider the container of medication to be contaminated and discard it.

Sterile eyedrops, fluids for washing contact lenses, and other solutions intended for use more than once are packaged in small bottles and contain chemical preservatives to help prevent bacterial or fungal contamination. Always inspect bottles before use for cloudiness or particulate matter in the liquid, indicating possible contamination. Cases have been reported of cracked BSS bottles being used in cataract surgery, with resultant fungal contamination discovered after the case is over. Diligence in inspecting these fluids is always necessary. Many bottles are not transparent enough to allow for this type of inspection, so instead be aware of expiration dates and consider dating bottles upon opening them if potentially they may be used for more than 6 months. If cloudiness or particulate matter is present, do not use the fluid, and discard the container. Single-dose vials of fluids are also available, and these are intended to be discarded after a single use. Storing or reusing such items after they are opened increases the risk of infection; the fluids contain no preservatives and should be considered contaminated.

Handling and Decontaminating Contaminated Materials

Any instrument, needle, swab, bandage, or other item that has come in contact with a patient's eye must be considered contaminated with potentially infectious microorganisms. Contaminated reusable objects must be decontaminated before they are used again; disposable items must be discarded. According to standard precautions, assistants should assume that fingers that have contacted a patient's eyes or face are contaminated and treat them accordingly. This means proper washing of the hands, even if contact occurred while wearing gloves.

Medical instruments and other reusable items are always first decontaminated by washing with soap and water to remove grease or protein matter, then stored and packed for later sterilization and reuse. Some offices require that these items be soaked in a chemical disinfectant before cleaning and sterilization. Check the preferred procedure in your office. Tonometers and some other reusable ophthalmic instruments with complex or delicate parts cannot be fully immersed or safely washed in this manner. Parts of such complex instruments that have touched a patient's eye should be disinfected with alcohol, bleach, or hydrogen peroxide after each patient contact. Follow the manufacturers' instructions (or check with the manufacturers) for proper disinfecting of such instruments. Be certain that the disinfectant has been rinsed off completely with sterile water or normal saline before it comes in contact with a patient's eye, to prevent eye irritation or damage to the ocular tissues.

Avoiding sticks with contaminated needles, sharp medical implements, and similar objects is an important office safety measure, especially in preventing the spread of HIV and hepatitis B. Take particular care in handling and disposing of scalpel blades, syringe needles, broken glass, and other sharp objects. Place these items, after using them, in a rigid, puncture-proof biohazard container (called a *sharps container*). When the container is full, close and dispose of it as biohazardous waste, according to the procedures used in your office.

Hygienic Practices in Potentially Infectious Situations

The ophthalmic assistant who has a common cold has the potential for transmitting the infection to a patient, particularly if the assistant is sneezing or coughing or has a runny nose. In these cases, the assistant should discuss with the physician the advisability of temporarily performing duties other than working directly with patients.

All medical professionals, including medical assistants, must take special precautions to prevent their own cuts and abrasions, even inapparent ones, from contacting the blood or body fluids of an infected patient, and vice versa. If the assistant has cuts, abrasions, or lesions on the hands, clean or sterile rubber gloves should be worn after washing the hands, to protect both the assistant and the patient. Health care professionals who have open lesions, dermatitis, or other skin irritations should avoid direct patient care activities or handling of contaminated equipment.

If a patient has a fever blister, ophthalmic medical assistants should avoid touching the patient's face near the lesion or the mouth with fingers or instruments. To protect themselves and other patients, assistants should wear gloves, carefully wash their hands after completing any tests, and be certain that any instruments used with the infected patient are properly sterilized, or disinfected when sterilizing is not possible.

Collecting Specimens for the Identification of Microorganisms

In many cases, the presentation and appearance of an eye infection helps the physician determine the type of offending microbe. For example, bacterial conjunctivitis often produces a white or yellow creamy discharge, while conjunctivitis caused by a virus generally produces a clear or yellowish watery discharge. If bacterial infection is suspected, rather than wait for the results of laboratory tests to identify the particular organism by culture and sensitivity testing, the physician may begin **empiric treatment**; that is, choose to prescribe an antibiotic with a broad spectrum of activity that is capable of destroying a wide range of bacteria.

At the same time, the physician may have a specimen of the discharge taken from the infection site and order laboratory tests to isolate and identify the causative microorganism. Further determination of its specific antibiotic susceptibility is very helpful in guiding more-effective treatments. This is done through microscopic observation of the microbes in specimen materials that have been stained or cultured (grown on specially prepared substances that promote recovery of the organism). In some viral, chlamydial, or protozoan diseases, stains may be the only method of confirming the presence of an infectious agent. Whenever possible, specimens should be collected for testing before empiric treatment is initiated, because the treatment might interfere with the ability to obtain a sample and identify the true disease-causing organism. Empiric treatment may then be employed and guided by the results from microbiologic testing when they become available.

Although ophthalmic medical assistants usually do not perform microbiologic testing, in some offices the assistant is responsible for receiving such specimens and forwarding them to a microbiologic laboratory. The sample of infectious material from the patient is obtained by swabbing or scraping the infected site, such as the conjunctiva or cornea, with a sterile swab or spatula (Figure 7.7). Materials taken this way from the site of infection are then transferred directly onto glass

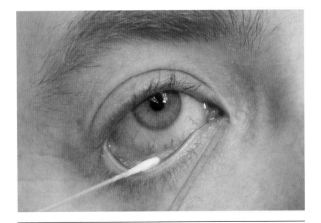

Figure 7.7 A sterile swab can be used to collect materials from the conjunctiva and lid margins for culture. *(Image courtesy of Brice Critser, CRA, Department of Ophthalmology and Visual Sciences, University of Iowa.)*

microscope slides (for staining), plated onto a culture media, or transferred into a container or sealable test tube filled with a substance, usually fluid, that preserves the sample until it can be used for testing. Assistants who are required to obtain and handle microbiologic specimens receive instructions from the physicians or technicians in their office; a more detailed discussion is beyond the scope of this book.

SELF-ASSESSMENT TEST

1. Name the 4 groups of microorganisms that commonly cause eye disease.

2. List the 5 principal means of transmitting disease-causing organisms from a reservoir to a host.

3. What is the practical purpose of microbial control (aseptic technique) in the medical office?

4. State at least 3 of the 6 basic infection control activities known as standard precautions.

5. Describe the special precautions to be taken to prevent infection when (1) the assistant has a herpes simplex lesion ("fever blister") and (2) the patient has a herpes simplex lesion.

6. Describe the basic hand-washing technique.

7. Distinguish between *disinfection* and *sterilization.*

8. Name the 2 principal methods of sterilization.

9. Describe the method of handling sterile items to maintain sterility.

10. List at least 2 aseptic precautions in the use of multidose containers of sterile eyedrops.

11. Describe the procedure for the handling and disposing of contaminated sharp objects such as scalpel blades, syringe needles, and broken glass.

SUGGESTED ACTIVITIES

1. Ask an experienced office staff member to show you the hand-washing technique and materials that are used in your office.

2. Ask a senior staff member to demonstrate the procedures for disinfecting office diagnostic and examination equipment.

3. Ask a senior office staff member to demonstrate the procedures for decontaminating instruments and disposing of contaminated waste materials.

4. Ask a senior staff member in your office to demonstrate the various procedures used to sterilize medical instruments, equipment, and other items in the office. Ask for a demonstration of how to handle sterile instruments and how to unwrap and handle disposable sterile items and bottles.

5. Ask to observe office procedures used to obtain microbial specimens from patients and to send them to the microbiology laboratory.

SUGGESTED RESOURCES

American Academy of Ophthalmology. Infection prevention in eye care services and operating area. Clinical Statement. 2009. http://one.aao.org/CE/PracticeGuidelines/ClinicalStatements_Content.aspx?cid=bfa87dce-adc9-4450-94a2-e49493154238. Accessed August 15, 2011.

Centers for Disease Control and Prevention (CDC). Bloodborne infectious diseases: HIV/AIDS, hepatitis B, hepatitis C. Universal precautions for preventing transmission of bloodborne infections. www.cdc.gov/niosh/topics/bbp/universal.html. Accessed June 27, 2011.

CDC. Health-associated infections. Website with numerous topics related to infection prevention. www.cdc.gov/hai. Accessed August 15, 2011.

CDC. Perspectives in disease prevention and health promotion update: universal precautions for prevention of transmission of human immunodeficiency virus, hepatitis b virus, and other bloodborne pathogens in health-care settings. *Morbidity and Mortality Weekly Report.* June 24, 1998;37:377–388. www.cdc.gov/mmwr/preview/mmwrhtml/00000039.htm. Accessed August 8, 2011.

DuBois LG. Sterile technique. In: *Fundamentals of Ophthalmic Medical Assisting.* DVD. San Francisco: American Academy of Ophthalmology; 2009.

Forbes BA, Sahm DF, Weissfeld AS, eds. *Bailey and Scott's Diagnostic Microbiology.* 12th ed. St Louis: Mosby; 2007.

Hill JE, ed. *Ophthalmic Procedures: A Nursing Perspective—Office and Clinic.* Rev ed. San Francisco: American Society of Ophthalmic Registered Nurses; 2001.

Rastogi N, Legrand E, Sola C. The mycobacteria: an introduction to nomenclature and pathogenesis. *Rev Sci Tech.* 2001;20:21–54.

Siegel JD, Rhinehart E, Jackson M, Chiarello L, and the Healthcare Infection Control Practices Advisory Committee. *2007 Guideline for Isolation Precautions: Preventing Transmission of Infectious Agents in Healthcare Settings.* www.cdc.gov/ncidod/dhqp/pdf/isolation2007.pdf. Accessed August 8, 2011.

Skilton R. Decontamination procedures for medical equipment. *Update in Anaesthesia.* 1997. www.nda.ox.ac.uk/wfsa/html/u07/u07_015.htm. Accessed August 15, 2011.

Stein HA, Stein RM. *The Ophthalmic Assistant: A Text for Allied and Associated Ophthalmic Personnel.* 8th ed. St Louis: Mosby; 2006.

Tabbara KF, Hyndiuk RA, eds. *Infections of the Eye.* 2nd ed. Boston: Little, Brown and Co; 1996.

Tortora GJ, Funke BR, Case CL. *Microbiology: An Introduction.* 9th ed. San Francisco: Benjamin Cummings; 2006.

United States Department of Labor, Occupational Safety and Health Administration. *Occupational Exposure to Bloodborne Pathogens* (OSHA 3127). Washington, DC: OSHA; 1996.

Versalovic J, ed. *Manual of Clinical Microbiology.* 10th ed. Washington, DC: American Society of Microbiology Press; 2011.

8 COMPREHENSIVE MEDICAL EYE EXAMINATION

Patients seek the help of an ophthalmologist for various reasons. They may have injured an eye or developed an infection. They may have noticed a sudden loss of vision or a gradual decline in their ability to see clearly. They may have been referred to the ophthalmologist by another physician because of a medical problem that might affect their eyesight. They may simply wish to confirm that their eyes are healthy and that their previous refractive correction is still appropriate. Even when no visual complaints are present, a periodic comprehensive ocular evaluation is a recommended precaution because some serious ocular disease may produce no symptoms until irreversible damage to sight has occurred.

The purpose of the comprehensive eye examination is to detect and diagnose abnormalities and diseases. This procedure includes an external and intraocular examination by the ophthalmologist with appropriate instruments, together with a series of tests and measurements. The ophthalmic medical assistant may be responsible for initiating the examination by taking the preliminary medical history. This narration consists of background information on the patient and details of the present illness. The doctor will use this information to arrive at a diagnosis and treatment plan for the patient. The assistant also participates by performing some tests. This chapter discusses the components of the eye examination, with particular attention to those aspects with which the assistant may be involved.

Overview of the Examination

The comprehensive medical eye examination is designed to reveal both existing and potential eye problems, even in the absence of specific symptoms. The procedure thus helps assure that the patient will receive timely and appropriate treatment to manage or prevent the development or progression of an abnormal condition. The examination may be divided into three major parts:

- patient history

- examination and testing to assess the anatomic and functional behavior of the eye and related structures

- evaluation of the findings; establishment of a diagnosis of the present illness, abnormality, or disease, if any; and selection of appropriate management or treatment plan

The ophthalmologist oversees all aspects of the comprehensive eye examination and performs a number of the individual tests. Evaluation of the results and decisions on further studies or treatment are the ophthalmologist's responsibility. The ophthalmic medical assistant is often responsible for taking the preliminary medical history and for performing several of the standardized test procedures, particularly those related to eye function. Most of the evaluations of anatomic status require the expertise and training of the ophthalmologist. In these procedures, however, the ophthalmic medical assistant helps the ophthalmologist by administering eyedrops, preparing and caring for ophthalmic equipment and instruments, and recording results.

The examination and testing procedures included in the comprehensive eye examination and the order in which they are performed may vary with the preference of the ophthalmologist and the needs of the patient. Nevertheless, 8 aspects of eye function and anatomy are generally evaluated in the comprehensive examination. The first aspects involve operation of the visual system: visual acuity examination, alignment and motility examination, pupillary examination, visual field examination, and intraocular pressure examination. The remaining aspects are concerned with the physical appearance and condition of the ocular structures: external examination, biomicroscopy, and ophthalmoscopy.

Visual Acuity Examination

Visual acuity tests measure the patient's ability to see fine detail. This test measures central vision. A more extensive evaluation of visual acuity includes **lensometry**, the measurement of the patient's current optical correction (eyeglasses or contact lenses); refractometry (refraction), a measurement to determine the type and amount of the existing refractive error, if any; and the selection of the proper optical eyewear. **Keratometry** or **corneal topography**, used to determine corneal curvature, are adjunctive tests that aid the refractive procedure and choice of the optical eyewear. Ophthalmic assistants perform the visual acuity test and related procedures.

Alignment and Motility Examination

Several procedures are used to confirm that the patient's eyes are correctly aligned and can move properly. Misalignment of the eyes or limited movement can interfere with normal vision. Experienced ophthalmic assistants often perform these tests.

Pupillary Examination

Reactions of the pupils under various light conditions provide the ophthalmologist with important information about specific eye conditions and general health. Basic pupillary screening procedures may be delegated to the ophthalmic assistant.

Visual Field Examination

A **visual field examination** tests the expanse and sensitivity of a patient's noncentral (peripheral) vision, that is, the perception of light and objects surrounding the direct line of sight. The basic assessment of the visual field is frequently delegated to the ophthalmic assistant. (See Chapter 9 for a more detailed examination of the visual field.)

Intraocular Pressure Measurement

Measurement of the pressure within the eye, a procedure called **tonometry**, is an important technique for the detection of glaucoma. Most ophthalmic medical assistants are expected to be able to perform this procedure.

External Examination

The ophthalmologist performs the external examination that includes a close inspection of the appearance of the patient's eyelids, lashes, and visible parts of the lacrimal apparatus and external globe. The ophthalmologist may include, or request the ophthalmic assistant to perform, some of these evaluations and certain additional procedures, such as tests for tear production.

Biomicroscopy

The **biomicroscope**, also called a **slit lamp**, consists of a microscope of low magnifying power (6× to 40×) and a light source that projects a rectangular beam that can be changed in size and focus. This instrument allows close examination of the eyelids, lashes, cornea, conjunctiva, iris, crystalline lens, and clear fluids within the eye in layer-by-layer detail. The ophthalmologist evaluates the structures to determine whether defects or abnormalities are present. Ophthalmic medical assistants may also use this instrument in performing some of these inspections and measuring the anterior chamber depth and intra-ocular pressure.

Ophthalmoscopy

In this procedure, the doctor uses an ophthalmoscope to examine the interior of the eye, particularly the vitreous and the **fundus** (a collective term for the retina, optic disc, and macula).

Frequency of Examination

Office policy and patient need dictate the frequency of a comprehensive eye examination; recommended intervals may be found in the Preferred Practice Patterns for adult and pediatric eye evaluations published by the American Academy of Ophthalmology (see "Suggested Resources" at the end of this chapter). Regardless of the precise frequency, a regular comprehensive eye examination by an ophthalmologist is of great benefit for three principal reasons. First, eye diseases may be present but exist with no noticeable symptoms (**asymptomatic**) until they are far advanced, when treatment may be less effective. Obviously, detecting a condition in its earlier stage will enhance the treatment outcome. Second, assessment of overall ocular health can be an important indicator of certain general health conditions. Third, some individuals—because of age, race, systemic health, or other factors—may not have existing eye problems but are at risk for developing certain eye diseases. For example, African Americans have a greater risk of developing glaucoma more frequently and severely than other races. Many individuals who have diabetes are more at risk for developing retinal disease. Patients in these categories will benefit from regular ophthalmologic monitoring and, if a problem does develop, they will be well served by early treatment.

Young adults, 20 to 39 years of age, are generally at low risk for ocular problems, unless they are African American. In that case a comprehensive eye examination every 3 to 5 years is recommended because of the reported higher incidence and more aggressive course of glaucoma in this population. Other patients in this age group require a comprehensive evaluation less frequently. Asymptomatic patients between 40 and 64 years of age should be examined every 2 to 4 years, particularly to check for the presence of presbyopia and glaucoma. After age 65, an examination every 1 to 2 years is recommended because of the variety of age-related and other eye abnormalities that may develop. Patients with medical conditions that may affect vision, such as diabetes, should be examined more frequently than healthy individuals of the same age. The frequency of such tests depends on the judgment and recommendations of the patient's ophthalmologist and primary care physician.

Most symptomatic patients and those with ocular abnormalities are usually diagnosed in the course of the comprehensive ophthalmologic examination and subsequently treated. Thereafter, follow-up examinations will vary depending upon the diagnosis. At any time, patients may warrant an interim appointment because of a specific ocular complaint. At that time a more focused ocular examination may be performed consisting only of certain parts of the comprehensive eye examination.

Ophthalmic and Medical History

Usually the ophthalmic assistant begins the comprehensive eye examination by taking a preliminary ophthalmic and general medical history of the patient. This information is entered in the patient's record and is reviewed by the physician before beginning the examination.

The purpose of the history is to determine the specific complaint that brought the patient to the office and to obtain information on any present illness or past ocular history that may help the physician in evaluating and diagnosing the patient's condition. Details of the patient's general medical history and that of the patient's family history may prove useful during the assessment and to help arrive at a diagnosis.

The ophthalmic assistant obtains the history by asking a specific series of questions and recording the information in the patient's file or chart. The type and amount of information to be gathered by the ophthalmic assistant may vary from one practice to another. Some offices have special forms for this purpose. Figure 8.1 shows a sample form that might be used in a general ophthalmology practice. Typically, the history interview usually includes questions in 5 principal areas: chief complaint and history of present illness; past ocular history; general medical and social history; family ocular and medical history; and allergies, medications, vitamins, and supplements. Table 8.1 summarizes these principal areas of the history and their related questions, which are described in detail in the following sections.

Chief Complaint and History of Present Illness

The **chief complaint** (in the patient's own words and placed in quotes) is the main reason for the patient's visit

EYE HISTORY

Name: _____ Date: _____

Thank you for choosing our office for your eyecare. To better serve you, please answer the following questions:

1. Do you wear glasses? ☐ YES ☐ NO

2. Do you wear contact lenses? ☐ YES ☐ NO

3. Do you have problems reading? ☐ YES ☐ NO

4. Are you currently experiencing any eye symptoms? Please circle all that apply:

| Eye pain | Blurred Vision | Eyelid Crusting | Flashes of Light | Halos |
| Discharge | Light Sensitivity | Double Vision | Decreased Vision | Floaters |

5. Have you ever had an eye injury? Please describe: _____
_____

6. Have you ever had eye surgery? Please list type, which eye and approximate dates:

_____ R/L _____

_____ R/L _____

7. Are you currently using any eye medications? Please list name and how often used: _____
_____

8. Are you being treated for any medical conditions? Please circle all that apply:

Diabetes   Heart Disease   High Blood Pressure

Stroke   Arthritis   Other: _____

9. What medications other than above are you taking? Please list: _____
_____

10. Are you allergic to any medications? Please list: _____
_____

11. Do you have any family history of eye problems? Please circle and list family relationship:

Glaucoma   Cataract   Retinal Disease   Macular Degeneration

12. Please circle any of the following that you would like more information about:

Radial Keratotomy   Contact Lenses   Cataract Surgery

Diabetic Eye Disease   Glaucoma   Other: _____

Figure 8.1 One type of form used for taking a preliminary ocular and medical history. *(Image courtesy of the Ophthalmic Medical Insurance Company.)*

to the doctor. In those cases where the comprehensive eye examination is for an evaluation of an asymptomatic patient, the chief complaint may consist of a statement "patient is here for a routine eye exam" or "screening for glaucoma."

For patients with a specific visual problem, define the chief complaint with the following questions:

- What are your symptoms?

- When did the problem start?

- Does the problem seem to be getting worse?

Depending on the patient's answers, you may have to ask additional questions in the following areas:

- *Status of vision:* Have both near and far vision been affected? Has vision been affected in one eye or both?

- *Onset:* Did the problem start suddenly or gradually?

- *Presence:* Are the symptoms constant or occasional, frequent or infrequent? (Ask the patient to specify the frequency in hours, days, weeks, or months.) Does a specific activity trigger the symptoms or make them worse?

- *Progression:* Has the problem become better or worse over time?

- *Severity:* Do the symptoms interfere with your work or other activities?

- *Treatment:* Have you ever been treated previously for this complaint? (If yes, ask how, when, outcome, and by whom.)

Table 8.1 Summary of Primary Areas of History Taking

Medical Area	Questions to Ask
Chief complaint and present illness	What is the main reason for your visit today? What are your symptoms? When did the problem start? Does the problem seem to be getting worse?
Past ocular history	Do you wear, or have you ever worn, eyeglasses or contact lenses? Have you ever had eye surgery? Have you ever been treated for a serious eye condition? Are you taking any prescription eyedrops or over-the-counter medications for your eyes?
General medical (present to past) and social history	Do you have a history of diabetes, pulmonary disease, bowel disorder, thyroid disease, hypertension, neurological disorder, or malignancy? Have you ever required surgical or medical treatment for any serious disease? Do you smoke, drink alcohol, use illegal drugs, or follow fad diets? What was or is your occupation? Do you work at or participate in risky activities?
Family ocular and medical history	Does anyone in your family have any significant eye or other health problems? Does anyone in your family use eyedrops on a regular basis? Did any members of your family lose their eyesight?
Allergies, medications, vitamins and supplements	Do you have any allergies to medications, pollen, food, or anything else? Are you taking any prescription or over-the-counter medications including vitamins, minerals, and herbal supplements?

Past Ocular History

The past ocular history describes any eye problems the patient has experienced before this initial office visit, usually in reverse chronological order, that is, from the present to the past. The following are typical questions used to obtain this information:

- Do you wear, or have you ever worn, eyeglasses or contact lenses? (If yes, ask at what age glasses or contacts were first prescribed and how old is the present prescription.) If contact lenses are worn, ask how often the patient removes them for disinfection and what disinfection method is used. Also ask how often the patient discards the lenses and replaces them with new lenses.

- Have you ever had eye surgery or laser treatment? (If yes, ask why, what type, when, and by whom.)

- Have you ever been treated for a serious eye condition? (Ask specifically about glaucoma, cataract, injury, or any other eye condition associated with visual loss.)

- Are you taking any prescription or over-the-counter eye medications, including eyedrops? (If yes, find out the purpose, duration of use, frequency of the eyedrop and when the last dose was administered.)

General Medical and Social History

A history of the patient's general medical health can be useful to the ophthalmologist because some health conditions can affect the eye and may influence the physician's choice of treatment (see Chapter 4). By the same token, appreciation of a patient's lifestyle and habits may affect treatment options or contribute to the development of ocular disease. Pursue the following line of questioning:

- Are you currently being treated for any disease? (If the answer is yes, ask the name of the condition and the treating physician.)

- Have you ever required surgery or medical treatment for any serious diseases? (Encourage the patient to think carefully about the question in order not to overlook a possible significant surgery or disease.)

- Do you have a history of diabetes, pulmonary disease, bowel disorder, thyroid disease, hypertension, neurological disorder, or malignancy?

Also include the following areas. Ask women if they may be pregnant or are nursing. Ask about social habits: smoking, alcohol use, drug use, and current diets. Determine the patient's occupation, exposure to hazardous substances, and dangerous recreational activities. Also, record the patient's marital status, children, highest educational degree, retirement status, and dates of military service.

Family Ocular and Medical History

Many health problems are hereditary, including ocular problems. For this reason, a history of the patient's family ocular and general medical health can be extremely useful. Obviously, only information about family members related by blood who share similar genetic information is required. Ask the following questions:

- Does anyone in your family have any significant eye or other health problems now or did anyone in the past? (Again, encourage the patient to think carefully.)

- Have any family members ever had glaucoma, cataract, crossed eyes, poor vision, or blindness?

- Have any diseases occurred in the family, such as diabetes, heart disease, hypertension, and cancer?

Allergies, Medications, and Supplements

Not only can allergies be a source of eye problems, but they also can affect the patient's ability to undergo certain diagnostic tests or use medications or other treatments safely. Obtain a complete list of the patient's prescription medications and over-the-counter vitamins, minerals, and herbal supplements. Ask women specifically about contraceptive pills because some patients don't think of them as a medication. Make this part of the patient's permanent record and update the list on each subsequent visit. Certain medications, like warfarin (Coumadin), have side effects that slow the blood-clotting mechanism and, therefore, before scheduling ocular surgery, the doctor should be aware of their use. Ask the following questions:

- Do you have any allergies to medications, pollen, food, or anything else? (If the patient answers yes, ask for specifics.)

- Are you taking any prescription medications for a health condition? (If yes, find out the purpose, dosage, and duration of use.)

- Do you take any over-the-counter drugs, vitamins, or herbal supplements?

History-Taking Guidelines

The ability to obtain a complete and accurate history is a valuable skill that is developed only with experience. The following are some general suggestions to help you develop this skill.

When you begin the history, introduce yourself to the patient with your full name and explain the purpose of the interview. Address the patient by surname and title, depending on office policy and patient preference (that is, Mr., Miss, Mrs., or Ms.). A simple approach is the following: "Mrs. _____, my name is _____ _____. I am Dr. _____'s assistant. I will be asking you some questions and performing certain tests to help the doctor with your examination." Remember, you are there to serve the patient. Be courteous and caring, but don't lose sight of the primary objective: to take an accurate history.

Be sure to find out whether the patient has been referred to your office by another person, especially by another doctor. Record the name of the person or doctor as part of the history. Ask if the patient has been seen previously as a patient by the ophthalmologist in your office.

Ask the name and relationship of anyone accompanying the patient, and determine whether the patient wishes these individuals to be present during the office visit.

When documenting the chief complaint, use the patient's words, not your own. Avoid substituting technical terms that the patient has not used. Stick to the facts as they are presented to you.

Patients may ask questions about their medical problem during the history interview. Handle these questions in a friendly manner but do not provide specific answers.

Always refer the patient to the ophthalmologist for a diagnosis or medical advice, even if you think you know the answer.

If the patient volunteers information you believe could be compromising (for example, drug abuse or sexual practices), write this information on a separate sheet of paper for review by the physician. If the doctor deems the information relevant to the patient's condition, it can be transferred to the permanent chart. Do not include nonmedical information in the history.

Keep details short and to the point. The interview should take 5 to 10 minutes. Don't rush the process. Do a careful, thorough job, and when you are finished, thank the patient. During the history taking and throughout the entire office visit, preserve the patient's privacy and confidentiality. For related information about privacy and confidentiality, refer to "Which Rules of Ethics Apply?" in Chapter 20 and "Health Insurance Portability and Accountability Act" in Chapter 16.

Visual Acuity Examination

Visual acuity refers to the ability to discern fine visual detail. To see fine visual detail, normal central vision is required. The primary acuity test performed as part of the comprehensive examination is the **Snellen acuity test**. This test reveals any loss of visual detail that may be due to a refractive error or other optical aberrations caused by an ocular disease. Ophthalmic medical assistants often perform this basic test and other visual acuity tests.

Distance Acuity Test

This procedure measures a patient's distance vision by testing the ability to read characters at a standard distance from a special target called the **Snellen chart** (Figure 8.2). Most people have seen this familiar eye chart in school or community vision-screening programs. The chart consists of Snellen optotypes, specially formed letters or numbers arranged in rows of decreasing letter size. The sizes are standardized so that the letters or numbers in each row should be clearly legible at a designated distance to a person with normal vision. Patients are placed at a specified distance, generally 20 feet, from the chart and asked to read aloud the smallest line they can discern. Adults who can read are usually tested with the alphabetic or number chart. Illiterate adults and young children may be tested with variations such as the "tumbling E" chart and the picture chart (Figure 8.3). (Chapter 16 discusses techniques for testing vision in children and infants.)

Visual acuity charts may be in printed form for wall display or projected onto a screen from glass slides inserted into a manual **projector** or by remote control of an automated projector. Projection with reflection of the image by mirrors permits use of a shorter actual viewing distance in a small office, although the characters appear to the patient as if viewed from the standard distance of 20 feet (Figure 8.4).

The viewing distance of 20 feet is used when testing vision because it approximates optical infinity.

Light rays coming from this distance and beyond are considered to be parallel, so that the emmetropic

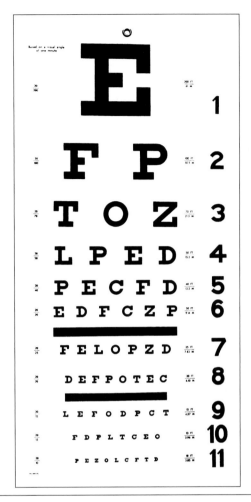

Figure 8.2 Example of a Snellen chart used for testing distance visual acuity.

eye (able to focus correctly without the need for optical lenses) need not accommodate to focus the rays on the retina. Depending upon the degree of myopia, a measurement taken at a shorter distance (less than 20 feet) may test normal (20/20).

At the left of each line of Snellen characters appears a numeric notation (for example, 20/50, 20/40, or 20/20). These values are used as measures of visual acuity. The first number (the top number as printed on the Snellen chart) represents the distance in feet at which the test was performed. The second number (the bottom number on the chart) corresponds to the distance at which the letters could be seen by a person with "normal" visual acuity. If the smallest letters a patient can read correctly are on the 20/60 line, the patient is able to read at 20 feet what the normal eye can read at 60 feet and the visual acuity

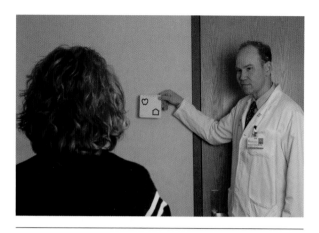

Figure 8.3 Example of a picture visual acuity chart used with patients unable to read. *(Image courtesy of Brice Critser, CRA, Department of Ophthalmology and Visual Sciences, University of Iowa.)*

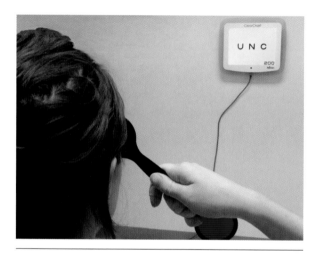

Figure 8.4 The projected visual acuity chart allows an actual testing distance of less than 20 feet. *(Image courtesy of Tina Newmark, RN, MS.)*

is recorded as 20/60. If the patient can read the smaller characters in the 20/20 line at 20 feet, the patient's visual acuity is equivalent to that of the normal eye. Actually, some patients are able to read even smaller letters at 20 feet. In this case, their acuity might be recorded as 20/15 or 20/10.

Some offices prefer to express the acuity values in metric terms. Equivalent metric values on some charts are listed on the right-hand side of the standard Snellen chart for this purpose. Since 20 feet equals about 6 meters, an acuity value of 20/40 would be expressed as 6/12. Although the Snellen acuity values are written as a fraction, they do not represent a proportion or percentage of normal vision. Rather, they simply *compare* the distance from which the patient can read a line of characters to the distance from which a person with normal visual acuity can read the same characters.

Visual acuity of 20/25 or even 20/30 may be acceptable for some patients but, generally, patients with below-normal visual acuity (20/30 or worse) due to refractive error will require optical correction (eyeglasses or contact lenses) for distance vision or, if that is not possible, some other form of visual assistance. Procedure 8.1 presents the basic distance acuity testing procedure. Because testing standards and procedures may vary from office to office, the ophthalmic medical assistant should consult the doctor or senior staff technician regarding the preferred methods of recording visual acuity notations, appropriate room lighting for viewing wall charts, and training in the use of the projector and target slides.

Pinhole Acuity Test

A below-normal visual acuity recording (20/30 or less) may be attributed to a refractive error or other cause. Procedure 8.2 describes the pinhole acuity test used to confirm whether a refractive error is the cause of below-normal visual acuity. In this text, the patient views the Snellen chart through a **pinhole occluder** (Figure 8.5). This handheld device completely covers one eye and allows the other eye to view the chart through one of the tiny openings. In most pinhole occluders, the central hole is surrounded by two rings of additional perforations. Some phoropters also include a pinhole device.

The pinhole admits only parallel rays of light, which do not require refraction by the cornea and lens. The patient is thus able to resolve fine detail on the visual acuity chart without an optical correction. If use of the pinhole improves a patient's below-normal uncorrected visual acuity to 20/20, or even 20/30, chances are the patient has a refractive error. If poor uncorrected visual acuity is not improved with the pinhole and the patient appears to be using it properly, the patient's visual problem is probably not due to an optical or refractive error. In this case, the ophthalmologist may wish to perform additional tests.

Near Acuity Test

The Snellen acuity test measures a patient's fine central vision at a distance. The procedure is sometimes referred to as a *distance visual acuity test*. A similar procedure may be used to test **near visual acuity**, the ability to see clearly at a normal reading distance (Figure 8.6). This test is performed if the patient has complaints about reading or other close work or if there is reason to believe the patient's ability to accommodate is insufficient or impaired. Some offices record a near vision test

Procedure 8.1 Performing the Distance Acuity Test

Patients who wear eyeglasses or contact lenses should wear them for the test. If a contact lens wearer is in monovision correction, where one eye (usually the dominant eye) is corrected with a lens for distance vision and the other eye is corrected with a lens for near vision, test the eye corrected for near by holding an appropriate minus (–) sphere lens (usually –0.50 to –2.50, depending on age) in front of that eye. On a first visit, patients may be tested both with and without optical correction. Test and record the visual acuity in each eye separately, beginning with the right eye. Less confusion results in recording information about the two eyes if the right/left sequence is followed habitually.

1. Position the patient 20 feet from an illuminated Snellen chart. If a projected chart is used, a shorter distance may be used, as specified for the particular projector. Sometimes the distance may be recorded in meters (m) where 6 m = 20 ft. When distance in meters is used, the denominator is in the same proportion as distance in feet (eg, 20/20 = 6/6, 20/40 = 6/12).

2. Have the patient cover the left eye with an occluder or the palm of the hand. Alternatively, you may hold the occluder over the patient's left eye. With either method, be sure that the eye is completely covered and that the occluder is not touching the eye. Observe the patient during the test to be sure the patient is not peeking around the occluder. This is especially important when testing children.

3. Ask the patient to read the letters from left to right on every other line down the chart until the patient misses more than half the letters on one of the lines. Alternatively, you may ask the patient

to begin reading on the smallest line legible. If a tumbling E chart is being used, ask the patient to identify the symbols visible on the smallest line by stating the direction or pointing the fingers in the direction the three spokes of the E point—left, right, up, or down.

4. Note the smallest line in which the patient read more than half the characters correctly, and record the corresponding acuity fraction (printed at the left or right of each line on the standard Snellen chart) in the patient's record, as well as the number of letters missed (for example, 20/30–2).

5. Repeat steps 2 through 4 for the left eye, with the right eye covered.

6. Record the acuity value for each eye separately, with and without correction, as shown in the following example:

$$V \quad \frac{OD\ 20/20}{OS\ 20/25}\ \overline{cc}$$

$$V \quad \frac{OD\ 20/200}{OS\ 20/100}\ \overline{cc}$$

The large V stands for "visual acuity" (sometimes written as a large VA). OD and OS are abbreviations of the Latin words for right eye (*oculus dexter*) and left eye (*oculus sinister*). The abbreviations *cc* and *sc* signify "with correction" (eyeglasses or contact lenses) and "without correction," respectively. Because recording methods may differ, check with the doctor or senior assistant for preferred methods of recording visual acuity in the patient's chart.

regardless of whether or not the patient complains about reading. All children should have their near vision tested.

As with the Snellen chart, numeric notations are printed next to each line on the near test card as a measure of near visual acuity. However, a near acuity card provides a choice of recording notations based on various units of measurements. One of the most commonly used is the *distance equivalent*, which assigns an equivalent Snellen acuity fraction to each line on the near vision card (for example, 20/20 for the smallest line). *Jaeger notation*, also commonly used, assigns each line on the card a single arbitrary numeric value corresponding to a Snellen value. For example, Jaeger 2, abbreviated J2 when recording in the patient's chart, is equivalent to the 20/30 Snellen distance-equivalent line on the near vision card. Other notation systems are the *point system* and the *Snellen M unit*. Ophthalmic medical assistants should follow

their office policy for the preferred testing procedures and proper notation for recording the patient's near visual acuity. Procedure 8.3 describes the general steps for performing the near acuity test.

Other Acuity Tests

Patients with severe low vision may not be able to see even the largest Snellen letter (usually, the 20/400 line) clearly at the standard 20-foot or equivalent distance. Repeating the distance visual acuity test at shorter distances is usually the next step in evaluating the patient's visual acuity. If this procedure is unsuccessful, the patient may be asked to count the number of fingers held by the examiner in front of the patient. Alternatively, the patient may be asked to indicate recognition of the examiner's hand motions or to detect light from a small penlight.

Procedure 8.2 Performing the Pinhole Acuity Test

1. Patients who wear corrective eyeglasses or contact lenses should wear them for the test. Position the patient as for the Snellen distance acuity test, and test each eye separately, starting with the right eye.

2. Have the patient cover the eye not being tested with the solid side of a pinhole occluder.

3. Have the patient hold the pinhole side in front of the eye that is to be tested.

4. Instruct the patient to look at the distance chart through any pinhole in the multihole device.

5. Instruct the patient to use very small movements to align the pinhole to produce the sharpest image.

6. Start the patient reading the line on the Snellen distance acuity chart with the smallest letters legible that were just read without the pinhole. Have the patient read the lines as far down the chart as possible.

7. Repeat steps 1 through 5 for the other eye.

8. Following the Snellen visual acuity data already recorded in the chart, record the pinhole acuity value for each eye. In the example that follows, ph = pinhole.

OD 20/80 ph 20/20
OS 20/100 ph 20/25

(Chapter 16 discussed these specialized acuity tests for visually impaired patients.)

Procedures Following Acuity Tests

If the results of testing indicate below-normal visual acuity, additional procedures may be performed to evaluate the source of the disability in an effort to help the patient achieve a visual acuity as close to normal as possible. For patients with eyeglasses or contact lenses, the first step is to determine whether the lenses the patient is wearing are providing appropriate correction for the patient's present refractive error. The optical correction of the patient's current lenses is measured by **lensometry**. The patient's present refractive state is then evaluated by **refractometry**, a group of optical tests to determine the type and amount of the patient's refractive error and the appropriate lens correction. If the prescription for the patient's existing lenses differs with the newly determined correction and the below-normal visual acuity is improved with this recent correction, a new spectacle lens prescription is warranted.

Keratometry and **corneal topography** are procedures for directly measuring a patient's corneal curvature. This information is useful as a measure for refractive errors and as a guide to fitting contact lenses. It may also be used for the calculation of intraocular lenses. These tests can reveal an irregular corneal surface contour, a sign of past or present corneal disease and a cause of decreased vision.

Lensometry, refractometry, and keratometry are discussed in detail in Chapter 5. Corneal topography is

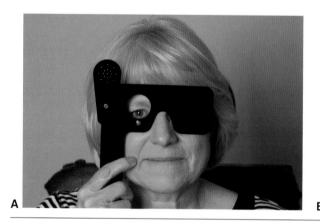
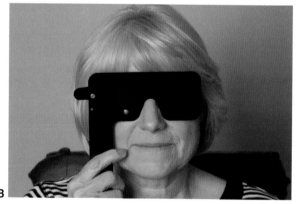

Figure 8.5 The occluder and pinhole. **A.** The occluder covers the right eye so that the left can be tested. **B.** The left eye views the chart through the pinhole. *(Image courtesy of Brice Critser, CRA, Department of Ophthalmology and Visual Sciences, University of Iowa.)*

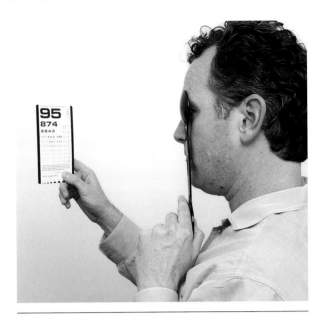

Figure 8.6   A printed card used for testing near vision at a normal reading distance of about 14 inches. *(Reprinted, with permission, from Wilson FM II, Blomquist PH,* Practical Ophthalmology, *6th ed, San Francisco: American Academy of Ophthalmology, 2009.)*

discussed in Chapter 9. Another test often performed at this stage of the comprehensive medical eye examination evaluates the patient's color vision. This procedure is discussed later in this chapter.

The ability to overcome glare from objects in the visual field and to discern various degrees of contrast is an important component of overall visual function. Measurement of these abilities, called *glare testing* and *contrast-sensitivity testing*, may be indicated by the patient's history or the results of the visual acuity examination. (Chapter 9 includes discussion of the exact purpose and principles of these tests.)

Alignment and Motility Examination

Proper alignment of the eyes and unrestricted function of the extraocular muscles are necessary for normal vision. If the eyes are misaligned or if the extraocular muscles are unable to move the eyes in a coordinated manner, the brain may not be able to merge the images received from the two eyes (**fusion**). Failure to achieve fusion produces **diplopia** (double vision) and in early childhood **suppression (ignoring one eye's visual input)** and amblyopia (decreased vision in an eye) with a resultant loss of **stereopsis**, the ability to perceive depth in three dimensions. While adult patients with ocular misalignment readily recognize their diplopia and seek medical help, children

---

Procedure 8.3 Performing the Near Acuity Test

Patients who wear eyeglasses or contact lenses for distance vision should wear them for the test. If a contact lens wearer is in monovision correction, hold an appropriate plus (+) power lens (+1.25 to +2.50) in front of the eye corrected for distance. Some ophthalmologists will also want each eye tested without correction. If the patient has reading glasses, bifocals, or other reading aids, the near vision should be tested with and without the near correction (at least on the first visit); after the first visit, the near vision with reading correction is usually enough.

1. Instruct the patient to hold the test card of printed letters, words, or numbers at the distance specified on the card, usually 14 inches. If the patient's near correction is for a distance other than 14 inches, then also test the near vision at the prescribed distance and record the distance used in the patient's record with the result (for example J2 at 10 inches).

2. Have the patient cover the left eye with an occluder or the palm of the hand. Alternatively, you may hold the occluder over the patient's left eye.

3. Ask the patient to read with the right eye the line of smallest characters legible on the card.

4. Repeat the procedure with the right eye occluded.

5. Record the acuity value for each eye separately in the patient's chart according to the notation method preferred in your office, as shown in the following examples:

near $\bigvee$ OD 20/25 $\overline{cc}$
         OS 20/25

near $\bigvee$ OD J2 $\overline{cc}$
         OS J2

---

with suppression and amblyopia may be totally unaware of their dependency on the vision of one eye and may be ignorant of their loss of stereopsis. For these and other reasons, evaluation of the alignment of the eyes and their motility, the proper movement of the extraocular muscles, is an important component of the comprehensive eye examination.

In an ocular alignment and motility examination, patients are observed and tested for three principal properties of the visual system: eye movement (motility), eye alignment, and fusional ability. Because these functions are physiologically complex, the methods used to test them are varied and at first glance complicated. Testing usually begins with a gross assessment of ocular motility, followed by additional tests if this screening evaluation indicates the presence of a potential alignment or motility problem.

For the initial, gross evaluation of ocular motility, the examiner holds a small object or displays a finger within the patient's central field of vision and asks the patient to hold the head still and to follow the object's movement with his or her eyes in the 6 **cardinal positions of gaze** (Figure 8.7):

1. right and up

2. right

3. right and down

4. left and up

5. left

6. left and down

Movements in these directions test the function of the 6 extraocular muscles and reveal possible weakness, paralysis, or restriction. However, detection of functional defects requires skill and considerable experience on the part of the examiner.

Several methods are used to assess alignment of the eyes (also known as **muscle balance**) and to detect the presence and measure the amount of **strabismus** (misalignment). Most tests are based on an observation of the position and compensatory movements of the eyes. These procedures are considered objective because no patient communication is needed. The principal objective test to detect eye misalignments, or strabismus, is the **cover–uncover test**. The principal method for measuring the extent of the eye's deviation is the **prism and alternate cover test**. (Both of these tests are discussed fully in Chapter 9.) Beginning ophthalmic medical assistants

are not usually required to perform these procedures, but they should have an understanding of the purpose and nature of the tests.

Worth 4-Dot Test

The **Worth 4-dot test** is designed to determine how a patient uses his or her eyes together. Three possible states may exist—fusion, diplopia, or suppression. If the images received by the eyes are normally aligned, the brain usually fuses the images into one visual perception. In the presence of an ocular misalignment or other abnormalities that interfere with fusion, the brain may ignore the image from one eye (**suppression**). If one image is not suppressed, then the patient will see double (diplopia). (Chapter 9 discusses the details of this test.)

Titmus Stereopsis Test

To perceive depth, both eyes must be able to fixate a visual target accurately and simultaneously. A marked defect in visual acuity, suppression of vision in one eye, or diplopia will interfere with depth perception. The **Titmus stereopsis test** determines whether the patient has fine depth perception, and quantifies it in terms of binocular cooperation. (Chapter 9 discusses the details of the Titmus stereopsis test.)

Pupillary Examination

Pupillary evaluation can reveal a variety of ophthalmic abnormalities, such as iris muscle or nerve damage, optic nerve or retinal pathology, and diseases affecting the visual pathway and the brain. Pupillary observation and testing may be performed by the ophthalmologist as

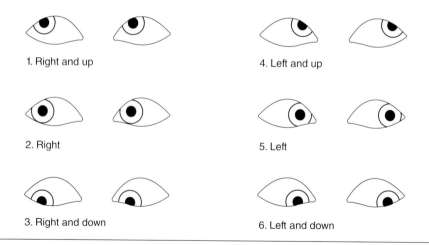

1. Right and up   4. Left and up

2. Right   5. Left

3. Right and down   6. Left and down

Figure 8.7 The cardinal positions of gaze used to evaluate eye movement.

part of the external examination, but certain elements of pupillary testing are sometimes delegated to the ophthalmic medical assistant.

Pupillary testing is scheduled before those portions of the comprehensive test that require diagnostic dilating drops (cycloplegic refraction, biomicroscopy, and ophthalmoscopy). This testing sequence is followed to prevent inaccuracies in evaluating pupillary responses.

Four procedures are used in pupillary evaluation. The first three include measurement of pupil size in dim illumination, speed of pupil constriction when a bright light is directed into the eyes, and pupillary response to a near fixation. The fourth evaluation, the **swinging-light test**, is used to quantify an important normal binocular pupillary response to light, called the **direct and consensual pupillary reaction**.

Normally, when light shines directly into an eye, the pupil of that eye constricts (direct reaction). Even when the light does not reach the other eye, the pupil of the fellow eye normally constricts as well (consensual reaction). In other words, the pupils react simultaneously to a light stimulus, even if only a single eye is directly stimulated by the light. The consensual pupillary reaction occurs even if the nonstimulated eye is blind and cannot itself react to light. Failure of the pupil in the nonstimulated eye to react consensually indicates abnormal function of the iris sphincter muscle or the nerve pathways to or from the brain. In an eye with normal function of the iris sphincter muscle, failure of the pupil to constrict in response to direct light stimulation suggests optic nerve or significant retinal damage. This response represents an **afferent pupillary defect** (**APD**), also called a Marcus Gunn pupil. When a fully demonstrable APD exists, the normal fellow eye's pupil does not constrict with the consensual response, but then constricts upon direct light stimulation.

The *swinging-light test* for direct and consensual reaction is a more subtle assessment that requires the final judgment of the ophthalmologist. In some offices the ophthalmic medical assistant might be required to perform a screening for the presence or absence of an APD. Procedure 8.4 describes the steps in checking direct and consensual pupillary reaction.

Visual Field Examination

The visual field examination measures the expanse and sensitivity of vision surrounding the direct line of sight, that is, peripheral vision. Unlike most losses of central vision, defects in peripheral vision can be subtle and are often unnoticed by a patient. Disturbances in peripheral vision are commonly due to diseases of the retina, optic nerve, or structures of the visual pathway in the brain. The **intracranial** (within the bony skull) diseases can be life-threatening as well as vision-threatening. Early

Procedure 8.4 Checking Direct and Consensual Pupillary Reaction

Seated opposite the patient in ordinary room light, have the patient look at a distant object and observe the patient's resting pupil size for both the right and the left eyes (Figure A). Pupils should be approximately equal in size (no more than 1 mm difference in diameter); some degree of inequality is normal (physiologic anisocoria).

1. In the patient's chart, record the resting pupil size for each eye in millimeters. To gauge size, you may either hold a millimeter rule close to the patient's eye or compare the patient's pupil size with relative pupil sizes printed on most near vision cards.

2. As shown in Figure B, in a dimly lit room shine a bright penlight (a small flashlight) into the patient's right eye and observe if the pupil constricts in response to the direct light stimulus. Look immediately at the left pupil to see if it constricts consensually.

3. Remove the penlight from the patient's vision briefly to allow the pupils to return to resting state and then repeat step 2 for the left eye.

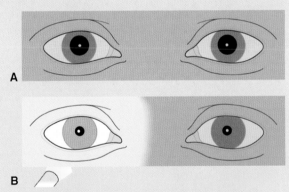

4. In the patient's chart, record the results for each eye. If the results are normal, record "Reactive to light, direct and consensual"; if the results are abnormal, record either "No direct response" or "No consensual constriction," whichever applies.

5. Report any abnormal pupillary response, such as dilation of a pupil with direct light (afferent pupillary defect), to the ophthalmologist before instilling dilating eyedrops.

detection of these abnormalities by a visual field examination permits treatment to be initiated that may halt further progression of the disease and prevent irreversible loss of central, as well as peripheral, vision.

The visual field examination consists of a number of different testing procedures. (See Chapter 11 for a detailed discussion.) Two relatively simple techniques are included in the comprehensive visual examination, however. One is the gross evaluation of the patient's peripheral vision, called confrontation visual field testing, and the other is the **Amsler grid test** that evaluates the central visual field. Performance of these tests is often the responsibility of the ophthalmic medical assistant. Positive results of these tests will indicate the need for more specific and detailed evaluations.

Confrontation Field Test

The **confrontation field test** compares the boundaries of the patient's field of vision with that of the examiner, who is presumed to have a normal field (Figure 8.8). Procedure 8.5 describes the steps in performing the confrontation field test.

Amsler Grid Test

The **Amsler grid test** determines the presence and location of defects in the central portion of the visual field. The Amsler grid is a printed square of evenly spaced horizontal and vertical lines in a grid pattern, with a dot in the center. The chart grid and dot may be either white on a black background or black on a white background (Figure 8.9). Procedure 8.6 gives step-by-step instructions for performing the Amsler grid test.

Intraocular Pressure Measurement

Pressure within the eye is maintained by a delicate balance between the continuous flow of aqueous fluid from the ciliary body and its steady drainage through the trabecular meshwork. Disturbance or malformation of any of the structures involved in this process can impede aqueous flow, causing intraocular pressure to rise, which leads to structural ocular damage. Continued elevation of intraocular pressure can permanently injure the retinal nerve fiber layer and the optic nerve. This scenario is defined as **glaucoma**.

Elevated intraocular pressure leading to glaucoma may be present long before a patient notices any symptoms such as visual loss. For this reason, early detection of the disease by measurement of intraocular pressure is a critical part of the comprehensive eye examination. If glaucoma is detected early, intraocular pressure can be reduced to normal or tolerable levels by medication or surgery, and the progression to blindness can be halted or significantly slowed. The examination to determine intraocular pressure is called **tonometry**; instruments used for this purpose are known as **tonometers**. Corneal thickness has been found to affect applanation tonometry readings and therefore, the management of glaucoma. A thinner cornea erroneously imparts lower intraocular pressure readings. The thickness of the cornea can be measured with a pachymeter. The use of this instrument is fully discussed in Chapter 10.

Principles of Tonometry

Tonometers measure intraocular pressure by principles of **applanation** or **indentation**. Applanation is the

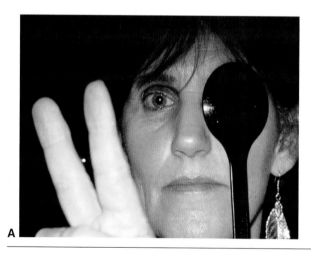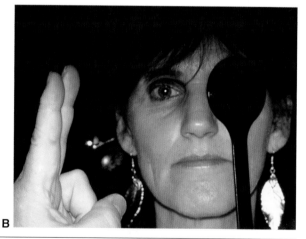

Figure 8.8 The confrontation field test. **A.** Correct position of fingers. **B.** Incorrect position of fingers. *(Reprinted, with permission, from Wilson FM II, Blomquist PH,* Practical Ophthalmology, *6th ed, San Francisco: American Academy of Ophthalmology, 2009.)*

Procedure 8.5 Performing the Confrontation Field Test

1. Seat the patient at a distance of 2 to 3 feet from you. Confront (face) the patient, cover or close your right eye, and have the patient cover the left eye (ie, test the patient's right eye first). You and the patient should fixate on each other's uncovered eye.

2. Extend your arm to the side at shoulder height and slowly bring one or two fingers just outside your peripheral vision toward the central area of your field of vision, midway between the patient and yourself. Ask the patient to immediately state how many fingers are visible.

3. Repeat the process of moving the extended finger(s) toward the central visual field from 4 different directions, randomly showing one or two fingers. If you picture a clock face in front of the patient's eyes, you start your hand with extended finger(s) outside 2 o'clock, 4 o'clock, 8 o'clock, and 10 o'clock, each time bringing the finger(s) toward the center of the clock face.

4. The patient should see the finger(s) at about the same moment you do in each of the 4 quadrants (upper-left, upper-right, lower-left, and lower-right quarters) of the visual field. (Note: A quadrant of vision is described from the patient's point of view.) If the patient does not see your finger(s) at the same time you do, the breadth of the patient's visual field in that quadrant is considered to be smaller than normal and additional perimetric studies will probably be required.

5. Record the patient's responses in the chart by indicating simply that the visual field is normal or full to counting fingers (VF full CF) or that it is absent or constricted in any one or more of the 4 quadrants for that eye.

6. Repeat the procedure with the patient's other eye and record the results similarly. Recording the result of this evaluation may be somewhat different in each office; therefore, check with your ophthalmologist to determine the method used in your office.

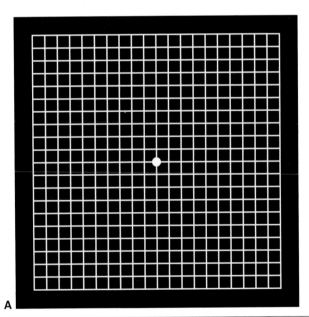
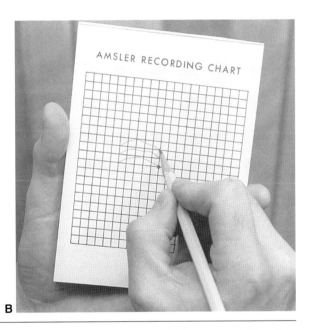

A   B

Figure 8.9 The Amsler grid test. **A.** The typical white-on-black Amsler grid. **B.** The patient marks the nature and location of his central field defect on the black-on-white grid paper.

measurement of the force required to flatten a small area of the central cornea. Indentation is the measurement of the amount of corneal indentation produced by a fixed weight. By convention, intraocular pressure is expressed in millimeters of mercury (mm Hg), the same units used in measuring blood pressure. Normal intraocular pressure ranges between 10 and 21 mm Hg.

The scales or indicators on some tonometers provide direct readings of intraocular pressure in millimeters of mercury. It is important to note there is no direct correlation to intraocular pressure and blood pressure. High blood pressure does not directly cause eye pressure to be elevated. Other tonometers indicate corneal resistance to applanation or indentation in values that

Procedure 8.6 Performing the Amsler Grid Test

1. Have the patient hold an Amsler test card about 12 to 14 inches away with one hand and cover one eye with the other hand, an occluder, or a patch. If applicable, the patient should be wearing his or her near correction.

2. Direct the patient to stare at the center dot and to report if any portions of the grid are blurred, distorted, or absent. The patient should not move the gaze from the center dot, so that the presence and position of any distortion can be specifically documented.

3. If the answer is yes, you may request that the patient record on a black-on-white Amsler sheet the location of the visual difficulties.

4. If test results are normal, state so in the patient's record. If abnormal, state so and include the Amsler recording sheet in the patient's record. If a central visual disturbance is noted, the patient will likely be a candidate for additional studies.

The patient can be instructed to perform this test in self-examination at home and report any changes to the ophthalmologist's office. The patient is to perform the test monocularly (one eye at a time), always at the same 14-inch distance and under the same illumination and with near correction.

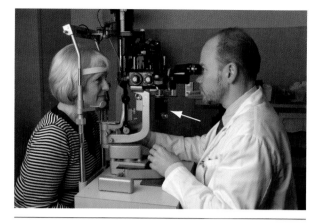

Figure 8.10 The Goldmann applanation tonometer is usually attached to a slit lamp (biomicroscope). Note the tonometer's black housing with the silver-colored force adjustment knob (arrow). *(Image courtesy of Brice Critser, CRA, Department of Ophthalmology and Visual Sciences, University of Iowa.)*

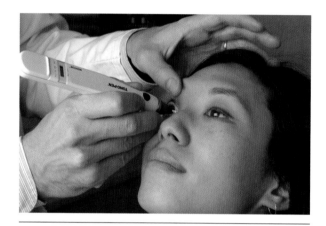

Figure 8.11 Applanation tonometry with the Tono-Pen tonometer. *(Image courtesy of Brice Critser, CRA, Department of Ophthalmology and Visual Sciences, University of Iowa.)*

are converted to millimeters of mercury by a simple calculation or the use of conversion tables.

While all methods and instruments used for tonometry produce satisfactory measurements of intraocular pressure, each system has advantages and disadvantages. Because almost all tonometers actually touch the highly sensitive cornea, anesthetizing eyedrops are used in patients before testing. Some tonometers also require instillation of **fluorescein**, a dye solution, to aid in the alignment and visualization of the images seen in the slit lamp.

Applanation Tonometry

The most commonly used instrument for performing applanation tonometry is the **Goldmann applanation tonometer** (Figure 8.10); the compact **Tono-Pen** (Figure 8.11) is also popular. Other devices include the handheld **Perkins tonometer** and the **iCare tonometer** (Figure 8.12), the electronic **MacKay-Marg tonometer**, and the **pneumatonometer**. The latter uses compressed air and a piston-like wand to applanate the surface of the eyeball and measure the intraocular pressure. The air-puff tonometer is a noncontact applanation device that employs a burst of air to applanate the cornea.

All applanation tonometers measure the force required to flatten a small area of the central cornea. The precise area to be flattened is predetermined and varies with the instrument used. The Goldmann applanation tonometer, for example, flattens a circle 3.06 mm in diameter. More force is required to flatten a circle on the cornea when intraocular pressure is high (a "harder" eye), and less force with lower intraocular pressure (a "softer" eye).

The Goldmann applanation tonometer is usually attached to a slit lamp (biomicroscope), shown in Figure 8.13A. The instrument consists of a double-prism head (the tonometer tip), attached by a rod to a housing that delivers measured force controlled by an adjustment knob. Positioning of the tonometer tip can be observed through the slit-lamp oculars (Figure 8.13B). Force is increased by turning the tonometer's force-adjustment knob until a circle of cornea 3.06 mm in diameter is

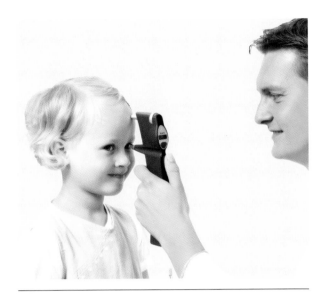

Figure 8.12 Applanation tonometry with the ICare tonometer. *(Image courtesy of Icare Finland Oy.)*

Procedure 8.7 describes the steps in performing Goldmann tonometry.

Pen-like in shape, the Tono-Pen portable electronic device consists of a stainless steel probe containing a solid-state strain gauge that converts intraocular pressure to an electrical signal. A protective, disposable latex membrane is placed on the tip of the Tono-Pen before use with each patient. Intraocular pressure is measured by lightly touching the patient's anesthetized cornea with the tip of the Tono-Pen. Four measurements are recorded for each eye, resulting in an average intraocular pressure measurement. Measurements can be taken with the patient either sitting or supine, which adds to the versatility of the instrument. Although the Tono-Pen is not as accurate as the Goldmann applanation tonometer, its size and versatility make it useful for screening purposes and with patients who are unable to cooperate for applanation tonometry.

Indentation Tonometry

Indentation tonometry provides a recording of intraocular pressure by measuring the indentation of the cornea produced by a weight of a given amount. The technique is commonly performed with a relatively simple mechanical device called a **Schiøtz tonometer**. This instrument consists of a cylinder, the bottom of which forms a concave footplate that contacts the cornea (Figure 8.14A). Surrounding the cylinder is a frame with a pair of handles by which the examiner holds the device while positioning it on the cornea. A plunger passes through the

flattened. The amount of force required is indicated by a number on the calibrated dial on the adjustment knob. This reading is simply multiplied by 10 to express the intraocular pressure in millimeters of mercury. Goldmann applanation tonometers are popular and common in ophthalmic practice because of the ease of alignment with the cornea, and they are highly accurate. In addition, intraocular pressure is directly related to the readings on the drum. The main disadvantages are their cost and nonportability. These devices also require a relatively normal corneal shape for accurate measurement.

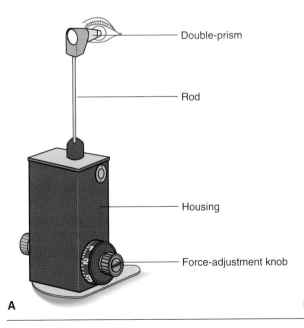

Double-prism

Rod

Housing

Force-adjustment knob

A

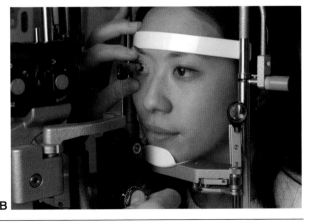

B

Figure 8.13 Primary parts of the Goldmann tonometer (**A**) and positioning of the tonometer tip (**B**). *(Part B image courtesy of Brice Critser, CRA, Department of Ophthalmology and Visual Sciences, University of Iowa.)*

Procedure 8.7 Performing Goldmann Applanation Tonometry

1. Ensure that the tonometer tip is clean and disinfected.

2. Instill an eyedrop of a local anesthetic and apply fluorescein dye into both of the patient's eyes. (Refer to Chapter 6 for information on these drugs and instillation techniques.) Instead of separate agents, some offices use a single solution containing both the anesthetic and the dye. Caution: Fluorescein dye can permanently stain soft contact lenses. Be sure a patient's soft contact lenses are removed before instilling fluorescein dye. Also remember to rinse the eye with irrigation solution prior to reinserting the soft contact lenses.

3. Seat the patient comfortably at the slit lamp with the forehead firmly against the headrest. Seat yourself opposite in the examiner's position, and instruct the patient to look straight ahead or to gaze steadily at your ear.

4. With the slit beam turned to a full circle of light turn the dial or lever that inserts the cobalt-blue filter in the beam's path and onto the tonometer tip. (The resulting cobalt-blue light causes the fluorescein dye on the patient's eye to fluoresce a bright yellow-green.) Using the magnification-adjustment knob on the slit lamp, set the magnification at low power. Adjust the arm of the slit lamp so that the cobalt-blue light shines on the tonometer tip at a wide angle, about 45° to 60°.

5. Looking from the side of the slit lamp, align the tonometer tip with the patient's cornea. Adjust the numbered dial on the force-adjustment knob to read between 1 and 2 (10 and 20 mm Hg). Instruct the patient to blink once (to spread the fluorescein dye) and then to try to avoid blinking. If it is necessary to hold the patient's lid open, push up on the skin of the lid with your thumb and secure the lid against the bony orbit; do not apply pressure to the globe.

6. Using the slit-lamp control handle (joystick), gently move the tonometer tip forward until it just touches the central cornea. Looking through the slit-lamp oculars, confirm that the tip has touched the cornea: the fluorescein under the tip will break into two semicircles, one above and one below a horizontal line. Raise or lower the vertical adjustment on the biomicroscope until the

semicircles are equal in size. You may also need to adjust the horizontal alignment slightly to the right or left if the semicircles are shifted off center.

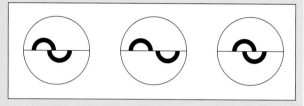

7. Slowly and gently turn the force-adjustment knob of the tonometer in the direction required to move the semicircles until their inner edges just touch, not overlap, as shown at the left in the figure. If the semicircles are separated, as shown in the center figure, the pressure reading will be too low. If the semicircles overlap, as shown in the right figure, the pressure reading will be too high.

8. With the slit-lamp joystick, pull the tonometer tip away from the patient's eye. Note the reading on the numbered dial of the tonometer's adjustment knob. Multiply the number by 10 to obtain the intraocular pressure in millimeters of mercury.

9. Record the pressure in the patient's record, followed by the abbreviation for the eye to which it applies, for example,

$$\text{TA} \begin{array}{l} 20 \text{ OD (A)} \\ 21 \text{ OS (A)} \end{array} \text{ or } \text{TA} \begin{array}{l} 20 \text{ OD} \\ 21 \text{ OS} \end{array}$$

TA stands for "applanation tension" or "tension by applanation." Also indicate the type of tonometer used, abbreviating the instrument as follows (or with the standard abbreviations used in your office): A = applanation (Goldmann) tonometer, S = Schiøtz (indentation) tonometer, P = pneumatonometer, AP = air-puff tonometer, TP = Tono-Pen. As always with ophthalmic data, record the measurements for the right eye (OD) first, and for the left eye (OS) second.

10. Clean and disinfect the tonometer tip as required in your office. (See Chapter 22.)

An incorrect pressure reading can occur from too much or too little fluorescein dye (semicircles too fat or too thin, respectively) or pressure from the examiner's fingers on the patient's eye when holding the eyelids open. Be sure the pressure from your fingers holding the eyelids open is against the orbital rim and not on the eye.

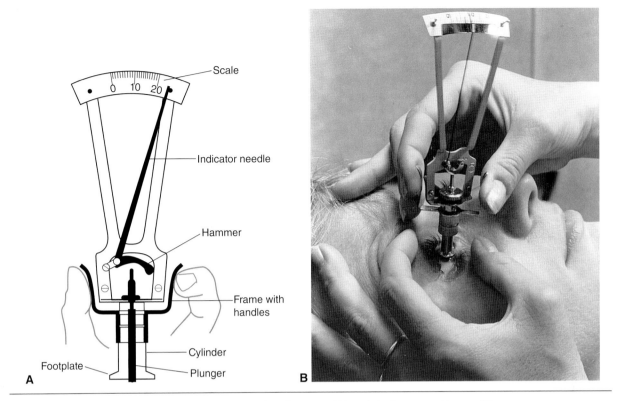

Figure 8.14 The Schiøtz indentation tonometer showing parts (**A**) and the instrument in use (**B**).

cylinder and at the upper end moves a hammer, which, in turn, moves a needle across a calibrated scale fixed to the top of the device.

The examiner chooses a weight of a given size (5.5 to 15.0 grams), attaches the weight to the top of the plunger, and gently lowers the device to rest on the patient's anesthetized cornea (Figure 8.14B). The amount of corneal indentation by a given weight is registered on the scale (for those who may be interested, each mm division on the scale corresponds to an indentation of 0.05 mm in the cornea) of the tonometer in increments of 0.5 scale units. The units are then converted to intraocular pressure in millimeters of mercury by the use of standard conversion tables supplied with the instrument. The examiner records the indentation units observed, the weight used in the test, and the conversion to intraocular pressure in millimeters of mercury in the patient's chart (for example, 6.0 units/5.5 weight = 15 mm Hg).

Applanation Versus Indentation Tonometry

Schiøtz indentation tonometry is used by nonophthalmologist physicians because it is easy to perform and does not require expensive instrumentation. Like Goldmann tonometry, the Schiøtz procedure requires relatively normal corneal curvature for accuracy. However,

the indentation technique assumes that **scleral rigidity** (resistance to stretching) is normal, which may not be the case with young subjects or patients with high myopia. If resistance of scleral tissue to stretching is higher than normal (ie, scleral rigidity is high), intraocular pressure will be overestimated; conversely, if scleral rigidity is low, the pressure will be underestimated.

Careless techniques can result in inaccurate readings by any tonometric method. For all methods, and particularly Schiøtz, patients must be relaxed and breathing normally, with tight collars loosened. Schiøtz tonometry also requires the examiner to hold the patient's eyelids apart, but done improperly, this maneuver can apply pressure to the globe and produce a false reading. Most inaccuracies in Schiøtz tonometry result in falsely low, rather than high, readings.

(See Chapter 22 for instructions on cleaning tonometers after each use to avoid the possibility of spreading infection.)

Pachymetry

Corneal **pachymetry** refers to the measurement of the thickness of the cornea. Pachymetry is measured in micrometers (μm). An average cornea is about 545 μm at the center and about 1000 μm thick at its outer edge.

Accurate measurement of the corneal thickness is necessary for diagnosis of many corneal diseases and aberrations such as corneal edema, keratoconus and irregular astigmatism. Pachymetry has been found to be an important parameter in the diagnostic evaluation of glaucoma. It is also essential in corneal refractive surgery so that incision depth and treatment parameters can be performed safely, avoiding perforations of the cornea.

There are many different acceptable methods for determining the corneal thickness. Optical pachymeters attach to the slit lamp and operate on optical principles to measure the distance between the epithelium (front or outer layer of cells) and the endothelium (back or inner layer of cells) of the cornea (see Figure 10.5). Ultrasonic pachymeters, which use reflected sound waves to measure corneal thickness, are used more commonly. Ultrasonic pachymeters may include corneal mapping display programs, which are used to provide information about the potential and actual results of refractive surgery procedures. Some ultrasonic probes are hard-wired to a tabletop instrument, and others are pen-like and portable. Although each instrument may be accurate variations in results exist between different instruments due to technical design reasons. Care must be taken to report multiple or average readings and indicate the device used to acquire the information.

Corneal pachymetry has become an important test in the evaluation of a patient for glaucoma or risk of developing glaucoma. (See Chapter 10.) The Goldmann applanation tonometer design assumed a standard central corneal thickness (CCT) but there is actually great variation in CCT. Thicker CCT overestimates real intraocular pressure and thin CCT underestimates real intraocular pressure.

External Examination

The purpose of the external eye examination is to provide an assessment of the ocular adnexa, external globe, and anterior chamber. During this evaluation, the examiner visually inspects the orbital soft tissues around the eyes, the eyelids, the lacrimal apparatus, the visible portions of the external globe, and the anterior chamber angle. **Palpation** (touching) and specialized measurement procedures may be used, as well as visual inspection. Together with the patient's history, the result of this examination provides numerous clues to the patient's general eye health and to some specific ocular complaints. Abnormalities revealed in the external examination may be further investigated in other portions of the comprehensive eye examination.

In examining the orbit, one looks for evidence of proptosis, inflammation of the orbital tissues, anomalous eyelid positions, and other visible abnormalities. The extent of proptosis may be measured by a special procedure called *exophthalmometry*, described later in this chapter. The examination includes observing the eyelids for general health, function, and abnormal positioning. If infection or abnormalities are found or the history suggests that they may be present, the eyelids may be further examined by biomicroscopy or other methods.

If the patient's history and a general examination of the lacrimal system suggest a tear deficiency, biomicroscopy may be employed for a closer inspection with the addition of **fluorescein** or **lissamine green** dye. *Schirmer testing*, described later in this chapter, is a specialized test of tear production that the ophthalmic assistant frequently performs. The pupillary examination, described earlier in this chapter, is sometimes performed as a component of the external examination.

Anterior Chamber Evaluation

The anterior chamber is the dome-shaped space between the back of the cornea and the front of the iris. In some individuals, this chamber is more shallow than normal. As these people age, the natural increase in the thickness of the crystalline lens may block aqueous flow through the pupil, causing the iris to bow forward in a convex shape and creating a narrow angle between the outer edges of the iris and cornea. When this happens, the flow of aqueous fluid out of the anterior chamber through the trabecular meshwork may be slowed and even eventually blocked, producing a sudden rise in intraocular pressure and, possibly, acute glaucoma. In addition, certain ophthalmic drugs commonly used to dilate the pupil for the fundus examination can cause a dangerous rise in intraocular pressure in a patient with a narrow chamber angle. Determining the patient's chamber depth and angle is an important part of the external examination in that it can reveal patients at risk for acute glaucoma and those in whom pupillary dilating drops should be avoided temporarily.

The **flashlight test** is a simple procedure used to estimate the depth of the anterior chamber and the chamber angle; it is often performed at the time of the pupil evaluation. This test, commonly performed by the ophthalmic medical assistant, helps screen for the presence of a shallow anterior chamber and if present the assistant can alert the physician who will then determine the appropriateness of using dilating drops. Procedure 8.8 describes this test.

Biomicroscopy

The **biomicroscope**, commonly called a **slit lamp** (Figure 8.15), consists of a magnification viewing system and a source of illumination that delivers an adjustable narrow beam, or slit, of light. The ophthalmologist uses this instrument to obtain a magnified view of the patient's ocular adnexa and anterior segment structures: eyelid margins, lashes, conjunctiva, sclera, cornea, tear film, anterior chamber, iris, lens, and anterior vitreous. The ophthalmic medical assistant may also use the slit lamp when performing applanation tonometry with the Goldmann applanation tonometer and other evaluations.

The ophthalmologist may also use the biomicroscope to examine the fundus: retina, retinal blood vessels and periphery, macula, and optic nerve head (Figure 8.16). A funduscopic examination is performed to determine the health and physical status of the posterior structures of the eye. A variety of handheld lenses (+90 and +78 D) and attachment lenses used in conjunction with the slit lamp are available. The **Hruby lens** (−55 D, see Figure 22.1), attached to the slit lamp, and the handheld lenses are all noncontact and are useful for examining the optic nerve head and small areas of the posterior retina and vitreous. A group of special contact lenses placed with a gel on the patient's anesthetized eye is also used with the biomicroscope for a magnified and detailed examination of the posterior pole and peripheral retina.

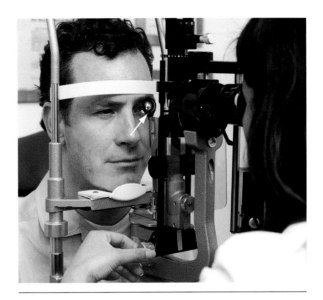

Figure 8.15 The biomicroscope, or slit lamp, with Hruby lens in use (arrow). *(Reprinted, with permission, from Wilson FM II, Blomquist PH, Practical Ophthalmology, 6th ed, San Francisco: American Academy of Ophthalmology, 2009.)*

Gonioscopy

A careful examination of the structures of the anterior chamber is important for the detection of conditions producing, or likely to produce, glaucoma. Because of the curvature of the cornea and its high index of refraction,

Procedure 8.8 Performing the Flashlight Test To Estimate the Depth of the Anterior Chamber

1. Hold a penlight near the limbus of the right eye from the temple side of the eye.

2. With the penlight parallel to the plane of the iris, shine the light across the front of the patient's right eye toward the nose.

3. Observe the appearance of the side of the iris closest to the patient's nose. In an eye with a normally shaped anterior chamber and iris, the nasal half of the iris will be illuminated like the temporal half (Figure A). In an eye with a shallow anterior chamber and narrow chamber angle, about two-thirds of the nasal portion of the iris will appear in shadow (Figure B).

4. Record your observations in the patient's record, and repeat the test on the patient's left eye. Consult the physician for the appropriate way to express your observations in the chart and to determine the appropriateness for dilating drops.

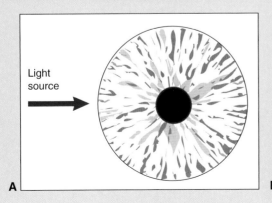

Light source

A

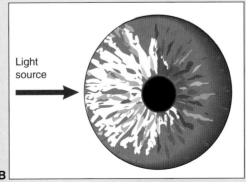

Light source

B

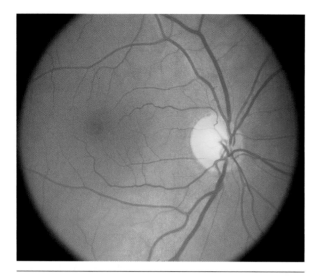

Figure 8.16 The normal fundus as seen through a slit lamp with a handheld lens in front of eye.

unaided examination of the chamber angle with the slit lamp is optically impossible. For these reasons, a specialized viewing method, called **gonioscopy**, is used. In this procedure, the ophthalmologist examines the anterior chamber angle through a special contact lens placed on the patient's anesthetized cornea. One type of gonioscopy, an indirect method, uses the **Goldmann goniolens** (a mirrored contact lens) to reflect the image of the anterior chamber angle which is viewed using the slit lamp. A water-soluble viscous gel is placed in the well of the lens before applying it to the cornea. Alternative goniolenses (Zeiss or Posner) are also indirect and mirrored lenses but these have attached handles or stems and are gently placed on the cornea without the use of a gel (Figure 8.17). Another, less common type of gonioscopy uses the **Koeppe lens** (a high-plus contact lens) to examine the angle structures as illuminated and observed directly with a handheld light

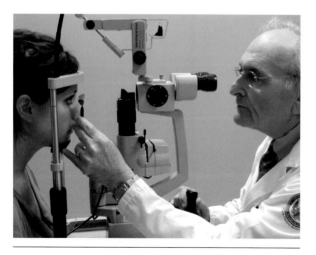

Figure 8.17 Preparing for gonioscopy with a slit lamp and a goniolens. *(Image courtesy of Tina Newmark, RN, MS.)*

source and microscope. After use, the contact lenses must be thoroughly cleaned by the ophthalmic assistant. (See Chapter 22 for procedures for cleaning.) Regardless of the goniolens utilized, the ophthalmic assistant should prepare the patient for the test and ready all the materials needed to perform the examination.

Ophthalmoscopy

Ophthalmoscopy is a method of examining the vitreous and fundus in great detail through the use of an ophthalmoscope. The procedure is sometimes referred to as a *funduscopic examination* or *posterior segment examination*. Ophthalmoscopy is performed exclusively by the ophthalmologist and usually requires the patient's pupils to be dilated with eyedrops to permit the viewing of a greater area of the retina and vitreous. Because pupillary dilation can alter the results of certain visual acuity and pupillary tests, dilation for ophthalmoscopy is usually performed after these procedures. The ophthalmic medical assistant is often responsible for instilling the dilating eyedrops. (Refer to Chapter 6 for information about these drugs and their administration.)

Direct and Indirect Ophthalmoscopy

The principal types of instruments used for this part of the comprehensive examination are the direct and indirect ophthalmoscopes. The **direct ophthalmoscope** is a handheld instrument with a light-and-mirror system that affords an upright, monocular survey of a narrow field but offers a 15-fold magnified view of the fundus (Figure 8.18). Rechargeable batteries located in the handle of the instrument supply power to the light source. Holding the instrument at close range, the ophthalmologist shines the light into the patient's eye and observes the fundus through the instrument's magnification viewing system.

The **indirect ophthalmoscope** is worn on the physician's head. The headset consists of a binocular viewing device and an adjustable lighting system wired to a transformer power source; the binocular system allows for a stereoscopic view of the fundus. The ophthalmologist holds one of a variety of condensing lenses (see Figure 22.2) a few inches from the patient's eye, and the ophthalmoscope headset provides both the lighting and the stereoscopic vision for the examination. Unlike the upright (direct), narrow and monocular view provided by the direct ophthalmoscope, magnified 15-fold, the view of the fundus with the indirect ophthalmoscope is inverted, stereoscopic, virtual, but has a wider field and is magnified only 2- to 4-fold (Figure 8.19). The indirect

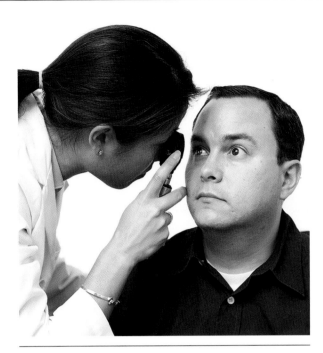

Figure 8.18 Ophthalmoscopic examination with the direct ophthalmoscope. *(Reprinted, with permission, from Wilson FM II, Blomquist PH,* Practical Ophthalmology, *6th ed, San Francisco: American Academy of Ophthalmology, 2009.)*

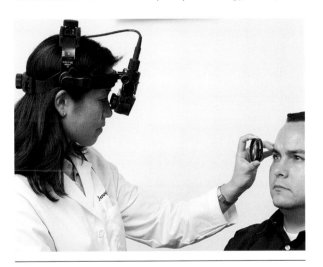

Figure 8.19 Ophthalmoscopic examination with the indirect ophthalmoscope. *(Reprinted, with permission, from Wilson FM II, Blomquist PH,* Practical Ophthalmology, *6th ed, San Francisco: American Academy of Ophthalmology, 2009.)*

ophthalmoscope remains the gold standard for examining the peripheral retina and identifying retina holes and retinal tears.

Additional Tests

Information from the patient's history and the results of any portion of the comprehensive eye examination may suggest an abnormality that requires further investigation. Conditions that may require specialized tests include color vision deficit; dry eye; corneal abrasions, lesions, or infections; and proptosis. Dozens of specialized ophthalmic diagnostic and measuring procedures are available. The following are a few of the common procedures that require the help of the ophthalmic medical assistant or become the assistant's sole responsibility.

Color Vision Tests

The impaired ability to perceive color is usually an inherited condition, passed from the mother to a son. Optic nerve or retinal disease may also cause defects in color vision. For the majority of patients with impaired color vision, the color red appears less bright than for normal individuals, preventing accurate perception of color mixtures that include red. While a deficit in color vision is not usually disabling, it can hinder individuals from pursuing certain specialized careers.

Evaluation of color vision is often performed with **pseudoisochromatic color plates** (Figure 8.20). Each eye is tested separately. Patients are instructed to look at a book of these plates, which display patterns of colored and gray dots. Patients with normal color vision can easily detect numbers and figures composed of, and embedded in, the multicolored dots. Patients with color vision deficits cannot distinguish the numbers and figures. Various combinations of colors are used to identify the nature of the color vision deficit.

The **15-hue test**, or **Farnsworth-Munsell D-15 test**, provides a more precise determination of color vision deficits (Figure 8.21). The test consists of 15 pastel-colored chips of similar brightness but subtly different hues, which the patient must arrange in a related color sequence. The sequence is obvious to patients with normal color vision, but patients with color deficiencies make characteristic errors in arranging the chips.

Tear Output Test

The patient's history and external and slit-lamp examinations may suggest the presence of a dry eye condition. The **Schirmer test** measures the patient's tear output and helps confirm the diagnosis. To perform this test, the examiner places one end of a strip of filter paper in the patient's outer lower fornix (Figure 8.22). After 5 minutes, the examiner removes the filter paper and measures in millimeters the extent to which the patient's tears have wet the strip. If performed with topical anesthetic, the test measures basic secretion of accessory glands; without anesthetic, the test measures tearing

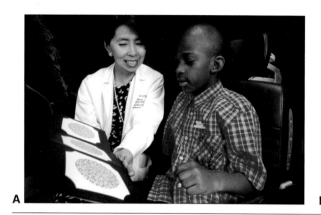
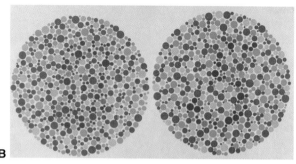

Figure 8.20 **A.** Pseudoisochromatic color plates used to test color vision. The patient must detect numbers or figures embedded in an array of colored dots. **B.** Pseudoisochromatic color plates in greater detail. *(Part A courtesy National Eye Institute, National Institutes of Health. Part B reprinted, with permission, from Regillo C. Basic and Clinical Science Course, Section 12, Retina and Vitreous. San Francisco: American Academy of Ophthalmology; 2004–2005.)*

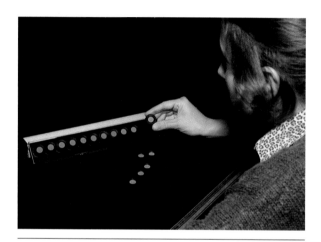

Figure 8.21 The 15-hue test of color vision.

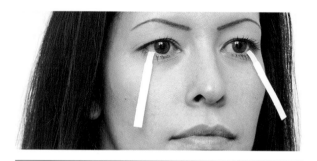

Figure 8.22 The Schirmer test, in which the amount of wetting of the paper strips is a measure of tear flow. *(Reprinted, with permission, from Wilson FM II, Blomquist PH, Practical Ophthalmology, 6th ed, San Francisco: American Academy of Ophthalmology, 2009.)*

from lacrimal glands (reflex tearing). Less than 10 mm of wetting indicates a dry eye.

Another commercially available test for assessing tear production is the **phenol red thread tear test**, which utilizes a cotton thread treated with the pH indicator phenol

red. In its dry acidic state, the thread is yellow; in contact with tears (basic pH), the thread changes to a light red. The test is performed without anesthesia. The folded 3 mm end of the thread is placed into the outer one-third of the lower eyelid. Each eye is individually tested for 15 seconds. The tread is removed and unfolded and the entire length of the red portion is measured in mm from the end of the thread. A reading less than 10 mm is considered to reflect a dry eye.

Evaluating the Corneal and Conjunctival Epithelium

Fluorescein, rose bengal, and lissamine green are dyes used to test the structural and physiologic integrity of the surface epithelium of the eyeball. These tissue dyes reveal areas of epithelial cell injury or loss as seen in dry eyes, corneal abrasions, and other corneal lesions. When a solution of one of the dyes or a moistened impregnated filter-paper strip is placed in the eye, the dye selectively stains abraded or diseased epithelium. Figure 3.7 shows rose bengal dye staining of an epithelial corneal defect in a dendritic pattern. A white light through the slit lamp reveals the abnormal epithelial cells present in dry eye disorders when stained with lissamine green and rose bengal dyes. A cobalt-blue light of the slit lamp, however, is needed to enhance the fluorescence and thereby the visibility of fluorescein. For essential information about these dyes and their use in ophthalmic testing, refer to Chapter 6.

Corneal Sensitivity Test

Certain diseases, such as herpes simplex infections of the cornea and some brain tumors, result in the loss of normal corneal sensitivity. Testing for the existence of corneal sensitivity can help confirm a diagnosis of these conditions. This test may be required by the patient's history or by the results of the external examination or slit-lamp examination. The test is simple but effective and must be performed before anesthetic is placed in the eye. The examiner merely touches the central portion of the cornea with a sterile wisp of cotton to determine whether or not the patient has a normal corneal sensation. A normal response is a blink. With decreased corneal sensitivity, the patient does not blink.

This test can easily be accomplished by twirling out a thin wisp from a cotton tip applicator and approaching the patient from the temple side in order to avoid a reflex blink that would occur as a defensive mechanism. During the test, the patient is asked to keep both eyes opened wide and to fixate upon a distant target. The examiner then gently touches the center cornea with the cotton wisp.

Exophthalmometry

Exophthalmometry measures the prominence of the eyeball in relation to the bony orbital rim surrounding it. The measurement is performed with an instrument called an **exophthalmometer**. The test is used to record the existence and extent of proptosis mainly caused by thyroid disease and orbital tumors (Figure 8.23).

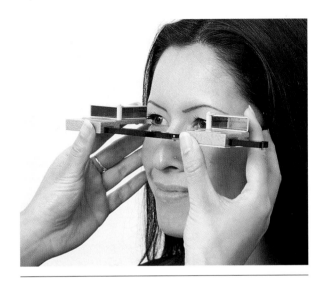

Figure 8.23 Measurements of proptosis with an exophthalmometer. *(Reprinted, with permission, from Wilson FM II, Blomquist PH, Practical Ophthalmology, 6th ed, San Francisco: American Academy of Ophthalmology, 2009.)*

SELF-ASSESSMENT TEST

1. State the purpose of the comprehensive medical eye examination.

2. Name 3 reasons why a regular comprehensive eye examination may be beneficial.

3. Name the 5 principal areas covered by the history-taking interview.

4. How should you respond to a patient's request for medical advice or a diagnosis of the patient's condition?

5. Define visual acuity.

6. A patient's visual acuity measures 20/40. What does the first number represent? What does the second number represent?

7. You have measured a patient's visual acuity without eyeglasses in place. The measurement was 20/60 in the right eye and 20/40 in the left eye. How would you write this patient's visual acuity in the office record?

8. What information is given by the pinhole acuity test?

9. Give 2 reasons for including the near acuity test in the comprehensive examination.

10. Which 3 principal properties of the visual system are evaluated by the ocular alignment and motility examination?

11. Name the 6 cardinal positions of gaze.

12. State the purpose of the prism and alternate cover test.

13. State the purpose of the Worth 4-dot test.

14. State the purpose of the Titmus stereopsis test.

15. What is the difference between a manifest and a latent deviation?

16. What important binocular pupillary response to light does the swinging-light test check?

17. State the purpose of the visual field examination.

18. During the confrontation field test, where do the patient and examiner fixate?

19. What does the Amsler grid test determine?

20. Why is the measurement of intraocular pressure a critical part of the comprehensive eye examination?

21. What are the 2 principles by which tonometers measure intraocular pressure?

22. Which of the 4 illustrations shows how the semicircles should appear through the slit-lamp oculars when intraocular pressure has been measured correctly with a Goldmann applanation tonometer?

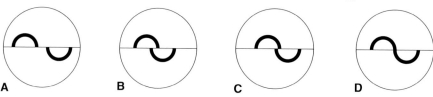

A   B   C   D

23. Why is pachymetry important?

24. State the purpose of the external eye examination.

25. Describe the purpose of the flashlight test and state the 2 principal reasons it is performed.

26. State 4 possible uses of the biomicroscope (slit lamp).

27. Describe the 78 D and 90 D handheld lenses and their use.

28. Define gonioscopy.

29. Name the 2 types of ophthalmoscopes. How do they differ?

30. Name 2 tests used to evaluate color vision.

31. What is the purpose of the Schirmer test?

32. What is the purpose of staining the ocular surface with dye?

33. Describe the corneal sensitivity test and its purpose.

34. Describe the purpose of exophthalmometry.

SUGGESTED ACTIVITIES

1. Discuss with the ophthalmologist or senior staff members in your office which tests will be your responsibility to perform or assist with. Request that you be permitted to observe trained members of the staff perform the tests and that you be allowed to practice the procedures under supervision.

2. Review the elements of the comprehensive medical eye examination with the ophthalmologist in your office. Ask specifically how much and what type of information you should discuss with the patient before the examination.

3. Confirm with the ophthalmologist the specific questions to be included when taking the patient's preliminary history.

4. With a senior staff assistant acting as a patient, role-play the taking of an ophthalmic patient history. Discuss your performance together afterward, and ask for specific tips to improve your technique.

5. Ask permission to observe a senior technician or the ophthalmologist performing the following procedures with patients: visual acuity testing; testing direct and consensual pupillary reaction; confrontation visual fields; applanation tonometry; and the flashlight test. Then, over a period of time, schedule sessions with the technician or doctor to train you in each of these procedures, using other assistants as volunteer "patients" before graduating to testing actual patients.

6. Ask permission to observe a senior technician or the ophthalmologist performing the following procedures with patients: alignment and ocular motility examination; visual inspection of the external eye; biomicroscopy; ophthalmoscopy; and other additional tests selected by the technician or doctor. In a later meeting with the training technician or doctor, go over the names and purposes of the types of instruments used, discuss the purposes of the tests, and determine whether and how you will participate in any of these procedures as a part of your job responsibilities.

SUGGESTED RESOURCES

American Academy of Ophthalmology. *Pediatric Eye Evaluations: Screening and Comprehensive Ophthalmic Evaluation.* Preferred Practice Pattern. San Francisco: American Academy of Ophthalmology; 2007.

American Academy of Ophthalmology. *Comprehensive Adult Medical Eye Evaluation.* Preferred Practice Pattern. San Francisco: American Academy of Ophthalmology; 2010.

Cassin B, ed. *Fundamentals for Ophthalmic Technical Personnel.* Philadelphia: Saunders; 1995: chaps 15, 19–22.

DuBois LG. Applanation tonometry, color vision screening, confrontation visual fields, evaluation of pupils, history taking, ocular motility, slit-lamp assessment of angles, visual acuity. In: *Fundamentals of Ophthalmic Medical Assisting.* DVD. San Francisco: American Academy of Ophthalmology; 2009.

Farrell TA, Alward WLM, Verdick RE. Fundamentals of slit-lamp biomicroscopy. In: *The Eye Exam and Basic Ophthalmic Instruments.* DVD. San Francisco: American Academy of Ophthalmology; 1993. Reviewed for currency: 2007.

Harper RA, ed. *Basic Ophthalmology.* 9th ed. San Francisco: American Academy of Ophthalmology; 2010: 165–182.

Lewis RA. Goldmann applanation tonometry. In: *The Eye Exam and Basic Ophthalmic Instruments.* DVD. San Francisco: American Academy of Ophthalmology; 1988. Reviewed for currency: 2007.

Movaghar M, Lawrence MG. Eye exam: the essentials. In: *The Eye Exam and Basic Ophthalmic Instruments.* DVD. San Francisco: American Academy of Ophthalmology; 2001. Reviewed for currency: 2007.

Stein HA, Stein RM. *The Ophthalmic Assistant: A Text for Allied and Associated Ophthalmic Personnel.* 8th ed. St Louis: Mosby; 2006.

Wilson ME Jr. Ocular motility evaluation of strabismus and myasthenia gravis. In: *Strabismus Evaluation and Surgery.* DVD. San Francisco: American Academy of Ophthalmology; 1993. Reviewed for currency: 2007.

9
OCULAR MOTILITY

Ocular motility can be defined as the evaluation of eye movements and their disorders. The evaluation of ocular motility involves observation of eye movement, identification of eye alignment abnormalities, and assessment of the patient's ability to use both eyes together. In order to understand the motility examination, it is important to understand the underlying anatomy and physiology of the extraocular muscles.

Anatomy and Physiology

Six extraocular muscles are attached to the eyeball in different surface locations (Figure 9.1). They are the 4 **rectus muscles** (**inferior**, **superior**, **lateral**, and **medial**) and the 2 **oblique muscles** (**inferior** and **superior**). The manner in which these extraocular muscles "grip" the eyeball allows it to move in 3 different planes: horizontal, vertical, and torsional.

Horizontal movement is lateral and medial (abduction and adduction). Vertical movement is up and down (supraduction and infraduction). Torsional movement twists the eye inward and outward (incyclotorsion and excyclotorsion). Figure 9.2 illustrates movements of the eye.

Horizontal movement of the eye is fairly straightforward. It is controlled by the medial and lateral rectus muscles with minor contributions from the other 4 extraocular muscles. The medial and lateral rectus muscles only function in the horizontal plane. Vertical and torsional movements are more complex. Vertical movements are primarily controlled by the superior and inferior rectus muscles, but the oblique muscles make a significant contribution. Torsional movements are primarily oblique muscle functions but the superior and inferior rectus muscles also help these movements. These movements have been sorted out to indicate their strongest (**primary**), intermediate (**secondary**) and weakest (**tertiary**) **actions** as shown in Table 9.1.

Within this complex interplay of actions, there are 6 positions of gaze wherein one muscle is the dominant mover of the eye. The examiner can observe the actions of the muscles in these 6 positions to evaluate the strength of a particular muscle. These are called the **cardinal positions of gaze** (Figure 9.3).

When eye movements are not equal in one of these cardinal positions, it implies a weakness or overaction of a specific muscle. A weak muscle does not pull the eye to its normal position in a field of gaze. It is said that the muscle "underacts." Overaction of the muscle means that it pulls the eye too strongly and the eye overshoots its usual position in a cardinal position.

An example would be a person with an overacting right inferior oblique muscle (Figure 9.4). In this example, note the right eye is elevated relative to the left eye, implying overaction of the right inferior oblique in its cardinal position. However, it is not always that simple. The muscle that moves the eye in a particular direction of gaze is called the **agonist**. The muscle of the same eye that opposes that action is called the **antagonist**.

> When one muscle *from each* eye works together
>
> to move the eyes in a particular direction,
>
> they are said to be "yoked" together.

One initially observes eye movements of both eyes together (**versions**). If there is an abnormality, observation of the movement of each eye separately (**ductions**) is necessary to determine which eye has the abnormality. In the example of the overacting right inferior oblique muscle, observation of versions alone would not totally isolate the abnormal muscle. It is not possible to tell if an

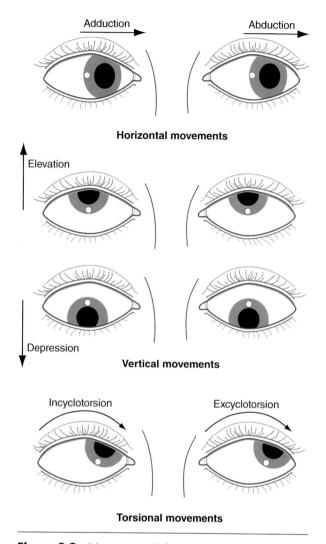

Figure 9.2 Movements of the eye. *(Illustration by Mark M. Miller.)*

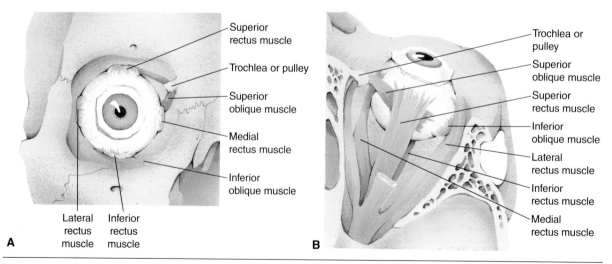

Figure 9.1 Anatomy of the extraocular muscles. **A.** Front view. **B.** View from above. *(Modified, with permission, from Jordan DR, et al. Ophthalmology Monographs 9: Surgical Anatomy of the Ocular Andexa, San Francisco: American Academy of Ophthalmology, 1996.)*

Table 9.1 Selected Actions of the Extraocular Muscles

Extraocular Muscle	1°	2°	3°
Medial rectus	Adduction	—	—
Lateral rectus	Abduction	—	—
Inferior rectus	Depression	Excyclotorsion	Adduction
Superior rectus	Elevation	Incyclotorsion	Adduction
Inferior oblique	Excyclotorsion	Elevation	Abduction
Superior oblique	Incyclotorsion	Depression	Abduction

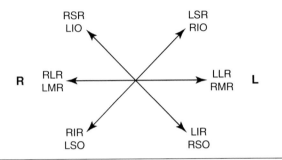

Figure 9.3 Cardinal positions of gaze and yoke muscles. RSR, right superior rectus; LIO, left inferior oblique; LSR, left superior rectus; RIO, right inferior oblique; RLR, right lateral rectus; LMR, left medial rectus; LLR, left lateral rectus; RMR, right medial rectus; RIR, right inferior rectus; LSO, left superior oblique; LIR, left inferior rectus; RSO, right superior oblique. *(Reprinted, with permission, from Wilson FM II, Blomquist PH,* Practical Ophthalmology, *6th ed, San Francisco: American Academy of Ophthalmology, 2009.)*

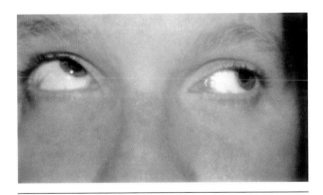

Figure 9.4 Overaction of the right inferior oblique muscle. *(Reprinted, with permission, from Basic and Clinical Science Course: Section 6,* Pediatric Ophthalmology, *San Francisco: American Academy of Ophthalmology, 2001–2002.)*

overacting right inferior oblique or its yoke, an underacting left superior rectus muscle, is causing the imbalance. By occluding one and then the other of the patient's eyes and observing each eye's movements separately, the examiner can determine the underlying abnormality. In this example, the right inferior oblique is elevating the right eye while the movements of the left eye are normal.

Nerve Control

The brainstem part of the brain coordinates movements throughout the body. There are 12 cranial nerves that extend from the brainstem to different parts of the body to control their actions. Three cranial nerves extend from the brainstem to the 6 extraocular muscles to power (stimulate) them (Figure 9.5). The **oculomotor or third cranial nerve** powers the superior rectus, inferior rectus, medial rectus and inferior oblique muscles. The **trochlear or fourth cranial nerve** powers the superior oblique muscle and the **abducens or sixth cranial nerve** powers the lateral rectus muscle. Unlike the trochlear and abducens nerves, the oculomotor nerve also powers the levator palpebral muscle that lifts the eyelid and connects also to an iris muscle that constricts the pupil. There is a complex interplay of nerve impulses that coordinate eye movements. Areas in the brainstem regulate **the distribution of power** to *yoke muscles* so that the right medial rectus muscle (cranial nerve III) and the left lateral rectus muscle (cranial nerve VI) are afforded equal nerve supply power to move the eyes smoothly and simultaneously to the left.

Eye Movements

Brainstem eye movement centers control smooth and equal movement of both eyes in both conjugate and disconjugate directions. When both eyes move in the same direction, the movements are said to be **conjugate**. Thus, when both eyes move to the left, a conjugate movement is taking place. **Disconjugate** eye movements are simultaneous movements of both eyes in opposite directions. The most important disconjugate movement is **convergence**, which occurs when both eyes move inward. It is used to align the eyes in near gaze and, as such, is a normal form of eye alignment.

Abnormal eye alignments, or **strabismus**, can be either comitant or incomitant. **Comitant** eye misalignments are constant in all fields of gaze. Most childhood

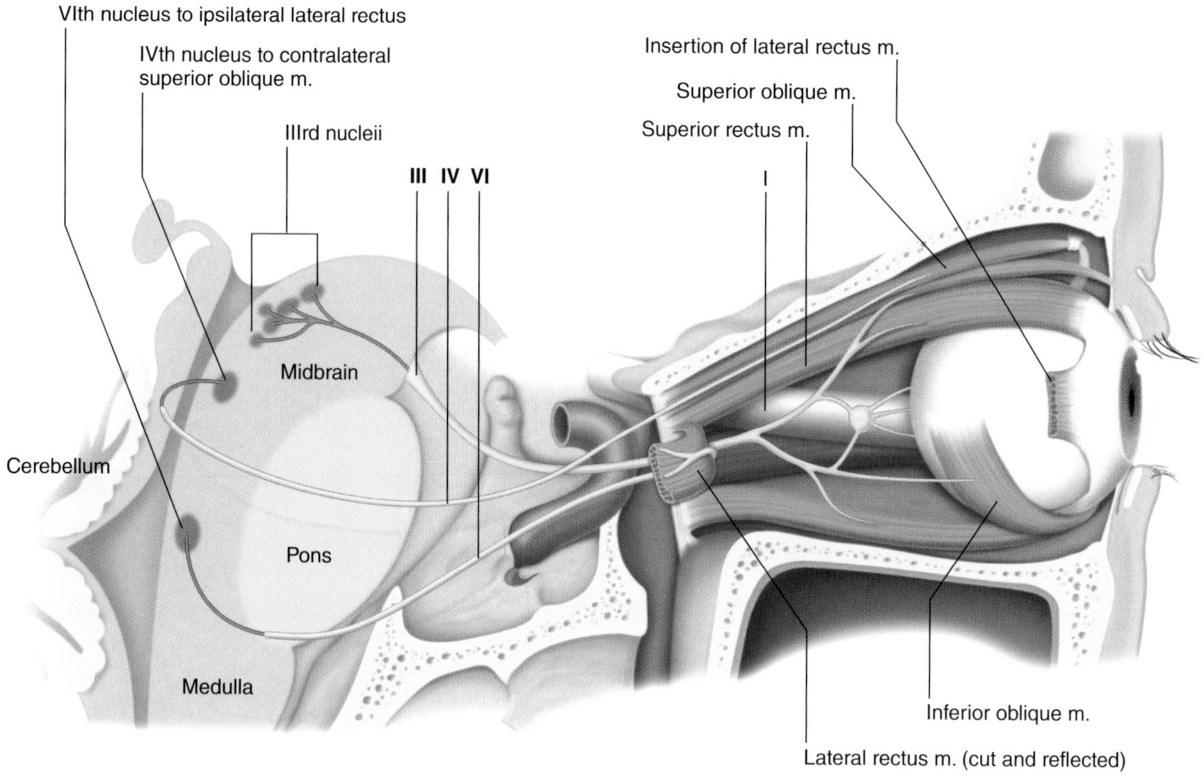

Figure 9.5 Brainstem anatomy of the cranial nerves involved in eye movement. *(Illustration by Mark M. Miller. Modified, with permission, from Yanoff M, et al, Ophthalmology, 2nd ed, New York: Elsevier; 2003:1324.)*

forms of strabismus are comitant. **Incomitant** eye misalignments have different amounts of deviation in different fields of gaze. They commonly arise from neurologic or mechanical problems. Strabismus is characterized as **eso-** (the eyes go in), **exo-** (the eyes go out), **hypo-** (one eye goes down) or **hyper-** (one eye goes up). Figure 9.6 illustrates types of strabismus. The condition can be **manifest**, consistently present, or **latent**, present only when fixation is interrupted. So, a person with a consistently in-turned eye (**esotropia**) would be said to have a manifest deviation. If that in-turning was not present under normal circumstances, but was brought out in the course of the examination by preventing both eyes from fixating on a target at the same time, that strabismus or abnormal eye alignment would be called an **esophoria** and considered a latent deviation. Hence, all tropias are manifest deviations and all phorias are latent deviations.

Motility Examination

The motility examination begins with observation of eye movements. The examiner holds a dim light or an interesting object, such as a toy (for a pediatric examination), in front of the patient. The examiner's finger can also be used as a fixation device, but it is less interesting for children. The general rule for examining children is "one look, one toy" as they lose interest quickly. Never use a bright light source for fixation as it is irritating to the patient. If you must use a light source, blunt the brightness by covering it with a finger or filter. See Procedure 9.1 for details.

Strabismus Tests

Eye movement deviations are assessed by strabismus testing. The primary tests used to evaluate eye movement abnormalities are **corneal light reflex** observation and cover testing. Corneal light reflex observations are rudimentary strabismus tests. They do not provide as much information as cover testing, but are easier to use and require less cooperation on the part of the patient. The Hirschberg and Krimsky corneal light tests use a light source that reflects off the cornea, producing the corneal light reflex.

Corneal Light Tests

The **Hirschberg test** involves observing the position of the corneal light reflex relative to the pupil. If the corneal light reflexes are centered in both pupils, the eyes are

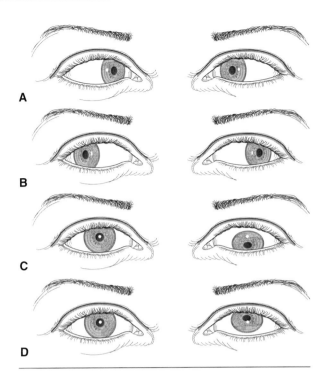

Figure 9.6 Types of strabismus. **A.** Esotropia.
B. Exotropia. **C.** Left hypotropia (right hypertropia). **D.** Left
hypertropia (right hypotropia). *(Illustration by Mark M. Miller.)*

Procedure 9.1 Conducting a Motility Examination

1. The motility examination begins with observation of eye movements. The examiner holds a dim light or an interesting object, such as a toy (for a pediatric examination), in front of the patient.

2. Instruct the patient to follow the object with his or her eyes while holding the head still.

3. Move the object into the 6 cardinal positions while observing the eye movements. If eye movements are normal in observed versions, there is no need to observe ductions.

4. If the versions are abnormal, ductions must be tested to determine the abnormal muscle. In this case, occlude one eye and direct the patient to move the other eye into the 6 cardinal positions (this is an observation of monocular eye movements). Test the other eye in the same manner.

---

aligned (Figure 9.7). If the light reflex is temporally displaced in one pupil, there is an esodeviation. If the light reflex is nasally displaced, there is an exodeviation. The light source provides a constant light reflex (reflection) off each cornea. If both eyes are aligned, that constant

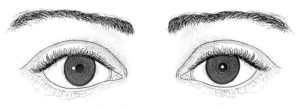

Figure 9.7 Hirschberg corneal reflex test. Every 1 mm displacement of the light reflex from proper position is estimated to represent 7° degrees on a round globe and equal to 15 prism diopters of deviation. *(Illustration by Mark M. Miller.)*

reflex should be centered in each pupil. However, if one eye is turned in, that reflex will rest on the outer part of the pupil and will be temporally displaced. If one eye is out-turned, its light reflex will land on the inner aspect of the pupil and appear nasally displaced.

The **Krimsky test** uses prisms to "balance" the light reflexes in the center of the pupils to more accurately measure the deviation (Figure 9.8). One observes the corneal light reflex. If one reflex is nasally or temporally displaced, a prism is placed over that eye in the appropriate direction to bring the displaced light reflex to the center of the pupil. The amount of prism that it takes to realign the light reflexes is a measurement of the deviation of the eye.

Cover Tests

Both corneal light reflex tests can be confounded by misshapen pupils and by abnormal retinal architecture. Because of this, cover testing is used whenever possible to assess strabismus.

COVER-UNCOVER TESTING   This kind of test involves the use of an occluder to cover one eye and thereby disrupt its fixation. The examiner then observes fixation and refixation behavior to determine if there is a strabismus. See Procedure 9.2 for details.

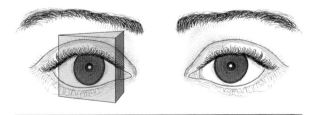

Figure 9.8 Krimsky test. Prism is placed in front of the deviating eye to correct the deviation of the corneal light reflex. The strabismus measurement is equal to the amount of prism necessary to center the corneal light reflex on the pupil of the deviating eye. *(Illustration by Mark M. Miller.)*

Procedure 9.2 Performing the Cover-Uncover Test

1. The cover-uncover test is used initially to assess eye misalignment. First, ask the patient to fix his or her gaze on a distant target as you observe both eyes open (Figure A). The distant target is usually a letter or line on the Snellen chart that is several lines above the smallest line that the patient can read.

2. To test the right eye, cover the left eye with an occluder and observe the uncovered eye for any movements (Figure B). The occluded eye is then observed for refixation movements as the occluder is removed (Figure C). This can be repeated several times for accuracy.

3. Then occlude the other eye and again watch for eye movement as the occluder is removed (Figure D).

4. Repeat the test in the up, down, in and out positions.

5. Test the patient while fixating a near target and repeat steps 2 to 4. If covering either eye produces a refixation movement, a **tropia**, or manifest deviation, is present.

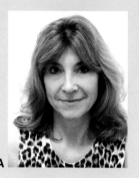 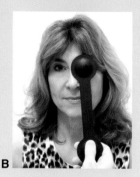 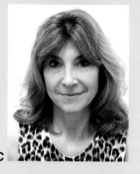 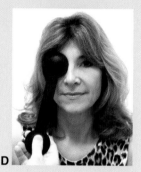

A   B   C   D

(Images courtesy of Tina Newmark, RN, MS.)

ALTERNATE COVER TEST If there is no movement observed in the cover-uncover test, then an **alternate cover test** is performed to detect a **phoria**, or latent deviation. Phorias are usually controlled by the patient's normal fusional ability. As long as both eyes are open and fixating on a target, the eyes are straight. However, when binocular fusion is disrupted, the eyes drift in or out or up or down. The alternate cover test disrupts the patient's ability to fuse by not allowing them to use both eyes at the same time. It is used after the cover-uncover test as it does not distinguish between a tropia and phoria. See Procedure 9.3 for details.

PRISM AND ALTERNATE COVER TEST When a strabismus is detected, the **prism and alternate cover test** is used to quantitate the amount of deviation. This test is basically an alternate cover test with prisms. The amount of prism necessary to neutralize an abnormal alignment is the measure of that deviation in **prism diopters**. A prism diopter is the unit of measurement of the refractive power of a prism. See Procedure 9.4 for details.

Additional Tests

Evaluation of eye alignment is an important component of the comprehensive eye examination. Strabismus prevents **fusion**, the ability of the brain to merge the 2 images received from each eye into a single binocular image. Adults complain of double vision (**diplopia**) when their fusion is disrupted. For example, the adult who develops a left sixth nerve palsy will note diplopia when she looks to the left, the field of action of the left lateral rectus muscle.

Children do not usually complain of diplopia because they have a compensatory mechanism available due to their developing brains. Young children can ignore the second image with an abnormal alignment preventing diplopia. The brain loses this ability to ignore an image as it matures and becomes less adaptable, so older children and adults cannot ignore or suppress the second image and therefore complain of diplopia. This brain mechanism is called **suppression**. Young children are also at risk of developing decreased vision due to visual deprivation called **amblyopia**. Decreased depth perception (**stereopsis**) can also develop from strabismus as the immature brains of children require stimulation from aligned eyes for their visual centers to develop normally. Depth perception requires good vision in both eyes. A child's inability to perceive an object in a 3-dimensional environment can be impaired directly from strabismus and indirectly from amblyopia.

Amblyopia, loss of vision in one or both eyes because of lack of visual stimulation of the developing brain, is

Procedure 9.3 Performing the Alternate Cover Test

1. The alternate cover test begins in the same manner as a cover-uncover test (Procedure 9.2). First, instruct the patient to fixate on a distant target.

2. Occlude one eye and observe movements in the uncovered eye (Figure A).

3. Slowly move the occluder to the other eye (Figures B and C). Slowness of movement is essential so that one eye is occluded before the other eye fully emerges from behind the occluder.

In this manner, the patient's ability to fuse latent deviations is disrupted.

4. Note any refixation movements.

5. Move the occluder back and forth between both eyes several times for accuracy of observation. Sometimes, the deviation may even become more apparent over several occlusions as the patient's ability to fuse is further disrupted.

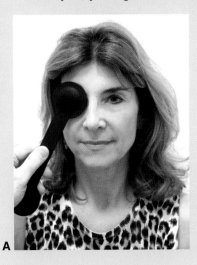
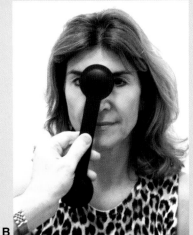
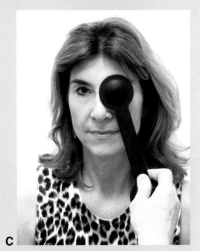

A   B   C

(Images courtesy of Tina Newmark, RN, MS.)

Procedure 9.4 Performing the Prism and Alternate Cover Test

1. When a strabismus is detected, the prism and alternate cover test is used to quantitate the amount of deviation. This test is basically an alternate cover test with prisms. First, ask the patient to fixate on a distant target.

2. Occlude one eye.

3. Observe refixation movements as you move the occluder back and forth in the manner of the alternate cover test.

4. An abnormal alignment is measured by standardized prisms with increasing degrees of power. Place a corrective prism in front of the deviated eye (figure). This will alter the apparent position of the fixation target, decreasing the amount of refixation movement necessary.

5. Adjust the amount of prism to the point where there is no refixation movement. When that happens, the strabismus is said to be "neutralized."

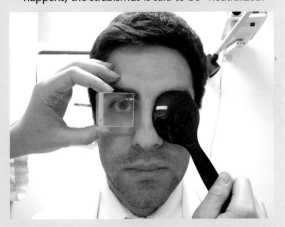

(Image courtesy of JoAnn A. Giaconi, MD.)

detected by visual acuity measurement. The techniques of visual acuity testing have been covered in other sections of this book. **Suppression**, a compensatory mechanism seen in young children when fusion is disrupted, can be measured by several different sensory tests.

WORTH 4-DOT TEST   This test is commonly used to assess fusion, diplopia and suppression. Several tests of depth perception are also available. See Procedure 9.5 for a description of the Worth 4-dot test.

STEREO ACUITY TEST   Stereo acuity testing is also part of the ocular motility examination in that the most refined degree of depth perception requires fusion. Poor vision in one or both eyes, suppression and diplopia all contribute to reduce the degree of stereopsis. Several screening tests for stereo acuity are commercially available, such as the **Titmus stereopsis test**, a simple screening test of depth perception. See Procedure 9.6 for a description of the Titmus test.

Summary

The evaluation of ocular motility involves several tests that require a certain level of skill in their execution. Attention to proper technique minimizes inaccurate results. Practice is important to maintain proficiency in performing these tests. The skilled performance of these tests contributes greatly to our knowledge of the patient's visual status.

Procedure 9.5 Performing the Worth 4-Dot Test

1. The Worth 4-dot test is commonly used to assess fusion, diplopia and suppression. The test involves an illuminated target and a pair of modified eyeglasses (figure). The flashlight target has 4 lighted dots: 1 white, 1 red and 2 green. The eyeglasses have a red filter on the right side and a green filter on the other side.

2. The patient wears the spectacles and views the 4-dot target. In this configuration, the right eye will see 2 red dots, the left eye will see 3 green dots.

   Patients capable of fusion will fuse the 2 images and report a total of 4 dots, with the fourth white dot perceived as either green or red. Sometimes it is perceived as alternating between red and green. Either way, the patient sees only 4 dots because he or she is "fusing" the white dot with both eyes.

   Patients with suppression will report either 2 dots (left eye suppression) or 3 dots (right eye suppression). Suppression causes the brain to ignore images from one eye. Therefore, patients with suppression will only see the dots with the nonsuppressed eye.

3. Five dots is the diplopic or double vision response unless the patient has alternating suppression. To distinguish between diplopia and alternating suppression, ask the patient if all 5 dots are seen simultaneously. A person with rapidly alternating suppression will see 3 then 2 then 3 then 2 dots.

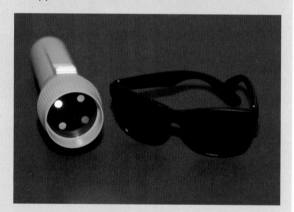

(Image courtesy of Brice Critser, CRA, Department of Ophthalmology and Visual Sciences, University of Iowa.)

Procedure 9.6 Performing the Titmus Test

The Titmus stereopsis test is a commonly used screening device for depth perception. It consists of a pair of light-polarizing spectacles and a booklet of stereo photographs (Figure A).

Each stereo photograph is actually 2 superimposed images that are polarized 90° degrees to one another. In some parts of the photographs the images are horizontally displaced. When the patient wears spectacles with polarizing filters, those horizontally displaced parts of the photographs appear to come forward off the page.

Basic Assessment

1. The patient wears the polarized spectacles and views the stereo photos at reading distance under good lighting conditions. With the current popularity of 3-dimensional movies, most patients understand the concept of depth perception and perform the test easily. However, some patients have to be instructed in how to recognize depth.

2. To help the patient understand the concept of depth perception, turn to the large stereo picture of a house fly on the inside cover of the Titmus testing book (Figure B). Show the patient the large photo of the fly and ask him or her to grasp the fly's wings. With the special polarizing spectacles the wings of this fly are normally seen to be coming forward in front of the plane of the page. This picture represents a gross degree of fusion or stereopsis. Fusing patients will grasp the wings several inches above the page. This will clue them into the desired response on the tests of finer degrees of stereoacuity.

3. If the patient has difficulty recognizing depth, ask if the image is flat or has a 3-D appearance. If the image is flat, the patient does not have stereopsis and the result is recorded as *fly negative*.

Assessing Finer Degrees of Depth Perception

1. If the patient does recognize depth, the finer degrees of depth perception can be quantified in the next section of the Titmus test plates. For young children, use the animal pictures; for adults, use the circle figures.

2. If working with children, ask the child to identify the animal that comes forward in each of the 3 columns of animals. Each column tests increasingly finer levels of stereopsis. If all the forward-appearing animals are successfully identified the result is recorded as *3/3*.

3. In the adult section, 9 groups of diamonds containing 4 circles each are tested. In each diamond of 4 circles, one circle is "raised" relative to the other 3. Again, the descending diamonds of circles test increasingly finer levels of stereopsis. The finest diamond wherein one circle can be correctly identified as raised represents the stereo acuity measurement of that patient. An individual with normal stereo acuity should be able to identify all 9 groups and is usually recorded as *9/9*.

4. Adequate lighting is important in optimizing performance on this test. A good reading light should be used. The examiner should hold the plates. The patient should not be allowed to jiggle the test plates as this can confound the results. Because the horizontal disparity is obvious in the first 3 groups of circles, these monocular clues to depth can also confound the results. Random-dot stereopsis tests resolve this problem by embedding the stereo figures in a background of random dots that disguise the horizontal disparities.

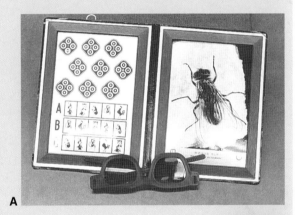

A

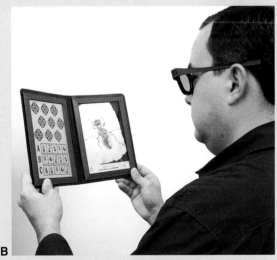

B

(Reprinted, with permission, from Wilson FM II, Blomquist PH, Practical Ophthalmology, 6th ed, San Francisco: American Academy of Ophthalmology, 2009.)

SELF-ASSESSMENT TEST

1. Name the 6 extraocular muscles and their primary actions.

2. What are the 6 cardinal positions of gaze?

3. How does the observation of ductions and versions differ?

4. Define *suppression.*

5. Define *amblyopia.*

6. What are the limitations of strabismus assessment with corneal light reflex testing?

7. Which cover test is performed first and why?

8. What is the name of the cover test that measures the amount of strabismus deviation?

9. What does the Worth 4-dot test assess?

10. What does the Titmus test assess?

SUGGESTED ACTIVITIES

1. Practice the observation of eye movements with your coworkers. Observe how the eyes move smoothly and symmetrically into the cardinal positions of gaze. Occlude one eye of the patient and then the other to practice observation of ductions.

2. Have one of your coworkers perform a Worth 4-dot test on you. Perform the test with both eyes open and observe how the fourth (white) dot can be either red or green or alternate between the 2 colors. Then close the right eye and observe how some dots disappear—you should see 3 dots. Open the right eye and close the left eye and observe how the number of dots that you see changes to 2. Open both eyes and place a large prism in front of one eye so that you can appreciate the double vision response of 5 dots. After that exercise practice the performance of the Worth 4-dot test on coworkers until you feel comfortable with its execution.

3. Have one of your coworkers perform the Titmus test on you with appropriate technique. Then remove the polarizing spectacles and observe the plates for stereoscopic cues. Note how the grosser measures of stereopsis have significant horizontal disparity. Then don the polarizing spectacles and perform the test with varying degrees of room lighting. Observe how your stereopsis degrades with poor lighting. After that exercise, perform the Titmus test on coworkers until you feel confident in its execution.

4. Observe the corneal light reflexes on coworkers. Place prisms in front of one eye and note how this changes the position of the light reflex relative to the pupil.

5. Practice cover testing on coworkers. Have your ophthalmologist or supervisor observe your technique.

6. Ask your ophthalmologist or supervisor to allow you to observe the motility examination of a patient with strabismus.

SUGGESTED RESOURCES

Cassin B, ed. *Fundamentals for Ophthalmic Technical Personnel*. Philadelphia: Saunders; 1995.

DuBois LG. Ocular motility. In: *Fundamentals of Ophthalmic Medical Assisting*. DVD. San Francisco: American Academy of Ophthalmology; 2009.

Ledford JK. *Handbook of Clinical Ophthalmology for Eyecare Professionals*. Thorofare, NJ; 2000.

Stein HA, Stein RM, Freeman MI. *The Ophthalmic Assistant: A Text for Allied and Associated Ophthalmic Personnel*. 8th ed. St Louis: Mosby; 2006.

vonNoorden GK, Campos EC. *Binocular Vision and Ocular Motility*. http://telemedicine.orbis.org. Accessed July 12, 2011.

Wilson ME Jr. Ocular motility evaluation of strabismus and myasthenia gravis. In: *Strabismus Evaluation and Surgery*. DVD. San Francisco: American Academy of Ophthalmology; 1993. Reviewed for currency: 2007.

10 ADJUNCTIVE TESTS AND PROCEDURES

Basic assessment and testing of the eye in 8 principal areas make up a comprehensive medical eye examination. The results of these basic assessments may reveal a deficiency or an ophthalmic condition that requires additional tests to determine the exact diagnosis and treatment. Dozens of adjunctive (additional) tests and procedures are available to complement the comprehensive eye examination. Ophthalmologists can perform the procedures, but many of these tests are delegated to the ophthalmic medical assistant.

This chapter describes several of the most common specialized adjunctive tests and procedures in 4 principal categories: (1) assessments of potential visual acuity and functional vision in patients with media opacities; (2) tests for corneal structure and disease; (3) photography of the external eye and fundus; and (4) ultrasonography. Most of the tests require the use of technical equipment; all of them require training, skill, and experience to be performed competently. For this reason, the ophthalmologist delegates the tests to an experienced technician and not to a novice ophthalmic medical assistant. Nevertheless, novice ophthalmic medical assistants should understand the nature and purpose of these tests in order to increase their effectiveness as members of the office team and to take the first step toward becoming skilled performers of these adjunctive procedures.

Vision Tests for Patients With Opacities

The term **ocular media** refers to the eye's transparent optical structures that transmit light: cornea, lens, and vitreous. **Media opacities** is the general term used to describe a variety of conditions that cloud, obscure, or otherwise affect these structures and may, ultimately, disrupt vision. The principal media opacities affect the lens (cataracts) and the cornea (edema or scars).

Patients with cataracts or cloudy corneas due to a variety of conditions may not have perfectly clear vision, but they are rarely significantly impaired because the other visual structures of the eye (eg, the retina) are normal.

Treatments such as cataract removal surgery with intra-ocular lens (IOL) implantation or corneal transplantation can often restore vision to an excellent functional level. Also low vision optical aids can often enhance vision to an adequate functional level.

Visual Potential Tests

Various testing procedures are used to determine the potential visual status of a patient with media opacity. The test results help the ophthalmologist determine the extent to which surgery or other types of therapy may potentially improve the patient's vision. With information about a patient's visual potential, the ophthalmologist can recommend the most appropriate treatment. In general, testing for visual acuity potential uses methods that essentially bypass the opacity, to measure the visual abilities of the retina and optic nerve. The result of this type of visual acuity testing provides information about the integrity of the visual system and about whether the vision will improve if the opacity is removed.

Four devices presently in use are the potential acuity meter, the occluder and pinhole, the interferometer, and the retinal acuity meter.

POTENTIAL ACUITY METER An older testing device in the presence of media opacities is the potential acuity meter (PAM). This device projects a brightly lighted miniaturized Snellen acuity chart through the least dense area of opacity onto the patient's retina (Figure 10.1). The advantage of this device is the familiar testing format. The patient is asked to read the chart just as he or she would do during standard vision testing. The disadvantage includes the need for the tester to find a clear "window" in the opacity to project the chart, and any movement by the patient may obscure that image. The PAM may not work well with dense media opacities. This device is no longer being produced.

OCCLUDER AND PINHOLE The pinhole acuity potential (PAP) test can help determine macular function in patients with opacities. In this test, the patient's pupils are dilated with eyedrops and the patient looks through pinholes in an opaque disc held before the eye (see Figure 8.5) at a near acuity chart illuminated by a Finoff light. By moving the pinhole disc around, the patient may be able to find tiny clearer areas in his or her cataract or corneal opacity through which potential vision can be assessed. Patients with a keen sense of awareness seem to be better candidates for this test.

INTERFEROMETER The interferometer uses the laser or other special light beams to determine visual acuity in

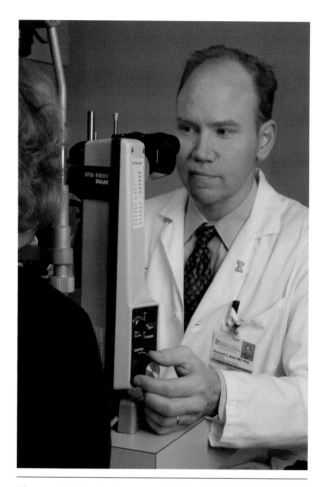

Figure 10.1 Testing with a potential acuity meter (PAM). *(Image courtesy of Brice Critser, CRA, Department of Ophthalmology and Visual Sciences, University of Iowa.)*

the presence of opacity such as a cataract (Figure 10.2). Sometimes attached to the slit lamp, this instrument measures visual acuity subjectively by projecting a target made up of parallel lines, through the least dense part of the opacity, onto the patient's macula. The targets vary in size, separation, and orientation of the lines. The patient is asked to report the orientation of the lines, and visual acuity is measured by the smallest separation of lines whose orientation is reported correctly.

RETINAL ACUITY METER The retinal acuity meter is a handheld, battery-powered device about the size of a digital camera. It consists of a brightly illuminated near card with Snellen letters or alternate symbols. The test measures the retinal acuity in eyes with opacities or a maculopathy. The illumination card is used in conjunction with a multiple pinhole frame at 40 cm or 16 inches and a near correction lens. Both patients and ophthalmic assistants find this device easy to use. It is commercially available and trademarked by AMA Optics (Miami Beach, Florida) as the RAM®.

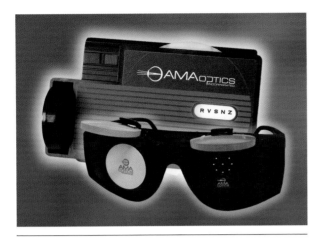

Figure 10.2 A retinal acuity meter. *(Image courtesy of AMA Optics, Inc.)*

Contrast-Sensitivity and Glare Tests

To perceive objects visually, some contrast of dark and light must be present between the object and its surroundings. Obviously, no one can see any object in absolute darkness. But even in dense fog or deep twilight, shapes at least can be discerned by their relative lightness and darkness. This ability of human vision is called *contrast sensitivity*.

Even if a patient's Snellen visual acuity is sharp, a cataract, corneal opacity, or some other disease can reduce an individual's contrast sensitivity. In these medical conditions, vision can become somewhat like viewing objects in fog or twilight. The **contrast-sensitivity test** is useful in determining whether a patient's visual complaints are caused by cataract, especially if the patient has shown good Snellen acuity. This testing method establishes an alteration in the patient's *functional vision* and aids the physician in determining the need for cataract surgery.

The simplest contrast-sensitivity test presents the patient with a printed chart showing letters or symbols in a faint gray print rather than the usual sharp, black-on-white characters of standard charts (Figure 10.3). Other types of charts exist for contrast-sensitivity testing as well as more technical methods involving the presentation of graded patterns or letters on an oscilloscope screen.

Glare can cause one's vision to be disturbed

and can also actually be painful.

Glare occurs when light from a single bright source, such as the sun or an automobile headlight, scatters across the entire visual field. Such scattering of light often dazzles the sight and markedly reduces the quality

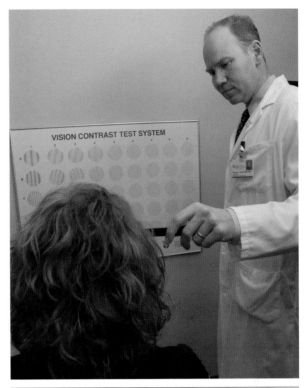

Figure 10.3 Contrast-sensitivity testing. *(Image courtesy of Brice Critser, CRA, Department of Ophthalmology and Visual Sciences, University of Iowa.)*

of image received by the retina. This phenomenon is easily demonstrated by driving toward the sun in a car with a dirty windshield.

Patients with cataracts or other ocular opacities often experience this type of optical disturbance. **Glare testing** assesses the patient's vision in the presence of a bright light to determine if sensitivity to glare is contributing to a patient's visual symptoms (Figure 10.4).

There are several methods of assessing glare disability. In all cases, the best corrected vision is determined in a darkened room, and then the vision is tested again while some device is used to introduce bright light from the periphery. Many autorefractors have built-in glare-testing capability. The simplest means of introducing glare is with a transilluminator (a small-tipped flashlight) held pointing into the eye from below at a 10° to 30° angle.

A common device is the **brightness acuity tester** (BAT). This instrument has a small cup with a hole, through which the patient views the standard eye chart. When the cup is illuminated, light surrounds the eye. Three settings simulate varying lighting conditions. A low setting simulates a brightly lit room; a medium setting, outdoor sunlight; and a high setting, sunlight reflected off concrete, beach sand, or water. Most patients with glare complaints will have a significant decrease in vision on medium intensity.

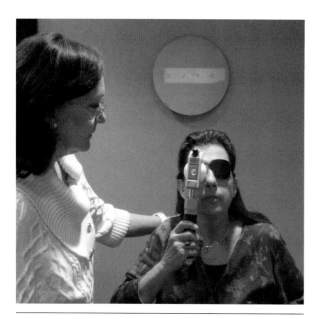

Figure 10.4 Glare testing.

Assessment of Corneal Abnormalities

Three tests for corneal abnormalities are commonly used: *pachymetry* measures corneal thickness; *corneal topography* maps the curvature of the cornea; and *specular microscopy/photography* allows the cells of the endothelial layer to be counted.

Pachymetry

The normal cornea is about 0.55 millimeters (mm) or 550 micrometers (1000th of a mm, noted with the symbol μm) thick at the center and about 1.00 mm thick at its outer edge. Several diseases, especially some inherited ophthalmic disorders called *corneal dystrophies*, create swelling and thickening of the cornea. The cornea then becomes cloudy, leading to visual disturbance.

Pachymetry (sometimes spelled *pachometry*) is a procedure for measuring corneal thickness. Pachymetry can help determine the extent of corneal dystrophies, allowing the ophthalmologist to provide timely treatment of the patient's symptoms. Pachymetry may be performed before cataract surgery and other surgical procedures to help estimate the cornea's ability to withstand the stress of an operation. Pachymetry is also being performed on glaucoma patients, and those suspected of developing glaucoma, to ensure accurate interpretation of their intraocular pressure readings. With commonly used applanation tonometers, above- or below-average corneal thickness affects the readings of intraocular pressure. A thicker-than-normal cornea creates an artificially

high pressure reading, and a thinner-than-normal cornea creates an artificially low pressure reading.

Optical pachymeters attach to the slit lamp and operate on optical principles to measure the distance between the epithelium (front or outer layer of cells) and the endothelium (back or inner layer of cells) of the cornea. **Ultrasonic pachymeters**, which use reflected sound waves to measure corneal thickness, are used more commonly (Figure 10.5). Ultrasonic pachymeters may include corneal mapping display programs, which are used to provide information about the potential and actual results of refractive surgery procedures. Some ultrasonic probes are hard-wired to a tabletop instrument, and others are pen-like and portable.

Corneal Topography

Corneal topography provides detailed information concerning the corneal curvature. It involves the use of a special camera that photographs a projected pattern of concentric lighted rings (Placido disk) onto the corneal epithelial surface. The distortions of the reflected rings are analyzed to produce a detailed map of the corneal curvature (power), showing steeper and flatter areas and irregularities (Figure 10.6). This information is used in calculations before refractive or other procedures that will potentially change the shape of the cornea. In addition, the test is useful for diagnosis and management of corneal disorders and transplants and the fitting of complex contact lenses. The Pentacam camera (Oculus, Lynnwood, Washington) can also be used to determine corneal topography by employing an alternate optical principle. The Pentacam camera can also determine the depth of the anterior chamber, corneal power, topography of the lens, and the density level of a corneal opacity.

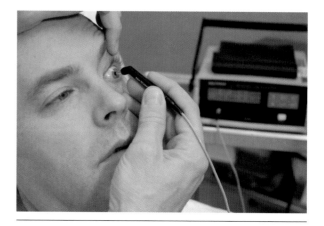

Figure 10.5 Ultrasonic pachymetry. *(Image courtesy of Brice Critser, CRA, Department of Ophthalmology and Visual Sciences, University of Iowa.)*

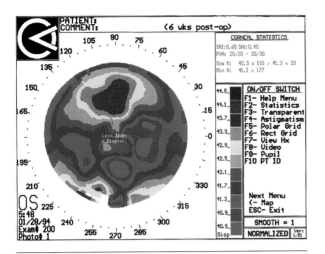

Figure 10.6 Corneal topography map showing a cornea needing additional refractive surgical correction.

Specular Microscopy/Photography

The cells of the corneal endothelium act as a pump to regulate the amount of fluid in the corneal layers, thereby maintaining the corneal clarity necessary for proper focusing of light rays. The number of cells in the endothelium serves as an important indicator of the health of the cornea. Too few, enlarged, or irregular endothelial cells can indicate the presence of disease and also may affect the ability of the cornea to withstand certain intraocular surgical procedures.

Specular microscopy/photography is a method of microscopically photographing the cornea's endothelial cells at great magnification and producing photographs from which the cells can be counted. Special slit-lamp attachments may be used to produce still photographs, or a video camera may be used to record and display the cells on a video screen. An image can be taken of the video screen to serve as a permanent part of the patient's medical record (Figure 10.7). Magnification of the photographs allows the cells to be counted visually and assists the surgeon in determining a treatment plan.

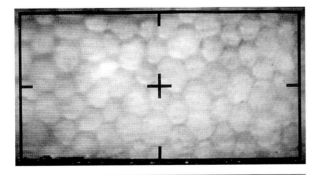

Figure 10.7 Specular photograph showing normal endothelial cells.

Ophthalmic Photography

Ophthalmic photography serves to document and diagnose ophthalmic conditions. Some knowledge of photography is required to perform most of these procedures, but a few highly automated photographic devices can be operated effectively, at least in part, by the ophthalmic medical assistant with a minimum of training.

The three general types of ophthalmic photography are *external photography*, *slit-lamp photography*, and *fundus photography*. All of these techniques use digital camera bodies. Color fundus images can be converted to color prints from digital format. Fluorescein or indocyanine green angiography uses digital format capability.

External Photography

External photography of the eye aids in documenting abnormalities of the eye's outer structures (eg, an eyelid tumor) that do not need high magnification to be seen. This method requires only a digital camera equipped with a close-up lens and electronic flash attachment.

Slit-Lamp Photography

A digital camera can be attached to the slit lamp to produce photographs that document abnormalities of the cornea, angle structures, iris, and lens (Figure 10.8). The optics of the slit lamp replaces the camera's normal lens, serving as a viewing and focusing system and providing the necessary magnification of these structures. The slit beam can be used to help determine the depth of a lesion within these structures.

Fundus Photography

Fundus photography encompasses the use of a fundus digital camera to take color images of the retina and optic nerve for future comparisons and to produce black-and-white images during fluorescein and indocyanine green angiography.

The modern **fundus camera** is, in effect, a large ophthalmoscope that can produce color images of the retina and optic nerve (Figure 10.9). A fundus camera consists of an optical system for viewing the retina, a light/flash system for illumination, and a digital camera. In order to allow the photographer the most encompassing view of the fundus, patients receive dilating eyedrops to enlarge the pupil before fundus photography.

Performed with the fundus camera, **fluorescein** and **indocyanine green angiography** makes it possible to view detail in blood vessels of the ocular fundus and

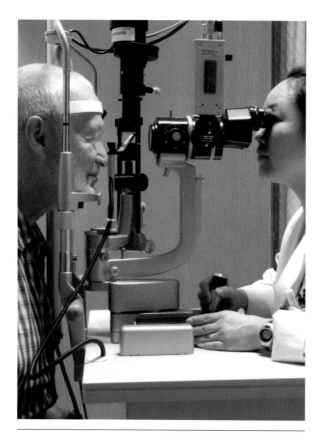

Figure 10.8 Slit-lamp photography of the anterior segment of the eye. *(Image courtesy of Tina Newmark, RN, MS.)*

occasionally the iris (Figure 10.10). In this procedure, a fluorescent dye solution of fluorescein or indocyanine green is injected into a vein in the patient's arm. The vascular system quickly delivers the dye to the ocular blood vessels. The fundus camera, equipped with special filters, highlights the dye as it courses through the vessels and finally fills the entire vascular tree. The images are taken in rapid sequence, thereby capturing the appearance of

the vessels at recorded time intervals. The images taken in this manner are called *fluorescein angiograms* or *indocyanine green angiograms*. **Fluorescein** dye is used for most routine angiograms. Indocyanine green dye is more specialized and is particularly used in studying the choroidal circulation and also when an overlying hemorrhage or exudate obscures the visibility of the choroidal vessels. The common abnormalities detected with fundus angiography include the presence of vascular obstructions, leakage, and **neovascularization** (the abnormal growth of new blood vessels).

Fluorescein dye can cause the patient to have momentary nausea or, rarely, a severe allergic reaction. Indocyanine green dye is better tolerated than fluorescein but should be avoided in patients with iodine or shellfish allergies. A physician and emergency equipment should be on hand during fundus angiography employing intravenous dyes. For more information about common dyes for ophthalmic use, refer to Chapter 6.

Tomographic Imaging

Several tomography devices have been developed to allow detailed mapping and analysis of the contours of the anterior chamber angle, optic nerve, and retina.

Optical coherence tomography (OCT) is a noninvasive, noncontact technique for obtaining images of translucent or opaque tissues of the eye with a result equivalent to a low-power microscope. It is essentially an optical ultrasound using image reflections of uniform light from within tissue to provide a cross-sectional view.

OCT provides an image of ocular tissue structure at a much higher degree (>10 μm) than other imaging methods such as magnetic resonance imaging or ultrasound.

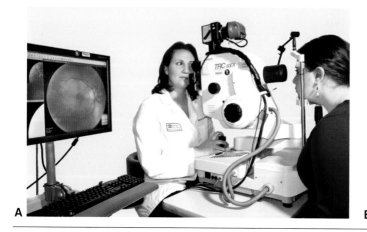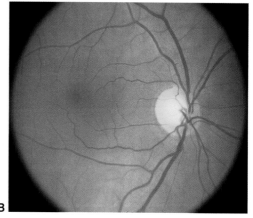

Figure 10.9 Retinal imaging. **A.** Fundus photography of the retina. **B.** Resulting photograph showing normal retina. *(Part A courtesy of National Eye Institute, National Institutes of Health.)*

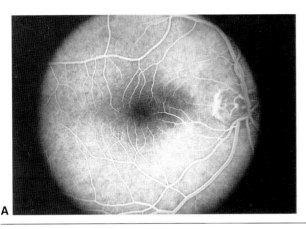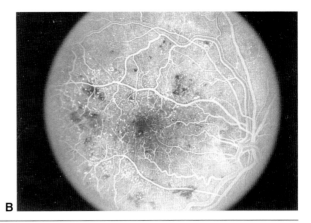

A

B

Figure 10.10 Fluorescein angiography. **A.** Fluorescein angiogram of a normal retina. **B.** Fluorescein angiogram of a diabetic patient. The numerous white dots are tiny outpouchings in abnormal capillaries (microaneurysms) that are filling up with dye.

The major components of an OCT system include a light source, a light detector, a beam splitter, and a movable mirror (Figure 10.11). A fundus camera may be included. There are several tomographic instruments commonly used, such as the Cirrus SD-OCT scanner (Carl Zeiss Meditec, Dublin, California), the Spectralis HRA+OCT system (Heidelberg Engineering, Carlsbad, California), and the OCT-2000 system (Topcon Medical Systems, Oakland, New Jersey). These instruments create 3-dimensional digital images of the anterior chamber angle, optic nerve and/or the retina. The digital data can be analyzed and compared to population-matched values or to previous images from the same patient. This data is particularly useful in glaucoma for evaluating the degree of change of the optic nerve, retinal ganglion cell layer, or retinal nerve fiber layer (RNFL) thickness. For retinal imaging, this technology captures superbly the presence of vitreoretinal, macular, and choroidal disorders

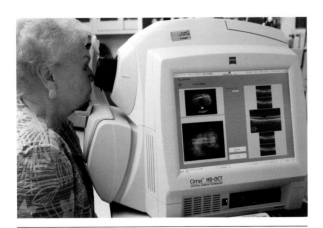

Figure 10.11 A detailed cross-sectional image of the back of the eye is obtained using an optical coherence tomography (OCT) system. *(Image courtesy of National Eye Institute, National Institutes of Health.)*

such as macular edema, drusen, vitreous traction, and macular holes. The image of the anterior chamber angle helps the ophthalmologist detect progressive narrowing of the angle in patients followed for anatomically narrow angles.

The GDxVCC scanning laser polarimeter with variable corneal compensation (Carl Zeiss Meditec) uses an alternate technology to analyze the RNFL and contour of the optic nerve head. It shines polarized light through the eye that is reflected off the retina. Because the RNFL splits the polarized light into two separate components, they can be independently captured by a detector and converted into a thickness measurement in micrometers.

Ultrasonography

Ophthalmic ultrasonography, or *biometry*, uses the reflection, or echo, of high-frequency sound waves to define the outlines of certain ocular and orbital structures and to measure the distance between structures. Ultrasonography also aids in detecting the presence of abnormalities such as tumors and in determining their size, composition, and position within the eye.

In an eye with dense media opacities, ultrasound may be the only nonsurgical method available to observe normal structures or tumors within the eye and to measure their relative or approximate position or their size. Ultrasound procedures are divided into two types: *A-scan ultrasonography* and *B-scan ultrasonography*.

A-Scan

A-scan (or **A-mode**) ultrasonography uses sound waves traveling in a straight line to reveal the position of and distances between structures within the eye and orbit.

This method is especially useful for measuring the **axial length of the globe**, a necessary value to properly calculate the power of an artificial intraocular lens (IOL). IOLs may be implanted into the eye either at the time of cataract extraction or later as a secondary surgery. Accurate and consistent measurements are extremely important, because small errors of measurement in axial length will produce large errors in the dioptric power of an IOL implant. About 0.30 mm of axial length inaccuracy results in 1 diopter of miscalculation. Consequently, the patient will have a postoperative hyperopic refractive error if the axial length measurement is erroneously too long and a myopic postoperative refractive error if the measurement is too short. Most patients expect to have a minimal need for glasses after cataract surgery, so an incorrect IOL calculation can result in an unhappy patient.

A-scan ultrasonography may be performed by placing the probe (handheld or attached to a slit lamp) directly on the eye (contact method) or into a fluid bath placed on the patient's eye (immersion method). The probe is connected to a device that delivers adjustable sound waves. The measurements are displayed as vertical spikes (peaks) on the screen of an **oscilloscope**, an instrument that determines the form of the wave. The appearance of the peaks and the distances between them can be correlated to structures within the eye and the distances between them (Figure 10.12).

B-Scan

B-scan (or **B-mode**) ultrasonography delivers radiating sound waves. This technique provides a 2-dimensional reconstruction of ocular and orbital tissues. B-scan ultrasonography is especially useful in detecting and measuring the size and position of tumors within the eye. It is also effective in providing an image of intraocular structures when media opacity interferes with the ophthalmologist's ability to view the interior of the eye.

As with A-scan ultrasonography, the B-scan method employs a probe tip that delivers sound waves when it is touched to the patient's eye. A gel must be used to eliminate air between the probe and the eye. The resulting 2-dimensional echo image is displayed on the screen of an oscilloscope (Figure 10.13).

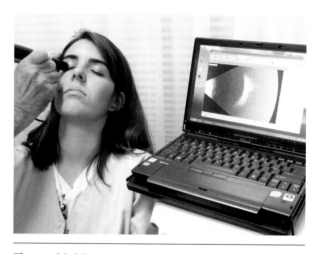

Figure 10.13 B-scan ultrasonography. *(Image courtesy of Tina Newmark, RN, MS.)*

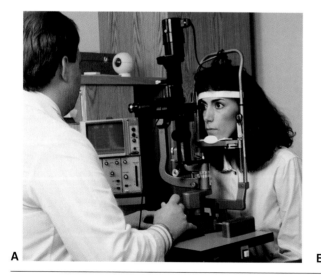

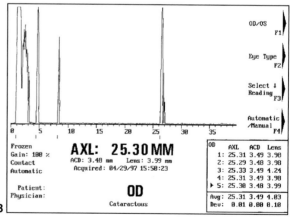

Figure 10.12 A-scan ultrasonography. **A.** A-scan ultrasonography performed with a probe attached to a slit lamp. **B.** Resulting measurement derived from A-scan ultrasonography.

SELF-ASSESSMENT TEST

1. What is the purpose of visual potential testing?

2. Name 4 methods used to measure visual acuity potential.

3. When are adjunctive ophthalmic tests indicated?

4. What are the 4 principal categories of adjunctive tests?

5. Why is contrast sensitivity tested?

6. Why is glare testing performed?

7. What does pachymetry measure?

8. State the purposes for performing pachymetry.

9. What is the main use for specular microscopy/photography?

10. The 3 principal types of ophthalmic imaging are which of the following?

    a. specular, pachymetry, and contrast-sensitivity

    b. external, slit-lamp, and fundus

    c. slit-lamp, pachymetry, and ultrasonography

    d. A-scan, external, and fundus

11. Fluorescein angiography is used for which of the following?

    a. counting the cells of the cornea

    b. documenting abnormalities of the eye's outer structures

    c. measuring the eye's contrast sensitivity

    d. viewing detail, such as blockages, in fundus blood vessels

    e. estimating the cornea's ability to withstand the stress of an operation

12. Briefly describe the procedure and process of fluorescein angiography.

13. Name 2 possible adverse effects a patient can experience during fluorescein angiography.

14. Describe the underlying principle and general diagnostic purposes of ultrasound procedures.

15. What is the chief purpose for measuring the length of the eye by A-scan ultrasonography?

    a. calculate the power of the artificial lens to be implanted at the time of cataract removal

    b. view the retinal blood vessels

    c. determine the size of the cataract for removal

    d. assess visual acuity

    e. construct 2-dimensional outlines of the retina

16. What is a principal diagnostic reason for performing B-scan ultrasonography?

   a. determine the size of the cataract for removal

   b. measure the distances between eye structures

   c. test for corneal opacity

   d. measure the distance between the corneal epithelium and endothelium to adjust for cataract surgery

   e. detect and measure abnormalities within the eye such as tumors or retinal detachment

17. What is a principal diagnostic reason for performing optical coherence tomography?

   a. determine the size of the vitreous base

   b. measure the retinal nerve fiber layer in glaucoma

   c. test for corneal clarity

   d. optically measure the corneal endothelium

SUGGESTED ACTIVITIES

1. Determine which of the procedures discussed in this chapter are performed regularly in your office. Ask the ophthalmologist or senior technician which of these procedures you may be expected to learn over time and obtain copies of office protocols for performance of these procedures.

2. Ask your ophthalmologist or senior technician for a "guided tour" of the technical instruments discussed in this chapter that are used regularly in your office. Note where these instruments are located in the office, their principal parts, and the purposes for which they are used in your ophthalmologist's practice.

3. Ask your ophthalmologist or senior technician when you may observe either of them performing as many of the procedures described in this chapter as possible. Take notes and meet afterward for questions and discussion.

SUGGESTED RESOURCES

Byrne SF. *A-Scan Axial Eye Length Measurements: A Handbook for IOL Calculations.* Mars Hill, NC: Grove Park Publishers; 1995.

Byrne SF, Green RL. *Ultrasound of the Eye and Orbit.* 2nd ed. St Louis: Mosby; 2002.

Cassin B, ed. *Fundamentals for Ophthalmic Technical Personnel.* Philadelphia: Saunders; 1995: chap 24.

Cunningham D. *Clinical Ocular Photography.* Basic Bookshelf Series. Thorofare, NJ: Slack; 1998.

DuBois LG. Pachymetry. In: *Fundamentals of Ophthalmic Medical Assisting.* DVD. San Francisco: American Academy of Ophthalmology; 2009.

Kendall CJ. *Ophthalmic Echography.* Ophthalmic Technical Skills Series. Thorofare, NJ: Slack; 1991.

Regillo CD, Maguire JI, Benson, WE. *Retina, Indocyanine Green Angiography.* In: Cohen, EJ. *Year Book of Ophthalmology, 1994.* St. Louis: Mosby; 1994: 181–187.

Stein HA, Stein RM. *The Ophthalmic Assistant: A Text for Allied and Associated Ophthalmic Personnel.* 8th ed. St Louis: Mosby; 2006.

11 PRINCIPLES AND TECHNIQUES OF PERIMETRY

Concerns with vision often emphasize central vision, that portion of eyesight that allows us to see clearly straight ahead in order to read, drive, sew, paint, and perform all the tasks requiring sharp vision. Visual acuity is our measure of central vision. However, many diseases of the eyes and visual system often affect the peripheral vision first, which is that part of our vision concerned with perception of objects and space that surround the direct line of sight. Peripheral vision provides the means to move safely within the environment by alerting the brain to potentially dangerous or interesting visual stimuli toward which the gaze (central vision) can be directed. For example, although central vision plays a large part in driving an automobile, it is the less sharp but all-important peripheral vision that alerts the driver to cars moving up on either side.

Chapter 5 discussed the nature, measurement, common defects, and correction of central vision. This chapter discusses the nature of peripheral vision and, most important, the principles of perimetry, the art of measuring the expanse and sensitivity of a patient's peripheral vision, called the visual field. Properly performed perimetry is crucial to the diagnosis and monitoring of a variety of ophthalmic conditions, especially those affecting the retina, optic nerve, and visual pathway. However, perimetry is a complicated, often highly technical process that requires not only concentration and time on the part of the patient but also skill and knowledge on the part of the person conducting the test. For this reason, this chapter presents only basic principles of perimetry that will introduce you to this complex topic. It includes information about the anatomic basis of the visual field, conventions used in "mapping" the visual field, the purpose and types of perimetry and the types of visual field defects perimetry can help measure. Also discussed are techniques that can help beginning perimetrists avoid measurement errors as they begin developing their skills. The technician must be thoroughly familiar with the visual field testing equipment being used, and so it is worthwhile to read and understand the manufacturer's manual before proceeding with testing patients.

Anatomic Basis of the Visual Field

The term **visual field** refers to everything that is visible to a person at a given time. The boundaries of this view are usually determined one eye at a time (monocularly), but the binocular visual field (ie, what the person sees with both eyes open) usually determines visual function. Vision originates in the retina, and the signal is processed and carried all the way to the occipital cortex in the brain. This visual pathway and the diseases that affect its components determine the extent of the visual field.

Collectively, the route of visual information from the retina to the occipital lobes is called the **visual pathway**. The retina is the beginning of the visual pathway; thus, it is important to understand its organization (Figure 11.1). The part of the image focused on the fovea, near the center of the retina, is seen in great detail because of the high concentration of cone cells in this area and the "one-to-one" wiring of the cones to the retinal nerve fibers. The parts of the image focused on the macula, which surrounds the fovea, and on other portions of the retina are seen slightly less clearly. This clarity gradually declines as the distance of the image from the fovea increases due to

a decrease in the concentration of photoreceptors and the way they are connected to the nerve fibers. The retinal nerve fibers converge at the optic disc to form the optic nerve, which exits the eye to take the image to the brain. Because there are no rods or cones in the optic nerve head, the tiny part of the visual image focused at this site is not visible. This "hole" in the normal visual field is called the **physiologic blind spot** (Figure 11.2). It is important to note that retinal nerve fibers are located both in the top (superior) and bottom (inferior) portion of the retina but neither group crosses over the horizontal midline. Therefore, any disease affecting the optic nerve or retinal nerve fiber layer will cause defects in the visual field that stop at ("respect") the horizontal midline.

The optic nerves from both eyes extend back and come together in a structure located just above the pituitary gland called the **optic chiasm**. The nerve fibers undergo an important reorganization within the optic chiasm. Fibers from the outer (temporal) half of each eye (carrying the image from the nasal portion of the visual field) travel back to the brain on the same side as the eye they came from. The fibers from the nasal side, however, carrying visual information from the temporal visual field, cross in the chiasm to go to the side of the brain opposite from the eye they came from. The result of this rearrangement is that visual information from the right side of the visual field (the nasal side of the right eye and the temporal side of the left eye) goes to the left side of the brain and vice versa. (This can be seen in Figures 11.21 and 11.22.) Visual field testing can therefore locate a lesion in the brain if it involves the visual pathways; visual field defects resulting from a lesion at the optic chiasm or farther back will respect the vertical midline (distinguishing them from retinal nerve fiber layer or optic nerve lesions).

From the optic chiasm, visual information is carried back to the occipital lobe of the brain through the optic radiations and optic tracts, where additional connections are made to bring the information to the frontal lobes for "interpretation."

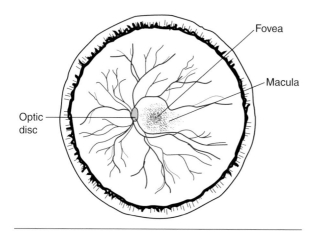

Figure 11.1 Locations within the retina of the left eye.

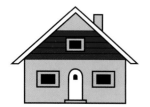

Figure 11.2 To demonstrate the physiologic blind spot, close your left eye and fixate on the house at a distance of about 14 inches. The black dot to the right disappears as it falls into the area of your blind spot.

Map of the Visual Field

The visual field has been likened to a 3-dimensional "island of vision in a sea of blindness" (Figure 11.3). It is the job of perimetry to draw a "map" of the island of vision for each eye. Visual field testing systems are designed to draw the map in different ways.

> The ability to draw the map of a patient's
>
> visual field is important in diagnosing diseases
>
> that cause defects in peripheral vision.

Locations at any point in both normal and defective visual fields can be qualitatively expressed in words (presence or absence of vision) as well as quantitatively expressed in numbers or color-coded (gray scale) for the location's level of sensitivity for seeing objects of light.

Viewed from directly above, the center of the island of vision may be considered to be the patient's point of central visual fixation, which corresponds to the fovea. Placing a series of concentric circles at equally spaced intervals of 10° from this central point provides coordinates that can be used as a reference for mapping the outer boundaries of this island, or, in other words, the extent of peripheral vision. These concentric circles are known as **circles of eccentricity** (Figure 11.4). Further dividing this circular mapping device into sections that radiate from the point of central fixation provides an additional point of reference for determining locations within the boundaries of the island of vision. These separations, known as **radial meridians**, divide the circular map much as cuts of a knife divide a pie into slices (Figure 11.5). The first cuts divide the pie, or circle, into quarters known as **quadrants**. These cuts, called the **horizontal and vertical meridians**, are the most significant

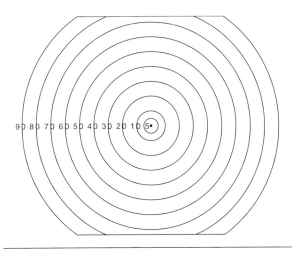

Figure 11.4 Circles of eccentricity in the standard chart form for plotting the visual fields.

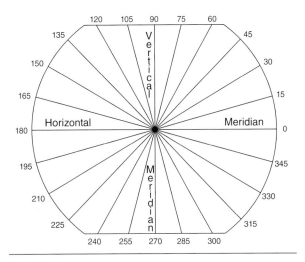

Figure 11.5 Radial meridians in the standard chart form for plotting the visual fields.

ones for diagnostic purposes. The circle can be subdivided by additional radial meridians into almost as many "thin slices," or sections, as needed.

Because a complete circle represents 360°, a specific meridian can be identified by the number of degrees, or angle, between the meridian and a baseline—as long as there is agreement on which point on the circle to begin. By convention, the 0° point on the charts for both the right and the left eye is on the extreme right of the horizontal meridian. Moving counterclockwise around the circle, the other meridians are marked in 15° or sometimes 30° steps identified by the angles they form with the horizontal meridian.

The resulting chart for plotting the visual fields of both eyes consists of a pair of adjacent circles with the meridians layered over the circles of eccentricity (Figure 11.6). Plots of the visual field represent the view as

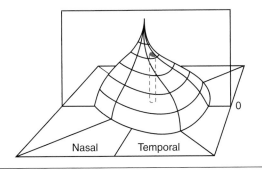

Figure 11.3 The 3-dimensional island of vision.

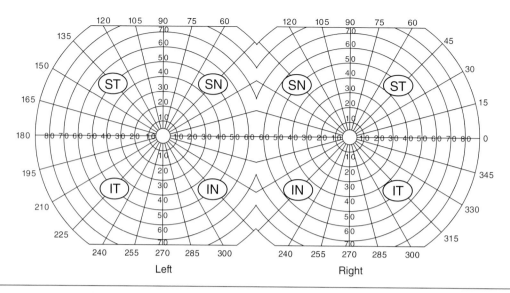

Figure 11.6 The standard chart form for plotting the visual fields, with the 4 quadrants labeled: SN (superior nasal), ST (superior temporal), IN (inferior nasal), and IT (inferior temporal).

seen by the patient. Thus, the circle on the right is used to plot the visual field of the right eye, and the circle on the left, the left eye. The inferior (lower) field is separated from the superior (upper) field by the horizontal meridian, and the nasal (inner) fields are separated from the temporal (outer) fields by the vertical meridian.

Any point in the visual field can be located by noting the number of degrees of eccentricity and the meridian. For example, the physiologic (normal) blind spot is usually located at 15° eccentricity on the 0° or 180° (horizontal) meridian. Can you locate the blind spot of the right and left eyes on Figure 11.6? This spot is always found temporal to fixation (that is, in the temporal field) and

serves as a handy reference point to identify which field belongs to which eye. In other words, the blind spot of the right eye will be found to the right of fixation and that of the left eye to the left of fixation.

Figure 11.7 depicts the concept of mapping the boundaries of the patient's visual field by showing the extent of a normal visual field on a standardized visual field "map." The boundary of the normal patient's island of vision—or, in other words, the visual field—extends on the circles of eccentricity to about 90° temporally and about 60° nasally, superiorly, and inferiorly. Objects appearing 110° temporally from the point of central fixation would obviously not be visible, for objects outside of the boundary

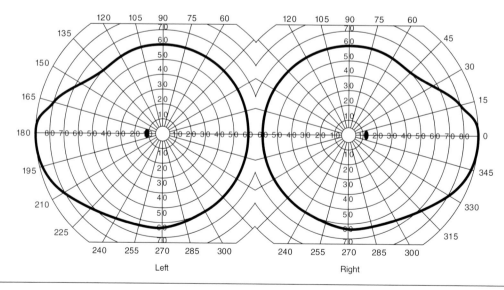

Figure 11.7 Boundaries of a normal visual field. The black spot in the temporal field of each eye represents the physiologic blind spot.

of the island of vision fall into the "sea" of blindness and cannot be perceived. The result of perimetry is an outline of the shape of the visual field and a map of defects within it.

In the island of vision analogy, the visual field is a 3-dimensional structure, with a peak at its center (corresponding to foveal vision) that slopes gradually to sea level (the outer, nonseeing area) at the boundaries of the island. The slope is steeper on the nasal side of the field and more gradual on the temporal side. The physiologic blind spot may be thought of as a deep vertical well that extends to sea level located temporal to the peak of vision at the fovea. This model of the visual field as an island illustrates how perimetry measures the extent and type of defect in the visual field. The height of the island at any point actually represents the "sensitivity" of the retina at that point.

Orientation of the Visual Field Map

Plotting of visual fields traditionally represents the view as seen by the patient. For example, parts of the field that appear to the patient on the temporal side are shown on the temporal side of the chart. When the fields from both eyes are drawn, the field from the patient's right eye is shown on the right. However, it is important to understand that a location in the visual field and the corresponding section of the retina that sees it do not share the same relative positions. The difference is due to the fact that images of objects focused on the retina are inverted and reversed by the optical system of the eye. In other words, the images appear upside down and backward on the retina. Thus, an object that the patient sees in the temporal visual field is actually focused on the patient's nasal retina. An object appearing in the superior visual field is detected by the inferior retina (Figure 11.8).

A defect in the patient's superior temporal retina, for example, will affect the patient's inferior nasal field of vision. An illustration of these relationships is the physiologic blind spot. Recall that the absence of photoreceptor cells at the head of the optic nerve is responsible for the absence of vision at this point. Although the optic nerve head is located on the nasal side of the eye, the blind spot appears in the patient's temporal visual field (see Figure 11.7).

The relationship between locations, sizes, and shapes of defects in the visual field and corresponding parts of the retina and other structures of the visual pathway is discussed later in this chapter. For the moment, the important point to remember is that the map or chart obtained by perimetry represents the visual field as seen by the patient.

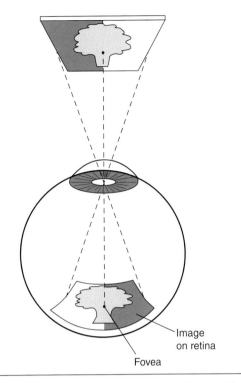

Figure 11.8 The image of an object in the visual field as focused on the retina.

Purposes and Types of Perimetry

Perimetry has two important functions. One is to detect abnormalities in the visual field, defects that are usually not perceptible to the patient. The other function is to monitor changes in the visual field that may indicate the development, progression, or improvement of diseases affecting the retina and visual pathway. Many diseases of the retina, optic nerve, and brain will affect the peripheral vision before they affect central vision. An accurate mapping of the visual field can help identify the nature and location of these diseases.

Many testing procedures have been devised to measure the visual field, each with certain advantages and drawbacks. However, all types of perimetry use a test object or target that must be seen by the patient against some specific type of background. The contrast between the test object and the background directly affects the measurements obtained by perimetry. The larger the object and the more it contrasts with the background, as well as the sensitivity of the retina at the point being tested, determines whether or not it will be seen by a particular eye at a particular location in the visual field. To illustrate this concept, consider how a small dark bird can be easily seen against a white cloud in daylight, while a large dark tree might be almost invisible when viewed against a dark mountain at dusk. Perimetric measurements are evaluated by taking into account the brightness of the background, which determines if the retina is light or dark adapted, as well as the size and brightness of the test object. In most types of perimetry, these qualities can be controlled by the examiner conducting the test.

The two basic methods employed to map the field of vision are **kinetic perimetry** and **static perimetry**. In general, kinetic perimetry uses a moving test object, usually of fixed size and brightness, while static perimetry uses an object of fixed size and varies its brightness at each test location.

The boundaries of the visual field are larger with brighter or larger targets and smaller with dimmer or smaller ones, because the less bright or smaller targets require more sensitive vision to be seen. A contour obtained with a single target of a particular size and brightness, such as with the tangent screen test described below, represents a line of equal or better sensitivity, called an *isopter*. A series of isopters of increasing sensitivity can be obtained through kinetic perimetry by using progressively smaller and/or dimmer targets. When these isopters are plotted on paper, they look like a stack of irregular ovals seen from the top (Figure 11.9). The shape of the ovals and their exact positions in relation to one another provide a surface contour map of the island of vision, that is, a 2-dimensional representation of the sensitivity levels of the visual field.

Drawing the boundaries and contours of the island of vision is only one objective of kinetic perimetry. Another

is to discover whether defects are present in the surface of the island and to determine their location and size. Perimetry searches for localized areas within the isopters of the visual field where the eye does not see as well as it should. Such an area of reduced sensitivity surrounded by an area of greater sensitivity is called a **scotoma**.

If the island of vision were observed from above, a **shallow scotoma** (mild defect) would appear as a depression in the island surface. A **deep scotoma** (more serious defect) would look like a pit or well. If the defect were so severe that the largest and brightest stimulus could not be seen, it would appear as a well that descends to the sea level of blindness. Such a defect is called an **absolute scotoma** (Figure 11.10). Remember that the term *absolute scotoma* does not necessarily mean "blindness"; it simply means the patient could not see the largest and brightest test object available with that testing method at that area of the visual field. Although it is normal and natural and not pathologic, the physiologic blind spot may be considered an absolute scotoma.

Kinetic Perimetry

A simple type of kinetic perimetry would be to move a hand or finger into the visual field of a patient who is fixating straight ahead, noting when the patient first sees the target. If the action were repeated from several directions around the visual field (that is, at several meridians), the examiner could obtain a rough idea of the boundaries of the patient's vision. This is the basis of the confrontation field test, in which the examiner compares the range of the patient's visual field with that of his or her own, which is presumed to be normal. Chapter 8 discusses the general principles of this test and describes how to perform it.

Although the confrontation field test is less sensitive than the perimetric methods described in this chapter, its simplicity makes it useful for screening patients for

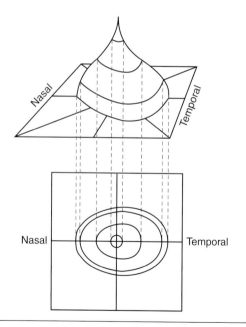

Figure 11.9 A series of isopters obtained by kinetic perimetry and the contours of the island of vision that they represent.

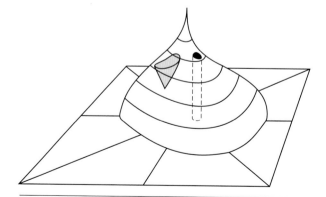

Figure 11.10 Defects in the island of vision. A deep scotoma (left) and an absolute scotoma.

major defects. The test is particularly useful with children, the very old, and the mentally impaired—indeed, for any patients physically or mentally unable to undertake the more complex tests.

TANGENT SCREEN TEST   A more detailed type of kinetic perimetry is the tangent screen test (Figure 11.11). In this procedure, the patient sits about 3 feet in front of a black felt or metallic gray screen. With one eye occluded by a patch, the patient fixates with the uncovered eye on a center dot on the screen while the examiner slowly moves a black wand with a small white or colored disc at its end into the field of vision. The patient indicates the moment the disc, or target, is seen, and the examiner marks the point on the screen. The process is repeated, moving the target into the field from various directions, each time at the same speed, until a number of points are marked. After the examination, the points are transferred from the tangent screen to a smaller paper chart and joined together by a continuous line. The result is a drawing of the boundaries of the visual field for the particular target used.

The tangent screen procedure is relatively simple to perform and, like the confrontation test, is often used to screen patients for visual field defects. It also remains popular in the specialty of neuro-ophthalmology, particularly for helping uncover "functional" visual loss. However, results obtained with the tangent screen are difficult to reproduce from one test to another, partly because neither the lighting of the screen nor the brightness of the test objects can be easily standardized. In addition, the tangent screen test measures only the central 30° of the visual field. (The flat screen would have to be excessively large to test the entire visual field.) It is useful for determining isopter boundaries, but very difficult to use for identifying shallow scotomata within those boundaries. For these reasons, the tangent screen was replaced for most purposes by a device called the **Goldmann perimeter** and subsequently by the automated perimeter.

GOLDMANN PERIMETER   Instead of a flat screen background, the Goldmann perimeter uses a large bowl that can be lighted accurately and reproducibly through a range of desired levels. The target is a projected light of adjustable size and brightness and moved over the entire visual field and beyond. Boundaries of the patient's visual field are measured in much the same way as described with the tangent screen. However, the Goldmann perimeter plots the isopters more easily and covers the entire visual field. Because the test conditions can be standardized and reproduced accurately, results obtained with the same patient at different sessions with a Goldmann perimeter are fairly, but not exactly, comparable, even if the tests are run by different technicians on different instruments.

In Goldmann perimetry, the patient is seated in front of a lighted bowl set at a specific light level (Figure 11.12). The technician is seated behind the device. The eye of the patient not being tested is occluded. Lenses are placed in front of the tested eye to correct for any refractive error plus the testing distance. The technician moves a small handle attached to a projector from outside the patient's expected visual field toward the center until the patient just sees the projected light. The patient indicates by knocking a key or coin on the table or by pressing a button connected to a buzzer when the light is seen. The handle is connected by a series of levers

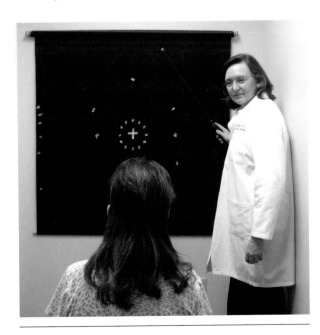

Figure 11.11   The tangent screen test.

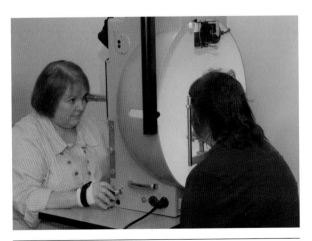

Figure 11.12   The Goldmann perimeter. *(Image courtesy of Brice Critser, CRA, Department of Ophthalmology and Visual Sciences, University of Iowa.)*

to the projector in such a way that a paper form representing the patient's visual field on the technician's side of the device and the actual visual field inside the bowl correspond. Thus, the technician can plot the visual field directly on the paper form.

The target can be varied by size and brightness. The targets come in 5 sizes and are indicated by Roman numerals I–V, representing a round light of sizes 0.25 mm^2 to 64 mm^2. The brightness is adjusted by a series of filters placed in the path of the projected light. The filters will dim the light in successive steps from the brightest available on the machine. The gross adjustment for brightness is the "1–4" scale. Each step is 0.5 log unit (1 log unit = a power of 10, equal to 5 decibels, abbreviated "dB") less intense than the previous, with 4 being the brightest. The fine adjustment for brightness is the "a–e" scale, with "e" being the brightest and the difference between each being 0.1 log units (1 decibel or 1 dB). The brightest test object would be the 1a, and the dimmest the 4e, which would be 1/1000 the brightness of the 1a. Commonly used targets, in ascending order of size and brightness, are I$_2$e, I$_4$e, and III$_4$e. This is the standard labeling for the isopters in Goldmann perimetry, with the size in Roman numerals and the intensity expressed with the subscripted Arabic numeral followed by the letter. Goldmann perimetry is a highly technical skill that, because of its complexity, has been mostly replaced by automated testing techniques. Unfortunately, the Goldmann perimeter is no longer manufactured. Devices such as the Octopus 900 perimeter (Haag-Streit, Mason, Ohio) provide Goldmann-type kinetic perimetry testing with manual and automated options.

OTHER DEVICES Devices other than the tangent screen and the Goldmann perimeter are also available for kinetic perimetry. The Autoplot, a refined version of the tangent screen, similarly measures only the central 30° of vision. Another device is the arc perimeter, which can test the entire field of peripheral vision one meridian at a time. Autoplots and arc perimeters are seldom used now and are mostly of historical interest.

ADVANTAGES AND DISADVANTAGES Kinetic perimetry has the advantage of being simple to understand for both the patient and the examiner. The procedure also produces a pictorial result that is easy to interpret. The disadvantage of kinetic perimetry is that accurate results depend on the capabilities of the patient and the examiner—human variables that can be difficult to control. For example, if the patient is slow to respond, because of either a long reaction time or a poor understanding of the test, the recorded field will be more constricted than the actual visual field.

A well-performed kinetic perimetric test requires considerable skill and experience and may be time consuming. The examiner has the difficult responsibility of moving the target at the same speed in each direction for accurate results. If the examiner moves the target too rapidly, by the time the patient signals that it has been seen the test object will have moved far beyond the true point of visibility, producing faulty results. If the examiner moves the target too slowly, the patient may become fatigued and unable to respond appropriately. Clearly, for accurate results, kinetic perimetry requires patience and cooperation on the part of the patient, and skill and experience on the part of the examiner.

Static Perimetry

Static perimetry tests the ability of the retina to detect a stationary target or light at selected points in the visual field. As with kinetic perimetry, the background can be varied but is usually left at the same levels as with kinetic perimetry. The two static methods used to estimate the light sensitivity of the retina are suprathreshold perimetry and threshold perimetry.

Some of the difficulties associated with any perimetric test can be minimized by giving the control of the test to a computer.

In **suprathreshold static perimetry**, a light or target of a specific size is chosen so that the patient should be able to see it when it is placed at a particular site in the visual field. If the patient does not see it, a defect probably exists at that point. If the brightness of the light or target is considerably above the normal minimal level of brightness for visibility, the defect is probably deep. Suprathreshold testing is typically used for screening the visual field for defects.

Suspicion of the presence and location of a visual field defect determines the placement of targets for exploration. The doctor may direct the examiner in choosing and placing the targets on the basis of a suspected defect or, in the case of computer-controlled devices, may direct the computer to certain locations. Automated static perimeters have programs with predetermined locations that are aimed at the kinds of defects expected in certain diseases. Although a shallow defect may be easily missed by suprathreshold static perimetry, the technique is useful as a screening procedure to find gross defects.

Static perimeters use the same test-object sizes as Goldmann kinetic perimetry and the same Roman numeral convention (I–V) to indicate that size (most tests are performed with the size III object). On the other hand, brightness of the test objects is indicated by a unit called a **decibel** (one-tenth [.10] of a log unit, a log unit being a power of 10). The decibel scale is a mathematical way of representing the brightness of the test object relative to the brightest test object available on a given machine. The higher the decibel number, the dimmer the test object is, indicating relatively better sensitivity. Thus, if a patient can see a size III test object at 38 decibels, the test point is more sensitive at that location than an eye that can see the same test object at 24 decibels.

Another, more specific, way of performing static perimetry is to place a target of a given size in the visual field and gradually increase its brightness until the patient just sees it. This procedure is called **threshold static perimetry**. The threshold is that level of brightness to which a patient will respond 50% of the time. If the threshold test is repeated at a series of points along one meridian, a cross-section of the island's contours, including the depth of scotomas and other depressions, can be obtained (Figure 11.13). This kind of cross-sectional mapping can be done with manual static perimetry (even on the Goldmann perimeter). However, to map multiple meridians, an automated perimeter is necessary (see the next section).

Several devices are available specifically for performing static perimetry, and new instruments and improved versions of existing units are being added to their

number continually. Devices designed for kinetic perimetry can also be used for measurements by static perimetry. Indeed, kinetic perimetry generally includes several suprathreshold measurements. However, such manual performance of the more comprehensive threshold static perimetry is very tedious for both the technician and the patient. For this reason, most static perimetry devices are automated with computer control and recording. These devices usually have the same lighted bowl as the Goldmann perimeter. The patient indicates with a pushbutton switch when a light (test target) is seen (Figure 11.14).

AUTOMATED THRESHOLD PERIMETRY This is the visual field testing procedure most commonly used today. The technique determines the sensitivity to light at each retinal location in numeric units (expressed in decibels). The computer converts these units into patterns of shades of gray (Figure 11.15A), resembling the isopter mapping of the visual field with kinetic perimetry (Figure 11.15B). The shades become increasingly gray as sensitivity is reduced. Black indicates lack of response to the brightest test object available on the machine.

The values generated by automated static threshold perimetry can be compared to those that might be expected in normal subjects of the same age. The figures can also be compared with the results of previous tests on the same patient. Analysis of multiple serial visual

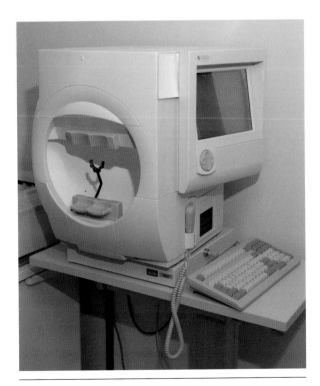

Figure 11.14 An automated perimeter. *(Image courtesy of Brice Critser, CRA, Department of Ophthalmology and Visual Sciences, University of Iowa.)*

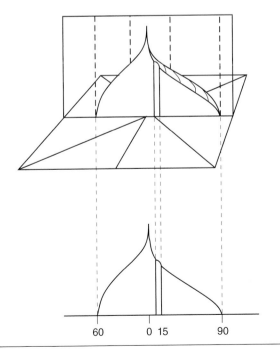

Figure 11.13 Cross-section of the island of vision obtained by static threshold perimetry.

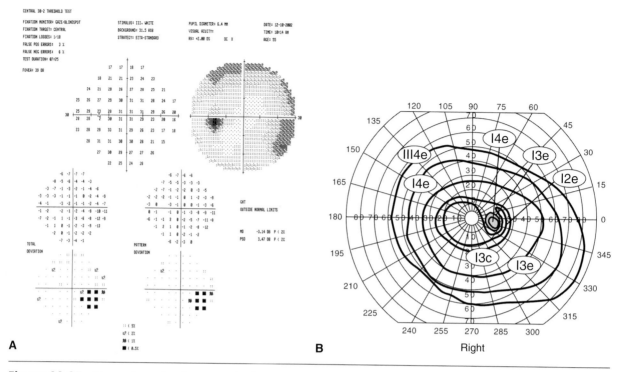

Figure 11.15 Comparison of perimetry methods. **A.** A computer-generated grayscale rendering of a left-eye visual field as measured by static threshold perimetry. **B.** A kinetic right-eye Goldmann plot.

fields with statistical methods is helpful in detecting trends of deterioration or improvement due to eye disease (Figure 11.16).

A visual field test performed on an automated static perimeter consists of an array of points ("the test pattern") and a strategy for testing them. Strategies are available for screening as well as threshold testing. Recent advances in threshold testing have been designed to shorten the time required for a patient to complete the examination. The most commonly used computer programs map the visual field with test points that are 6° apart. With such programs, scotomas 6° in size and smaller can be missed. Generally, these scotomas are not clinically significant, unless they are close to the macula. If a scotoma is suspected near the macula, another computer program can be selected to concentrate test points in this area.

Some computer programs are designed strictly for screening purposes, others are intended to monitor visual field defects caused by glaucoma, some are directed to macular problems, and still others monitor visual defects resulting from pathology in the brain. Obviously, it is important to know what the doctor is looking for in a particular patient in order to select the program most likely to provide the needed information. As beginning ophthalmic medical assistants work with the perimeter and their ophthalmologist or technical supervisor, they

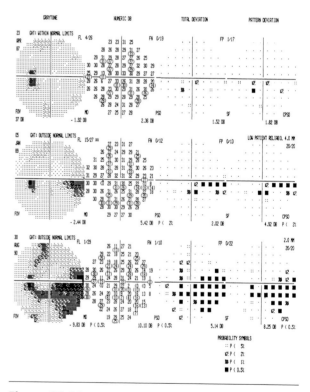

Figure 11.16 A series of static visual fields showing progression of glaucoma. Notice the increasingly darker areas at right, denoting progressive visual field loss.

will become familiar with available and newly developed computer programs and their applications.

ADVANTAGES AND DISADVANTAGES Automated static threshold perimetry is more sensitive than kinetic perimetry at detecting small or shallow defects in the visual field. The automated procedure also has the advantage of eliminating the burden on the technicians for actually performing the test. However, patient or examiner errors can still occur and may be even more frequent than with kinetic perimetry because, despite automation, computerized threshold perimetry takes longer to perform and is more tedious. In addition, the procedure is more difficult for patients to understand. For patients with limited mobility or attention span and for those with limited understanding of the language spoken by the examiner, Goldmann perimetry may yield more reliable results.

Miscellaneous Visual Field Tests

Occasionally, the technician may be asked to perform some form of specialized visual field testing, depending upon the equipment available in the office or clinic and the types of patients encountered. One type of test utilizes the standard computerized static perimeter but changes the color of the background illumination and test stimulus. This test is called **short-wavelength automated perimetry** (SWAP) and uses a blue stimulus on a yellow background. Check the user manual for the equipment available in your office to see if this test is available. SWAP isolates the blue cone portion of the visual system and may be able to detect optic nerve–based damage (usually from glaucoma) earlier than the standard (white-on-white) test. This test is usually utilized when glaucoma is suspected but the standard visual field is normal. This test may be very difficult for some patients and can take up to 20 minutes per eye, so it is important for the technician to be supportive and help the patient complete the test. Because of the uncertainty of its value, difficulty, and length of time for testing, the SWAP test is being replaced by **frequency doubling technology** (FDT).

The FDT test requires special equipment that may not be available in your office. The test is used for screening for glaucoma and utilized when glaucoma is suspected but the standard visual field is normal. It is able to detect optic nerve–based damage (usually from glaucoma) earlier than the standard (white-on-white) test. It is very easy to perform; a screening test may take only 1 minute per eye and a full examination 4 minutes. The patient is presented with targets consisting of alternating black and white stripes. The black and white stripes are alternated

(flickered) while the contrast between the black and the white is increased. When the contrast reaches "threshold," the patient will perceive twice as many stripes as there actually are; this is the frequency-doubling illusion. FDT is very sensitive to early glaucoma damage and correlates well with established glaucoma damage, making it very useful for screening. Because of the small number of test points, the screening version of this test is not useful for following patients with glaucoma. However, a version of FDT is available that is capable of testing out to 30° and can generate threshold data in patterns identical to those available on the standard computerized static threshold perimeters. This machine also has built-in age-related normative data and a hard drive for data storage and can perform serial analysis to detect change over time.

Defects Shown by Perimetry

Pathologic changes in the visual field can be divided into two main types: **generalized defects** and **focal defects**. Visual field defects due to disease usually fall into recognizable patterns, and may involve one or both eyes. Remember, the defects will correspond to the anatomy of the visual system and indicate to the doctor how the disease has affected the patient.

Generalized Defects

A generalized defect (**depression**) occurs when all of the test points in the visual field are reduced in sensitivity by approximately the same amount. This may also be thought of as the field of vision shrinking symmetrically (to the same extent from all directions) or becoming depressed evenly across the entire surface. When a generalized defect is present, the visual field is said to be contracted or constricted. Generalized defects can be pictured as the whole island of vision sinking into the sea of blindness (Figure 11.17). In Goldmann perimetry, a general defect appears as a symmetric contraction or depression (inward movement) of each isopter; that is, the isopters shrink toward the fixation point. In threshold perimetry, the threshold values at each tested point are reduced.

Generalized depression of the visual field can result from several disease conditions, including glaucoma, retinal ischemia, optic nerve atrophy, and media opacity, such as a cataract or corneal scar. A gradual, but usually not significant depression of the visual field can also occur with age, due to the natural loss of retinal sensitivity. The normal values stored with most computerized static perimeters account for the age-related changes. A

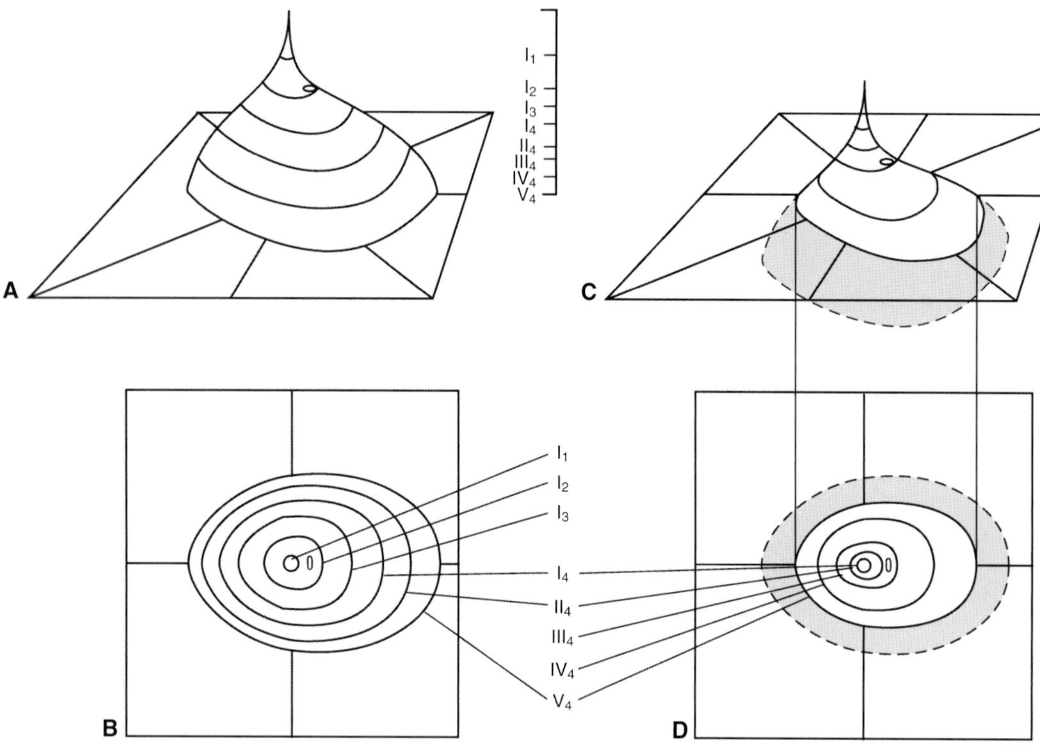

Figure 11.17 Normal "island" and visual field (**A, B**) compared with an island and visual field that evidences generalized depression (**C, D**).

visual field that has generalized depression will probably be of a normal "shape" but its overall height will be lower.

Apparent visual field contraction can also result from poor testing technique. Examples in kinetic perimetry include too rapid movement of the test object, poor understanding of the test by the patient, and slow patient reaction time in signaling that the target has been seen. Small pupils, interference with vision by the edge of the correcting lens holder, uncorrected aphakia, or a target that seems to be out of focus due to refractive error will also produce generalized depression as measured by perimetry.

Focal Defects

The presence of scotomas indicates localized changes in the contours of the island of vision and the visual field is said to contain focal defects or depressions. They may be thought of as holes or a loss of small portions of the island of vision. Small, shallow focal defects can be caused by refractive error, but most are due to an abnormality in the retina, optic nerve, or brain. The size, shape, location, and depth of these visual defects can be helpful in identifying the nature and location of the abnormality. Most scotomas, like the physiologic blind spot, are not noticed by the patient.

A *focal depression* or *scotoma* is an indentation in the surface of the visual island (Figure 11.18A), and represents an abnormality in the expected shape of the island of vision. On a kinetic field, a scotoma may appear as an inward shift of a portion of several isopters (Figure 11.18B). On a static field, the retinal sensitivity will be reduced at one test point or cluster of points relative to other sensitivities at the same circle of eccentricity. A scotoma may also be thought of as a pit or well in the island (Figure 11.19A), represented on the kinetic visual field chart as a circumscribed area in which one or more targets are not perceived (Figure 11.19B). On the static field, a scotoma appears as an area of decreased sensitivity within the outer boundaries of the field (Figure 11.20). Focal depressions may be characterized by their depth, depending upon the amount of loss compared to expected normal values, and are sometimes classified as mild, moderate, severe, or absolute.

When a visual field defect is mapped, 5 main features are noted. These are location, size, shape, depth, and slope of margins. The general concepts of location and size were discussed earlier in this chapter. The shape of a visual field defect depends a great deal on the target size and brightness used to map the defect. One important consideration related to shape and location is

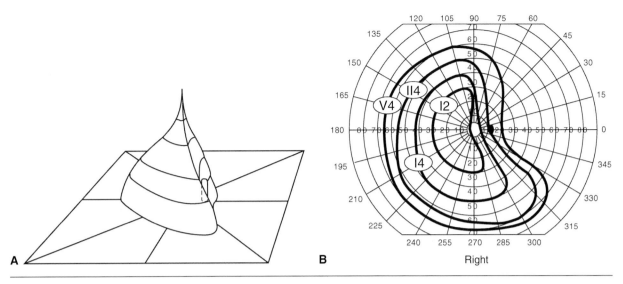

Figure 11.18 Depression, a focal defect that appears as (**A**) an indentation of the island of vision or (**B**) an inward deviation of a portion of several isopters, as measured by kinetic perimetry. The closeness of the isopters at the border of the defect characterizes it as steep rather than gradual.

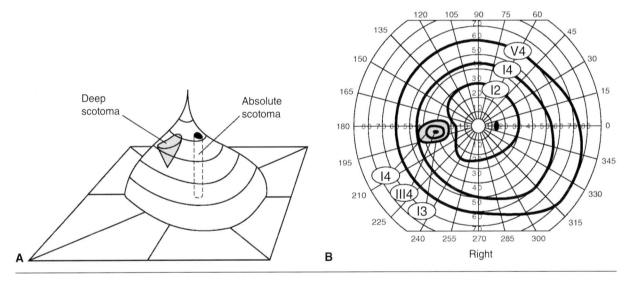

Figure 11.19 Scotoma, a focal defect that appears as (**A**) a pit or well in the island of vision or (**B**) a circumscribed area in which one or more targets are not perceived, as measured by kinetic perimetry. The pit represents a relative defect; the well, an absolute defect. The well in this illustration is actually the normal physiologic blind spot.

whether a defect is aligned with the vertical or horizontal meridian. Due to the anatomy of the visual pathways, defects that respect (don't cross) the vertical midline suggest a neurologic cause (at or behind the optic chiasm); defects that respect the horizontal midline are related to the retinal nerve fiber layer or optic nerve. Visual field defects that do not respect the vertical or horizontal midline may originate in the retina. The distinction can be helpful in assisting the ophthalmologist in locating the source of a visual field defect.

The depth of a defect is the extent to which it "excavates" the island of vision. If the largest and brightest target of the testing device used cannot be seen in a portion of the defect, that part of the defect is said to be absolute; less severe defects are considered relative (see Figure 11.19A and B).

The slope of the margins of a defect is determined by how close the defect's borders of different isopters are to one another. For example, if all of the isopters crowd together at the border of the defect, the margins of the

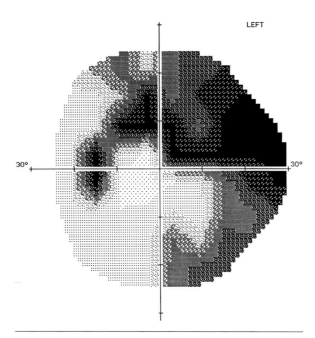

LEFT

30°   30°

Figure 11.20 A large scotoma as measured by static perimetry. The smaller oval dark area on the left is the blind spot. The remaining dark area is the scotoma.

defect are said to be steep (see Figure 11.18). Steep defects tend to be associated with conditions caused by blood vessel closure such as strokes, or brain tumors. On the other hand, if the isopters showing the defect are widely spaced, the slope of the margin is said to be gradual. Gradual slopes tend to be associated more with slowly progressive conditions such as glaucoma. In automated perimetry, slope is determined by differences in sensitivity values of adjacent points.

Hemianopic and Quadrantanopic Defects

Another example of abnormal visual fields is a condition in which the right or left half (**hemianopia**) or quarter (**quadrantanopia**) of the field is missing. If the right or left half of the visual field is defective or missing in both eyes, the defect is called a **homonymous hemianopia**. This visual defect results from damage to the optic tract or optic radiations in the visual pathways due to a stroke or brain tumor (Figure 11.21). A **bitemporal hemianopia**, missing or defective temporal field vision in both eyes, is often due to a tumor or other lesion in or near the optic chiasm (Figure 11.22).

A quadrantanopia may occur as a result of damage to the optic radiations in the visual pathways of the brain. In this condition the right or left upper or lower quadrant of the visual field shows a defect.

Detection of hemianopic or quadrantanopic defects is of critical importance because they suggest the presence of a lesion within the brain that may be life threatening as well as vision threatening. Early detection increases the chances of recovery because many lesions are treatable.

Other Defects

Glaucoma may produce various kinds of defects in the visual field, depending in part on the stage of the disease. Three common types are the **Bjerrum scotoma**, **paracentral scotoma**, and **nasal step** (Figure 11.23). The Bjerrum scotoma is a small area of reduced sensitivity that appears at about 15° of eccentricity in the upper or lower field. As glaucoma progresses, the Bjerrum scotoma may become enlarged to form an arc-shaped area called an *arcuate scotoma*. A paracentral scotoma is a defect occurring above or below the horizontal midline near the center that is smaller than a Bjerrum scotoma. The nasal step is so called because, when plotted, it appears as a step-like loss of vision at the outer limit of the nasal field. A nasal step and an arcuate scotoma may join and enlarge to cause loss of the entire upper or lower visual field; this type of defect is called an altitudinal scotoma or hemianopia (Figure 11.24). Advanced glaucoma also may result in large visual field losses that limit vision to small islands, especially on the temporal side of the eye (Figure 11.25).

Damage to the optic nerve or lesions involving the macula can produce a **central scotoma**, a defect in the very center of the visual field (Figure 11.26). In contrast to most of the visual field losses already discussed, these defects are usually associated with decreased visual acuity.

Conditions for Accurate Perimetry

A visual field test is a complicated procedure regardless of the method or the device used. Many conditions must be controlled to secure an accurate result. Conditions that can lead to errors are usually related to one or more of 4 factors: the environment, the device, the patient, and the examiner.

Environment-Related Factors

It is the examiner's responsibility to ensure that the testing environment facilitates the test procedure. The room

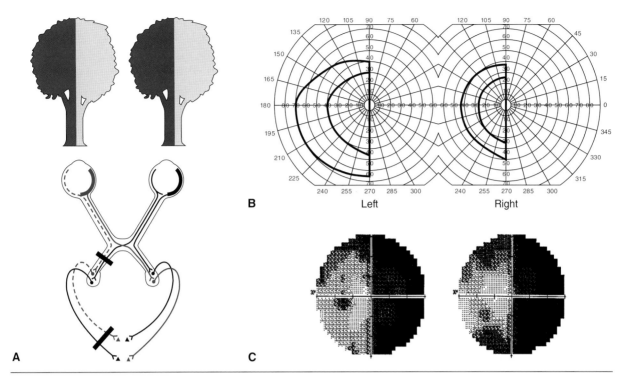

Figure 11.21 A right homonymous hemianopic defect resulting from a lesion in the optic tract or in the optic radiation of the visual cortex. **A.** The lesion (black rectangles) has destroyed fibers of the optic tract or optic radiation from the temporal retina of the left eye (dotted line) and the nasal retina of the right eye (solid line). As a result, objects in the right half of the visual space (gray part of the tree) are not seen. **B.** A Goldmann visual field chart of a right homonymous hemianopia. **C.** A static chart of a right homonymous hemianopia.

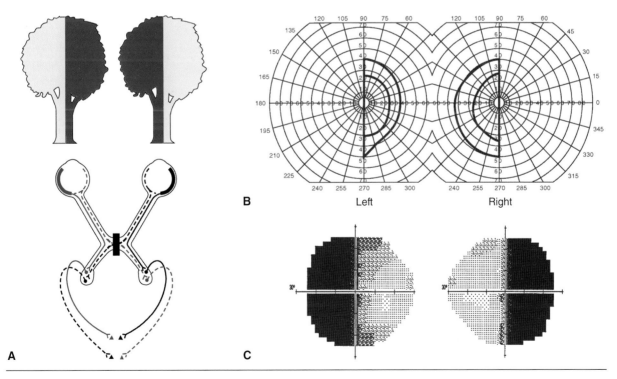

Figure 11.22 A bitemporal hemianopia due to a lesion (black rectangle) of the optic chiasm. **A.** The lesion has destroyed chiasmal crossing fibers from the nasal retinas (dotted lines). As a result, objects in the temporal half of the visual space (gray part of the tree) are not seen. **B.** A Goldmann visual field chart of a bitemporal hemianopia. **C.** A static chart of a similar defect.

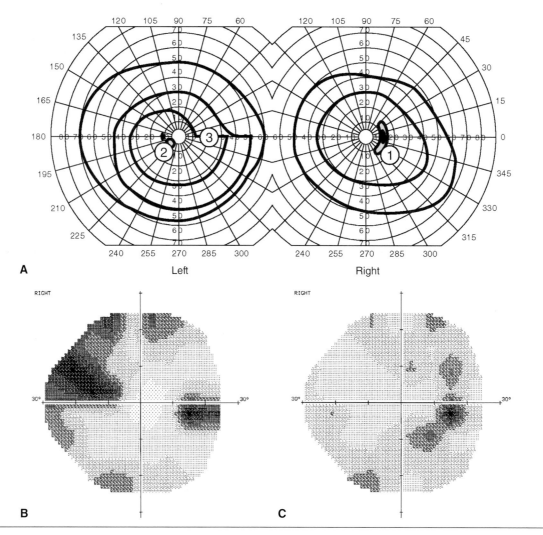

Figure 11.23 Glaucoma field defects. **A.** In early glaucoma, defects may include (1) an enlarged blind spot called a Siedel scotoma (shown in the right field), (2) a paracentral scotoma, or (3) a nasal step (both shown in the left field). **B.** A static chart of a nasal step. **C.** A static chart of a Bjerrum scotoma.

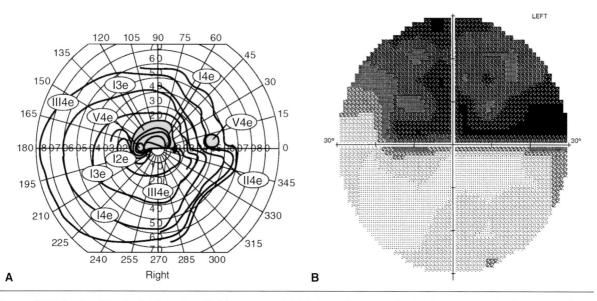

Figure 11.24 An altitudinal defect. **A.** A Goldmann visual field chart of an altitudinal defect. **B.** A static chart of a defect in the same patient.

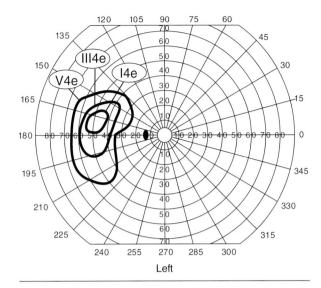

Figure 11.25 In advanced glaucoma, the visual field may be limited to small islands, especially on the temporal side.

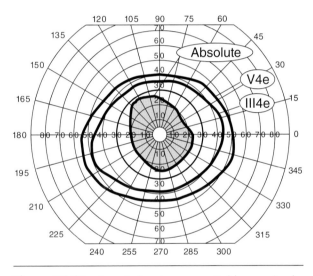

Figure 11.26 A central scotoma on a Goldmann visual field chart.

temperature must be neither too warm, which may make the patient drowsy, nor too cold, which can make the patient uncomfortable. The room lighting should be adjusted to the level best suited for the particular test device or method being used. Room lights that are too bright or that change during the test will affect illumination of the background and that of the test object and, consequently, the results of the test.

Intrusion, movement, and noise should be minimized, so that the patient can concentrate on the test. A crying child in a nearby room can distract both the patient and the examiner. The test should not be interrupted. Even with automated equipment, the examiner should remain in the room in case the patient has questions, grows restless, requires further instructions, or needs encouragement. A useful visual field test cannot be expected from a patient who has been seated at an automated perimeter, instructed on its use, and left alone during the test.

The patient should be made physically comfortable during visual field testing. The chair should be comfortable but not too soft. The chair should not permit the patient to sink in as the test progresses or to squirm around. The height of the chair, the table on which the perimeter sits, and the chin rest must be adjusted so that the patient is in a comfortable position and the head is straight, without an up or down tilt or a right or left swivel. The patient's forehead must remain against the headrest for the entire test. If the table is too high the patient's head will tend to move away from the machine.

Device-Related Factors

A perimetric instrument must be calibrated before use every day to obtain the desired amount of illumination for both the background and the test object. Often performed by the examiner, **calibration** consists of testing the illumination against a known standard to ensure that the level indicated on the device is in fact the actual level desired. Some automated devices also have automatic calibration. The Goldmann perimeter has a specific calibration protocol, which should be followed at least daily. Calibration may need to be rechecked if a particular patient's clothing is very dark or very light, because these qualities can affect the relative brightness of the background illumination.

Each device has its own checklist of items to monitor and procedures to follow before beginning the test. Some items are common to most devices:

- Are the room lights at the right level of brightness?

- Is the room door closed to avoid noise, which may distract the patient, and light, which might affect background levels?

- Is paper in the right place or in the printer?

- Are pencils or other markers present?

- If the perimeter is computer-controlled, is the correct disk for storing patient information in the disk drive?

Patient-Related Factors

Several factors concerning the patient can affect the success of visual field testing. These include the patient's comprehension of the test, reaction time, physical condition, distractibility, boredom, anxiety, comfort, pupil size, visual acuity, and refractive error. With any kind of perimetry, the results will be most accurate if the patient fully understands the test procedure. The technician should not assume that the patient knows what to do simply because the patient has done the test before. Both very young and very old patients may have forgotten how to do the test or may not have understood fully on the previous occasion. The safest course of action is to underestimate what the patient knows or remembers and to explain the purpose and methods of the test, at least briefly, each time. To overcome any awkwardness associated with repeating the information, the examiner might introduce the topic in the following manner: "I know that you have done a visual field test before, but I'm going to repeat the instructions just to be sure we both understand what is going to happen."

Patient anxiety can lead to error and faulty test results.

The examiner can help set the patient's mind at ease by a sympathetic, understanding, and gentle manner. Showing impatience and irritation when a patient seems slow to learn or gives inappropriate responses is counterproductive and unacceptable. Some patients approach a visual field test as if taking a final exam and are anxious not to "make a mistake." The examiner must explain that there is no right or wrong and that the patient is expected not to see the test object all the time. Reviewing the purpose of the test and making a brief trial run can do much to relieve patient anxiety before beginning the actual test. It is also useful to tell a patient that during the course of a threshold test there will be periods during which the stimuli will be too dim to be seen. This helps allay patients' fears that they are "blind."

Patient fatigue can also lead to errors in testing the visual field. Patients younger than 20 and older than 60 years tend to tire more quickly than others, but anyone can tire in a dark room with a tedious test. The examiner should be alert for signs of fatigue, such as frequent loss of fixation, distractibility, unresponsiveness, and intermittent drooping of the eyelids. Rest periods may help the patient overcome fatigue. If several lengthy tests are required, it may be possible to schedule some of them for another session.

Some patients have severely drooping eyelids (ptosis) that can cut off the upper visual field. In patients with ptosis, the eyelids may need to be held up with tape to get an accurate picture of the upper visual field. Droopy lids

should be noted on the test results as well as any other patient problems like lack of fixation or cooperation. during the test.

The size of a patient's pupil should always be recorded at the time of perimetry because a pupil 2 mm or smaller will produce a contraction of the visual field independent of any other condition that might be present. The person interpreting the field chart must take into account the pupil size at the time of the test. Recording pupil size is particularly important in patients with glaucoma because these patients may have smaller than normal pupils, either because of medications that cause the pupil to constrict (not very common) or the nature of their disease. Some ophthalmologists will dilate pupils that are less than 3 mm to avoid this problem.

When the central 30° field of a presbyopic or aphakic patient is tested, the patient's near add or correction must be in place. Because the rims of a patient's eyeglasses can interfere with accurate test results, most perimeters include a special lens holder for this purpose, into which the examiner inserts the appropriate corrective lens or lenses from the trial lens set. The near correction helps the patient properly focus on the target in the perimeter bowl, which is about 33 cm from the eye. In addition, if the image is blurred, the patient may not see the test object, thereby falsely suggesting the presence of a scotoma. The amount of correction needed for different refractive conditions can be determined by the use of printed tables that suggest the amount of add for a given age. These will usually be found in the instrument's instruction manual.

To avoid errors when testing with a correction in place, the lens should be as close to the eye as possible without touching the eyelashes when the patient blinks. This precaution avoids the possibility that the patient may be distracted or that the lens may become smeared when the lashes touch the lens. On the other hand, if the lens is too far from the eye, the lens edge may interfere with the patient's vision. Because it is easy to select the wrong lens in the darkened testing room, the examiner should ask the patient to confirm that the test object can be seen clearly once the chosen lens is in place.

Examiner-Related Factors

As suggested by the foregoing discussions, the examiner contributes to accurate test results by ensuring that the patient is comfortably seated, understands the procedure, and is not worried or anxious about the test. The examiner calibrates the testing device and ensures that the environment is free of distractions, adequately heated, and properly lighted. The examiner also makes sure the eye not being tested is covered with a specially made disinfected patch or other occluder.

The patient should be instructed to look steadily at the fixation point and not search for the test object. In automated static perimetry, the computer randomizes the location of the test target. In kinetic perimetry, the examiner can vary the order of presentation so that the patient cannot anticipate where the target will appear.

In kinetic perimetry, the examiner must pay careful attention to the speed of movement of the test object. The usual suggested speed is 2° per second, but this rate should be reduced if the patient's reaction time is slow, as may be the case with elderly patients. On the other hand, moving the test object too slowly will lengthen the test and tire both the patient and the examiner. Presenting test objects too rapidly or too slowly in automated static perimetry can have similar negative effects.

SELF-ASSESSMENT TEST

1. Define *perimetry*.

2. Why is the part of the visual field focused on the fovea seen in such great detail?

3. Describe the anatomic location of the physiologic blind spot and state why no sight is possible there.

4. Describe briefly the purpose of a mapping system for measuring the visual field.

5. What structure of the eye corresponds to the center of the island of vision?

6. Name the 2 types of reference coordinates used for mapping the visual field.

7. Where is the physiologic blind spot located in a map of the right and left visual fields?

8. State in degrees of eccentricity the approximate boundaries of the 4 quadrants of the normal visual field.

9. A person sees an object in the superior temporal quadrant of the visual field. In what quadrant of the retina is the view focused?

10. Name the 2 principal functions of perimetry.

11. Name the 2 basic methods used to survey the field of vision, and describe how the targets used differ between them.

12. Define *isopter*.

13. Define *scotoma* and explain the difference between shallow, deep, and absolute scotomas.

14. Name the 3 main tests used for kinetic perimetry, and describe the advantages of each.

15. Describe the 2 advantages of kinetic perimetry.

16. Describe 2 sources of human error in kinetic perimetry.

17. Name 2 methods of static perimetry.

18. Describe 2 advantages of computerized static threshold perimetry over kinetic perimetry.

19. Describe at least 2 disadvantages of computerized static threshold perimetry in comparison with kinetic perimetry.

20. Name the 2 main types of pathologic changes in the visual field.

21. Name 4 disease conditions that may produce generalized depression of the visual field.

22. Give at least 3 examples of factors that may cause an apparent contraction of the visual field.

23. Name the 5 main features of a focal defect that may be noted in mapping a visual field.

24. Define *hemianopia* and *homonymous hemianopia*.

25. Name 3 common types of visual field defects produced by glaucoma.

26. Describe the visual field defect known as an *altitudinal scotoma* or *hemianopia*.

27. Name the 4 types of factors that can lead to errors in visual field testing.

28. List at least 2 examples of each of these 4 factors.

SUGGESTED ACTIVITIES

1. To gain a better understanding of perimetry from both the examiner's and the patient's standpoint, ask your ophthalmologist or the perimetrist in your office to perform, over time, several different perimetric measuring procedures on you: confrontation field test, tangent screen test and automated perimetry. Ask questions as the procedures are being performed.

2. Ask your ophthalmologist or technical staff manager to tell you which perimetric measurements you may be required to perform. Request that regular sessions be scheduled for training in the use of specific techniques and equipment.

3. Read the instruction manuals that accompany the various perimetric devices in your office. Pay close attention to calibration techniques and any information or tips offered for avoiding measurement errors with each device.

4. Request that you be allowed to observe while an examiner in your office conducts a variety of perimetric measurements with different patients. Take notes and schedule a meeting with the examiner to review the test results (the visual field plots) and discuss your questions.

5. Practice administering the test under the supervision of an experienced examiner, first on a volunteer, such as someone who works in the office, then on patients.

SUGGESTED RESOURCES

Cassin B, ed. *Fundamentals for Ophthalmic Technical Personnel*. Philadelphia: Saunders; 1995: chaps 16–18.

Choplin NT, Edwards RP. *Visual Fields*. Basic Bookshelf Series. Thorofare, NJ: Slack; 1998.

Choplin, NT, Edwards RP. *Visual Field Testing With the Humphrey Field Analyzer*. 2nd ed. Thorofare NJ: Slack; 1999.

Heigl A, Patella VM. *Essential Perimetry: The Field Analyzer Primer*. 3rd. Dublin, CA: Carl Zeiss Meditec; 2002.

Harrington DO, Drake MV. *The Visual Fields: Text and Atlas of Clinical Perimetry*. 6th ed. St Louis: Mosby; 1990.

Movaghar M, Lawrence MG. Eye exam: the essentials. In: *The Eye Exam and Basic Ophthalmic Instruments*. DVD. San Francisco: American Academy of Ophthalmology; 2001. Reviewed for currency: 2007.

Stein HA, Stein RM. *The Ophthalmic Assistant: A Text for Allied and Associated Ophthalmic Personnel*. 8th ed. St Louis: Mosby; 2006.

12 FUNDAMENTALS OF PRACTICAL OPTICIANRY

Opticianry is a specialized area of eye care that includes the making of corrective lenses from refractive prescriptions and the fitting of both the lenses and the eyeglass frames for proper visual correction. It combines the science of lenses, frame materials, and styling with the trends of fashion. An ophthalmology office may have an optician on staff to support the doctor's patients; however, opticianry services frequently are located elsewhere. Whatever the case, ophthalmic medical assistants are often required to perform certain tasks related to opticianry.

Ophthalmic medical assistants may be called upon to answer patients' questions or solve problems concerning the proper fit or correction of their eyeglasses, serving as an intermediary between the ophthalmologist's office and the optician who filled the prescription. This chapter provides information about types of corrective lenses and materials used in lens manufacture. It introduces you to special optical measurements and techniques used to determine the proper fit and correction of eyeglasses. Frame design, eyeglass care, and adjustments are also discussed. Although opticianry frequently concerns contact lens manufacture and fitting, these subjects are covered in depth in Chapter 14.

Types of Corrective Lenses

Two principal types of eyeglass lenses may be manufactured to correct vision. Single-vision lenses provide correction for only one distance (that is, far or near). Multifocal lenses (bifocals, trifocals, and progressive addition and occupational multifocals) combine two or more corrections in a single lens to provide sharp vision at more than one distance. As part of the process of refraction, the doctor recommends which type of lens would most benefit a particular patient. Alternatively, the optician may have the responsibility of explaining the lens options and helping the patient decide.

Single-Vision Lenses

Generally speaking, a single-vision lens can focus at only one distance. Single-vision lenses are used to correct a refractive error, such as myopia, hyperopia, or astigmatism, for one working distance, usually either far or near. Figure 12.1 demonstrates how a convex lens corrects hyperopia and Figure 12.2 demonstrates correction of myopia with a concave lens. Patients receiving a prescription for single-vision lenses to correct a vision problem can select from many different lens materials, styles of eyeglasses, and frame designs.

Multifocal Lenses

Many people, especially those over 40 years of age, need lenses that will focus not only at far distances but at near or intermediate distances as well. One solution is to have two or three single-vision eyeglasses for each working distance. This solution works for some patients, but is inconvenient for most. A more practical solution for most people is a multifocal lens.

Multifocal lenses are used to correct vision for two or more distances. A **bifocal lens** has two powers, usually one for correcting distance vision and one for correcting near vision. A **trifocal lens** has three power zones: one for correction of distance vision, one for intermediate range of sight, and one for near vision. The terms *segment*, *add*, and *near add* are used interchangeably to describe the portion of the multifocal lens (usually the lower part) that provides near vision.

PLACEMENT AND TYPES OF SEGMENTS Segments of various shapes can be placed at different locations within a lens. An **executive** bifocal lens consists merely of a top distance band and a bottom near band, which divide the entire width of a lens into two parts. This same principle may be applied to manufacture a trifocal lens as

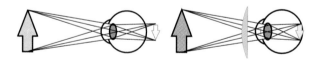

Figure 12.1 Convex lenses and how they correct far-sightedness. *(Image courtesy of Mark Mattison-Shupnick, ABOM, Jobson Medical Information LLC.)*

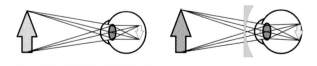

Figure 12.2 Concave lenses and how they correct near-sightedness. *(Image courtesy of Mark Mattison-Shupnick, ABOM, Jobson Medical Information LLC.)*

well. Executive bifocal lenses are rarely used today, but it is helpful to know about this older lens style.

The biggest benefit of lined bifocals is that the line "directs" a patient where to look for the optimum power for the task at hand. The patient merely looks over the line for distance vision and under the line for near vision. Because of the visible line, it is also the easiest type of multifocal for the optician to fit.

Figure 12.3 shows examples of 5 different types of multifocal lenses. **Round-top segments** are portions of circles fused or ground into the distance lens. Round-top segment lenses are seldom used anymore, but you may still see them in practice and should be familiar with them. The straight-top, or flat-top, **D segment** is so called because it is shaped like the capital letter D lying on its side, and it is the most popular of the lined multifocals. The D segment may be used in bifocals and trifocals. They can be manufactured in a variety of widths that provide adequate field of vision for desk chores and other near work. A drawback of lined bifocals is the visibility of the line and its association with aging. Moreover, as the patient ages, the addition power required for reading increases. In a bifocal, this causes a vision gap at mid-range or intermediate distances, because the loss of accommodation results in difficulty in focusing on objects at arm's length. As a result, lenses that provide an intermediate power (trifocal) are indicated. Most patients think that the trifocal is even less attractive than the bifocal, and that probably explains why trifocals have little usage. The solution has been **progressive addition multifocal lenses**, which give clear vision at all distances (Figure 12.4). They do this with increasingly steep curves designed on the front surface, which causes the plus power to increase as the eyes look down and converge.

PROGRESSIVE ADDITION LENSES These have become the most popular multifocal in recent years, due to lens design and manufacturing improvements. Older-style progressive addition lenses had distortions and design limitations that created relatively low patient satisfaction rates. Modern progressive lenses have an over 90% satisfaction rate, much higher than lined bifocals, and have been clinically proven to work for most patients, even those previously wearing lined multifocals. There are progressive addition lenses designed exclusively for previous lined-multifocal wearers, and "short corridor" progressive addition lenses that can be fit in small, fashionable frames with fitting heights as low as 14 mm.

Progressive lens technology continues to evolve. The newest progressive lens designs can be personalized for the patient's prescription, frame style, tilt of the lens, and position of the lens in front of the eye. In addition to fitting in the traditional flat frame, progressive addition

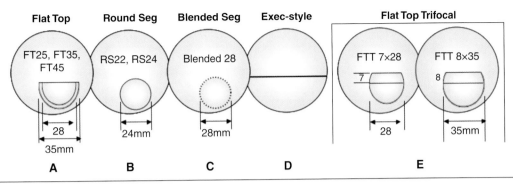

Figure 12.3 Different types of multifocal lenses. **A.** Flat top. **B.** Round segment. **C.** Blended segment. **D.** Executive style. **E.** Flat top trifocal. *(Images courtesy of Mark Mattison-Shupnick, ABOM, Jobson Medical Information LLC.)*

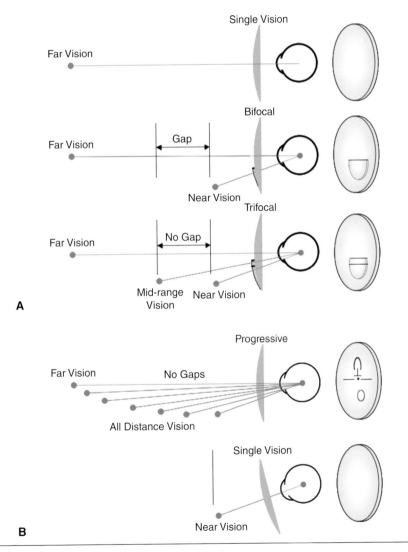

Figure 12.4 Different forms of vision correction. **A.** Distance vision correction with single-vision lens, distance and near correction with bifocal, and far, mid-range, and near correction with trifocal lens. **B.** All distance vision correction with progressive lens and near vision correction with single-vision lens. *(Images courtesy of Mark Mattison-Shupnick, ABOM, Jobson Medical Information LLC.)*

lenses can now be used in highly curved sports frames. Many sports eyewear companies have lab programs that offer snorkel masks, swim and ski goggles, and other optics for sports tailored to the patient's prescription. Fitting techniques for progressive addition lenses are more exacting than for lined bifocals. For this reason, you should make sure that the referral optician is knowledgeable in fitting and dispensing progressive addition lenses.

Neutralization (lensometry) of progressive addition lenses is a little more complicated than with lined bifocal lenses. Progressive addition lenses have reference marks laser engraved on the lenses to use in the verification process. These engravings are located 34 mm apart nasal and temporal on the 180° line and are visible when viewed under a bright light against a dark background. Special instruments are available that help locate these engravings, such as the Essilor PAL-ID progressive lens identifier (Figure 12.5). The engravings commonly include a symbol of some sort with the lens add power underneath temporal, and the company logo underneath nasal (Figure 12.6). These are used with a manufacturer's "layout" chart to mark up the lenses for lensometry.

Many brands of progressive addition lenses are available today. If you are required in your office to neutralize progressive addition lenses, contact the manufacturer of the lenses that are most commonly used in your area for in-service training on how to neutralize and troubleshoot their lenses. Prescription lens laboratories can also supply a copy of the Progressive Lens Identifier, distributed

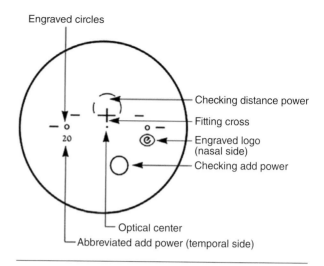

Figure 12.6 Progressive addition lens markings.

by Optical Laboratories Association (Alexandria, Virginia). This guide is a complete reference for progressive lenses. See Procedure 12.1 for the steps in verifying the prescription and fit of progressive addition lenses. These lenses should not be confused with **invisible bifocals** (also called *blended* or *seamless* bifocals). This type of lens provides a blended transitional zone between the segment and the distance portion and displays no observable dividing line. This blended transitional zone is merely cosmetic and gives the wearer no intermediate viewing area. These lenses are rarely used anymore, due to their poor optical performance. Figure 12.7 shows various multifocal lens designs.

No single solution is right for every multifocal wearer.

CUSTOMIZING THE CORRECTION The choice of a particular type and configuration of multifocal correction often depends on the patient's work or avocational interests. For example, a house painter, auto mechanic, or other tradesperson may need to see through the middle of a lens for distance, through the bottom for near, and through the top for intermediate overhead work at arm's length. The solution for this type of problem might be a **double-D segment** multifocal lens (Figure 12.8), also known as an occupational lens, with the distance correction in the middle of the lens, a traditional near-power D segment at the bottom, and an intermediate-power inverted D segment at the top of the lens so that the wearer can see a ceiling or a portion of an automobile undercarriage at arm's length while looking up.

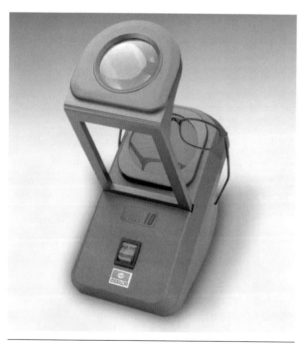

Figure 12.5 Essilor PAL-ID (progressive addition lens identification device).

Assistants are often asked to neutralize eyeglasses of new patients for the medical chart or to check an existing patient's new glasses to make sure they have been fabricated with the correct prescription.

1. Locate the laser-engraved markings (circle or other symbol) on the front surface of the lens. This can be done by holding the lenses up in a brightly lit area against a dark background or by using a PAL-ID (Figure 12.5).

2. "Dot" the manufacturer's markings with a water-soluble marking pen and use the lens manufacturer's "mark-up" chart to re-mark reference points. When the reference points have been remarked, the fitting cross should be directly in front of the patient's pupil center.

3. Note the first two numbers of add power engraved temporally. Engraved circles are 34 mm apart, 17 mm on either side of the pupil. Note that 1.7 refers to an add of 1.75, 2.2 to 2.25, and so on.

4. Note the prescription and any relevant information in the patient's chart.

If a patient spends more than 2 hours a day in front of a computer, special computer glasses may be indicated. People with presbyopia find these lenses of great help. Standard progressives provide intermediate power but they are usually narrow in higher add lenses or require the wearer to raise the chin to see clearly, resulting in neck and backaches. Computer progressives are

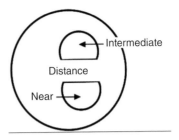

Figure 12.8 Double-D segment occupational lens. *(Image courtesy of Mark Mattison-Shupnick, ABOM, Jobson Medical Information LLC.)*

designed to maximize reading and intermediate vision with a wide intermediate area specifically designed for computer use. The lenses are ordered for a specific range of vision, typically limiting distance vision, and instead increasing intermediate and near. This provides the right powers for the location of the computer monitor, desktop, or laptop, for the width of either screen. Lenses can also be ordered for the choir director, hobbyist, or sports enthusiast, who may require distance vision and intermediate vision but no near correction. The key to satisfying these patients is for the ophthalmologist, optical dispenser, and ophthalmic medical personnel to determine each individual's unique visual needs.

Types of Lens Materials

Patients requiring eyeglasses have many lens materials to choose from today. Each material has its own refractive index, which is the ratio of the speed of light in a vacuum to that in the given material. The closer the index

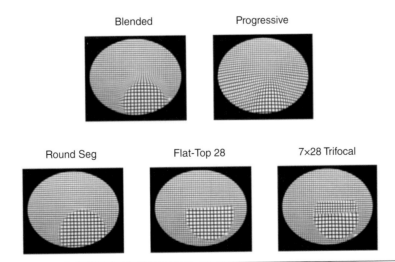

Figure 12.7 Different patterns of add in different multifocal lenses. The larger pattern indicates magnification. *(Image courtesy of Mark Mattison-Shupnick, ABOM, Jobson Medical Information LLC.)*

of refraction is to 1.0 (the refractive index of air), the less the material or medium bends, or refracts, the light passing through.

The index of refraction of the particular material determines the thickness of the lens made from the material. In general, the higher the index of refraction, the thinner the lens will be. Examples of common lens materials (and their respective indices of refraction) include **CR-39** plastic (1.49), high-index plastic (1.54 to 1.74), glass (1.52 to 1.7), Trivex (1.53), and **polycarbonate** (1.59). Although very scratch resistant, glass is heavier than newer plastic materials and its usage in eyewear has declined significantly—glass now accounts for about 2% of all lenses sold. CR-39 plastic is declining in use as well, in favor of newer, higher-index lens materials and impact-resistant polycarbonate lenses. New scratch-resistant lenses and antireflective lenses (plastic, polycarbonate, Trivex and high index) have improved scratch resistance, some with virtually the same abrasion resistance as glass.

Lens Safety Standards

The American National Standards Institute (ANSI) has determined standards for the quality control of eyeglass manufacturing. The latest specification for safety (ANSI Z87.1-2003) requires that all prescription safety protective lenses have a minimum edge thickness or center thickness of 2.0 to 3.0 mm, depending on the material.

Standards for eyeglasses designated as dress eyewear (nonsafety but impact-resistant eyewear) are specified by ANSI Z80.1-2011. ANSI provides quality control standards for the optician; that is, how much a manufactured lens may deviate from a doctor's refractive prescription. Table 12.1 summarizes tolerances. for the single vision/bifocal lens standard. Table 12.2 summarizes tolerances for the progressives standard.

For dress (nonsafety) eyewear, there is no actual thickness standard. Instead, the impact resistance of lens materials governs thickness—or rather the lens thinness in which patients are more interested. An impact test of the lens in its final form must meet U.S. Food and Drug Administration standard 21CFR801.410, implemented in 1971 and amended from time to time. The standard requires that lenses pass a "drop ball test" in which a five-eighth-inch steel ball is dropped onto the lens from a height of 50 inches. If the lens does not fracture or release lens material visible to the eye, it passes. All plastic, high-index and polycarbonate lenses can be batch sampled, so laboratories and manufacturers have sampling programs

Table 12.1 General Tolerances for Single Vision and Multifocal Lenses

Measurement	Power Range	Tolerance
Highest meridian[a] power	≥ 0.00 D, $\leq \pm6.50$ D	±0.13 D
	$> \pm6.50$ D	$\pm2\%$
Cylinder power	≥ 0.00 D, ≤ 2.00 D	±0.13 D
	> 2.00 D, ≤ 4.50 D	±0.15 D
	> 4.50 D	$\pm4\%$
Cylinder axis	> 0.00 D, ≤ 0.25 D	$\pm14°$
	> 0.25 D, ≤ 0.50 D	$\pm7°$
	> 0.50 D, ≤ 0.75 D	$\pm5°$
	> 0.75 D, ≤ 1.50 D	$\pm3°$
	> 1.50 D	$\pm2°$
Add power	$\leq +4.00$ D	±0.12 D
	$> +4.00$ D	±0.18 D
Unmounted prism and PRP	≥ 0.00 D, $\leq \pm3.37$ D	$0.33\,\Delta$
	$> \pm3.37$ D	1.0 mm
Vertical prism imbalance	≥ 0.00 D, $\leq \pm3.37$ D	$\pm0.33\,\Delta$ total
	$> \pm3.37$ D	±1.0 mm difference
Horizontal prism imbalance	≥ 0.00 D, $\leq \pm2.75$ D	$\pm0.67\,\Delta$ total
	$> \pm2.75$ D	±2.5 mm total
Vertical segment height		±1.0 mm each
Vertical segment difference		1.0 mm difference
Horizontal segment location		±2.5 mm total
Horizontal segment tilt		$\pm2.0°$

[a] The *highest meridian* applies to the principal meridian (Sphere or Sphere + Cylinder) with the strongest absolute power. For instance, the highest meridian of a prescription calling for -2.00 DS – 1.00 DC × 180 is: -2.00 + (-1.00) = -3.00 D.

Table 12.2 General Tolerances for Progressive Addition Lenses

Measurement	Power Range	Tolerance
Highest meridian[a] power	≥ 0.00 D, ≤ ±8.00 D	±0.16 D
	> ±8.00 D	±2%
Cylinder power	≥ 0.00 D, ≤ 2.00 D	±0.16 D
	> 2.00 D, ≤ 3.50 D	±0.18 D
	> 3.50 D	±5%
Cylinder axis	> 0.00 D, ≤ 0.25 D	±14°
	> 0.25 D, ≤ 0.50 D	±7°
	> 0.50 D, ≤ 0.75 D	±5°
	> 0.75 D, ≤ 1.50 D	±3°
	> 1.50 D	±2°
Add power	≤ 4.00 D	±0.12 D
	> 4.00 D	±0.18 D
Unmounted Prism and PRP	≥ 0.00 D, ≤ ±3.37 D	0.33 Δ
	> ±3.37 D	1.0 mm
Vertical prism imbalance	≥ 0.00 D, ≤ ±3.37 D	±0.33 Δ total
	> ±3.37 D	1.0 mm difference
Horizontal prism imbalance	≥ 0.00 D, ≤ ±3.37 D	±0.67 Δ total
	> ±3.37 D	±1.0 mm each
Vertical fitting point height		±1.0 mm each
Vertical fitting point difference		1.0 mm difference
Horizontal fitting point location		±1.0 mm each
Horizontal axis tilt		±2.0°

Additional Mechanical Tolerances

Measurement	Comment	Tolerance
Center thickness	When specified	±0.3 mm
Base curve	When specified	±0.75 D
Segment size	For multifocals	±0.5 mm
Warpage		1.00 D

[a]The *highest meridian* applies to the principal meridian (Sphere or Sphere + Cylinder) with the strongest absolute power. For instance, the highest meridian of a prescription calling for -2.00 DS – 1.00 DC × 180 is: -2.00 + (-1.00) = -3.00 D.

that verify impact strength. Also, manufacturers publish minimum thinness guidelines based on results of impact testing various forms of prescriptions. Every glass lens dispensed must have been individually dropball tested prior to being glazed in the frame. Typically, the thinnest center for glass and CR-39 lenses is 2.0 mm, for high-index lenses is 1.3 to 1.5 mm, and 1.0 mm for polycarbonate and Trivex lenses. The reduced center thickness is the result of the increased impact resistance of those materials.

For the complete standards, contact the American National Standards Institute (www.ansi.org), the Optical Laboratories Association (www.ola-labs.org), or your local optical laboratory.

CHOOSING A LENS WITH SAFETY IN MIND More than 40% of disabling eye injuries occur at home or

during sports and outdoor activities. This high rate of injury occurs because most people are unaware of the potential hazards that surround them. Polycarbonate and Trivex have become the material of choice for safety lenses because of their impact resistance. Polycarbonate materials were used in the face shields of headgear for astronauts, motorcyclists, and firefighters long before these compounds became available for use in eyeglass lenses. In the past, manufacturing problems with polycarbonate caused the lenses to look dingy or have optical aberrations. Advances in the manufacturing process, driven by the manufacturers of music compact discs, have created crystal-clear polycarbonate lenses. Trivex lens material, made by a variety of manufacturers in their own lens designs, is widely available.

Although polycarbonate and Trivex are more expensive than plastic, ophthalmic professionals should always insist on polycarbonate or Trivex lenses for children and monocular patients due to the high impact resistance of these lenses. Monocular patients may not have received the message that losing vision in 1 eye makes the other eye more susceptible to injury. Using your position to encourage monocular patients to protect their good eye, even if they do not have a refractive error, is good preventive medicine and a service to your patient.

Sports enthusiasts who engage in potentially high-impact activities like tennis, racquetball, and squash should also use polycarbonate lenses in protective eyeglasses or shields (Figure 12.9). Individuals who do not require prescription eyewear should protect their eyes with nonprescription polycarbonate lenses in the wrap-around type of frame during sports activities. Polycarbonate and Trivex lenses also offer 100% protection from ultraviolet A and B, the wavelengths of ultraviolet linked to damage from sunlight.

Lens Treatments, Tints, and Coatings

Special lens treatments, tints, and coatings aid eyeglass wearers in normal daily activities or in particular situations. These include **photochromic lenses**, **polarized lenses**, and **antireflective lens treatments**.

Photochromic lenses (lenses that darken when exposed to the ultraviolet in sunlight) were once available only in glass. Today, plastic photochromic lenses are as clear as regular glasses inside and as dark as sunglasses in very bright light. Photochromic lenses are a good choice for all-purpose lenses. The lenses rely on ultraviolet light to activate to a darkened state; therefore they do not completely darken behind a windshield. Patients who are sensitive to bright light may need a separate and darker pair of sunglasses. Photochromic lenses are available in

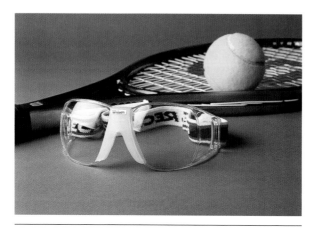

Figure 12.9 Wraparound goggles for a variety of sports.

most lens designs and plastic materials and they protect the eyes from harmful ultraviolet A and B rays.

Polarized lenses, the most effective sunglass lens choice, help reduce or eliminate glare from horizontal, reflective surfaces like water, snow, or any shiny surface. Eliminating this type of glare can reduce eye fatigue and increase visual comfort. Polarized lenses also protect the wearer from harmful ultraviolet A and B rays.

Antireflective lenses eliminate nearly all reflections from lenses, improving both appearance and vision. Technology breakthroughs have improved antireflective coatings, reducing or eliminating past problems such as peeling, cracking, crazing, and cleaning difficulties. Modern hydrophobic (resists water), oleophobic (resists oils), and antistatic (resists airborne dust and dirt) topcoats greatly improve the ease of cleaning, durability, and scratch resistance of plastic lenses. All high-index and polycarbonate lenses benefit from antireflective treatments. No lens transmits 100% of light, and all lenses lose 8% to 14% of light, depending on the index of refraction. The higher the index of refraction, the less light the lens transmits to the eye. An antireflective coating increases light transmission up to 99%—higher than any untreated lens, thus improving vision.

Key Measurements in Fitting Eyeglasses

For eyeglasses to be effective, patients must feel satisfied with the prescription and the overall fit of the lenses on the face. Eyeglasses that fit improperly may cause vision problems. To help determine the source of a patient's dissatisfaction or discomfort with eyeglasses, ophthalmic medical assistants may need to measure interpupillary distance, vertex distance, and the base curves of the lenses. For other ways to ensure a patient's satisfaction with eyeglasses, see the sections on fitting and adjusting eyeglasses later in this chapter.

Interpupillary distance (commonly called *PD*, *PDs*, or *IPD*) is the distance between the lines of sight. The line of sight exits the pupil near its center but is typically nasal to it, so an instrument like a corneal reflection pupillometer is preferred for measuring accurate PDs. PDs are important to the laboratory technician who makes eyeglass lenses because it indicates where to place the optical centers in the finished lenses so that they lie directly in front of the patient's pupils. The **optical center** of a lens denotes the point of optimal vision; it is the single point through which light may pass without being bent or changed, its optical axis (Figure 12.10).

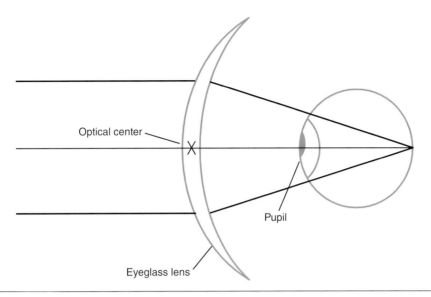

Figure 12.10 Relationship of the optical center of the eyeglass lens to the pupil.

The **vertex distance** is the distance from the back surface of an eyeglass lens to the front surface of the patient's cornea. This measurement can be an important factor, because at higher powers the distance from the eye can change the effective power of a lens. The **base curve** is the front curve of the lens surface, from which the other curves necessary for sight correction are calculated.

Interpupillary Distance

Interpupillary distance, the distance between the pupils, is measured in millimeters. This measurement should be obtained both at near and at distance for each patient. Both a *binocular* measurement (a single recording of the total distance from pupil to pupil) and a *monocular* measurement (the individual distance from the center of the bridge of the nose to the center of each pupil) should be recorded (Figure 12.11).

In **orthophoric** (normal alignment) patients, the eyes look straight ahead when they focus on an object directly in front of them at a distance of 20 feet or more. Eyes that are straight in the primary gaze (straight ahead) will have virtually parallel visual axes when they fixate on a distant object. However, when the same pair of eyes focuses on a near object, the eyes converge (turn in slightly) to allow fixation of the object. Because of this convergence, the near PD measurement will be less than the distance PD.

The distance PD measurement is required to manufacture single-vision and multifocal eyeglasses. The near PD measurement is required when single-vision or multifocal

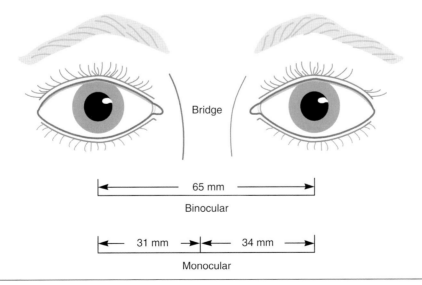

Figure 12.11 Relationship of binocular and monocular measurements for interpupillary distance.

eyeglasses are prescribed for reading or other close-up activities. The accurate measurement of both distance and near PD ensures the appropriate placement of the optical centers of the eyeglass lenses. If the **distance between optical centers** does not correspond to the patient's PDs, the patient can experience pulling or, in extreme cases, double vision. Therefore, the ophthalmic medical assistant should verify the correct PDs and measure the distance between lens optical centers for all eyeglasses whether they are new prescriptions or eyeglasses brought in by patients with vision complaints.

METHODS OF MEASURING PD Several methods exist for measuring distance or near PD. In addition, either binocular or monocular measurements may be chosen. Monocular measurements of PDs are considered more accurate than binocular measurement because the monocular recording takes into consideration any facial asymmetry that might be present.

A binocular distance PD requires just one pupil-to-pupil measurement made with a millimeter ruler. For the patient with very dark eyes, a limbus-to-limbus measurement can be used. For a monocular distance PD measurement, the distances between each pupil and the midline of the bridge of the nose are measured separately, and the results are added together to yield a single measurement. Simple and relatively accurate monocular PD measurements may be made with a specially calibrated ruler and a penlight. Specific instructions for both of these distance PD measuring techniques are presented in Procedure 12.2 and Procedure 12.3. PD measurements can also be made with a corneal reflection pupillometer, discussed later.

Both binocular and monocular near PDs may be measured or calculated. Table 12.3 presents the approximate near PDs corresponding to a range of common monocular distance PDs. Measuring the binocular or monocular near PD requires both the millimeter ruler and the penlight. Procedure 12.4 contains step-by-step instructions for measuring binocular near PDs. The monocular measuring technique for near PD is essential for patients with

---

Procedure 12.2 Measuring Binocular Interpupillary Distance PD

Determining the precise center of a patient's pupils can be difficult, especially if the pupils are large. A reasonably accurate measurement can be obtained by measuring from the temporal limbus of one eye to the nasal limbus of the other eye.

1. Position yourself about 16 inches in front of the patient. Make sure your eyes are level with the patient's eyes.

2. Close your right eye and ask the patient to look at your left eye.

3. Rest the millimeter ruler lightly on the bridge of the patient's nose.

4. Line up the zero point on the temporal limbus of the patient's right eye (Figure A).

5. Holding the ruler in this position, close your left eye and open your right eye. Have the patient fixate on your right eye.

6. Observe the number on the millimeter ruler that is directly under the nasal limbus of the patient's left eye (Figure B).

7. Close your right eye, open your left eye, and check the zero point of the ruler, making sure it is at the temporal limbus of the patient's right eye.

8. Check the measurement on the ruler for the patient's left eye and record it on the patient's chart or form as appropriate.

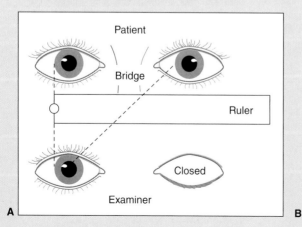

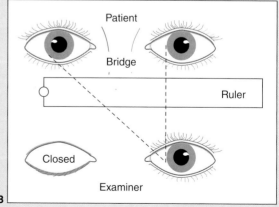

Procedure 12.3 Measuring Monocular Distance PDs

1. Position yourself 14 to 16 inches in front of the patient. Make sure your eyes are level with the patient's eyes. Hold the millimeter ruler lightly over the bridge of the patient's nose.

2. Hold a penlight under your left eye, aiming the light at the patient's eye. Note the position of the spot of light reflection called the corneal reflex on the patient's right eye (see the figure), and record the number on the ruler just below the reflex. This represents the number of millimeters from the patient's right corneal reflex to the center of the bridge of the nose.

3. Hold the penlight under your right eye, aiming the light at the patient's eye. Observe the corneal reflex on the patient's left eye. Record the number of millimeters from the left corneal reflex to the center of the bridge of the nose.

4. Add the two numbers together and record the sum on the patient's chart or form as appropriate.

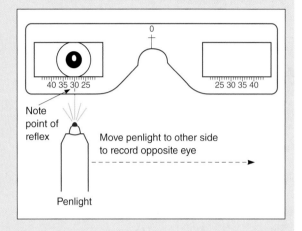

Table 12.3 Monocular Distance PD With Corresponding Average Near PD (mm)

Distance	Near	Distance	Near
24.75	23.00	31.00	29.00
25.25	23.50	31.50	29.50
25.75	24.00	32.00	30.00
26.25	24.50	32.75	30.50
26.75	25.00	33.25	31.00
27.25	25.50	33.75	31.50
27.75	26.00	34.25	32.00
28.50	26.50	34.75	32.50
29.00	27.00	35.25	33.00
29.50	27.50	36.00	33.50
30.00	28.00	36.50	34.00
30.50	28.50	37.00	34.50

Procedure 12.4 Measuring Binocular Near PDs

1. Place your dominant eye in front of the patient's nose at the patient's near working distance, which is usually 14 to 16 inches.

2. Close your other eye and have the patient fixate on your open eye (your dominant eye).

3. Rest the millimeter ruler lightly on the bridge of the patient's nose and line up the zero point at the center of the patient's right pupil.

4. Record the reading from the ruler marking at the center of the patient's left pupil.

5. Hold the penlight directly under your right eye and shine the light toward the patient's nose. A crisp corneal reflection on both eyes will be seen. This may help you in making these measurements because the light reflex is the center of the cornea (and almost the center of the pupil), and you can determine a reading on the millimeter scale by reading from the ruler at the corneal reflex.

an asymmetric face. To obtain a monocular near PD, instruct the patient to fixate at the bridge of your nose and then, as you did when taking the monocular distance PD, alternately close each of your eyes and record the distance on the ruler separately.

The accurate measurement of both distance and near PDs ensure that the optical centers of the patient's eyeglass lenses are correctly placed in front of the patient's pupils. If the distance between optical centers does not correspond to the measured PDs, an optical distortion known as **prismatic effect** may occur. Prismatic effect causes incoming light rays to deviate inappropriately when they strike the lens (Figure 12.12), leading to eye

discomfort or distorted or double vision for the lens wearer. The direction of the prismatic effect can vary depending on whether a plus-power lens or minus-power lens is involved and on whether the distance between the lens centers is wider or narrower than the PD.

Several common errors can occur when using the millimeter ruler to measure distance and near PD. Some errors in measurement relate to a patient's strabismus or

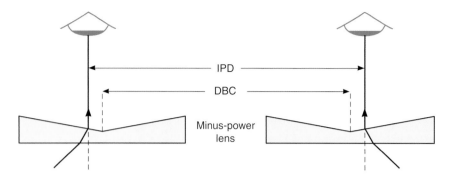

Figure 12.12 Prismatic effect in a minus-power lens for which the distance between optical centers (DBC) is narrower than the interpupillary distance (PD).

asymmetric face. The most common cause of error in assessing PD is *parallax*, an optical distortion that occurs when the measurer's and the patient's lines of sight are not parallel. Parallax can result in the measured PD being significantly different from the patient's actual PD. It can result from the measurer standing closer to the patient than 14 inches, from head movement by the measurer or patient, from improper eye fixation by the patient during the measurement, or from the examiner's line of sight being higher or lower than the patient's.

INSTRUMENTS FOR MEASURING PD Special instruments, such as the Essilor **digital corneal reflection pupillometer** (**DCRP**) and other metering devices, are used to measure PDs (Figure 12.13). Opticians use them routinely because these meters correct for parallax error. In addition, the instruments provide a monocular reading that avoids errors due to facial asymmetry or strabismus. The Essilor DCRP is a very reliable method of taking PDs. Using a pupillometer is relatively easy, but due to model differences, ophthalmic medical assistants should read in detail the user's manual for the particular instrument available in their practice and request practical instruction in its use from the ophthalmologist or a senior staff assistant.

Vertex Distance

The distance between the back of an eyeglass lens and the front of the eyeglass wearer's eye is the vertex distance (Figure 12.14). A vertex distance of 13.5 mm is considered average, but vertex distance can range from 5 mm to more than 26 mm. The most effective fit for eyeglasses usually is obtained by fitting the frame as close to the eye as possible without the eyelashes touching the lenses.

Positioning a patient's eyeglasses at a vertex distance other than that used during refractometry will change the effective power of the lenses. The amount of change depends on the power of the lens. For low-powered

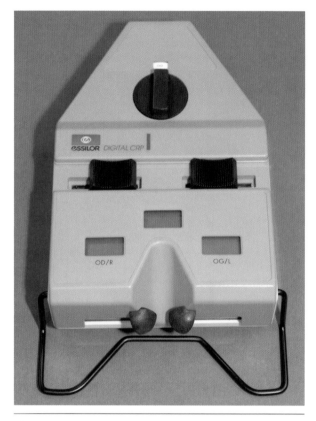

Figure 12.13 Essilor pupillometer used to measure interpupillary distance. *(Image courtesy of Brice Critser, CRA, Department of Ophthalmology and Visual Sciences, University of Iowa.)*

lenses, the patient will not notice a difference in vision correction. For high-powered lenses, however, a small alteration in vertex distance makes a considerable and noticeable change in the effective power of both the spherical and the cylindrical components of the lens. For example, if a patient's refractive prescription is less than or equal to minus or plus 5 diopters (or up to 7 diopters, according to some authorities), an accurate assessment of vertex distance is not required to ensure proper eyeglass prescription. If the prescription calls for more than

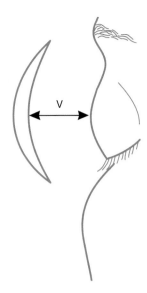

Figure 12.14 Vertex distance (V).

minus or plus 5 (or 7, please check your doctor's preference) diopters, the vertex distance should be measured during refractometry to avoid refraction errors that could lead to vision difficulties with the eyeglasses.

INSTRUMENTS FOR MEASURING VERTEX DISTANCE
A specially designed instrument called a **distometer** (vertometer) is used to measure vertex distance accurately. Instructions for measuring vertex distance with a distometer appear in Procedure 12.5. Some pupillometers also allow for accurate vertex distance measurements.

> When recording the ophthalmologist's refractive prescription for a patient, the ophthalmic medical assistant should always include a vertex distance on prescriptions with higher powers.

Base Curve

The base curve of a lens is the curve on the front surface of a lens "blank" supplied by a manufacturer. Using this curve as a basis for measurement, the laboratory technician grinds additional curves on the lens back surface to achieve the final power and refractive correction of the lens. The power of a lens equals the algebraic difference between the power of the front curve and that of the back curve, and many different combinations of base curves and other curves can be used to arrive at the same power.

ADVANTAGE OF ASPHERIC LENS DESIGN Changing the base curve of a lens, either flatter or steeper away from the best form (or "corrected curve"), will increase

Procedure 12.5 Using a Distometer

1. Ask the patient to close both eyes.

2. Gently rest the fixed arm of the distometer caliper on the closed eyelid and carefully place the movable caliper arm against the back surface of the trial lens or eyeglass lens (see the figure).

3. Record the separation distance between these two surfaces from the millimeter scale on the distometer. (Note: Check the instrument instructions. The scale may allow for an average eyelid thickness, or the user may need to add 1 mm for lid thickness.)

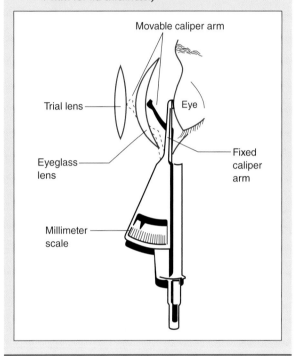

aberrations. Modern lens designers have been able to use an aspheric lens design to minimize or eliminate these aberrations. Typically, aspheric surfaces are designed to flatten from the center to the periphery in plus prescriptions and steepen from center to edge in minus prescriptions, resulting in thinner and lighter lenses, with the added advantage of better peripheral vision. Figure 12.15 compares the thickness of spherical and aspheric designs.

Patients can become accustomed to wearing lenses ground with a particular base curve. Occasionally, changing the base curve when a new pair of lenses is prescribed can cause the patient mild visual discomfort, if the lens surface is not aspherical. When ordering replacement lenses or supplying the patient with a second pair of glasses, the optician should take into account the base curves for both pairs of eyeglasses. The ophthalmic medical assistant may be required to measure the base curve

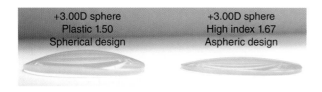

Figure 12.15 Comparison of thickness of spherical and aspheric lenses. *(Image courtesy of Mark Mattison-Shupnick, ABOM, Jobson Medical Information LLC.)*

of lenses as part of a comprehensive measurement of new and previously worn spectacles to help determine the source of a patient's visual complaints.

MEASURING THE BASE CURVE The **Geneva lens clock** is used to measure the base curve of an eyeglass lens. The lens clock is calibrated in diopters and has three blunt pins at its foot, the outer two fixed and the central pin movable (Figure 12.16). When the pins are held against a flat surface, the indicator hand of the lens clock points to zero. When the instrument is placed against a concave lens surface (the back of the lens), the indicator will point to minus (–), or red, numbers; placed against a convex lens surface (the front), the indicator will point to the plus (+), or black, number scale. Some Geneva clocks may show + or – without color. The base curve is shown in quarter-diopters steps (ie, +6.25, +6.50, +6.75). When measuring a multifocal lens, always keep the pins of the lens clock away from the multifocal segment; if the pins impinge on the multifocal segment, an error in base curve measurement could result (Figure 12.17). Other possible reasons for errors in base curve measurements include an aspheric front lens surface, measurement of a progressive lens, or measurement being taken with the

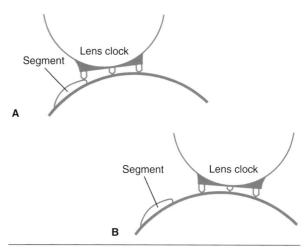

Figure 12.17 Placement of the Geneva lens clock onto a multifocal lens. **A.** Incorrect placement. **B.** Correct placement.

pins at an angle other than 90° or perpendicular to the surface. Lens clocks are calibrated for an index of refraction of 1.53 and lens manufacturers list the true lens base curves of lens fronts by converting the value to a 1.53 equivalent regardless of lens material index.

> Using the Geneva lens clock to measure the base curve in the patient's new and previous glasses can avoid costly remakes.

Fitting, Care, and Adjustment of Eyeglasses

Eyeglass frames come in a wide variety of sizes, shapes, styles, and materials. Naturally, most patients try to choose frames that they feel are becoming to their appearance. However, opticians, ophthalmic medical assistants, and others who help patients choose frames and wear them comfortably also must consider frames from the aspects of their tilt and curve in relationship to the wearer's face and their overall size and shape (both of which can affect proper peripheral vision), as well as their comfortable fit.

Fitting of Eyeglasses

Figure 12.18 shows the principal parts of a typical frame. The **pantoscopic angle** of an eyeglass frame is the angle by which the frame front deviates from the vertical plane when the glasses are worn on the face. The pantoscopic

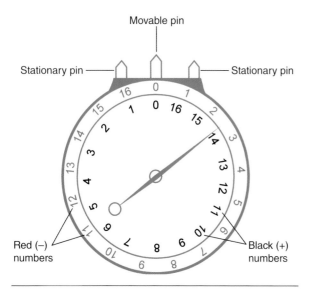

Figure 12.16 The Geneva lens clock for measuring the base curve of a lens.

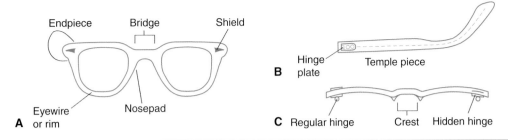

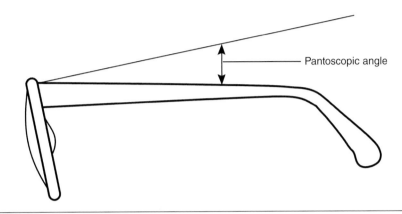

Figure 12.18 Anatomy of an eyeglass frame. **A.** Front view of frame. **B.** Side view temple piece. **C.** Top view of frame front.

Figure 12.19 Pantoscopic angle estimated by viewing the eyeglasses on the face from the side.

angle is estimated by viewing the eyeglasses on the face from the side (Figure 12.19). The lower rims of the frame front normally are closer to the cheeks than are the upper rims. A usual pantoscopic angle ranges from 4° to 18° (the average pantoscopic angle is 12° to 15°), although an individual with protruding eyebrows may exceed this range. The term **retroscopic tilt** is used to describe eyeglasses that are adjusted so that the lower rims tilt away from the face; this rarely happens by design but can occur in error.

A proper pantoscopic angle allows the eye to rotate downward from the distance gaze to the near gaze while maintaining a similar vertex distance. Patients can have visual problems that may prompt an office visit if a retroscopic tilt is present or if the pantoscopic angle is incorrect; patients with moderate cylinder powers and above-average refractive errors have more problems and notice this improper tilt.

RESTRICTIONS RELATED TO FRAME SIZES AND SHAPES Some patients' choice of frame sizes and shapes may be restricted because of their lens prescriptions. If the eyeglass prescription is moderate to high (that is, approximately 3 diopters or more of myopia or hyperopia), lens base curve, frame size and shape play a significant role in altering peripheral vision. This problem primarily relates to the increase in vertex distance

from the center of the lens to the edge of the lens. For larger lenses, the increase in vertex distance at the edge of the lens compared to the center may dramatically change both the spherical and the cylindrical components of the optical prescription. Moreover, the farther the eye views through the lens from the center, the greater the optical distortion. Large lenses may cause significant optical aberration in the peripheral parts of the lens. A good general rule is to make sure that the eye is well centered in the eyewire (the metal that encircles each lens), in addition to recommending a smaller frame.

EFFECTS ON PATIENT COMFORT A patient who requires eyeglasses will not consistently wear them if the frames do not fit well, even though the prescription may be correct. Misaligned frames or improper frame size can cause the following problems:

- Frames slide forward (this can also be caused by heavy glass lenses).
- Frames fit loosely.
- Frames must be positioned awkwardly to see properly.
- Frame temples create pressure on the side of the head or at the ears.
- Eyelashes or eyebrows touch the lenses.

When fitting or adjusting the fit of a pair of eyeglasses, pay special attention to the physical structure of a patient's face. Because most of the weight of the eyeglasses is placed on the bridge of the patient's nose, the weight should be evenly distributed. One ear may be slightly higher than the other ear; therefore, the fit over or behind each ear should be carefully made. The nature of the individual's skin (for example, the degree of oiliness) may cause some types of frames to slip down from the bridge of the nose. No easy formula exists for adjusting a pair of glasses so that the patient will wear them, but thorough observation and listening carefully to what a patient says will allow you to help the patient choose frames appropriately and wear them comfortably.

When checking the fit or assessing other problems, take special care when putting the eyeglasses on the patient or taking them off. Always cover the tips of the temple pieces (also called *temples*) with your fingers until you have moved them past the patient's eyes. This procedure avoids poking the patient in the eye with the pointed ends of the frame temples.

Care of Eyeglasses

Eyeglass lenses and frames, especially those worn daily, are subject to considerable wear and tear. Although most frames and lenses are designed to take a certain amount of abuse, patients can get longer, more satisfying wear out of their eyeglasses if they receive instructions in proper cleaning and handling.

CLEANING THE LENSES A variety of cleaning sprays and special cloths exist for cleaning eyeglass lenses. Patients can keep their glasses clean without damaging lens surfaces by using proper cleaning methods and materials. Conventional glass or plastic lenses can be cleaned simply with a solution of mild dish soap and water, then dried with a soft, 100% cotton cloth. Unless using a specially designed lens cloth, lenses should be cleaned while wet. Rubbing a cloth or tissue, which contains wood fibers, over dry lenses may drag dirt across the lens surfaces and scratch them, resulting in blurry vision.

When appropriate, the ophthalmic medical assistant should instruct patients in the proper method of cleaning their eyeglass lenses. Patients should also be instructed to protect their eyeglasses from impact or pressure by storing them in the eyeglass case when not in use, being sure the temple tips to not touch the back of the lenses. The assistant may also caution patients that when placing eyeglasses on a hard surface, they should place the side with the temple pieces down so that the lenses will not be scratched.

Adjustment of Eyeglasses

Ophthalmic assistants are often asked to make minor adjustments to the frames, such as tightening screws, measuring optical centers, and, for multifocals, measuring segment heights to ensure that they are properly placed and not a source of patient complaint.

FRAME SCREWS Plastic frames usually have a single screw holding each temple piece to the frame front (Figure 12.20). Most nonrimless metal frames have two screws on each side, one to hold the eyewire together and one to keep the temple piece in place. Loose eyeglass frame screws are a common problem. To adjust or tighten these screws, a jeweler's or optician's screwdriver and a small bottle of clear nail polish are needed. For instructions, see Procedure 12.6. Remind the patient to come in for routine adjustments to tighten screws before they loosen and fall out.

OPTICAL CENTERS The ophthalmic medical assistant may need to check the optical centers of the patient's eyeglass lenses to determine whether the placement of the optical centers matches the measured interpupillary distance. Measuring the optical center or distance between centers of eyeglass lenses requires using the marking, or dotting, device on a lensmeter. Procedure 12.7 describes

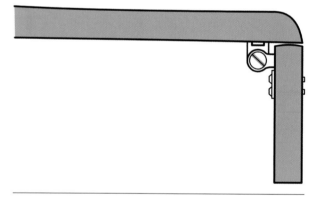

Figure 12.20 Typical frame screw for a plastic frame.

Procedure 12.6 Adjusting Frame Screws

1. Tighten the screws with a jeweler's or optician's screwdriver so that the temple piece moves freely without binding.

2. Apply a small drop of clear nail polish to the screw head. Alternatively, back the screw out, add a drop of polish in the hinge, then tighten the screw. When the nail polish dries, the screw will not loosen easily. Do not attempt to tighten screws with fingers if the screwdriver slips off.

Procedure 12.7 Checking Optical Centers

1. Place the lens against the lens stop of the lensmeter.

2. Make certain the eyeglass frame sits squarely on the spectacle table.

3. Focus the mires and center them within the focused eyepiece target (figure). Use the dotting device to mark the lens while it is held in this position. The center mark (usually of three) is the optical center of the lens. If the lensmeter does not have a marking device, use a nonpermanent marker pen to record the approximate center of the lens.

4. Use a millimeter ruler to measure the distance between the center dots; this measurement should correspond to the patient's distance PDs unless a prism has been prescribed.

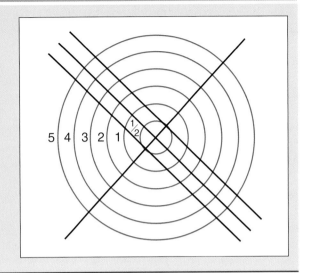

these steps. (See Chapter 5 for instructions on operating a lensmeter.)

SEGMENT HEIGHTS The **segment height** is the distance between the lowest part of the rim and the top of the multifocal lens segment (Figure 12.21). The correct segment height for a multifocal lens has a direct effect on the patient's satisfaction with the eyeglasses. In determining segment heights, remember that each patient has different vision requirements and must be treated individually with respect to these special requirements. Most opticians recommend fitting the top of a bifocal segment level with the patient's lower lid margin, which is the area where the lid touches the eyeball (Figure 12.22). Some patients prefer the bifocal line at a slightly higher or lower level than at the lower lid margin, but the segment height usually will not vary more than 1 or 2 mm higher or lower. Trifocals are usually fit about 7 mm higher than the lower lid margin.

Progressive addition lenses should be fit at the patient's pupil center. The lens is designed for the intermediate area to begin as the eye moves down the lens and the patient's eyes converge. Fitting progressive addition lenses takes more skill than lined bifocals. Properly fit progressive addition lenses have a very high patient satisfaction rate; therefore most patient complaints are usually the result of poor fitting and dispensing techniques. Always check to determine the patient's previous segment height, if any, and whether it was satisfactory.

Figure 12.21 The segment height is the distance between the lowest part of the rim and the top of the segment. **A.** Incorrect measurement. **B.** Correct measurement.

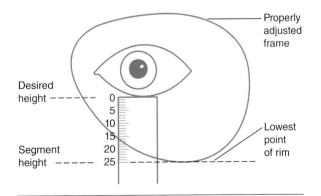

Figure 12.22 Placement of bifocal segment.

SELF-ASSESSMENT TEST

1. Choose the single lettered description that best matches each type of lens listed.

   _____ bifocal

   _____ trifocal

   _____ progressive addition

   _____ single-vision

   a. corrects for 1 distance

   b. corrects for 2 distances

   c. corrects for 3 distances

   d. corrects for 2 or more distances by increasing optical power in a transitional zone

   e. corrects for near and intermediate distances only

   f. corrects for near vision in a single eye only

2. Choose the single lettered task that is best associated with each instrument listed.

   _____ lensmeter

   _____ millimeter ruler

   _____ distometer

   _____ Geneva lens clock

   a. measures interpupillary distance

   b. determines the optical center of a lens

   c. determines the pantoscopic angle of a frame

   d. determines the base curve of a lens

   e. measures vertex distance

   f. identifies a plastic lens

3. Prescription safety, occupational protective lenses must have a minimum edge or center thickness, depending on the material of the lens, of which of the following?

   a. 1.0 mm

   b. 1.0 mm or 1.5 mm

   c. 2.0 mm or 3.0 mm

   d. 2.5 mm or 3.0 mm

   e. 3.0 mm

4. Which lenses are more commonly used—glass or plastic?

5. Lenses that darken when exposed to ultraviolet light are described as which of the following?

   a. ultraviolet

   b. photochromic

   c. safety

   d. polycarbonate

6. Define *base curve.*

7. Which color scale on a Geneva lens clock is used when the instrument is placed against a convex surface?

8. Define *pantoscopic angle.*

9. Label the parts of the eyeglass frame that are pointed out in the illustration below.

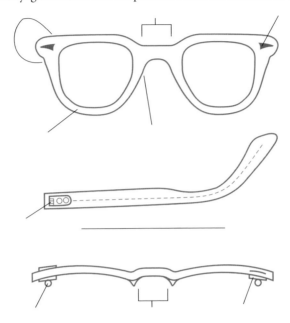

10. Describe the precaution taken to avoid poking a patient when placing eyeglass frames on the patient's face.

11. When the fit of bifocals is checked, the top of the near segment generally should be level with the patient's _____.

12. Label the multifocal lenses listed with the letter corresponding to the correct illustration.

_____ round-top segment

_____ straight-top D segment

_____ round-top invisible bifocal

_____ progressive addition bifocal

_____ executive trifocal

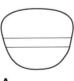

A   B   C   D   E

SUGGESTED ACTIVITIES

1. Schedule a time for your ophthalmologist or a senior staff member to supervise your practice in using the following tools: millimeter ruler, Geneva lens clock, optician's screwdriver, and pupillometer. Use discarded or sample eyeglasses or frames when they are necessary.

2. Do the following tasks several times to gain practice:

    a. Measure the segment widths of various multifocal eyeglasses to become familiar with the different multifocal styles, always measuring segments at their widest point.

    b. Measure the segment heights. Note that sometimes they will be dissimilar. Consider why this is so.

    c. Use the Geneva lens clock to measure the base curves of a patient's new and old pair of glasses. Compare these sets of readings.

    d. Ask those in the office who wear eyeglasses if you may check the tightness of the temples on the frames. With their permission, use the technique described in this chapter to tighten the frame screws.

3. Arrange with several of your coworkers to measure their distance and near interpupillary distance, using the procedures outlined in this chapter. Have your ophthalmologist or senior technician check your work.

4. Arrange with coworkers who wear eyeglasses to measure their vertex distance with a distometer, using the procedure outlined in this chapter.

5. Ask a local optician if you may have samples of old single-vision and multifocal lenses that are chipped, undersized, crooked, or otherwise not useful (not chipped glass as it is unsafe to handle). Use them to perform the following tasks for practice and learning. Ask your ophthalmologist or senior technician to check your work.

    a. Practice using the lensmeter to dot the various lenses for optical center.

    b. Measure the segment heights of the multifocals with a millimeter ruler.

    c. Use the Geneva lens clock to measure the base curves of all sample lenses.

    d. Locate the markings on the front surface of a progressive addition lens and use the manufacturer's chart to "re-mark" the lenses.

SUGGESTED RESOURCES

Brooks CW, Borish IM. *System for Ophthalmic Dispensing.* 3rd ed. St Louis: Butterworth-Heinemann/Elsevier; 2007.

Milder B, Rubin ML. *The Fine Art of Prescribing Glasses Without Making a Spectacle of Yourself.* 3rd ed. Gainesville, FL: Triad; 2004.

Opticians Association of America, Guild of Prescription Opticians of America. *Professional Dispensing for Opticianry.* 2nd ed. Newton, MA: Butterworth-Heinemann; 1996.

PDR Network. *PDR for Ophthalmic Medicines (Physicians' Desk Reference for Ophthalmic Medicines).* Montvale, NJ: PDR Network; updated annually.

Stein HA, Freeman MI, Stenson SM. *Residents Curriculum Manual on Refraction, Spectacles and Dispensing.* Metairie, LA: Contact Lens Association of Ophthalmology and Gerber Communications; 2001.

13

LOW VISION

Worldwide, there are many more people with low vision than there are people who are blind. Approximately 90% of blindness and low vision occurs in the developing world, and approximately 80% of blindness is "avoidable"; that is, it can be prevented or corrected. As a matter of public health and well-being, low vision services should be integrated into all eye care programs. Awareness, recognition, and correction of low vision should be promoted among eye care workers, public service organizations working for prevention of blindness, and health agencies. In addition to refraction and treatment of an underlying disease, there are other simple interventions that can assist people with low vision and significantly improve their eyesight and their lives.

Loss of vision or the fear of vision loss adversely changes a person's life and is a devastating experience at any age. People who lose sight later in life still relate to the world as sighted persons and require visual information. They want to know the visual details of people and their surroundings. Providing this information is an important aspect of assisting patients with visual impairments.

People with unimpaired vision sometimes erroneously categorize all persons with visual impairments as blind. They also may assume persons who are blind to be in complete darkness when, in fact, only 10% of all "legally blind" persons are totally without sight. **Legal blindness** is often defined as a best-corrected visual acuity of 20/200 or less or as a visual field reduced to 20° or less in the better-seeing eye. It is of utmost importance that those who work with people with visual impairments appreciate the great differences in an individual's degree of deficit and the varying abilities of those with visual impairments to cope and maneuver in the "sighted world." Any of the following common deficits, either singly or in combination, can impair vision: no peripheral vision but good central vision, no central vision, less than 20/200 visual acuity, only portions of the visual field perceived, light perception only, no light perception, or fluctuations in vision.

The ophthalmic assistant should be careful not to treat visually impaired or blind patients as if they were deaf or mentally defective. Although visually impaired and blind patients may not see as well as others, they usually hear, speak, and think as well as the average individual. Patients with poor vision often rely on their hearing to understand activity around them. Be careful not to startle these patients, which can happen unintentionally if you approach them noiselessly in a carpeted room. Try always to face these patients and use their name when speaking to them, or gently touch their elbow when speaking to them. It is never appropriate to shout at any patient. (Refer to Chapter 16 for additional information and office policies on working with and assisting an individual with a visual disability.)

Educational services, low vision optical devices, and social support all help to maximize an individual's visual potential. Many organizations around the world can provide further information on low vision services. Some of these organizations are further described here, and Appendix B contains a broader list of international resources in this area.

Visual Acuity and Low Vision

Visual acuity is a measurement of the eye's capacity to see detail. Distance visual acuity is a measurement of the ability to read standard figures on a chart at 6 m (20 ft). *Near visual acuity* is a measurement of the ability to read standard figures on a card at 40 cm (16 in). *Vision* is the sense of sight as a whole, which includes visual acuity and peripheral, or side, vision (visual field). The term *vision* is not equivalent to visual acuity. *Functional vision* is visual acuity and peripheral vision sufficient for the person to carry out his or her normal activities.

Low vision, or *functional visual impairment*, is a significant limitation of visual capability resulting from disease, trauma, or a congenital condition that cannot be corrected to a normal range with refraction, medical treatment, or surgery. Such impairment may be manifested by insufficient visual resolution, inadequate field of vision, or reduced peak contrast sensitivity. Even after therapeutic measures are taken, the patient may still remain with visual impairment or low vision.

Definitions of blindness and low vision vary from country to country. The World Health Organization definition of low vision is a visual acuity of less than 6/18 (20/60) and equal to or better than 3/60 (20/400) in the better eye. A person who has better than 6/18 (20/60) visual acuity in the better eye, but whose peripheral vision is less than 20° is considered also to have low vision. See Chapter 21 for a more detailed discussion of definitions of vision impairment and blindness worldwide.

Common Causes of Low Vision

There are numerous causes of low vision. Cataract that is not surgically treated is the single most common cause of blindness or low vision in the world. Ocular traumas, including surface injuries and penetrating intraocular injuries, are significant causes of low vision. Other causes, include high refractive errors, corneal scarring, macular degeneration, glaucoma, onchocerciasis (river blindness), diabetic retinopathy, congenital causes, and retinopathy of prematurity (ROP). Fortunately, a large percentage of people with impaired vision can be helped. Their total vision may not be fully restored, but their visual level can be improved.

Uncorrected high refractive errors—high myopia of more than −6.00 diopters or high hyperopia of more than +3.00 diopters—are common causes of low vision. The chapter on community medicine provides information on the international prevalence of low vision due to a lack of corrective lenses. It is important to provide refractive services to all people with low vision. Visual acuity can often be improved with a spectacle correction, although not always to normal visual levels.

Xerophthalmia (due to vitamin A deficiency), corneal ulcer, or injury can produce various degrees of scarring and irregularity of the cornea leading to distortion and low vision. More severe corneal scarring from trachoma and other diseases is common in many regions of the world and is a major cause of low vision. Corneal tissue replacement (transplantation) for corneal scarring from trachoma is not recommended because of poor surgical results.

Degeneration of the macula is most commonly related to aging (age-related macular degeneration) and is usually bilateral. This is a more serious problem in countries where life expectancy is high and a large percentage of the population is elderly. An inherited type of macular degeneration may occur in young adults, but it is a less common condition. Macular degeneration will become an increasing problem in the developing world in the coming decades as their population and life expectancy rise.

Both angle-closure glaucoma and open-angle glaucoma may be responsible for low vision. Peripheral vision (used for moving about and finding things in the larger environment) is initially lost in glaucoma. Because visual acuity (central macular vision, used for reading and detail work) may be good until late in the disease course, a person with glaucoma (particularly open-angle glaucoma) may not even be aware that the disease is present until central visual acuity is affected. When central acuity becomes affected in glaucoma, usually the peripheral vision loss has already been severely compromised.

Secondary uveitis, corneal scarring, and glaucoma from onchocerciasis (river blindness) are major causes of low vision in western and central African nations. Worldwide this is a significant cause of loss of vision but is uncommon in the western world. For more information, see Chapter 7.

Diabetic retinopathy, a retinal vascular complication of diabetes mellitus, is a common cause of low vision in industrialized countries. At present, diabetic retinopathy is not a common condition in most developing nations, but it will become more common as insulin and other treatments become more available and diabetic patients live longer.

Low vision may be due to inherited congenital causes. An infant or young child with a congenital visual defect should be treated as soon as the condition is diagnosed and the patient referred for special educational assistance.

Premature infants subjected to high oxygen levels in incubators may develop neovascularization (abnormal fragile new blood vessels) of the retina, resulting in damage to the retina, macula, vitreous, and lens, a condition called *retinopathy of prematurity* (ROP). It is usually bilateral and the visual acuity may be severely affected. It is anticipated that ROP will become a more common cause of low vision in developing nations as premature infant care improves and neonatal mortality decreases.

Increasing Awareness

Professional eye care workers are often unaware of the possibilities for detecting usable vision in their patients with low vision and for providing assistance that will allow them to function more effectively. All too often, a patient with a degenerative disease or an inoperable condition and low vision is not evaluated properly by medical and nonmedical eye care practitioners. If low vision cannot be improved by an accurate refraction or by medical or surgical treatment, the patient should be considered for fitting with a low vision aid.

If their vision is impaired but cannot be improved by medical treatment or routine refraction, patients should be informed that they can be helped by a low vision specialist or an ophthalmic assistant specially trained to dispense low vision devices under the supervision of the ophthalmologists. If someone is not available to dispense low vision aids in your practice patients should be referred to an experienced low vision specialist for examination and treatment. Technicians can help in the identification of these patients and determination of low vision services utilized by the patient.

Public health information and educational materials on low vision should be included in comprehensive national, regional, and local blindness prevention and sight restoration programs. Organizations working with blindness prevention and cataract programs should also refer people with low vision for further evaluation and treatment. Community leaders should know the value of screening for low vision and blindness and medical personnel should encourage the support of these programs. (See Chapter 21 for additional information on community health eye care.)

Low Vision Care

To determine the extent of vision loss, the examiner should test visual acuity and the visual fields. Visual acuity is tested with both eyes together and then by testing each eye separately. Patients should have their vision tested both without and with their spectacles. Visual field screening is tested by the confrontation field test. (Chapter 8 outlines this procedure.) Accurate visual acuity measurements in each eye—together with the comprehensive eye examination—are necessary to determine if low vision is present and how it may be improved. (See Chapter 8 for the method for visual acuity measurement and Procedure 13.1 for a procedure for low vision testing.)

Low Vision Aids

MAGNIFIERS AND READING GLASSES A careful refraction is the first step in any evaluation of aids in low vision. Presbyopic people who wear spectacles for distance require a second lens for reading because of loss of accommodation. Bifocal lenses are usually prescribed for this purpose. A +3.00 diopter bifocal add is customarily the maximum effective power for near vision in a normally sighted individual who is greater than 60 years of age or has hyperopia. Single-vision spectacles of greater than +3.00 diopters (6- to 10-diopter magnifying glasses) are prescribed for people with low vision. However, reading matter must be held closer to the face to be seen with high-plus spectacles. (Also see Chapter 12.)

Kestenbaum's rule is used to calculate the magnification needed to read standard newsprint (20/60 or J5 level) by low vision patients. In Kestenbaum's rule, one divides the denominator of the Snellen acuity by the numerator.

Procedure 13.1 Testing Acuity for Patients With Low Vision

Test and record the visual acuity in each eye separately, beginning with the right eye. Make sure that the eye not being tested is well covered.

1. If the patient is unable to resolve the largest optotype on the distance acuity chart from the standard testing distance, ask the patient to stand or sit 10 feet from the well-illuminated test chart. A projected chart is less desirable to use in this situation than a printed wall chart. A low vision test chart, if available, is preferable for these patients.

2. Repeatedly halve the testing distance (up to 2.5 feet) and retest the distance visual acuity at each stage until the patient successfully identifies half the optotypes on a line.

3. Note the corresponding acuity measurement shown at that line of the chart. Record the acuity value for each eye separately, with correction and without correction, as would be done for standard distance acuity testing, recording the distance at which the patient successfully reads the chart as the numerator of the Snellen acuity designation; for example, 5/80.

4. If the patient is unable to resolve the largest optotypes on the chart from a distance of 2.5 feet, display 2 or more fingers of 1 hand and ask the patient to count the number of fingers displayed. Record the longest distance at which counting is done accurately; for example, CF at 2 ft.

5. If the patient cannot count fingers, move your hand horizontally or vertically before the patient at a distance of approximately 2 feet. Record the

distance at which the patient reported seeing your hand movement; for example, HM at 2 ft.

6. If the patient cannot detect your hand motion, shine a penlight toward the patient's face from approximately 1 foot and turn it on and off to determine if light perception is present. If the patient cannot see the light, dim the room lights and shine the brightest light available (usually the indirect ophthalmoscope) toward the patient's eye again. If the patient cannot see even the brightest light, record the response as NLP (no light perception). If the patient can see the light, record the response as LP (light perception). No record of distance is required.

7. If light is perceived from straight ahead, move the light sequentially into each of the 4 quadrants of the visual field. Turn the penlight on and off in each field, and ask if the patient can see the light.

8. If the patient correctly identifies the direction from which the light is coming, record the response as LP with projection. Specify the quadrant(s) in which light projection is present. If the patient is unable to identify any direction but is able to discern light in the straight-ahead position, record the response as LP without projection.

9. If the light can be seen from straight ahead, colored filters can be placed in front of the light and the patient is asked to identify the color of the light. Record whether or not color perception is present.

10. Repeat steps 1 to 9 for the fellow eye, as appropriate.

For example, a person with 20/200 vision would require a +10 (200/20) diopter lens to read J5 print. This +10.00 near spectacle requires the low vision patient to hold the print about 4 inches from their face or 10 cm for sharpest focus; however, if you chose a focal length of 25 cm (0.25 meters) or 10 inches the magnification achieved with a +10 diopter lens would be 2.5×. This is calculated by multiplying the reading distance in meters (0.25) by the power of the lens (+10 D) or 10 × 0.25 = 2.5. Hence, a +8 D lens has 2× magnification and a +20 D lens 5× magnification. The corollary is to divide the power of the lens by 1/4 (the fraction of 0.25) or 10 ÷ 1/4 = 10/4 = 2.5×. Thus, at a focal length of 25 cm, the degree of magnification achieved would be 10/4 or 2.5×.

APPROPRIATE LIGHTING AND GLARE REDUCTION For reading, low light (dim illumination) does not bring out contrast in the printed matter. A brighter light source (higher illumination) will produce greater

contrast between the background (paper) and the target (printed numbers or letters) and make reading easier. A low-intensity light source may be placed close to the reading material for greater contrast if brighter ambient lighting is not practical.

The position of the light source for reading is very important. The light should be placed in a position that will not produce glare for the reader. Glare is overly bright light or reflection from a smooth surface that interferes with vision. Glare can decrease reading ability of people with low vision. To prevent glare, the light source can be positioned behind the reader or obliquely from the side so that light does not reflect directly off the page into the reader's eyes. Bright light from an overhead source causing glare may be reduced by having the patient wear a hat with a brim. Tinted spectacle lenses may also reduce glare, create greater contrast, and make reading easier. However, darker tints are to be avoided as they decrease the transmission of light into the eye.

Low Vision Devices

SPECTACLES   High plus reading spectacles with prismatic correction may be helpful as an inexpensive and convenient appliance. These spectacles have the disadvantage of requiring the reader to hold the printed material closer to their face.

HANDHELD MAGNIFYING LENSES   The patient may find a handheld or stand magnifying lens (Figure 13.1) more convenient than magnifying spectacles. Generally, the larger the area of the magnifying glass, the easier it is for the patient to read the printed material.

The disadvantage is that magnification usually decreases with broader [wider] hand lenses. Larger size magnifying lenses offer wider fields of view but less magnification. This increased ease of reading occurs because of the larger field resulting from the larger area of glass. A larger field of view is usually more helpful to a patient with low vision than a smaller-size magnifying lens (Figure 13.2). For patients with low vision who are only minimally affected by their disease, a small pocket magnifier may be useful for reading the smaller font sizes (Figure 13.3).

TELESCOPES   Small telescopes that fit on spectacle lenses may be helpful and convenient for some people with low vision who require improved distance vision. Most telescopes are handheld, however, and are difficult to use because of their small field of view (Figure 13.4). Telescopes are more expensive than handheld magnifiers and magnifying spectacles (for near vision correction) and are difficult to fit onto spectacles. Because of their expense and limited usefulness most people with low vision in developing nations are not using this device.

Nonoptical Aids

Nonoptical aids include enlarged print material and a variety of projection devices.

ENLARGED PRINT MATERIAL   Practical nonoptical aids are large-print books, newspapers, and magazines. One can also increase the font size on computer screens and use larger computer screens to accommodate the enlarged print. Enlarging printed numbers, figures, and words allows for easier reading in the presence of low vision. Many literate people with low vision find enlarged printed material readable with ordinary near corrective lenses.

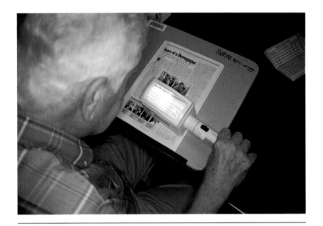

Figure 13.2   Patient using a halogen lighted hand magnifier to read a magazine. Bright illumination often enhances benefit of magnification. With this magnifier, complete width of column can be viewed without moving magnifier. The tilted reading stand allows the reader to have his hands free. *(Reprinted, with permission, from Fletcher DC, Ophthalmology Monographs 12: Low Vision Rehabilitation, San Francisco: American Academy of Ophthalmology, 1999.)*

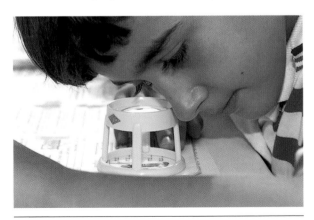

Figure 13.1   This child is using a stand magnifier, which allows him to read while keeping his place and his hands free. *(Reprinted, with permission, from Fletcher DC, Ophthalmology Monographs 12: Low Vision Rehabilitation, San Francisco: American Academy of Ophthalmology, 1999.)*

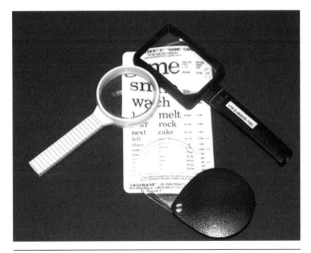

Figure 13.3   Hand magnifiers.

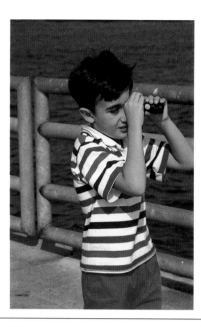

Figure 13.4 A monocular telescope can assist a visually impaired child to explore his environment. It is portable and, for most children, easy to use. *(Reprinted, with permission, from Fletcher DC,* Ophthalmology Monographs 12: Low Vision Rehabilitation, *San Francisco: American Academy of Ophthalmology, 1999.)*

One can also enlarge the print on handwritten text by printing in large block letters with a thick black felt tip pen on white paper. The enlarged print and enhanced contrast make handwritten notes easier to read.

PROJECTION DEVICES Many of the low vision devices available in industrialized countries are too expensive to be practical for developing countries at present and are not widely available. Not only are these devices expensive, but they require reliable electrical power and maintenance which may not be available in all countries. In the industrialized world, these devices include (1) talking machines, (2) scanning machines that read aloud,

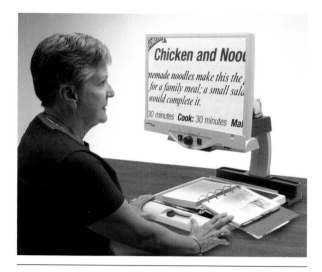

Figure 13.5 A portable, closed-circuit television (CCTV) provides magnification as well as contrast enhancement. *(Image courtesy of Enhanced Vision.)*

(3) television monitor screens that display magnified images, and (4) closed-circuit television (CCTV) that uses a video camera to project a magnified image of the printed material onto a television screen (Figure 13.5). CCTV can achieve higher degrees of magnification and one can also adjust brightness and contrast.

Other Services

Nonophthalmic personnel can play an important role in caring for the low vision patient. Occupational therapists help patients adapt to their disability both at work and in the home. Psychological counselors help to combat the loneliness, isolation and depression associated with low vision. In addition, the incorporation of a pet into the lives of the visually impaired has been found to be therapeutic and useful.

SELF-ASSESSMENT TEST

1. What is the World Health Organization's definition of low vision?

2. Name 5 common causes of low vision.

3. Using Kestenbaum's rule, determine the degree of magnification needed for a person with 20/100 vision to read J5 newsprint with a focal distance of 25 cm.

4. When reading, the low vision patient should avoid which of the following?

   a. direct sunlight

   b. fluorescent light

   c. glare

   d. high contrast reading sources

5. Describe 3 low vision devices that can be worn or carried in the pocket of a low vision patient for convenient use.

SUGGESTED ACTIVITIES

1. Review low vision information and services available in your office.

2. Visit websites that provide information on low vision services.

3. If there is a low vision specialist in your office, ask to shadow this person when he or she evaluates and treats low vision patients.

SUGGESTED RESOURCES

Brown B. *The Low Vision Handbook for Eyecare Professionals.* 2nd ed. Thorofare, NJ: Slack; 2007.

DuBois LG. Formal visual fields. In: *Fundamentals of Ophthalmic Medical Assisting.* DVD. San Francisco: American Academy of Ophthalmology; 2009.

Fonda GE. *Management of Low Vision.* New York: Grune & Stratton; 1981.

Journal of Visual Impairment and Blindness. Special issue on low vision. 2004; 98 (10).

Schwab L. *Eye Care in Developing Nations.* London: Manson Publishing; 2007.

Wilson ME, Morese SE, Hoxie J. Rehabilitation of the low vision patient. In: *Refinements.* Module 34, July 2001. Now available through JCAHPO, www.jcahpo.org.

14 PRINCIPLES AND PROBLEMS OF CONTACT LENSES

Prescribing and fitting contact lenses have become an integral part of today's comprehensive ophthalmology practice. More than 30 million people in the United States wear contact lenses, with the majority using them for cosmetic purposes. Other reasons for wearing contact lenses include occupational preferences, sports, and therapeutic uses.

Beginning ophthalmic medical assistants may function in a contact lens practice by taking a patient history, obtaining basic preliminary refractive measurements, and performing lensometry and keratometry. With experience, responsibilities may include assistance in the fitting of the contact lenses, confirming contact lens parameters, and suggesting contact lens modifications. In addition ophthalmic medical assistants often teach and instruct patients on insertion and removal of their contact lenses. as well as help educate patients in the proper use and care of their contact lenses and help assess patients' related problems. Hence, it is important for the ophthalmic medical assistant to have a basic understanding of contact lens principles, types of contact lenses, appropriate use, and possible complications.

This chapter describes how contact lenses work to correct vision and how they differ from eyeglasses. We will also discuss the different types of contact lenses available and their uses. Contact lens care is emphasized because improper care can lead to problems and complications. Procedures for inserting and removing contact lenses are presented, as well as a discussion of commonly encountered wearing problems. We will also describe the types of patients who may be unable to wear contact lenses successfully.

Although you can read extensively on the subject of contact lenses, the most productive and practical knowledge will come from observing contact lens fittings, talking to patients who have worn contact lenses, and actually trying on contact lenses yourself. When in doubt about your role in the ophthalmologist's office, exercise caution, never assume diagnostic responsibility, and always readily and appropriately discuss a patient's symptoms and signs with the ophthalmologist.

Basic Principles

The contact lens places a new refractive surface (the contact lens) over the surface of the cornea. The contact lens itself rests on a thin liquid cushion, the tear layer, and not on the eye. With rigid gas-permeable contact lenses, this fluid lying between the back surface of the contact lens and the front surface of the cornea fills out corneal irregularities (the amount and type depends on the contact lens material and design), converting the interface between the contact lens and the cornea into a smooth, spherical surface. In principle, the contact lens then alters the refractive power of the eye by providing a radius of curvature (the front of the contact lens) different from that of the cornea. This new front curvature is able to correct the optical error of the eye and allow light to focus on the retina, thereby correcting the patient's spherical and astigmatic refractive error to the extent possible by a given contact lens material (Figure 14.1).

A complete medical and ocular history and ophthalmic eye examination must be performed in order to fit the most appropriate contact lens. The following procedures are specifically required to arrive at a contact lens prescription:

- determination of the refractive error (refraction/refractometry)

- determination of the flattest and steepest corneal meridians and the axis (in degrees) in the central visual axis of the eye (keratometry) (In some cases a corneal topography test [detects aberrations of the corneal contour] may be desirable.)

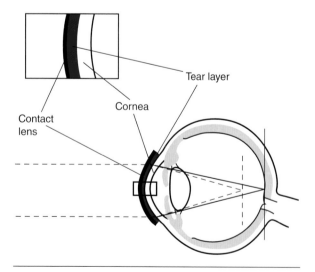

Figure 14.1 Physiology and refractive result of contact lens. Dotted line: focal point/plane without contact lens; solid line: focal point/plane with contact lens.

- choice of contact lens type based on the medical and ocular history, ocular examination, and patient's specific contact lens requirements

The refractive state of the eye (the type of refractive error) and keratometry measurements provide a starting point from which to choose the type of contact lens as well as the appropriate base curve, the diameter, and the power of the contact lens.

According to their experience and office policy, ophthalmic medical assistants may perform some of these procedures as well as take a contact lens patient's history and instruct patients in contact lens care and wear.

Characteristics of Contact Lenses

The contact lens must allow adequate oxygen to reach the cornea and allow the metabolic waste products under the contact lens to be removed so that normal corneal metabolism is not compromised. Depending on the type of contact lens material used, oxygen reaches the cornea either directly through the contact lens or indirectly by the *tear pump*. The tear pump results from blinking; the movement of fresh tears under the contact lens carries oxygen to the cornea and pushes out the old tears with their metabolic wastes. In addition to maintaining corneal metabolism and promoting waste removal, the contact lens must also sustain the integrity of corneal epithelium and normal corneal temperature. Three kinds of contact lenses meet these objectives: **soft lenses**, **rigid gas-permeable (RGP) lenses**, and polymethylmethacrylate (**PMMA**) lenses.

Soft or hydrophilic contact lenses provide oxygen and carbon dioxide diffusion through the lens material itself with a minimal tear pump. High-oxygen-transmissible silicone hydrogels were introduced in 1998 for 6 nights of extended wear and were approved for up to 30 nights of continuous wear in 2001. They are also available for daily-wear use. RGP contact lenses provide oxygen and carbon dioxide diffusion through the contact lens material and the tear pump. PMMA contact lenses were introduced in 1948 and provide oxygen diffusion only by means of the tear pump and, therefore oxygen and carbon dioxide do not diffuse through the lens. These contact lenses are prescribed very rarely today.

Contact Lenses Versus Eyeglasses for Vision Correction

Contact lenses are useful for cosmetic purposes. They can enhance one's self-esteem, avoid the need for thick and heavy or unsightly eyeglasses, cosmetically conceal a disfigured eye, or achieve a fashionable or different eye color. They are also useful in sports. Contact lenses can be a real boon for patients whose eyeglasses irritate or actually inflame their ears or nose.

ADVANTAGES Some advantages of contact lenses over eyeglasses are that they do not impair or distort peripheral vision; do not fog or become easily dislodged during work, sports or under adverse environmental conditions; permit better correction of certain types of refractive errors that occur with high power errors, keratoconus, nystagmus, congenital albinism, and irregular astigmatism caused by corneal scars; provide a normal retinal image size, especially in those who have high refractive errors or who have had cataract surgery without an intraocular lens implant; and can provide 24-hour vision (with extended-wear contact lenses).

DISADVANTAGES Some disadvantages of contact lenses over eyeglasses are that they require fastidious, continuous, careful maintenance; carry a small risk of infection and other adverse physiologic effects on the cornea and conjunctiva; are inappropriate in some environments, such as in the presence of dust, smoke, or caustic agents; may cost more than eyeglasses, particularly because contact lenses can be lost or damaged more easily during cleaning and handling than eyeglasses and therefore, require replacement more frequently; and require help with insertion, removal and maintenance in young children and disabled adults.

Contact Lens Specification Versus Eyeglass Prescription

The specification for a patient's contact lenses differs from a prescription for eyeglasses. A prescription for eyeglasses includes such information as the refractive error expressed as sphere and cylinder (either plus or minus), with bifocal or prism included if required and vertex and pupillary distance as appropriate. When indicated, the lens material (polycarbonate or high-index glass) should be noted as well as a tint or transitions. In contrast, a contact lens prescription can only be determined after the contact lens is successfully fit on the patient's eye. A contact lens prescription (specification) requires the details outlined here:

- spherical equivalent of refractive error (power) or the sphere, cylinder, and axis if a toric (spherocylindrical) contact lens is required

- diameter of contact lens

- base curve of contact lens

- lens thickness (for an RGP lens)

- material, polymer or brand name of the contact lens

- edge blends or peripheral curves (for an RGP lens)

- lens tint (if any for an RGP lens) or lens color (if any for a soft contact lens)

- wearing instructions

- care regimen instructions

- schedule of follow-up appointments

Types and Materials of Contact Lenses

After determining the preliminary specifications for a patient's contact lenses, the ophthalmologist chooses the contact lens type and material that will provide the best vision and fit and meet the physiologic and comfort needs of the patient. Ophthalmic medical assistants may be called upon to educate patients in the advantages and disadvantages of the different types of contact lenses, help instruct patients in the insertion and removal of their contact lenses, the wearing schedule, and contact lens care regimen.

More than 85% of those wearing contact lenses today wear soft contact lenses. The presently available soft contact lenses are made of flexible, gel-like materials (hema or hemacopolymers) that contain between 38% and 74% water. The high **oxygen-permeable** silicone contact lenses (sometimes called *high-Dk silicone lenses*) contain between 23% and 47% water. The silicone is combined with conventional hydrogel monomers, forming a copolymer that combines silicone with hema. The silicone increases the oxygen permeability of the contact lens (Figure 14.2A).

Approximately 10% to 15% of contact lens users wear RGP contact lenses made of materials that bend or flex only slightly (Figure 14.2B). The RGP contact lenses allow direct passage of oxygen and carbon dioxide through the lens materials and allow oxygen to reach the cornea via the tear pump. Between 3 and 4 million individuals use soft or RGP contact lenses for extended wear; of these extended-wear contact lenses, a significant number are disposable soft contact lenses or high-Dk silicone contact lenses. The availability of high-Dk silicone hydrogel contact lenses has regenerated interest in extended or continuous contact lens wear.

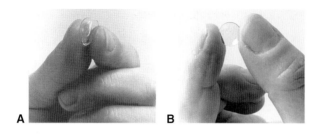

Figure 14.2 Contact lens materials. **A.** Soft contact lenses are made of flexible, gel-like materials. **B.** Hard contact lenses comprise rigid gas-permeable and polymethylmethacrylate lenses.

PMMA and RGP Contact Lenses

Polymethylmethacrylate (PMMA) was the plastic material originally used in hard contact lenses. Today only a very small number of contact lens wearers use these lenses on a daily-wear basis. The non–gas-permeable PMMA material allows oxygen to reach the cornea only by the pumping of oxygenated tears around and under the lens.

RGP contact lenses, however, are made from materials that permit oxygen and carbon dioxide to diffuse through their semi-flexible plastic structure (Figure 14.3). These kinds of rigid contact lens materials include silicone acrylates, fluorosilicone acrylates, fluorosilicate acrylic, strylsilcone, fluorosiloxane acrylate, butylstyrene silicone acrylate, and fluorosiloxanyl styrene.

ADVANTAGES The RGP contact lens materials are easier to adapt to and provide better comfort than PMMA lenses. RGP lenses maintain improved corneal physiology because of their oxygen and carbon dioxide permeability. They have applications for difficult visual problems, such as in keratoconus, large amounts of astigmatism, or irregular corneas, compared to soft contact lenses. They offer better vision potential because of the availability of larger optical zones. They minimize **spectacle blur** (temporary blurred vision upon switching from contact lenses to eyeglasses), compared to PMMA

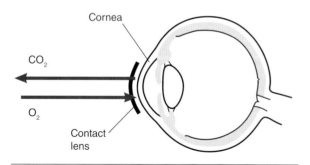

Figure 14.3 Rigid gas-permeable contact lenses permit oxygen and carbon dioxide to diffuse through their semiflexible plastic structure.

lenses. Finally, RGP lenses may be modified after manufacture to alter fit, size, or power.

DISADVANTAGES RGP contact lens materials are more fragile, compared to PMMA. They may warp (especially thinner or higher-oxygen-permeable RGP lenses) and may scratch easily or craze (silicone acrylate). They may require special solutions or have other increased requirements for cleaning. They are more susceptible than PMMA contact lenses to protein deposits that can blur vision or irritate the eye. Finally, RGP lenses may cost more than either PMMA or soft contact lenses.

Soft Contact Lenses

Soft contact lenses can be classified into the low-Dk hydrogels and the high-Dk hydrogels. The low-Dk group is predominantly made from hydroxyethylmethacrylate (HEMA) polymer that can be cross-linked or copolymerized with other polymers. The resulting material often has improved properties that can solve problems of wettability, comfort, stability, and durability. In this group oxygen transmissibility (how much oxygen passes through the contact lens to reach the cornea) is determined largely by the water content of the material and to a lesser extent the thickness of the lens. The high-Dk group is composed of silicone monomers that are copolymerized with hydrogel material to give the material significantly higher oxygen permeability. In this group the oxygen transmissibility is inversely proportional to the water content and directly related to the amount of silicone; the thickness of the contact lens is of secondary importance. These contact lenses have between 3 and 6 times the oxygen transmissibility as non–silicone-hydrogel contact lenses.

ADVANTAGES Soft lens materials are comfortable, and thus easy to adapt to and wear. They rarely cause spectacle blur (the patient can easily switch from contact lenses to eyeglasses), and so they can be worn intermittently, and they rarely become "lost" or dislodged from the eye. Soft contact lenses have reduced incidence of overwear symptoms (especially the high-Dk contact lenses), and they are a useful alternative for patients who were unsuccessful in wearing rigid contact lenses. Soft lenses can be inexpensively and accurately mass-produced, and they are available as disposable lenses. The high-Dk silicone contact lenses can be worn for extended or continuous wear for up to 30 nights. Silicone hydrogels worn on a daily basis may be better for patients with dry eyes and those who had previous contact lens problems.

DISADVANTAGES The major disadvantages of soft contact lenses are that the lenses can cause variable vision due to dehydration of the contact lenses and can become dirty because of improper care. Soft contact lenses are less durable than rigid contact lenses. They are more prone to deposit formation. They cannot be modified after manufacture, as RGP contact lenses can. They require meticulous and somewhat expensive care, cleaning, and disinfecting (except for the daily disposable contact lenses). Finally, soft contact lenses may not be able to correct all refractive errors, especially in cases of high astigmatism and irregular corneas.

Extended-Wear Contact Lenses

Extended-wear contact lenses include soft contact lenses that have increased oxygen permeability/transmissibility and certain RGP contact lenses of high oxygen permeability that have been approved by the United States Food and Drug Administration (FDA) for overnight wear for up to 6 nights (conventional hydrogels) and up to 30 nights for the high-Dk silicone hydrogels. Some patients choose to wear their extended-wear contact lenses on a flexible schedule of just 1 or 2 nights of extended wear, while others opt for wearing their contact lenses for the FDA-recommended maximum without contact lens removal.

Extended-wear contact lenses are associated with increased incidence of adverse corneal effects and corneal ulcers, and it is especially important that patients receive and follow instructions in the care and wearing schedules of their contact lenses. It is also important for these patients to have follow-up examinations at regular intervals. High-Dk silicone contact lenses appear to be associated with fewer adverse ocular effects and less severe corneal ulcers than low-Dk contact lenses worn on an extended-wear schedule. Because of their high oxygen transmissibility, the high-Dk silicone contact lenses are the preferred contact lens for extended or continuous wear.

Daily-Wear Contact Lenses

Daily-wear contact lenses comprise both rigid and soft contact lenses that are intended to be worn for fewer than 24 consecutive hours, while awake. Significant corneal problems can occur if a contact lens approved only for daily wear is worn overnight. Injury can result from the deprivation of oxygen to the cornea under the closed eyelid and/or from mechanical trauma of the contact lens.

Disposable Contact Lenses

Disposable contact lenses refer to a group of contact lenses that are worn and cared for in the following ways.

Daily disposable contact lenses consist of contact lenses that are worn on a daily basis and then discarded. Two-week disposable contact lenses are worn daily, cleaned and disinfected each night and replaced at 2-week intervals (in some cases they are replaced weekly). Disposable contact lenses for extended wear are contact lenses approved by the FDA for extended wear for 6 or 7 nights, at which time they are removed from the eye, discarded, and a new contact lens is inserted onto the eye for the next week of contact lens wear. The high-Dk silicone contact lenses also fit into this group, of which certain high-Dk contact lenses (approved by the FDA) can be worn for up to 30 nights and then discarded.

As noted here, disposability serves as a way to categorize these contact lenses rather than as an indication of a specific contact lens material. Because they are worn for only a short time and then discarded, disposable contact lenses usually require minimal care. However, if the contact lens is to be reused it must be cleaned and disinfected after removal and before reinsertion. Many contact lens wearers feel that the time and money they save in maintenance offsets the added cost of disposable contact lenses.

Planned-Replacement Contact Lenses

Planned-replacement contact lenses, also referred to as programmed-replacement contact lenses or frequent-replacement contact lenses, are soft contact lenses that are replaced at intervals of 1, 2, 3, or 6 months. In planned replacement, contact lenses are replaced before the contact lens material is significantly degraded. (In clinical practice, 2-week disposable contact lenses that are worn on a daily basis and replaced every 2 weeks can be considered frequent-replacement contact lenses.) The ophthalmologist determines the frequency of replacement based on the response of both the contact lenses and the patient's eyes and wearing conditions. Planned-replacement contact lenses require contact lens care, including cleaning and disinfecting after each use. Enzyme cleaning may be required, depending on how long the contact lenses are worn and how the patient's eyes respond to wearing the contact lenses.

Contact Lens Designs for Special Purposes

Contact lenses can meet the special needs of individuals who require a prosthetic device to conceal ocular disfigurement or treatment for certain ophthalmic disorders.

Some of the possible uses for unique contact lens designs are described below.

Cosmetic Fashion Contact Lenses

Soft contact lenses can be tinted to enhance or change the color of a person's iris (Figure 14.4). Although changing the color of the eyes usually serves no therapeutic purpose, tinted contact lenses may offer some relief from photophobia in glare-sensitive individuals. In addition, contact lenses with a handling, or visibility, tint may help patients, especially those with hyperopia or presbyopia, to find their contact lenses more easily than they could colorless contact lenses. This light-colored handling tint does not affect the eye color. Cosmetic tinted contact lenses can have a clear pupillary area or a total overall color. The tint itself may eventually fade ("weather") over time. Some cleaning solutions promote this fading process.

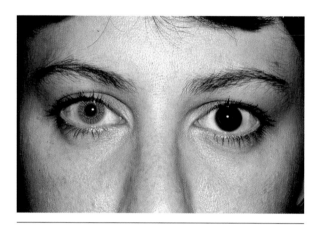

Figure 14.4 This patient is wearing a cosmetic opaque fashion lens in the right eye that is tinted to alter her normal iris color from brown to blue.

While all contact lenses require a prescription, non-prescription cosmetic contact lenses, which are illegal, can be obtained in some retail stores as well as through the Internet. These illegal contact lenses have been associated with severe eye disorders and infection that can lead to permanent ocular damage. It is important for the ophthalmic medical assistant to understand and convey to their patients that a contact lens is a medical device and must be fitted by or under the supervision of a licensed eye care professional.

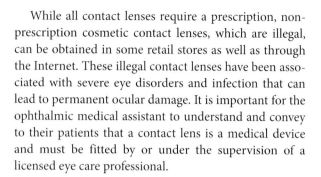

Over-the-counter sales of nonprescription cosmetic contact lenses, sometimes called decorative contact lenses, have been illegal in the United States since 2005.

Cosmetic Restorative Contact Lenses

Contact lenses can serve a cosmetic restoring function, such as being used as a prosthetic device for eyes disfigured by trauma, infection, or other conditions (Figure 14.5). These contact lenses can have a sclera, iris, or pupil painted, printed, or laminated onto them. They also can be used in eyes with limited or no visual potential.

Toric Contact Lenses

Toric contact lenses have two different radii of curvature on their anterior and/or posterior surfaces. This type of contact lens corrects the vision of patients whose astigmatism cannot be adequately masked by spherical contact lenses. Toric contact lenses correct for astigmatic errors in the same way eyeglasses do (correcting the refractive error in each meridian). In special cases,

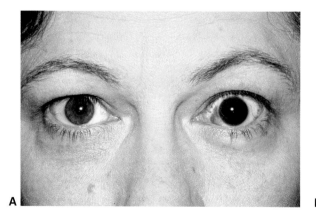
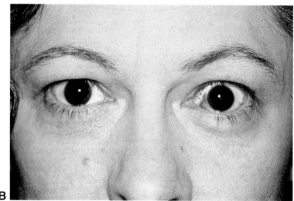

Figure 14.5 A patient with hyperpigmentation of the iris and sclera of the left eye (**A**) can wear an opaque soft contact lens as a cosmetic restorative lens on the right eye to equalize iris color (**B**).

a toric design may help center the lens on the cornea. These contact lenses are available as both soft and rigid contact lenses.

Bifocal Contact Lenses

Bifocal contact lens design attempts to provide individuals with correction for both near and distance vision. These contact lens designs are based on alternating vision or simultaneous vision. Alternating design contact lenses have two separate areas—one for near, usually at the bottom of the contact lens, and one for distance, over the central area of the contact lens. As the individual looks down toward the reading position, the lower

lid pushes the contact lens up and the near segment is over the pupil. As a result, by the individual's eye position, the contact lens wearer "chooses" either distance or near (Figure 14.6A).

With the simultaneous vision design, light rays from near, intermediate, and distant objects enter the eye and are focused on the retina. The brain selects the image—near or distant—it wants and suppresses the other images. There are various simultaneous lens designs. The central concentric area can correct distance vision and the surrounding concentric area correct near vision (Figure 14.6B) or the central concentric area can correct near vision and the surrounding concentric zone corrects distance vision. A variation on this design involves

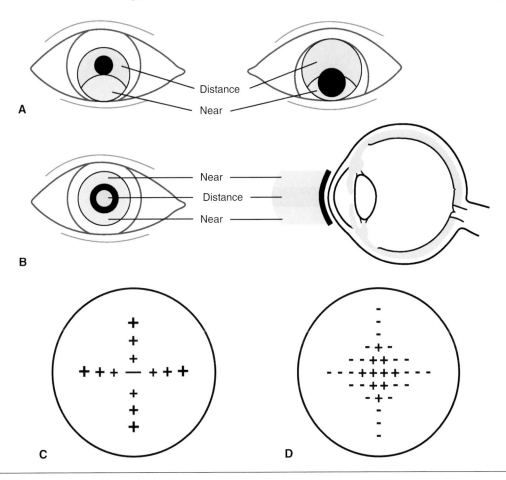

Figure 14.6 Bifocal, progressive, and degressive contact lenses. **A.** For alternating vision in a bifocal lens, the distance segment is positioned over the pupil (left); as the patient looks down toward the reading position, the lower lid pushes up the contact lens so that the near segment covers the pupil for reading (right). **B.** For simultaneous vision in a bifocal lens, the distance (or near) optical portion of the lens is made smaller than the pupil so that light rays from both distance and near pass through the pupil simultaneously. The lens wearer chooses either the central portion of the contact lens for distance vision or the peripheral portion for near vision. This can also be designed so that the central optical portion of the contact lens can correct near vision and the peripheral portion of the contact lens can correct distance vision. **C.** In a progressive aspheric design, the central area of the contact lens corrects distance vision. There is a progressive increase in power toward the periphery of the contact lens. When the individual looks through the peripheral part of the contact lens, intermediate and near vision is corrected. **D.** In a degressive aspheric design, the central area of the contact lens corrects near vision and the power of the contact lens decreases towards the periphery of the contact lens. As the individual looks through the peripheral aspect of the contact lens, intermediate and distance vision is corrected.

5 concentric rings in which distance correction is alternated with near correction.

Most soft bifocal contact lenses are of the aspheric design. In this design the contact lens can have an increasing power from the center of the lens to the periphery (called a *progressive* aspheric design, Figure 14.6C) in which case the central area of the contact lens corrects distance vision. As the individual looks through the peripheral part of the contact lens, the power of the contact lens gradually increases to correct near vision. The lens can also be designed so that the central part of the lens has the most power, thus correcting near vision (called a *degressive* multifocal design, Figure 14.6D) with the power decreasing toward the peripheral part of the contact lens (distance correction).

Both the progressive and degressive designs provide correction for the intermediate range in addition to the correction for near and distance vision. For patients whose needs for intermediate vision are not met with the previously described contact lenses, a design with the center of the contact lenses corrected for intermediate vision and the periphery of the contact lenses with either distance or near vision can be prescribed. This is important for patients who have intermediate visual needs such as working on a computer.

Presbyopic correction with bifocal contact lenses has improved over the years. The numerous soft and RGP contact lenses available have rekindled a new interest in fitting these contact lenses. However, the vision correction with bifocal contact lenses is still a compromise. Not everyone will achieve the near, intermediate, and distance vision that they want or require with these contact lenses. Patients may experience unacceptable near or distance vision, ghosting of images and halos or flaring around headlights at night. The newer designs have helped solve some of these problems. Thus proper patient selection is important for successfully fitting bifocal contact lenses. This includes a discussion of the benefits and limitation of bifocal contact lenses with respect to their design, the patient's needs, as well as physiological and optical limitations that may be present.

Another successful option in the correction of presbyopia is **monovision** in which one eye (usually the dominant eye) is corrected with a contact lens for distance vision, and the other eye is corrected with a contact lens for near vision. Monovision is useful for the correction of early presbyopia, but as the power difference between the two eyes increases patients experience difficulty with this modality of vision correction. In addition monovision interferes with binocular vision and stereopsis. Such patients can benefit from driving glasses in which the near eye is corrected with a spectacle lens (to be worn with the contact lens) to improve distance vision. Using a bifocal contact lens in one eye and a single distance vision contact lens in the other eye is also an option.

Keratoconus Contact Lenses

Keratoconus is a progressive thinning and cone-like protrusion of the cornea. This results in an irregular corneal surface that produces an irregular astigmatism. This condition most often affects both eyes, but one eye can have a more advanced cone than the other eye. Most patients with keratoconus are fitted with specially designed RGP contact lenses. These lenses help correct the irregular astigmatism associated with the condition, thus giving significantly better vision than can be achieved with glasses. Over 80% of patients with keratoconus can be managed with contact lenses.

Therapeutic Contact Lenses

Soft contact lenses can serve as therapy for various ocular problems. Soft contact lenses can be used as "bandage contact lenses" to cover damaged or painful corneas and to help in the healing of epithelial defects of the cornea. They provide therapeutic covers for recurrent corneal epithelial breakdowns and protect exposed nerve endings present in **corneal bullous edema** (profound corneal edema causing various size epithelial blisters). They are useful after corneal transplant or refractive surgery to treat epithelial defects. Both rigid and soft contact lenses have been used for occlusion and patching to treat amblyopia or to eliminate diplopia.

Care of Contact Lenses

In order for patients to wear their contact lenses safely and comfortably and to maintain clear vision, contact lenses that are removed and then reinserted onto the eye require cleaning and disinfection. It is important to minimize bacterial contamination (disinfection) and keep the contact lens surface free of mucus and other debris (cleaning). In some cases lubricating ("wetting") and soaking solutions are also required. Patients must understand that the contact lenses should feel comfortable when placed on the eye after a suitable period of adjustment. Discomfort may signal a poor contact lens fit or may be caused by a contact lens that needs cleaning or lubrication, or that is torn, chipped, or spoiled beyond repair. Numerous cleaning, disinfecting, and lubricating solutions exist. Most popular brands are multipurpose solutions with "no rub" labeling. Contact lens wearers should be instructed in appropriate contact lens care and urged to read their contact lens manufacturer's printed recommendations or physicians' instructions as well as the labels of contact lens care solutions carefully to ensure that the solutions they use are compatible with the type of contact lens they wear.

Cleaning

Contact lenses can become coated with substances from the tear film (the 3-layer moist coating that covers the anterior surface of the globe), from the environment, or from handling the contact lens. The substances that can contribute to contact lens deposits and spoilage can consist of organic elements, such as proteins, mucins, environmental pollutants, and microbial contamination; inorganic elements such as calcium; and mixed elements such as mucoprotein lipid complexes. If the coating is advanced, the patient may see it; however, it is often invisible (Figure 14.7). If not removed by cleaning, the deposits can become thick, blur vision, or irritate the eye when the contact lenses are worn and can serve as a reservoir for microorganisms. Some people develop deposits on their contact lenses rapidly; others rarely do.

Contact lens cleaning requires using **surfactant cleaners** (specially designed detergents) and rubbing the contact lens with clean fingers. Surfactant cleaners are designed to help remove surface deposits by solubilizing the organic debris on the contact lens (interacting with the deposits and displacing them away from the lens surface, where they can be washed away in the rinsing step), thereby increasing clarity of vision and reducing irritation caused by coated contact lenses.

Because foreign-matter deposits can interfere with the disinfecting step of contact lens care, **enzyme cleaners** have been specifically developed to remove accumulated deposits. These agents consist of **proteolytic** (remove protein) and **triphasic enzymes** (remove protein, lipid, and mucoid deposits) that hydrolyze debris into water-soluble products that can be rinsed or rubbed away. Enzymatic cleaners are used less frequently with contact lenses that are replaced at weekly or monthly intervals than with contact lens that are replaced at greater intervals. Part of cleaning the contact lens is the physical step of rubbing the lens between the index finger and thumb to remove the debris on the contact lens surface.

Disinfecting

Disinfecting is a critical step in contact lens care because it prevents organisms such as bacteria, viruses, fungi, and protozoa from growing on the contact lens. Any of these organisms may cause a potentially blinding infection of the cornea. Two methods are used for disinfecting contact lenses: chemicals and ultraviolet (UV) radiation. Heat was the first approved disinfecting method for soft contact lenses but is rarely used today.

Examples of chemicals with antimicrobial action include hydrogen peroxide; thimerosal, no longer used in major brands of solutions but may be found in generic products; chlorhexidine, no longer used; quaternary ammonium compounds; benzalkonium chloride (BAK), not for soft lenses; and paraaminopolybiguanide (PAPB). Presently the chemical-care systems for soft contact lenses can be divided into 2 groups. The first is a preservative-free oxidizing system, which uses hydrogen peroxide as the disinfecting agent. After appropriate time in hydrogen peroxide, the hydrogen peroxide is neutralized before the contact lens is inserted on the eye. The second group consists of multipurpose solutions, which contain in a single solution all the components necessary for cleaning, disinfection, and storage.

UV radiation is an effective method of disinfecting contact lenses. With the "hands-free" PuriLens system (PuriLens, Inc, Wall Township, New Jersey), subsonic agitation in preservative-free saline cleans the contact lens. In the next step, germicidal UV-C (a subtype of UV radiation) light kills any microorganisms present.

Some patients have sensitivity reactions to at least one, but usually not all, of the preservatives or disinfectants used in contact lens solutions. In these patients, the use of a hydrogen peroxide nonpreserved care system may be indicated.

Sensitivity reactions are discussed later in this chapter. Both PMMA and RGP contact lenses are less susceptible than soft lenses to contamination and are easier to clean and disinfect.

Ophthalmic medical assistants who handle trial contact lenses in the office should keep abreast of current procedures for the care of contact lenses with

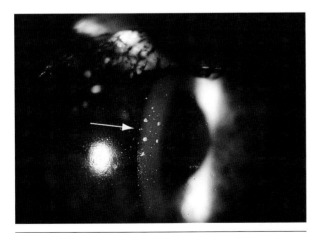

Figure 14.7 Deposits that collect on a contact lens surface (arrow) may not be visible to the patient but they show up when the ophthalmologist views the lens in place by the light of a slit lamp.

reference to persons infected with the human immunodeficiency virus (HIV), which causes acquired immunodeficiency syndrome (AIDS). (See "Suggested Resources" at the end of this chapter.)

Lubrication

Contact lens wearers use lubricants, or wetting/cushioning solutions, to keep the contact lens surface hydrophilic. This helps to decrease complaints of dryness and increase the comfort of the contact lens. These solutions act like a cushion between the contact lens and the cornea and between the contact lens and the eyelid. Patients may wish to use lubricants when they insert their contact lenses, but usually their own tears perform the cushioning function. A patient's saliva should never be used to wet contact lenses because of the possibility of infection.

Storage

The ophthalmic medical assistant should make certain the contact lenses stored in the office remain in a clean, ready-to-wear condition. Contact lenses that have been tried on but not dispensed should be cleaned, disinfected appropriately, and returned to the fitting sets. Rigid contact lenses should be stored in individual containers with the proper storage solutions or in a dry state, according to the ophthalmologist's instructions. Soft contact lenses should be cleaned with surfactant cleaners, disinfected, and kept in individual sealed containers. With the introduction of disposable and planned replacement contact lenses, most ophthalmologists are able to fit from a trial contact lens set. After fitting the patient, the doctor either dispenses the contact lens set to the patient or discards it. Be sure that patients understand the appropriate methods for storing their contact lenses at home. Patients should store contact lenses in the contact lens case that the ophthalmologist recommends. The assistant should instruct the patient to clean and dry the case daily and replace it at intervals recommended by the doctor.

Insertion and Removal of Contact Lenses

An important part of the dispensing of both soft and rigid contact lenses is the instruction to the patient, by the ophthalmic medical assistant, on how to insert and remove the contact lenses. The insertion and removal of soft and rigid lenses require different techniques. These methods are best learned by experience, but the basic

principles for insertion and removal apply. Clean hands, appropriate solutions, near-sterile techniques, and clean containers are prerequisites for both contact lens types.

Soft Contact Lenses

Although there are variations in technique, in general the soft contact lens is placed below the cornea on the lower white of the eye (sclera) and gently positioned onto the cornea by closing the eye and looking at each hour on a clock. A second way is to place the contact lens on the index finger concave side up. The patient will look slightly down, the upper and lower lid will be retracted, and the contact lens placed onto the cornea. To remove the soft contact lens, the contact lens is decentered by sliding it with the index finger to the lower sclera while looking up and is then gently pinched off the eye with the thumb and index finger. Procedures 14.1 and 14.2 describe these actions in detail. Many equally effective techniques appear in contact lens booklets accompanying solution kits.

Rigid Contact Lenses

As opposed to most soft contact lenses, which are placed on the sclera, rigid contact lenses must be placed directly on the cornea. Because they are not flexible, rigid contact lenses are removed by pulling aside an eyelid and blinking, which makes them pop out. Procedure 14.3 and Procedure 14.4 describe how to insert and remove rigid contact lenses.

An alternative method for inserting and removing a rigid contact lens uses a special suction cup. This procedure is best performed by the ophthalmic medical assistant rather than by the patient, because the patient could accidentally apply the suction cup to the cornea and cause an abrasion. An ophthalmologist or a senior technician in your office can demonstrate the use of the suction cup to you. The ophthalmic medical assistant should at all times conduct these procedures with thoroughly washed and dried hands, making sure hands are free of hand lotions, oils, and soap residues. Also be sure to keep fingernails trimmed.

Problems With Contact Lenses

Because the ophthalmologist treats problems that can occur with the use of contact lenses, the ophthalmic medical assistant, in order to assist the ophthalmologist,

Procedure 14.1 Inserting Soft Lenses

Instruct the patient to insert a soft contact lens as follows:

1. Wash your hands and dry them with a lint-free towel. Be sure all traces of soap are rinsed off.

2. Remove the clean lens for the right eye from the case with your clean finger or pour the contents of the contact lens vial into the palm of your hand, allowing the solution to drain between your fingers into the sink.

3. Rinse the lens with an FDA-approved saline solution. If you do this over a sink, placing a stopper or drain plug perforated with small holes over the drain opening can prevent the lens from being accidentally lost down the drain.

4. Place the lens on the tip of a dry index finger or middle finger of your dominant hand. Check the lens contour to be sure it is not inside out. You may allow the lens to dry for 10 to 20 seconds in the air until it "rounds up"; thicker lenses require little or no drying.

5. With small lenses, look up, pull down the lower lid with the middle or third finger of the hand holding the lens, and, while looking upward, place the lens onto the lower sclera (figure). Larger lenses are best placed directly on the central cornea by holding the upper lid up with the opposite hand.

6. Express any air under the lens by pressing gently, remove your index finger, and gently release the lower lid.

7. Carefully close your eyes and center the lens by lightly massaging the closed upper eyelid over the contact lens.

8. Repeat steps 1 through 7 for the left lens.

Insertion and Removal by Assistant

When inserting or removing a soft lens from a patient's eye, the ophthalmic medical assistant should follow all steps outlined above while the patient performs the ocular movement; that is, the patient looks up or straight ahead and opens the eye widely, and the ophthalmic medical assistant holds the lens and places it on the sclera or cornea. To remove the lens, the assistant moves the lens downward off the cornea and compresses the lens between the thumb and index finger, and removes it. At all times, both patient and assistant should conduct these procedures only with thoroughly washed and dried hands. In addition, ophthalmic medical assistants should keep their fingernails short and their hands free of lotions, oils, and soap residues in order to avoid tearing or soiling the contact lens and possibly causing injury to the patient's eye.

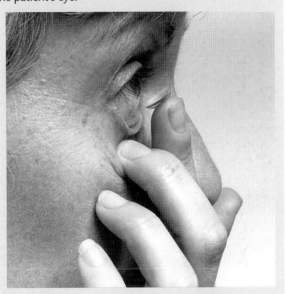

should recognize and understand the symptoms and causes of the difficulties that are typically seen in contact lens wearers. Ophthalmic medical assistants play an important role in educating patients in the prevention of these problems, in alerting patients to the danger signals of potential problems, and in encouraging patients to comply with appropriate contact lens care and wear.

The ophthalmic medical assistant should instruct all patients to remove their contact lenses and call the ophthalmologist's office whenever they experience the following symptoms: redness in the eye, increased light sensitivity, watery or tearing eye, discharge from the eye, blurred or decreased vision, or pain or burning.

Allergy

About 10% to 20% of contact lens wearers have sensitivity reactions to at least one (but usually not all) of the preservative or disinfectant chemicals used in contact lens solutions. Such allergic reactions occur more often among soft contact lens wearers. In a hypersensitivity reaction, the patient may complain of irritation, fogging, redness, tearing, light sensitivity, and decreased wearing time within weeks to months after using the solution containing the offending chemical. The preservative thimerosal most commonly causes this type of allergic reaction. Other preservatives implicated in solution sensitivities include sorbic acid, chlorhexidine, and ethylenediaminetetraacetic acid (EDTA). The diagnosis of a

---

Procedure 14.2 Removing Soft Lenses

Instruct the patient to remove a soft lens as follows:

1. Wash your hands and dry them with a lint-free towel. Be sure all traces of soap are rinsed off.

2. To make certain the lens is in place on the cornea, check that the eye's vision is clear by gazing at a distant object with the opposite eye covered.

3. Begin with your right eye. Look up, then pull down the lower lid with your middle or third finger and place your index finger on the lower edge of the lens.

4. Move the lens down to the sclera.

5. Compress the lens between your thumb and index or middle finger to break the suction.

6. Remove the lens from your eye (figure).

7. Clean the lens appropriately and place it in the case for disinfection. Be sure to place the right contact lens in the compartment of the lens case marked "right."

8. Repeat steps 1 through 7 for the left lens.

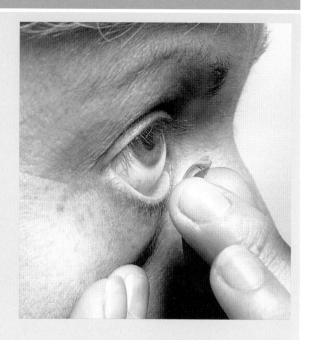

---

sensitivity reaction to a preservative agent is confirmed when the signs and symptoms disappear after the patient uses a solution free of the offending chemical. Currently, many soft contact lens saline solutions are sold as "preservative-free," but these should be used as rinses since they are not "disinfecting" agents.

Solution–Contact Lens Interaction

Not all contact lens solutions are compatible with all materials used in contact lenses. The ophthalmic medical assistant must help ensure that each patient uses the proper and compatible solutions for the particular contact lens being dispensed. In addition, heat and certain chemical disinfectants may not work well together for a specific kind of contact lens. Chemical incompatibility can result in binding of the chemical to the contact lens materials, changes in contact lens parameters or oxygen permeability, discoloration, and other deleterious effects. Improper combinations of contact lenses and solutions can lead to ocular irritation, itching, tearing, hazy vision, redness, and a gritty feeling. The package inserts that come with the contact lenses and contact lens solutions explain in detail which contact lenses and which solutions are compatible. Always consult the contact lens and solution manufacturers' instructions before giving the patient information.

Overwearing Syndrome

Overwearing syndrome, as its name suggests, usually results from wearing a contact lens longer than recommended and is caused by inadequate amounts of oxygen reaching the cornea. Symptoms and signs of the overwearing syndrome include moderate to severe eye pain, eyelid swelling, tearing, and marked light sensitivity. The pain can be very intense, usually occurring 2 to 3 hours after removal of the lens. Upon examination with fluorescein, the cornea of the affected eye may show diffuse fluorescein staining over its central area. Topical anesthetic drops instilled by the ophthalmologist into the eye immediately stop the pain but are never given to patients to use on their own, because patients may unknowingly allow severe injury or even permanent damage to occur to the anesthetized eye.

Overwearing syndrome usually responds within about 24 hours to an analgesic for pain, and a short-acting cycloplegic eyedrop to relieve **ciliary spasm** (painful contractions of the ciliary muscle). Nonpreserved lubricating drops are often necessary to treat the keratitis. The eye is not patched. Although symptoms can resolve overnight or within a day, the actual healing can take up to several days. Overwearing syndrome can be largely avoided by ensuring that patients are properly instructed in their contact lens wearing schedule.

Procedure 14.3 Inserting Rigid Lenses

Instruct the patient to insert a rigid contact lens as follows:

1. Wash your hands and dry them with a lint-free towel. Be sure all traces of soap are rinsed off.

2. Begin with the right eye. Using an approved solution, rinse off the disinfecting solution from the clean rigid lens and wet it with the appropriate wetting solution. (Many approved solutions are now multipurpose.)

3. Use your right hand for inserting the right contact lens and your left hand for the left lens, or, if more comfortable and natural, use your dominant hand for both eyes.

4. Position the lens concave side up on the tip of your index or middle finger.

5. Look straight down, place your chin on your chest, and keep both eyes open.

6. Hold your upper lid at the eyelash margin with the finger of the opposite hand, pressing up against the brow. Hold the lower lid at the eyelash margin with the third or fourth finger of the hand that is holding the lens and press down against the cheek (figure).

7. Bring the finger holding the lens directly up to the eye until the lens comes in contact with the cornea of the eye (figure). This is facilitated by staring with the other eye at a convenient straight-ahead target and keeping the eye open.

8. Immediately release the lower lid and then slowly release the upper lid.

9. Cover the opposite eye and check vision to be certain the lens has been inserted.

10. Repeat steps 1 through 9 for the left lens.

Insertion and Removal by Assistant

As with soft lenses, when the ophthalmic medical assistant inserts or removes a rigid contact lens from the patient's eye, all steps of each procedure should be conducted with the patient performing the ocular movements and the ophthalmic medical assistant's fingers placing the contact lens on the cornea or, in the case of contact lens removal, moving the eyelid and retrieving the lens into the cupped hand as the patient blinks.

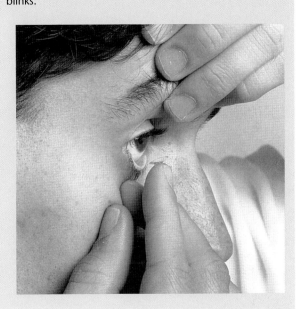

A similar complication is **contact lens-induced acute red eye** (**CLARE**), which has been observed in patients wearing extended wear contact lenses. Patients complain of ocular discomfort, foreign body sensation associated with a red eye that occurs upon awakening. Conjunctival injection (redness), conjunctival edema, and corneal infiltrates are present. Signs and symptoms will resolve after contact lens wear is discontinued.

Improper Contact Lens Fit

A contact lens that fits improperly can produce discomfort and blurred vision. It may even lead to corneal abrasions and/or corneal edema, both of which can promote corneal infections.

A loose-fitting contact lens may cause variable visual acuity because the contact lens moves too much and thus the optical portion of the contact lens may not always cover the visual axis. A loose-fitting contact lens can be corrected by providing the patient with a contact lens that is larger, has a steeper curvature, or both. Excessive movement of a loose-fitting rigid contact lens can also result in a corneal abrasion.

Alternatively, a tight-fitting contact lens causes a stagnation of tears because of lack of movement of the contact lens. This can lead to corneal edema from oxygen deprivation. The signs and symptoms can be similar to those seen in the patient exhibiting overwearing syndrome. The tight-fitting lens syndrome does not occur immediately after placement of the lens but after the contact lens has been on the ocular surface for a while. The syndrome is associated with conjunctival injection and punctate corneal staining. In addition epithelial defects and corneal infiltrates may occur. The patients experience symptoms of ocular irritation, discomfort or pain, blurred vision, and light sensitivity. A tight-fitting

Procedure 14.4   Removing Rigid Lenses

Instruct the patient to remove a rigid contact lens as follows:

1. Wash your hands and dry them with a lint-free towel. Be sure all traces of soap are removed.

2. Begin with your right eye.

3. To be sure the lens is centered on the eye, check for clear vision by gazing at a distant object. If not centered, manipulate the lens gently through the lid to center it on the cornea.

4. Look down and cup your left hand under your right eye to catch the lens (figure).

5. Place your right forefinger on the outer corner of the eyelid and pull the upper lid aside toward the upper ear as you blink. The lens will pop out (figure). If it slides off the cornea, slide it back before again attempting removal.

6. Clean the lens and place it in an appropriate disinfectant solution in the case or store it clean

and dry in a cleaned case. Be sure to place the right lens in the compartment of the contact lens case marked "right."

7. Repeat steps 1 through 6 for the left eye.

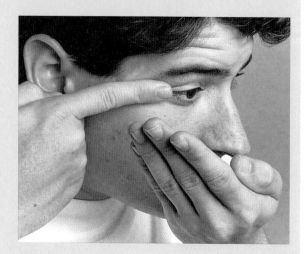

contact lens should be replaced with a lens that is smaller, flatter in curvature, or both. With a steeply curved contact lens, vision is usually clear right after a blink and then fades. The examiner may see an indentation on the white of the eye in a patient wearing a tightly fitting soft contact lens. The contact lens does not move easily and the eye becomes irritated as the patient continues to wear the contact lens.

An improperly fit rigid contact lens and rarely a soft contact lens can result in a semipermanent change in the corneal curvature, called *corneal warpage*. Refitting the contact lens correctly can treat this problem.

Giant Papillary Conjunctivitis

Giant papillary conjunctivitis (GPC) is characterized by large raised bumps called *papules* on the upper tarsal conjunctiva (Figure 14.8). Associated mainly with soft contact lenses, GPC can occasionally occur with rigid contact lenses. This condition can develop months to years after seemingly successful contact lens wear. Symptoms include ocular itching, foreign-body sensation, redness and mucus, and decreased contact lens wearing time. Considered an autoimmune response to the patient's own proteins on the contact lens or to the "trauma" of contact lens wear, GPC is treated by discontinuing contact lens wear for 2 to 4 weeks. Additional treatments with a preservative-free lubricating drop and/or a topical mast cell stabilizer may be indicated. The patient should then be refitted with a new type of contact

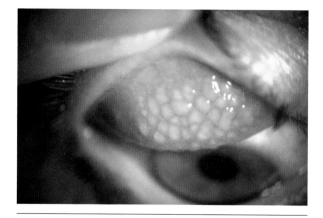

Figure 14.8   Giant papillary conjunctivitis. This condition occurs in patients who wear soft contact lenses, and occasionally occurs in patients who wear rigid gas-permeable contact lenses. *(Reprinted, with permission, from Schwab IR, External Disease and Cornea: A Multimedia Collection, San Francisco: American Academy of Ophthalmology, 1994.)*

lens. The use of daily disposable contact lenses has been found to be very effective in controlling GPC. Patients should be instructed on the importance of keeping their lenses clean and replacing them at frequent intervals.

Irritation and Tearing

Irritation, often described by the patient as "the eye doesn't feel right," may be due to early contact lens deposits or tiny particles trapped by the contact lens. A contact lens patient reporting occasional mild eye irritation or tearing can often safely be instructed to remove and clean the contact lens, then reinsert it. If the irritation was due to dust, particles, or something temporary, the symptoms probably will not recur. If the symptoms persist, an examination by the doctor may be warranted.

Corneal Problems

The principal causes of most contact lens problems are wearing contact lenses too long, or wearing lenses that have been improperly cleaned and disinfected, damaged, spoiled, or do not fit properly. Acting singly or together, these factors as well as others (solutions, contact lens polymer, and environmental pollutants) can lead to a variety of corneal problems.

CORNEAL EDEMA   Corneal edema, or swelling, occurs because of a lack of oxygen to the cornea (Figure 14.9). In addition to overwear and improper contact lens hygiene and fit, the use of a contact lens material that does not allow sufficient corneal oxygenation will cause edema. Improving tear exchange or oxygen penetration can help reduce or overcome this problem. With rigid contact lenses, flattening the contact lens curve can allow better tear exchange; with soft contact lenses, changing the fit to a contact lens that is flatter, smaller, thinner, or of higher oxygen permeability may help. Refitting the patient to a high-Dk silicone contact lens will often eliminate this condition. Corneal edema needs to be remedied promptly before it leads to permanent corneal injury. Corneal edema is usually visible with a slit-lamp examination, but early cases may require pachymetry (corneal thickness measurement) for diagnosis.

CORNEAL VASCULARIZATION   This is an ingrowth of superficial or deep blood vessels into the cornea. It may be a serious sign of corneal oxygen deprivation or mechanical trauma from an improperly fit contact lens (Figure 14.10). Many soft contact lens wearers may have .5 to 1.5 mm of vessel ingrowth into the peripheral superficial cornea. If the ingrowth does not progress, this is acceptable. If the vascular ingrowth is greater or involves the corneal stroma, the ophthalmologist needs to determine and remedy other causative factors (fit, oxygen transmissibility of the contact lens). Stromal or deep neovascularization can result in corneal scarring and intracorneal hemorrhage that may lead to decreased vision.

CORNEAL INFILTRATES   They can occur in patients wearing contact lenses and can be either sterile or infectious. Sterile infiltrates are also called **contact lens peripheral ulcers**, or CLPUs (Figure 14.11). They typically occur in the anterior stroma of the peripheral cornea and are small (2 mm or less). There is associated

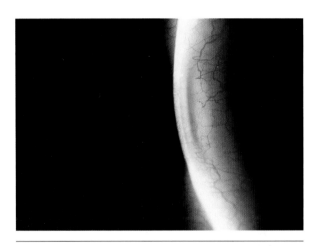

Figure 14.10   Slit-lamp view of corneal vascularization occurring from oxygen deprivation due to a poor-fitting soft contact lens. *(Image courtesy of Thomas D. Lindquist, MD, PhD.)*

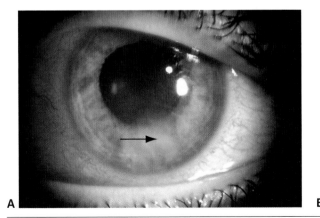
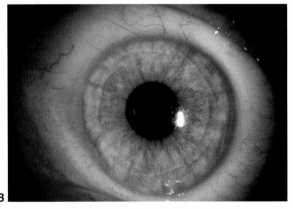

A   B

Figure 14.9   Corneal edema (swelling) occurs from poor oxygenation under the contact lens. Compare the swollen area of the cornea (arrow, **A**) with the appearance of a normal cornea (**B**). *(Part A courtesy of Thomas D. Lindquist, MD, PhD.)*

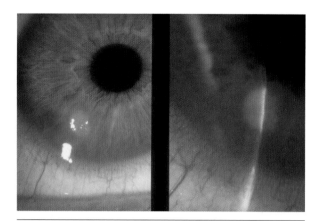

Figure 14.11 Contact lens peripheral ulcer. *(Reprinted, with permission, from Schwab IR,* External Disease and Cornea: A Multimedia Collection, *San Francisco: American Academy of Ophthalmology, 1994.)*

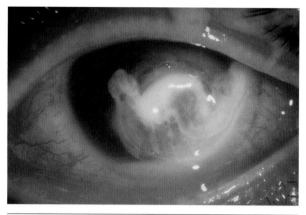

Figure 14.12 Infectious corneal ulcer. *(Reprinted, with permission, from Schwab IR,* External Disease and Cornea: A Multimedia Collection, *San Francisco: American Academy of Ophthalmology, 1994.)*

ocular discomfort but not severe pain, mild conjunctival inflammation, and minimal anterior chamber evidence of inflammation. The management of this condition consists of discontinuing contact lens wear and treatment with a topical antibiotic. While CLPUs are probably not due to a microbial infection it may be difficult to distinguish their presenting clinical picture from an infectious corneal ulcer and thus a topical antibiotic is often prescribed. If the peripheral ulcer does not respond to topical antibiotics then the condition may be due to an organism that is resistant to the prescribed antibiotic. The ulcer would have to be cultured and a new antibiotic (fortified) would be instituted. Once a CLPU resolves the individual may wear contact lenses but the type of contact lens, the wearing schedule, and the frequency of follow-up visits would be evaluated.

INFECTIOUS CORNEAL ULCER The most serious complication of improper contact lens wear is an infectious corneal ulcer (Figure 14.12). Symptoms may include severe pain, redness, irritation, tearing, and diminished vision. On examination there is a grayish white opacity with a defect in the corneal stroma. Anterior chamber inflammation is usually present and a **hypopyon** (inflammatory white cells layered in the anterior chamber) may be present. The ophthalmologist may scrape the corneal ulcer to obtain specimens for smears and cultures and send them to the laboratory. This can help identify the offending organism and aid in determining the correct antibiotic therapy for the patient. *Pseudomonas aeruginosa* is the most common bacteria associated with corneal ulcers in patients wearing soft contact lenses for daily or extended use. These infections can progress rapidly, thus early recognition, diagnosis,

and appropriate antibiotic treatment are imperative. Initial therapy with frequent topical instillation of fortified antibiotics (gram-positive and gram-negative coverage) or fourth-generation fluoroquinolones are indicated, depending on the clinical condition.

FUNGAL AND PROTOZOAN INFECTIONS These infections can also occur as a complication of contact lens wear. Fungal corneal ulcers are more common in warm humid climates where the organism is more prevalent. *Acanthamoeba*, a free-living type of protozoa, is found commonly in soil, contaminated water, and dusty environments. This organism has been responsible for severe painful corneal infections in contact lens wearers using homemade saline solution (rather than the commercial saline solution called for in heat disinfection of soft contact lenses, an older process rarely used today), rinsing contact lenses with tap water, or wearing contact lenses while swimming or soaking in hot tubs. Therefore, contact lens wearers must understand that they should never use homemade saline solutions, tap water, or distilled water to care for their soft or rigid contact lenses. In addition, they should avoid wearing their contact lenses in hot tubs or swimming pools, where this organism is found.

CORNEAL ABRASION A corneal abrasion may occur not only from overwear or improper hygiene or fit but also from foreign material lodged between the contact lens and the cornea. This condition is extremely painful for rigid contact lens wearers, but the effects of the abrasion can be masked in soft contact lens wearers by the "bandage" effect of the soft contact lens itself. A corneal abrasion has the potential to become infected.

Because reports have appeared in the ophthalmic literature of *Pseudomonas* corneal ulcers developing after a patch for what seemed to be a simple corneal abrasion in a contact lens wearer, today ophthalmologists consider all abrasions to be potentially infected and treat them with frequent topical antibiotics and do not patch the eye.

REDUCING THE RISK OF INFECTION   Corneal infections are severe complications of improper use of contact lenses, but the risk of infection can be reduced by ensuring that patients are properly instructed in careful contact lens handling and maintenance and that scrupulous contact lens hygiene is also followed in the office. Preventing contact lens infections is the responsibility not only of the patient but also of the ophthalmologist and the ophthalmic medical assistant.

Inability to Insert or Remove Lenses

Patients may have difficulty inserting or removing their contact lenses, especially during the initial trial period of contact lens wear. Sometimes patients become panicky if their first attempts fail, making the situation worse. The ophthalmic medical assistant can best assist the patient by providing calming advice. For most individuals, taking a few minutes to rest and relax before retrying leads to success. When teaching patients proper contact lens insertion and removal techniques, remind them to remain relaxed and not to panic. If patients are truly unable to remove the contact lens, they should immediately notify their ophthalmologist or seek care in the emergency room.

Lens "Lost" in the Eye

It is impossible for a contact lens to be truly lost in the eye because the conjunctiva, which lines both the globe and the inner lid, prevents the contact lens from disappearing behind the eye. On rare occasions, a patient may displace a contact lens into the cul-de-sac or to the side of the eye. In the office, fluorescein drops may aid in locating a "lost" soft contact lens. If the "lost" contact lens is a rigid type, careful office examination and double eversion of the upper lid will assist in finding the contact lens. Rigid contact lenses can often be located and removed by the patient, but soft lenses may fold or tear in the eye and become lodged in the superior cul-de-sac, requiring in-office removal.

Contraindications for Contact Lenses

The term **contraindication** describes any condition that renders a particular treatment, medication, or medical device inadvisable because complications or adverse effects may result. Patient-related complications from contact lens wear can be overcome by considering the possible complications and taking steps to prevent them before fitting the patient with a contact lens. A thorough ocular history and a total ocular examination by the ophthalmologist must be completed, with special emphasis on the lids, conjunctiva, cornea, and tears, as well as inquiries into the possible history of allergies, medications, occupation, and the success or failure of previous contact lens wear. Emphasis should be placed on inquiring about the patient's commitment to compliance and dedication to proper contact lens wear and care.

Even with meticulous care to avoid

complications, some patients who desire

contact lenses may be unable to wear them.

The ophthalmologist may choose to discourage some patients from wearing contact lenses in order to avert potentially serious eye problems. The following list of contact lens contraindications lists conditions and characteristics of patients who are likely to have a lower rate of success in contact lens wear:

- certain ocular pathologic conditions (for example, severe allergies, chronic blepharoconjunctivitis, pterygium, seventh nerve palsy, lid abnormalities, or anesthetic cornea)

- inappropriate "nervous" and emotional temperaments

- poor or no blink reflexes

- moderate to severe dry eyes (because all contact lenses require adequate tear production)

- disabling conditions such as parkinsonism (tremor) or arthritis (deformed hands), which make insertion and removal of contact lenses difficult

- certain occupations that expose workers to dusty, dirty, or particulate environments or to caustic chemicals in the air

- seizure disorders

SELF-ASSESSMENT TEST

1. Briefly describe how a contact lens provides a new refractive surface for the cornea and corrects refractive error.

2. Name the 4 objectives that a contact lens must meet to maintain the health of the cornea.

3. Name at least 5 elements that may be required in determining the specification of a contact lens.

4. Match the type of contact lens with the most appropriate possible use.

    _____ cosmetic restorative   a. corrects astigmatic error

    _____ cosmetic fashion   b. acts as a prosthetic device for a disfigured eye

    _____ therapeutic   c. enhances or changes iris color

    _____ toric   d. corrects irregular astigmatism associated with keratoconus

    _____ bifocal   e. corrects both near and distance vision

                                     f. "bandages" a damaged or painful cornea

5. Briefly describe the different methods by which soft contact lenses, polymethylmethacrylate contact lenses, and rigid gas-permeable contact lenses provide oxygenation to the cornea.

6. Briefly compare the purpose of contact lens cleaning with the purpose of contact lens disinfection.

7. Name 2 methods of disinfecting contact lenses.

8. What are the purposes of a contact lens lubricant, or wetting solution?

9. What is the first step to take in inserting a contact lens?

10. Name at least 5 symptoms that may indicate an allergic or sensitivity reaction to a contact lens solution.

11. Define and state the cause of warping caused by contact lenses.

12. Name the 5 principal types of corneal problems that may occur in contact lens wearers.

13. Why is it impossible for a contact lens to become "lost" behind the eye?

14. Name at least 3 possible contraindications for contact lens use.

SUGGESTED ACTIVITIES

1. Ask permission to observe several contact lens fittings for a variety of types of patients. Take notes and ask questions in a later meeting with the ophthalmologist or the technician overseeing the fitting.

2. Talk to friends, family, or patients who wear or have worn contact lenses to understand the advantages and disadvantages of their use.

3. With your ophthalmologist's permission and under supervision, try on a set of contact lenses yourself to appreciate your patients' reactions. Follow the steps for insertion and removal outlined in this chapter.

4. On your next trip to a pharmacy, visit the contact lens solutions section. Discuss the many choices of contact lens solutions with the pharmacist or your ophthalmologist so that you can better advise patients.

5. Under supervision of the ophthalmologist or an experienced technician in your office, practice cleaning and disinfecting the trial lenses used in your ophthalmologist's practice.

SUGGESTED RESOURCES

Bennett ES, Henry VA. *Clinical Manual of Contact Lenses.* Baltimore: Lippincott Williams & Wilkins; 2008.

Cassin B, ed. *Fundamentals for Ophthalmic Technical Personnel.* Philadelphia: Saunders; 1995: chap 23.

Donshik PC, guest ed. Contact lenses. *Ophthalmol Clin North Am.* 2003;16:305–494.

Extended Wear of Contact Lenses. Information Statement [downloadable from www.aao.org]. San Francisco: American Academy of Ophthalmology; 2008.

Freeman MI. Selecting rigid versus soft contact lenses. *Ophthalmol Clin North Am.* 1989;2:229–234.

Horn MM, Bruce AS. *Manual of Contact Lens Prescribing and Fitting.* 3rd ed. With CD-ROM. St Louis: Butterworth-Heinemann/Elsevier; 2006.

JCAHPO/CLAO Contact Lens Learning Systems Series 1 & 2. An interactive training CD that covers basic information on soft contact lenses material and properties, fitting techniques for soft spherical, soft toric, RGP contact lenses, presbyopia and the irregular cornea. It also contains information on insertion and removal techniques, and contact lens care. Visit www.jcahpo.org for more information.

Kastl PR, ed. *Contact Lenses: The CLAO Guide to Basic Science and Clinical Practice.* 3rd ed. Dubuque, IA: Kendall/Hunt Publishing; 1995.

Key JE, ed. *The CLAO Pocket Guide to Contact Lens Fitting.* New Orleans: Contact Lens Association of Ophthalmologists; 1994.

Millis EAW. *Medical Contact Lens Practice.* Boston: Butterworth-Heinemann; 2005.

Minimizing Transmission of Bloodborne Pathogens and Surface Infectious Agents in Ophthalmic Offices and Operating Rooms. Information Statement [downloadable from www.aao.org]. San Francisco: American Academy of Ophthalmology; 2002.

Stein HA, Freeman MI, Stein RM, Maund LD. *Contact Lenses: Fundamentals and Clinical Use.* Thorofare, NJ: Slack; 1997.

Stein HA, Slatt BJ, Stein RM. *Fitting Guide for Rigid and Soft Contact Lenses: A Practical Approach.* 4th ed. St Louis: Mosby; 2002.

Stein HA, Stein RM. *The Ophthalmic Assistant: A Text for Allied and Associated Ophthalmic Personnel.* 8th ed. St Louis: Mosby; 2006.

15 PATIENT INTERACTION, SCREENING, AND EMERGENCIES

The ophthalmic medical assistant is frequently the first professional contact the patient has when telephoning or visiting the ophthalmologist's office. In this role, assistants represent the doctor's office to the patient and therefore are responsible for acting in a manner that is caring and courteous as well as technically proficient. Assistants not only greet patients but also screen patients by asking a specific series of questions to determine the urgency of their need to see the doctor and to schedule a visit appropriately. Assistants also must be able to deal confidently and quickly with patients who call the office with a medical emergency or who experience an emergency during an office visit. In these capacities, assistants are required to be aware of certain ethical and legal concerns to avoid compromising the rights or proper treatment of patients.

This chapter discusses how to greet patients courteously in person and by telephone, screen patients and schedule appointments, process patients referred by other physicians, and handle a variety of emergency situations in a professional manner.

Patient–Assistant Interaction

Patients telephoning or arriving at the ophthalmologist's office often are frightened or apprehensive. In addition to exercising common courtesy in office greetings and telephone conversations, you should also convey your concern for the patient as an individual by talking calmly and quietly and showing genuine compassion, understanding, and, when necessary, reassurance. The ability to gain the patient's trust and respect will greatly enhance the gathering of the necessary information for diagnosis and treatment and will ease the patient's concerns.

Patient Greeting

Whether in person or on the telephone, always address adult patients as Mr., Mrs., Miss, Ms., or according to their preference. When meeting patients in the office, introduce yourself by name and identify your role in the office (for example, "I am _____, Dr. _____'s assistant"). Let patients who seem concerned know that your interaction with them is not delaying their seeing the ophthalmologist but is, in fact, facilitating their meeting with the physician.

The caring and concern that you exhibit over the telephone help put patients at ease and assure them that they will be treated with courtesy and respect. Office personnel who answer the telephone must remember that callers who seem aggressive or even rude may simply be masking fear and worry. Maintaining your composure and assuring patients that you understand their situation is the best way to respond to their anxiety. Chapter 16 presents specific tips for dealing with patients who require special attention because of age, health conditions, or life situations. That chapter also provides the knowledge to help patients having medical emergencies.

Although general office procedures may vary from practice to practice, the requirement for good telephone manners applies to all areas of health care. Basic efficient office telephone protocol includes the following:

- Determine which callers should be transferred immediately to the ophthalmologist and under what circumstances.

- When the telephone rings, answer it as promptly as possible.

- Answer the telephone by stating your doctor's name or the name of the practice; then identify yourself and ask, "How may I help you?"

- Project an attitude of patience and helpfulness, and always answer the telephone with a "smiling" and pleasant (not tense) voice. The individual calling may need a calm person to talk to, and although your face cannot be seen over the telephone, the caller can easily sense your mood by your tone of voice.

- Handle all telephone calls efficiently by forwarding to the correct individual quickly. Ask for a return telephone number in case the call is inadvertently disconnected.

- Try not to put the callers on hold unless it is absolutely necessary. If it is necessary, ask for permission to put the caller on hold and wait for his or her response. Also consider the option of returning a call. If available, you can suggest the use of a voice mail message system for routine matters.

- Write all messages, including the name, date, time and return telephone numbers on a message pad

kept beside the telephone. Ask the callers to spell their name if you are not sure about the spelling.

- Ask the caller to repeat information if you are uncertain about something you have heard.

- At the end of the call, thank the person for calling. End the conversation gently and without abruptness.

- Always return a call if you have told the caller you would do so.

- Refer patients to the practice's web page, if available, for further information.

Patient Screening

In many offices, one of the ophthalmic medical assistant's major responsibilities is to perform a preliminary interview with patients to determine the urgency of their situation and to schedule their visit with the ophthalmologist appropriately. This important screening, known as **triage**, ensures that patients with the most serious complaints are seen promptly. Triage most frequently takes place on the telephone when the patient calls the office, but it may apply when a patient appears in the office requesting to see the doctor without calling beforehand. In either case, the basic triage procedure (determining whether a patient's complaint is an emergency, an urgent problem, or a routine situation and scheduling an office visit accordingly) is the same.

The triage situations and procedures presented in this chapter are intended mainly as illustrations and general guidelines; ophthalmic assistants should verify the precise triage situations, steps, and policies followed in their office. Assistants have an important responsibility to perform triage exactly as their ophthalmologist or senior staff instructs or as their office policy dictates. Failure to do so could result in a disservice to the patient's health and vision.

Triage

The aim of triage is initially to assess and classify patients' signs and symptoms according to their severity and urgency. This process aids the ophthalmic medical assistant in deciding if the patient's difficulty is an emergency or urgent problem, which should be seen relatively soon, or a routine case, which can be seen at a later time.

Triage does not include an in-depth evaluation of the patient's dilemma or a complete medical history. Rather, it is a brief gathering of essential data, beginning with the date and time of the call and the name and telephone number (and possibly the address) of the caller. Thereafter, the urgency for an appointment depends on the nature, origin, and duration of the patient's complaint or symptom. To determine this, the assistant must ask the patient a series of questions that focus on what, when, how, and where:

- What is the basic medical complaint or symptom? Examples: What is the nature of your vision loss? What was sprayed into your eye causing the pain? Is it in one eye or both?

- When did the complaint or symptom start? For example: When did you lose vision from your right eye? If the patient does not know the exact time, ask if it was minutes, hours, days, or weeks ago.

- How did the complaint or symptom start? Examples: How did you know there was something wrong with your eye? Did it start suddenly or slowly? When were you exposed to the chemical agent?

- Where were you at the onset of your complaint or symptom? Examples: Where were you when your left eye was injured? Where were you when the vision loss started and what were you doing?

As with history-taking procedures, occasionally some prompting is required to elicit a complete answer, and sometimes an answer to a general question leads to more specific questions. To ensure proper scheduling, assistants performing triage must be certain they completely understand the patient's complaint. It may be necessary to ask patients to restate or rephrase their complaint to obtain this information. The patient's own mental state or sense of emergency should also be taken into consideration when scheduling the visit with the doctor.

In general, the more recent the onset of the patient's symptom, the more urgent the situation.

When any doubt exists about the nature or urgency of a patient's situation or how to schedule a patient, assistants should either consult the ophthalmologist or allow the patient to speak to the ophthalmologist directly. Sometimes you may find it helpful to speak with a family member during triage or have that person present during the patient's office visit. He or she may be able to provide details about the injury or problem that the patient may have overlooked or forgotten. If you do not speak the language of a patient who calls or if you cannot understand someone's speech, try to identify a family member, friend, or neighbor who can clarify the situation and/or accompany the patient to the office.

Eye trauma may be the result of child abuse or domestic violence. For medical-legal considerations, the ophthalmic medical assistant should be alert for discrepancies between the history of the trauma and the injury itself. Any dissimilarity in the details of an injury should be brought to the attention of the ophthalmologist, in private and isolated from the patient and those accompanying the patient. (Symptoms of abuse can be similar to those exhibited by patients who require extra attention due to withdrawal, irritability, anxiety, physical symptoms, and vague complaints. See "Patients Who May Be Suffering from Abuse" in Chapter 16 for more information.)

EMERGENCY SITUATION Ophthalmic **emergencies** are those situations that require immediate action. Assistants who determine that a patient has a medical emergency should advise the patient to come into the office immediately if that is appropriate or go to the nearest medical or emergency facility capable of treating ophthalmic problems. Many offices have protocols in place that help to determine appropriate triage. When in doubt, consult the ophthalmologist. (See Table 15.1 for a summary of situations that constitute emergencies.)

URGENT SITUATION An **urgent** situation requires that the patient be seen within 24 hours of contacting the ophthalmologist's office. Some offices define this time period as up to 48 hours. In general, however, patients with urgent conditions should be seen before the next available routine appointment time.

Patients with urgent conditions may report a variety of symptoms, some of which may suggest an emergency condition while others, although not as serious, may nevertheless deserve prompt attention. It can be difficult to distinguish an urgent situation from an emergency. When you have any doubt, the safest course of action is to consult with the ophthalmologist, perhaps with more regularity than you would for an emergency or routine situation. Obviously, erring on the side of safety and completeness is preferred to the possibility of patients losing vision or even an eye because a physician did not promptly see them. (See Table 15.1 for a summary of situations that are generally considered to be urgent situations.)

ROUTINE SITUATION The **routine** situation usually includes conditions that have been present for several weeks or more. Patients with routine conditions do not normally have problems that pose an immediate threat

Table 15.1 Assessing and Classifying Signs and Symptoms

Level of Urgency	Signs and Symptoms
Emergency: requires immediate action, either in the office or another medical or emergency facility	Chemical burns: alkali, acid, or organic solvents in the eye (Important detailed instructions for dealing with chemical burns both over the telephone and in the office appear later in this chapter.) Sudden, painless, severe loss of vision (This suggests an acute vascular occlusion such as a central retinal artery or vein occlusion that frequently causes permanent loss of sight.) Sudden loss of vision in an elderly patient associated with headache and/or scalp tenderness (This is indicative of temporal arteritis, also known as cranial or giant cell arteritis.) Sudden painful loss of vision associated with nausea and vomiting (This is indicative of an acute attack of angle closure glaucoma.) Trauma in which the globe has been or is likely to be lacerated, ruptured, or penetrated from a high-velocity-projectile object such as a nail, screw, or piece of concrete or wood Any trauma that is associated with visual loss or persistent pain Severe blunt trauma, such as a forceful blow to the eye with a fist or high-velocity object such as a tennis ball or racquet ball A foreign body in the eye or a corneal abrasion caused by a foreign body or blunt object Acute, rapid onset of eye pain or discomfort Sudden onset of diplopia, ptosis, pain and a dilated pupil Any emergency referral from another physician
Urgent situation: requires the patient to be seen within 24 hours of contacting the ophthalmologist	Loss of vision that has evolved gradually over a period of a few days to a week (Ask the patient whether the vision loss is now persistent or intermittent.) Sudden onset of diplopia or other distorted vision Recent onset of light flashes and floaters Acute red eye, with or without discharge (Some patients, such as contact lens wearers, may need an emergency appointment.) Blunt trauma, such as a bump to the eye, that is not associated with vision loss or persistent pain and where penetration of the globe is not likely Double vision that has persisted for less than a week Photophobia (sensitivity to light) Progressively worsening ocular pain or discomfort Loss or breakage of glasses or contact lenses needed for work, driving, or studies (Not all physicians consider losing or breaking glasses urgent.) Acute swelling of eyelids and tissues of the globe with eye pain, mucous discharge, blurring of vision, or double vision (This is indicative of orbital cellulitis.)
Routine situation: scheduling of next available routine appointment time, unless symptoms worsen or vision becomes impaired	Discomfort after prolonged use of the eyes Difficulty with near work or fine print Mild ocular irritation, itching, burning Tearing in the absence of other symptoms Lid twitching or fluttering Mucous discharge from the eye Mild redness of the eye not accompanied by other symptoms Persistent and unchanged floaters whose cause has been previously determined

to vision. However, because their condition may cause considerable concern, these patients should be shown an appropriate level of attention. When assessing a routine situation, take the patient's mental state into account. Their state of mind may require a more urgent visit, even though their medical condition would normally be scheduled for a routine appointment.

Schedule patients with routine complaints for the next available routine appointment time, which might be within a few days or a week or two. However, the assistant performing the triage should instruct patients to contact the office if their symptoms worsen or if vision becomes impaired before their scheduled office visit. (See Table 15.1 for a summary of situations that may represent routine appointments.)

Appointment Scheduling

Whether as a part of performing triage or simply filling the role of office receptionist, ophthalmic medical assistants should follow these basic guidelines for scheduling appointments efficiently and courteously:

- Be sure the patient knows the exact location of the office.

- Provide details about parking facilities or access to public transportation if necessary.

- Let patients know if their condition, tests, or treatments they will be receiving require that a companion or family member assist them to or from the office.

- Especially in a multiple-physician office, it is important for patients to know which physician will be seeing them.

- Remind patients to bring their glasses and/or contact lenses with them. They should also bring all medications they are using, especially those for the eye.

- Advise contact lens patients who desire a spectacle correction to stop wearing the lenses for an appropriate time prior to the examination. Ask your ophthalmologist for his or her appropriate recommended time.

- Advise patients of the approximate length of time for their entire office visit. Diabetics may wish to bring a snack with them. Parents of infants may wish to bring formula and diapers.

- Inform patients to bring referral forms, insurance cards, and other necessary business papers.

- Inform the patients of possible side effects of dilating eyedrops causing blurry vision and light sensitivity, and the need for someone to drive them home.

- Inform patients of the office hours, and ask if they have any special considerations related to their office visit for transportation, work or school. Accommodate the patients' needs as much as possible for time and day of the appointment.

Referred Patients

Each medical practice has specific office procedures for handling patients referred by other physicians. Upon joining the ophthalmologist's office, you should familiarize yourself with these protocols. Follow these general guidelines when receiving a telephone call from a referring physician or referred patient. First, obtain the referring physician's name and, if possible, the reason for the referral, especially if a letter from the referring doctor is not available. If it is routine in your office after the patient's examination, assure the patient that the referring physician will be informed of the results of the examination and any treatment recommendations.

Emergencies in the Office

The assistant's competence in handling an emergency calmly and capably is a skill most appreciated in the ophthalmology office. In general, assistants will encounter two common types of ophthalmic emergencies in the office: chemical burns and trauma. However, many patients will present with other eye problems, ranging from corneal abrasions to vitreous floaters, which are also emergent eye conditions requiring prompt attention. Nonophthalmic emergencies that may occur during the patient's office visit include fainting, falling, and, on rare occasions, seizures, respiratory distress, heart attack, and stroke.

In any emergency, if you are uncertain about what to do lose no time in summoning someone nearby—either the doctor or a senior staff member—whom you think will be able to assess the situation and administer appropriate aid. Before an emergency happens, take the time to familiarize yourself with office policy and the location of emergency medications, instruments, and materials. After the initial administration of the emergency first aid, you may be asked to assist with further evaluation and care of the patient. You can also be helpful to the patient or accompanying family member or friend by explaining what is happening, what can be expected next, and about how long the patient will be detained.

Burns

Burns from chemicals, heat, and ultraviolet rays are among the emergencies encountered in the office.

CHEMICAL BURNS A chemical burn can cause severe eye damage very rapidly. Ophthalmic medical assistants should know whether their office policy allows them to initiate first aid for chemical injuries. These burns are true emergencies and assistants need to know what to do when the doctor is out of the office.

Any patient who telephones the office to report a chemical in the eye should be instructed to irrigate (wash out, or flush) the affected eye immediately by holding it open either under a continuous flow of running tap water or in a basin filled with water for at least 15 to 20 minutes before coming to the office or proceeding to an emergency facility. Remind the patient to take along the bottle of offending agent, if possible. Once the patient arrives in the office, chemical burns must be treated *immediately* by washing out the eye with large amounts of sterile irrigating solution (if available) or tap water. Hold the patient's eyelids open or use an eyelid speculum or a Morgan irrigating contact lens that facilitates continuous irrigation. Absorb the run-off fluid with a towel or an emesis basin. Topical anesthetic drops may be needed. The irrigation is directed into the conjunctival fornices and over the cornea with large amounts of sterile saline solution, balanced salt solution, or tap water. Identification of the offending chemical agent may be found on the product label. Its pH and concentration are very helpful pieces of information because they give the physician an idea of the severity of damage to the eye. Irrigation is continued until the tear film records a pH between 7.0 and 8.0 (neutral) as tested by litmus paper or pH dip strip.

An **alkali burn**, the most destructive type of chemical injury, requires especially prompt irrigation even before the patient comes to the doctor's office. Alkali chemical exposure causes rapid tissue destruction with deep ocular penetration, causing tissue death and subsequent intense scarring that results in blindness. Therefore, alkali compounds such as calcium hydroxide or lime (which is found in plaster, cement, and whitewash), household ammonia, and agricultural anhydrous ammonia can rapidly penetrate ocular tissues. These substances also may leave particles in the eye, which can cause further damage if they are not completely washed out. Alkali burns, because of their destructive nature, may require prolonged irrigation in the office, possibly exceeding 30 minutes.

Like alkali burns, **acidic burns** require immediate irrigation because they too can lead to blindness, especially with delay in treatment. Acids damage tissues by destructive coagulation necrosis (tissue death). Acid burns usually result from exploding car batteries, industrial products, household bleach, and other sterilizing products. Although they tend to be less injurious than alkali burns, they nevertheless require thorough and prompt irrigation. Irrigation should continue for 20 to 30 minutes nonstop.

Organic solvents include such common household substances as kerosene, gasoline, alcohol, and cleaning fluids. Although some organic solvents may not be as destructive to the eye as alkali or acid, they nevertheless require both home and office irrigation, as with other chemical injuries.

Treatment of chemical injuries includes topical antibiotics, cycloplegic agents, lubricants (artificial tears and gels), and corticosteroids. The ophthalmologist is the best judge of the specific treatment and the necessity for irrigation and the length of time it should be performed. Even when irrigation is necessary, care must be exercised, as profuse or forceful irrigation can cause damage to the cornea. The ophthalmologist will decide what topical medications and anesthetic drops to use prior to irrigation. The ophthalmic assistant's role will be to administer the topical agents as well as to perform the irrigation. Procedure 15.1 presents the steps of this office procedure.

After irrigation, the assistant may be asked to help gather important data, including the following:

- the patient's visual acuity measurements, when possible

- an accident summary (Worker's compensation cases require very specific information, often including time, place, and other details.)

- the name or type of chemical involved—for example, a household cleaning product that contains chemicals such as bleach, ammonia, or lye (Some of this information may have been gathered in the initial telephone assessment, but it is important to ensure that the medical record notes are complete.)

- the extent of exposure to the chemical—for example, a large quantity splashed directly into the eye or a small amount of chemical residue transferred from the finger to the eye

THERMAL BURNS   Thermal injuries usually involve the face, eyelids, cornea, adnexa, and scalp areas. Such injuries commonly occur from house fires, industrial explosions, gasoline fires, hot liquids, and electrical mishaps. Special care must be taken when examining these patients, with the supervision from your doctor, in order to avoid additional damage to the eye.

ULTRAVIOLET BURNS   Ultraviolet radiation can cause keratitis and skin burns in patients who fail to properly protect their eyes and skin from irradiation. These patients fail to protect their eyes while skiing, boating, using an arc welding light, or tanning in commercial booths. An ultraviolet burn is commonly a bilateral corneal problem that responds favorably to topical eyedrops and ointments. The "bandage effect" of a therapeutic soft contact lens aids in healing and pain relief. Keep in mind that although topical anesthetic drops work well to relieve pain, they also retard the corneal epithelial healing process; therefore, they should not be used repeatedly or given to the patient.

Procedure 15.1 Irrigating the Eye

1. Immediately upon arrival, ask the patient to lie down on a stretcher, sofa, examining table, or a chair with a tilted back.

2. If the ophthalmologist requires and permits and if the patient has no known allergy to anesthetic medication, instill 1 drop of topical anesthetic solution. (See Chapter 6 for information about instilling eyedrops.)

3. Holding a gauze pad to help you keep your grasp, use your gloved fingers to separate the lids of the affected eye. Gently, but firmly, hold the lids open to counter the spasm and forceful closure of the eye during irrigation. A lid speculum may also be used to hold the lids open.

4. Give the patient a towel to hold against the face to absorb the excess fluid. In addition, you can position a basin next to the patient's face to catch the fluid.

5. Perform irrigation with a bottle of ready-made balanced salt solution (Figure A). If available, a continuous–rapid-drip bottle (suspended like an intravenous drip) is easier because you don't have to keep squeezing the bottle; you just have to direct the stream into the patient's eye. Direct the irrigating stream away from the nose to avoid contaminating the other eye.

6. You may need to evert (turn out) the upper lid while irrigating to wash away particles of chemical that may have become lodged there. To evert the lid:

   a. With the thumb and forefinger of one gloved hand, grasp the lashes of the upper lid and pull it out and down slightly (Figure B).

   b. Using your other hand, place the stick portion of a cotton-tipped applicator horizontally on the upper eyelid, approximately one-half inch above the margin of the eyelid (Figure C).

   c. Rotate the lid up and over the applicator stick to expose the conjunctival surface (Figure D).

7. After irrigation has been completed. check with the ophthalmologist before patching the eye. It is contraindicated in alkali exposures and certain other situations. (For information about patching the eye, see Chapter 17.)

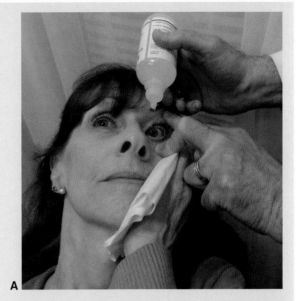

A

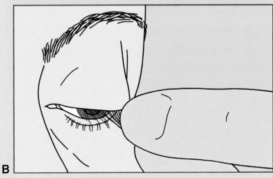

B

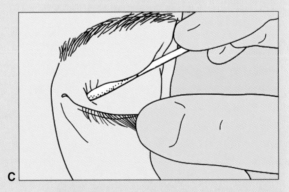

C

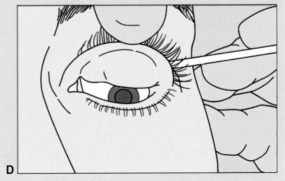

D

Trauma

Because of the seriousness of the possible consequences of trauma, the ophthalmologist takes principal responsibility for assessing and treating patients who appear in the office with eye trauma. However, assistants may be requested to help in the following ways:

- Take the patient's medical history.

- Check visual acuity to establish a baseline measure; this should always be done unless further trauma or injury could result from forcefully opening the eyelid or disrupting traumatized tissue.

- Ask questions to gather details of the accident and identify the nature of the injury. Determine if a foreign body is suspected.

When assisting the doctor with a patient who has a traumatized eye, it is important to remember the following points:

- Never unnecessarily touch or handle an eye that has a laceration or rupture.

- Never apply pressure to the globe while attempting to open the lids.

- Never administer drops or other medications without authorization from the physician and instruction on the proper methods.

- Never use a previously opened bottle of eyedrops for a patient who may have a penetrating eye injury (always use a new, unopened, sterile bottle) or touch the dropper to the eye.

TYPES OF TRAUMA INJURIES Assistants should know that trauma patients may present with a variety of injuries. Several common examples follow.

Blunt trauma to the orbital region shows *contusion* (bruising) and *edema* (swelling) of the eyelids with varying degrees of **ecchymosis** (hemorrhage into skin tissue). These patients often have orbital bone fractures with orbital **emphysema** (air escaping from the nasal sinuses and entering the tissues of the orbit). It is important for these patients to be instructed not to blow their nose as that could increase the orbital emphysema with pronounced swelling of the eyelid tissues.

Penetrating injury from small projectile objects can cause intraocular tissue damage. This is likely to occur when patients are exposed to particulate debris from explosions. Hammering a nail, using a grinding wheel, and striking metal-to-metal or metal-to-stone are other common sources of small projectiles.

Lacerations of the eyelid and facial areas often occur with blunt and penetrating trauma. When superficial they may heal without suturing, but more-extensive lacerations require surgical repair. It is not uncommon to find embedded foreign bodies in the wound margins, requiring exploration and irrigation by the doctor. Lacerations often involve deeper-lying eyelid structures such as the levator muscle complex, which when unable to function causes ptosis (drooping of and inability to raise the upper eyelid). A medial extension of a laceration may sever the tear duct canalicular system, which can possibly lead to chronic tearing.

Traumatic iritis and hyphema are frequently associated with blunt trauma. The presenting history, signs, and symptoms are described below. Both iritis and hyphema are associated with all types of head, orbital, and eye trauma, such as that caused by foreign bodies, motor vehicle crashes, or school playground injuries.

Traumatic hyphema is characterized by bleeding into the anterior chamber from trauma to the iris and/or ciliary body muscles. An associated rise in intraocular pressure from mechanical blockage by red blood cells can occur.

Traumatic iritis occurs when there is damage to the iris. The patient usually presents with light sensitivity and pupil miosis (pupillary constriction) or mydriasis (pupillary dilation). Ocular trauma is the most common cause of a dilated pupil. Other causes of a dilated pupil are cranial third nerve palsy and ruptured aneurysm (a thin localized area of an arterial wall), and also pharmacological agents.

Traumatic iridoplegia develops from concussive blunt trauma that damages the iris sphincter muscle and the nerves and leads to a fixed dilated pupil.

Posterior vitreous detachment and **retinal tears** and/or **detachment** can result from blunt trauma to the forehead, face, or orbit. The most common injuries are posterior vitreous detachment, presenting as central floaters associated with flashing lights, or a vitreous hemorrhage noted by many "spots" or a "spider web" in the field of vision. Retinal breaks, tears, detachment, and choroidal ruptures are less common and are associated with flashing lights, floaters, vision distortion, and central or peripheral vision loss.

Commonly, with acute retinal trauma, a patient will complain of vision loss that occurs from **retinal edema** (**Berlin's edema**) caused by damage to retinal photoreceptor cells. Vision will slowly improve depending on the extent of the edema.

Traumatic optic neuropathy occurs with blunt trauma to the head, orbit, and globe from forces transmitted posteriorly, through the orbit to the optic canal, involving the optic nerve. Invariably this shearing effect (deformed by force) of the optic nerve develops nerve tissue edema resulting in vision loss.

Retrobulbar hemorrhage is a serious complication of orbital trauma that occurs with orbital bone fractures and direct eyelid or globe trauma. The injury precipitates a rupture and bleeding of orbital, eyelid, and eye muscle vessels within the confines of the orbit. Patients with this type of injury have pronounced eyelid swelling, the lids closed shut or the eyeball protruding (proptosis), "frozen globe" (without movement), and severe hemorrhage into the eyelids and conjunctiva. This condition requires immediate surgical intervention to release the orbital pressure.

Orbital bone fractures are frequently associated with blunt trauma and are characterized by obvious swelling over the involved orbital and facial area, with facial numbness commonly seen when the orbital floor is fractured (blowout fracture).

General Emergency Assistance

Be alert to patients, who are in pain, feel faint, need to lie down, or feel nauseated. These symptoms may require immediate aid or may signify an impending emergency. Ophthalmic medical assistants should have access to emergency telephone numbers of hospitals, clinics, or a community emergency number (eg, 911). The telephone number of the nearest poison control center should also be immediately available. All assistants should also be able to administer first aid and cardiopulmonary resuscitation (CPR) in an emergency. First aid or CPR may be needed to treat a patient who has fainted or fallen or who develops respiratory distress or an adverse reaction to medication. To become certified as an ophthalmic medical assistant, one must obtain CPR certification through local chapters of the American Red Cross or other community service organization.

Learn where the emergency first aid kit for minor injuries is kept in your office. If your office has an emergency cart, know its location. This portable, wheeled device usually contains oxygen, intravenous glucose, and medications, such as epinephrine or adrenalin, used to revive a patient (Figure 15.1). The cart may also include intravenous syringes, CPR instructions, and cortisone, which may be required to manage a severe allergic reaction. In addition, some offices keep a supply of juice on hand to give to patients with diabetes who experience an unexpected low blood sugar level. (Procedure 15.2 presents steps to take in helping a patient who feels faint. Also see "Treatment of a Hypoglycemic Reaction" in Chapter 16.)

GUIDELINES FOR HANDLING A PATIENT FALL   The first step in handling a patient fall is to notify the doctor

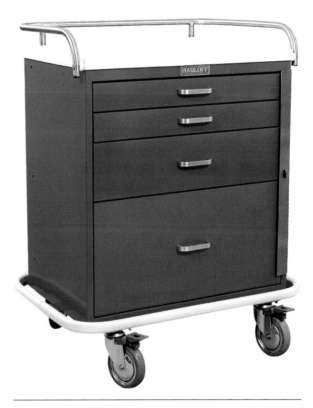

Figure 15.1 An office emergency cart. *(Image courtesy of The Harloff Company.)*

or other staff of the fall immediately. If you witness the fall or if the patient is on the floor when you arrive on the scene, do not move the patient until the doctor has assessed the patient for any injury. If you do not witness the fall and the patient has since become able to stand, do not allow the patient to leave the office until the doctor has assessed the patient for any injury.

A fall may be the result of a serious medical condition such as a stroke, heart attack, heart arrhythmia, or a fainting spell from many different causes. Patients should be asked about any chest pain or tightness, headache, weakness, shortness of breath, or heart palpitations. Breathing rate, heart rate, and blood pressure should be taken as soon as possible after the doctor is notified to come assess the patient. Special care should be taken if the patient is cyanotic (looks pale) or diaphoretic (sweating profusely). These signs indicate serious illness and/or injury.

Hospital Admission

Ophthalmic medical assistants may be called upon to help arrange emergency hospital admission for a patient who is not only ill but also possibly confused, scared, and upset. In addition, you may be asked to contact family

Procedure 15.2 Assisting a Patient Who Feels Faint

1. If possible, get the patient's head below the heart; if the patient is sitting, do this by bending the patient's head forward and down toward the knees (Figure A). Figures B and C show other ways to position a patient who feels faint.

2. Loosen the patient's collar or tight clothing.

3. Break the capsule of smelling salts or ammonia from the first aid kit or emergency cart and hold it under the patient's nose to revive the patient.

4. Heart rate, blood pressure and breathing rate should be assessed. Pulse should be assessed to see if it is regular or irregular. Notify the ophthalmologist immediately of any irregularities.

5. Insist the patient remain seated until the faintness has completely subsided; be prepared to steady patients when they stand.

6. Reassure the patient, who may be disoriented or embarrassed by the fainting incident.

7. Notify the doctor of the patient's fainting episode.

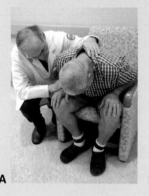
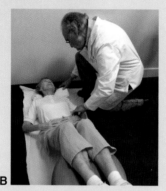
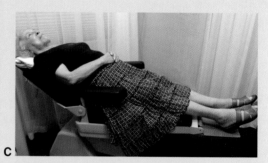

A B C

(Images courtesy of Tina Newmark, RN, MS.)

members or work associates for the patient. The following tips can help you make the process go smoothly:

- Let the patient know the plan of action; repeat it as necessary.

- Provide the patient with written directions to the hospital.

- Provide the name of the ophthalmologist, the office address, and phone number for the patient to keep on hand for admission to the hospital.

- If the patient is alone and proceeding immediately to the hospital, ask for (and write down) the name of the nearest family member or friend to notify.

SELF-ASSESSMENT TEST

1. Define *triage*.

2. What 3 basic questions should be answered during the triage process?

3. Triage is a very important part of screening patients. When do we begin the triage process?

4. Triage includes which of the following? (Check all that apply.)

   a. involves an in-depth evaluation of the patient's complaints

   b. is conducted via a series of questions to the patient

   c. alerts the medical assistant for possible eye trauma caused by domestic violence

   d. helps distinguish emergencies from routine eye care

5. Which of the following guidelines provide for a more efficient office? (Check all that apply.)

    a. When the telephone rings, answer it promptly.

    b. Record all telephone messages.

    c. Always thank the person for calling your office practice.

    d. Always display a pleasant attitude in answering the telephone.

    e. Use patients' first names to make them feel more comfortable.

6. Name the 3 main types of substances that may cause a chemical burn in the eye.

7. What is the first instruction to be given to a patient calling to report a chemical burn to the eye?

8. Which of the following are considered eye emergencies? (Check all that apply.)

    a. chemical alkali burns

    b. penetrating dart injury

    c. profuse tearing, eyelid fluttering and twitching

    d. acute painless loss of vision

    e. difficulty reading fine print

9. Which of the following might probably be scheduled as routine situations? (Check all that apply.)

    a. photophobia

    b. progressively worsening ocular pain

    c. mucous discharge from the eye

    d. difficulty with near work or fine print

    e. sudden onset of diplopia or other distorted vision

10. What is the first step to take in assisting a patient who feels faint?

11. Which of the following statements is incorrect?

    a. Mucous discharge from the eye without pain represents a routine appointment.

    b. Recent onset of flashes and floaters is an urgent situation.

    c. Photophobia (sensitivity to light) represents a routine appointment.

    d. Acute onset of pain and double vision is an emergency situation.

12. When is it okay to apply gentle pressure to a potential penetrating eye injury?

    a. always okay

    b. only gentle pressure with finger tips

    c. only gentle pressure with cotton-tip applicator

    d. never

13. Which of the following are associated with blunt eye trauma? (Check all that apply.)

    a. hyphema

    b. traumatic ptosis

    c. corneal abrasion

    d. double vision

    e. blurred vision

14. Medical assistants should be aware of the following guidelines for a patient who has fainted or develops respiratory distress. (Check all that apply.)

    a. Be aware that first aid or CPR may be needed in an emergency.

    b. Know the location of the emergency cart should oxygen or cortisone be required.

    c. Be prepared to give orange juice or glucose to a patient with diabetes for low blood sugar.

    d. Help the patient to stand and allow the patient to leave the office without being seen by the doctor.

Patient Screening Exercises

Complete the following patient screening exercises, which are intended to help you learn to clarify the patient's symptoms systematically:

1. A 54-year-old office worker calls complaining of blurred vision. Select from the questions listed below all those that would be most appropriate in screening this call.

    a. Do you have a history of hypertension?

    b. How long have your symptoms been present?

    c. Was your vision change rapid or gradual?

    d. Do you see well at night?

    e. Are both eyes involved?

    f. Has your vision decreased or worsened?

    g. Do you have a family history of cataracts?

    h. Do you have other eye problems of recent onset?

2. A 22-year-old woman calls to say she has splashed a cleaning solution in her eye. Select from the questions listed below all those that would be most appropriate in screening this call.

    a. Have you flushed your eye with running water for at least 15 minutes?

    b. Were you wearing glasses?

    c. When did the accident occur?

    d. Is your vision impaired?

    e. Do you know what the chemical was?

    f. Do you have glaucoma?

    g. Are your eyes tearing?

    h. Which eye was involved?

    i. Do you have transportation to the doctor's office available?

3. A 67-year-old patient calls to complain that his eyes are burning. Select from the questions listed below all those that would be most appropriate in screening this call.

    a. Do you use reading glasses?

    b. How long have your eyes burned?

    c. When do your eyes burn the most?

    d. Do you have cataracts?

    e. Are your eyes red?

    f. Do other symptoms accompany the burning?

    g. Are you seeing double?

    h. Does anything you do relieve the burning?

4. A 73-year-old patient calls to report episodes of transient visual loss (vision that seems to come and go). Select from the questions listed below all those that would be most appropriate in screening this call.

    a. When did the episodes of visual loss begin?

    b. Is the visual loss in 1 eye or both?

    c. Do you have any tearing or discharge?

    d. For how long is your vision impaired when the losses occur?

    e. Do you have other symptoms preceding or occurring with the episodes of visual loss?

    f. Is there a family history of blindness?

    g. Do you have headaches?

SUGGESTED ACTIVITIES

1. Review the triage and emergency procedure guidelines presented in this chapter with your ophthalmologist or senior staff member. Determine in what ways your office's protocol is similar or different.

2. Discuss with the ophthalmologist and the office manager how appointments are made in your office, especially covering how emergency appointments are handled.

3. Tour your office in the company of a senior staff member to learn where emergency supplies are kept and how to use them.

4. Set up a time to role-play some patient screening and emergency procedures (handling an emergency phone call, performing eye irrigation, and assisting a patient after falling or fainting) with an experienced member of the office staff. Afterward discuss the accuracy of your performance.

SUGGESTED RESOURCES

Davis CM. *Patient Practitioner Interaction: An Experiential Manual for Developing the Art of Health Care*. 5th ed. Thorofare, NJ: Slack; 2011.

Herrin MP. *Ophthalmic Examination and Basic Skills*. Thorofare, NJ: Slack; 1990: chap 11.

Kliegman RM, Behrman RE, Jenson HB, Stanton B. Evaluation of the sick child in the office and the clinic. In: *Nelson Textbook of Pediatrics*. 19th ed. Philadelphia: Saunders; 2011: chap 60.

Purtilo RB, Haddad AM. *Health Professional and Patient Interaction*. 7th ed rev. Philadelphia: Saunders; 2007.

Stein HA, Stein RM. *The Ophthalmic Assistant: A Text for Allied and Associated Ophthalmic Personnel*. 8th ed. St Louis: Mosby; 2006.

Wilson FM II, Blomquist PH, eds. *Practical Ophthalmology: A Manual for Beginning Residents*. 6th ed. San Francisco: American Academy of Ophthalmology; 2009.

16

PATIENTS WITH SPECIAL CONCERNS

Ophthalmic medical assistants have an important role in assuring that patients are satisfied with their eye care. Often, the way a patient is treated in the physician's office is as important to that individual as the medical care itself. The ophthalmic medical assistant who can communicate with individual patients in a compassionate and courteous manner is more effective by earning the patients' trust and cooperation. Assistants should consider the individual patient and any extra care or attention they might need because of their age, health condition, or life situation. Being able to recognize those patients who have special concerns and conditions will help you serve the patients in a more professional, supportive, and empathic manner.

The goal of this chapter is to aid you in understanding patients' emotions and learn how to assist patients with the following special concerns: disruptive patients, visually impaired or blind patients, infants and young children, elderly patients, physically handicapped patients, and patients with diabetes. In this chapter you will also learn to recognize the stresses, complaints, and difficulties all patients experience and the importance of awareness and compassion. In addition, you will learn to provide the special assistance and perform the special testing or care some patients require because of their situation or disability.

All Patients Considered

By considering all patients as individuals and attempting to understand and anticipate their needs, you can make each patient's office experience more pleasant and aid the ophthalmologist in effective treatment. Considering patients as individuals requires that you view patients as people, not as diseases. In any conversation, whether in the presence of patients or not, always discuss their problem or condition in terms of the individual. For example: "Mrs. _____, our patient with the cataract," not "the cataract in examining room 3"; "Mr. _____, who has his eyelid sutured," not "the lid suture we did last week." When addressing patients in a public area, you need to consider the privacy and confidentiality standards discussed in this chapter.

Do not avoid patients who speak a foreign language or who have physical disabilities. Try to overcome any personal discomfort or apprehension you may feel and give these individuals the same quality of attention you would convey to any other patient. Working with patients of different cultures will help you become a better communicator and patient advocate.

Learn to be aware of your own communication style and watch the body language of the patient to help you assess a need to change your approach. Facial and eye expression, gestures, physical appearance, and the tone of your voice all play a critical role in the overall responsiveness of your patients, their satisfaction with your level of service, and your success in obtaining accurate medical histories and measurements.

Patients and Their Families

Many times a family member will accompany the patient to the office visit, either out of concern or in the capacity of a caregiver, especially in the case of an elderly patient or a patient with visual or other physical disabilities. These family members are often greatly concerned about the patient's condition and may ask for specific information about the patient. In such situations, politely inform them that you are not permitted to share information about the patient and request that they refer their questions to the doctor. Federal law discussed in the next section prevents the sharing of patient information without specific written consent. Relatives or other caregivers who are present in the examination room with the patient have an implied permission to receive the information. By the same token, try to accommodate family members who may not want to voice their concerns in front of the patient but may want an opportunity to talk with the doctor in private. After obtaining a patient release, you can suggest a later time to call the doctor or have the doctor call them.

Health Insurance Portability and Accountability Act

Patients may wish to keep their medical conditions confidential, and for both ethical and legal reasons we must honor those requests. Both state and federal laws protect patients' rights to privacy and confidentiality. One of the most prominent is the Health Insurance Portability and Accountability Act (HIPAA). HIPAA was signed into law in 1996 and is administered by the Department of Health and Human Services at the federal level. HIPAA is intended to improve efficiency throughout health care and requires that health care providers adhere to standardized national privacy and confidentiality protections. There are severe penalties for not following these standards. It is imperative that you talk to your office manager or supervisor to become knowledgeable about office policies and procedures regarding these patient privacy regulations. (Also see "Communication With Patients" in Chapter 20 and "Compliance" in Chapter 17.)

Office Waiting Periods

Waiting for any reason can be frustrating, but it can be especially so for patients who may be anxious about their illness and fearful about an upcoming procedure or diagnosis. Most people are sympathetic about delays, however, especially if they have received a logical explanation of the circumstances and do not feel they have been forgotten or ignored.

Because ophthalmic medical assistants frequently help manage the daily flow of patients through the office, they are often required to communicate with patients if an unusually long delay occurs.

The following guidelines can help avoid waiting-room situations that tend to distress patients:

- Be sensitive to the valuable time a patient may have lost in waiting excessively for an examination. Assure patients that you do think their time is important.

- Whenever possible, tell patients when the doctor will actually see them or how long a test might take.

- Tell patients how long you will be gone when you leave them alone in the examination room or waiting area.

- If one patient must be seen out of turn ahead of others, explain the situation to those who are waiting in a manner that assists them in understanding and accepting the occurrence.

- If a child becomes fussy, try to have the doctor see the family member quickly or suggest they take a walk and come back in a specific amount of time. If the family member is seen ahead of others, explain the situation to those waiting and convey the doctor's appreciation for their understanding. Many offices have a small play area with books and toys to entertain children. Direct family members to utilize this area.

- Be alert to patients who say they feel sick or are in pain. They may need to be seen by the doctor promptly or be rescheduled if their situation is less urgent. (Chapter 15 covers triage situations and procedures.)

- If an appointment time is excessively delayed, offer to reschedule an appointment or invite the patient to use the telephone to call home or work.

- Patients who are in the office for more than one type of procedure or examination may be required to wait for periods between tests. Be sure these patients know what to expect and why and how long they will be waiting. Do not assume that anyone else has explained this already.

Disruptive Patients

The sheer stress of illness, fear of an unknown diagnosis or procedure, a previous bad experience in a doctor's office, or just the office wait occasionally can make some patients speak loudly and become irritable, hostile, or disruptive. Patients scheduled for office surgery may be anxious, fearful, and impatient, which can cause them to overreact to a comment or question. Some patients may also react this way if they are just overwhelmed by problems, whether associated with their medical condition or with an unrelated situation, such as a financial or family problem. Unfortunately, you may be the person on whom the patient decides to vent anger or frustration.

Ophthalmic medical assistants should be aware of the reasons for these kinds of patient reactions and resist the temptation to react impatiently or angrily to a distressed patient. All patients, no matter what their situation, deserve your compassion and understanding. The following guidelines can help you deal with patients who are irate or disruptive:

- Take the patient out of the reception area or waiting room to avoid upsetting other patients.

- Listen to the patient. Often your caring attention alone will defuse the patient's anger, and listening may help you understand the origin of the patient's hostility. (Chapter 19 discusses communication skills in more detail.)

- Try to identify the problem or perceived problem by restating or paraphrasing what the patient has said to you.

- Explain the delay but offer alternative solutions.

- Apologize when appropriate, even if you believe the patient is unreasonable or wrong. An apology is often sufficient to defuse anger.

- Never argue and never respond aggressively or offensively.

Aggressive, hostile, angry patients may be individuals who communicate ineffectively with everyone, including their family or friends. They may be overwhelmed or feel they are a burden to those around them. Talking with someone who knows and understands his or her medical circumstances, but is removed from the daily situation, can be a comfort.

During your encounter with an irate or hostile patient, you may learn of some nonmedical reason for the behavior. While respecting the patient's confidences and right to privacy, the ophthalmic medical assistant may be able to alert the doctor that the particular patient has a troubling nonmedical problem. It may then be appropriate for the doctor to refer the patient to a social service agency or support group for help.

Visually Impaired or Blind Patients

Chapter 13 covers the topic of low vision. To follow are some specific suggestions on ways to work with and assist an individual with a visual disability.

Patient Greeting and History-Taking Guidelines

When first encountering a patient who is visually impaired or blind, approach the patient, introduce yourself, and use the patient's name as well as your own; for example: "Hello, Mr. _____. My name is _____ _____ and I work with Dr. _____, who will be examining you today. Let's go on back to the examining room now." Or "Hello, Ms. _____. I'm _____ _____; I saw you last time you were in. Are you ready to get started?"

A smile may not be seen, but it can be "heard" when you speak in a friendly, cheerful manner. Another important point is to speak directly to the patient, not to an accompanying companion or, worse, to others in the waiting room.

Look for an extended hand to shake but do not make a point of insisting on a handshake if none is offered. Do not stumble over expressions like "How nice to see you!" or "I look forward to seeing you again soon." Generally, you may be more apologetic or overly sensitive about the use of such words than the person you are addressing.

Ask the patient whether the accompanying family members or friends should be invited to come along to the examining room. Some patients welcome the company, but others prefer to be alone with the doctor during the examination so they can ask their own questions. You can help smooth over any awkwardness by telling the family you will call them in when the testing is over and the doctor is ready to talk to everyone. When you arrive at the examining room, introduce the patient to the people who are in the room as you enter as well as to those who enter later.

Some special questions are usually included when taking the history of a patient with low vision. These include questions to ascertain the onset of visual loss; the patient's use of low vision aids; any problems or goals related to the low vision; and the nature of any home, family, or community support that the patient may have. A functional history includes questions about the patient's ability to perform a variety of specific daily living activities, everyday near-vision and distance-vision tasks such as reading a newspaper, mending, watching television, or reading an overhead menu at a fast-food restaurant. Also included are questions about the patient's orientation and mobility skills such as the ability to ambulate within the home and yard, or to go to and maneuver within a grocery store. Such a functional history is useful to help document progressive visual loss. It reveals how the patient is using his or her remaining vision and what accommodations the patient is making to the low vision. It also allows the patient to relate fears and concerns that may not be communicated during routine eye care.

Offering Assistance

If you have been able to observe how the patient navigated into the office or in the waiting room, you may know what kind of help, if any, the person needs in maneuvering around the office. If you have not noted this, offer assistance as unobtrusively as possible. Do not push yourself on patients or hurry them along.

When guiding a patient with a visual impairment, you may find it useful to ask gentle questions such as "Would you like some assistance?" or "Would you like to take my arm?" Patients who want to take your arm will usually do so above the elbow or around your lower arm. The patient may prefer to walk slightly behind you, which allows you to guide them and enables the patient to anticipate your directional changes. You can keep your arm relaxed and at your side unless the patient has balance problems and needs support in addition to guidance (Figure 16.1).

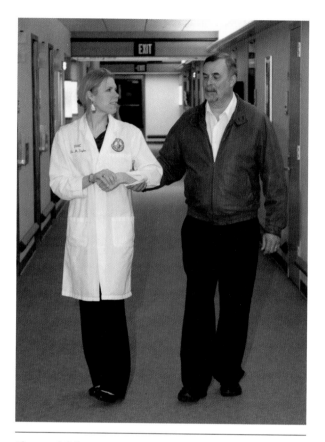

Figure 16.1 Guiding a visually impaired patient. *(Image courtesy of Brice Critser, CRA, Department of Ophthalmology and Visual Sciences, University of Iowa.)*

Never push or pull visually impaired patients, even gently. Always ask for patients' permission before touching them.

Think ahead and remove unnecessary chairs or obstacles in the hallway to avoid any embarrassment or accident to the patient who might bump into something. Verbally describe the path you will be taking to the patient: "We will be turning right and going along a narrow corridor" or "The chair is just to the left of the door; I'll put your hand on the armrest (or the back of the chair) so you can seat yourself." If you are called away while guiding a patient to a room, do not leave the patient stranded in the hallway. Either proceed to a room with the patient or have another member of the office staff take over for you.

When interacting with any patients who have severe visual impairment, give verbal information whenever possible. For example, you can say "I am reading through your chart and also making some notes" or "I will leave you alone in the room now while you wait for Dr. ____. She should be about 10 minutes" or "Dr. ____ is not quite ready to see you. I'd like you to come with me to another waiting area while your pupils are dilating." Tell the patient what is planned: "This next test will take about 20 minutes." If you must leave the patient, do not just quietly leave the patient alone. Instead say, "It was nice talking with you. I have to go now, but someone will be in to check (what they are waiting for) in just a few minutes."

Visual Acuity Assessment

The term *legal blindness* can be misleading, carries an unfortunate stigma, and offers little information about how the individual functions. One person who is visually impaired may work, study, and function in society, while another may be totally handicapped and dependent on others.

Patients with severe low vision may be referred to a low vision specialist. However, the ophthalmic medical assistant may first be required to estimate visual acuity. To begin, perform the visual acuity test using the standard Snellen chart and procedure. (See Chapter 8.) If the patient cannot see the largest (20/200) Snellen letter from the standard distance, ask the patient to move toward the chart or move a portable chart toward the patient yourself until the largest optotype can be seen.

In the visual acuity record, the numerator will then indicate the distance from the chart and the denominator, the largest line seen; for example, 10/200 means the patient could see the 200 optotype at 10 feet; 5/200 means the patient was tested at 5 feet. If a patient cannot see the largest Snellen letters at 3 feet, test the patient's ability to see and count fingers, detect hand movements, or perceive light. (See Procedure 13.1 in Chapter 13.) However, standard testing distances and performance procedures may differ between ophthalmology offices. Be sure to check the preferred procedure used in your office for testing the visual acuity of patients with visual impairment.

Infants and Young Children

In physical development, behavior, and needs, children differ greatly from adults. They should be approached and examined in a different manner than adult patients. When assisting and testing children, be aware of their short attention span and be understanding of their keen interest in exploring items around them. You should be prepared to protect any valuable instruments and lenses in the examination room that may be within a child's inquisitive reach. Offer a toy as an alternative to the instrument.

Parents want and need to understand their child's condition and to help the child comply with the treatment that the doctor prescribes. Parents are often fearful of the possibility of medical disorders in their children and are anxious. They are also usually uncomfortable if they sense that their child is feeling any type of discomfort or pain. Be sensitive to these needs and fears when assisting both the parent and child in order to have a successful and worthwhile visual examination that yields useful information.

Patient Greeting

Introduce yourself to the child as well as to the accompanying adult. For children older than 3, you might ask who they brought along with them today, but do not assume it is a parent. Explain who you are and what you will be doing both to the adult and, in simpler terms, to the child.

Be flexible enough to change the order of your examination. You might wish to start with taking a medical history, but you may find this procedure bores children, causing them to become inattentive or uncooperative for the duration of the examination. Be prepared to obtain pieces of the child's medical history throughout the examination or during testing. Explain this approach to accompanying adults, so that they do not feel you are ignoring them or are disorganized in your history taking.

Patient Positioning

Be sure the child is comfortable. Some small children may be more comfortable on the adult's lap, while others will feel important if they can sit alone in the chair (Figure 16.2). Ask children what they prefer, then respect

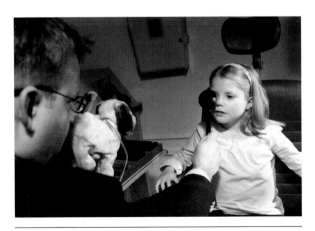

Figure 16.2 A child may prefer to sit alone for the examination, rather than on an adult's lap. *(Image courtesy of National Eye Institute, National Institutes of Health.)*

the answer. Adults should be requested to hold infants and babies in the lap, over the shoulder in the burping position, or in some other way that facilitates the examination and keeps the child quiet and comfortable.

A **papoose board** may be needed to immobilize an infant during an ophthalmologic evaluation, and the ophthalmic medical assistant may be asked to help out. Basically, the papoose board is a padded board with Velcro straps that fasten around the baby, holding arms and legs still and out of the way. The board is then placed on a stretcher.

Alternatives to a papoose board include the use of sheeting wrapped around the infant's arms and legs in mummy fashion or placement of the infant on the adult's lap with the head on the adult's knees and legs around the adult's waist. In this second method, the adult holds the baby's arms outstretched or snugly against the baby's own head. The infant thus feels the warmth and security of the adult.

Visual Acuity and Ability Testing

Visual acuity can be measured in toddlers and older children. However, infants and handicapped children, such as those with Down syndrome or cerebral palsy, frequently do not have the verbal and motor skills required to participate in a routine visual examination. For these children, it may only be possible for you to assess their general visual function by observing their response to a light stimulus or how they grab a toy in monocular testing.

Assessing visual function in infants, in children with mental or physical disabilities, and in children with severe visual impairment is difficult even for the most experienced examiner. The ophthalmic medical assistant will probably not be asked to make such an assessment alone, but may be asked to help with a child who is being evaluated. Checking visual function or acuity can be divided into 3 general examination groupings: infants, toddlers, and school-age children, with some overlap.

INFANTS   Infants do not undergo testing for visual acuity but rather for visual function, which is considered the ability to fixate a visual object and to follow the movement of that object with the eyes. Most babies without visual impairment display this capacity to "fix and follow" by age 2 months.

Procedure 16.1 provides step-by-step instructions for testing an infant's visual ability. When testing an infant, keep the following guidelines in mind.

Many infants do not want a stranger nearby or their head touched by someone they do not recognize. Always approach babies slowly to avoid frightening them.

Procedure 16.1 Testing an Infant's Visual Ability

1. Seat the infant on the adult's lap.

2. Select an object that stimulates sight only, such as a handheld spinning top or a sparkler-type toy.

3. Hold the object about 1 to 2 feet from the baby's face and slowly move it horizontally to the left, then to the right. Watch the infant's eyes for fixation eye movements.

4. If you discern no visual response, repeat step 3 in a darkened room with a small penlight.

Generally, the younger the patient, the less precisely you can estimate visual acuity; therefore, ask the accompanying adults how they think the child sees. Ask for examples of the baby's visual behavior, such as the ability to reach for toys or recognize familiar faces.

Check for a difference in the baby's response when either eye is covered. Some infants will object to the examination only when the better-seeing eye is covered.

TODDLERS AND SCHOOL-AGE CHILDREN   As part of the clinical team, ophthalmic medical assistants should learn the office protocol for working with young patients. Try to determine which charts and testing routines are preferred, whether you should check acuity with and without glasses, and whether you should check both distance and near vision.

Toddlers and school-age children are tested for visual acuity with standard charts. Children in these age groups, however, can present some special challenges. They may play, peek, guess the letters with a straight face, memorize with lightning speed, suddenly become very shy and uncooperative, and often need extra encouragement.

Toddlers as well as school-age children thrive on praise; they need to be told that they are doing a good job and that it is all right when they do not know the answer to a specific question or cannot see a test symbol. It is especially important that you tell them they are doing a good job not only when they answer correctly, but also when they are trying hard and cooperating—even if they cannot see or they make an error.

Children thrive on praise and fun. Encourage them by telling them they are doing a good job. Use toys to help in the examination.

A principal goal is to assess visual acuity without intimidating the child. Allow the child to read from right to left in order to avoid confusion of common letters. You are not being asked to teach letter recognition, to diagnose reading problems, or to administer an intelligence test.

During your visual acuity testing and in general observations of a toddler or school-age child, make a note of any unusual head positions, jiggling eye movements (nystagmus), excessive squinting, or closing one eye when both eyes should be opened.

The following charts are most often used to test the visual acuity of toddlers and school-age children:

- Snellen charts

- charts with silhouetted pictures to identify

- tumbling E or E game chart

- letter matching tests

- Teller Acuity Cards

Standard Snellen charts can be used with children who know the alphabet or numbers. Charts with silhouetted pictures to identify are called *Allen charts* (Figure 16.3A). The figures used on the Allen charts are also available on small 4 × 4-inch "Allen cards" for near vision testing or to use when the distance charts are not available.

The tumbling E or E game chart shows the capital letter E turned on its various edges (Figure 16.3B). The child points the hand in the direction that the spokes of the E are pointing for the letter you indicate.)

In letter-matching tests, you point to one of several letters on a chart, and the child selects the matching letter from a handheld card (HOTV-type test). Children do not need to know letters in order to be able to match the shapes in this test. Teller Acuity Cards test infants' and preverbal children's visual acuity by means of gratings (vertical black-and-white stripes).

All of these visual acuity testing charts have advantages and disadvantages. As you become experienced in conducting visual acuity examinations, the ophthalmologist or senior staff assistant who helps with your training can give you specific instructions in using these specialized charts with children and recording the visual acuity measurements.

TIPS FOR TESTING TODDLERS Some toddlers do better with number charts; others seem to prefer letter charts. If a child seems hesitant with one kind, try the other. Do not be surprised if children seem to have difficulty identifying images on an Allen picture chart. Some of the images are so schematic and old-fashioned that many are not readily recognizable today.

The E game can present problems unrelated to visual ability. Preschoolers may not readily understand that a letter or a symbol turned in other directions is a "new" letter; they frequently interpret an E that is upside down and an E on its side as the same. They may be able to point up and down but often cannot twist their hands to demonstrate fingers pointing right or left. In this case, you might try testing using just the up and down E. Correspondingly, a plastic E on a handle can be held by a nonverbal toddler and turned to mimic the orientation of the E on the chart.

TIPS FOR TESTING SCHOOL-AGE CHILDREN When working with children in general, do not assume that at a given age all children are able to recognize and name letters of the alphabet. If embarrassed, they may become very shy and not cooperate at all. It is preferable to ask "Do you know some letters?" rather than "Can you read?" It is not uncommon for children to struggle over the word OFLCT because you have asked them to "read" the chart. Until you tell them to say each letter separately, they may not understand that this is what you really wish them to do. Some children will say they know the letters and, when shown the line, will brightly say "A, B, C, D, E" instead of naming the letters on the chart.

Be sensitive about embarrassing children who stumble when trying to read a chart. Some 2-year-olds know how to read letters but some 8-year-olds do not. When children act timid in the beginning or reach a line that is smaller than they feel confident to try, you can begin to do it together by each saying a letter in turn along the line. This sort of game often gets the child started. When a letter is read incorrectly, skip over it and recheck it later so as not to lose the child's cooperation out of fear of criticism.

Often children stop at the "small" 20/30 line at the bottom of a chart projected on a screen, but if you isolate that line they can read it easily. Also, if you make it the

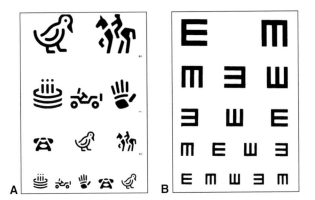

Figure 16.3 Charts for testing the visual acuity of toddlers and children. **A.** Allen chart. **B.** E chart.

top or biggest of several smaller lines, they often do not hesitate in identifying the letters.

Do not be too concerned if the letters are read in a scattered order rather than from right to left. Allow errors if consistently stated; for example, the child may repeatedly call a V an A or a P a B. When examining children in these age groups for visual acuity, do not give up: be creative.

Elderly Patients

It is important not to draw conclusions about patients based on their age alone or their medical condition. However, elderly patients seen in the ophthalmology office often have special age-related health problems and emotional needs, which ophthalmic medical assistants should consider. Elderly patients are often anxious and fearful of losing their independence and financial security. They may be facing limitations of mobility that may cause them not to relate well or be difficult to examine. An elderly person may also be particularly worried about declining health and may notice or complain about subtle changes in vision. Examiners should not overlook or downplay these observations. Make note of the symptoms so that the doctor can follow up.

In elderly patients as well as in others, worry may manifest itself in the form of crossness, unreasonable blaming of others, or anxiety. The ophthalmic medical assistant needs to treat elderly patients with special consideration, keeping in mind the following:

- Healing may be slower.

- Understanding may be slower.

- Apprehension about their condition may be greater than with younger patients. Some elderly patients fear impending blindness, even with relatively minor eye problems. Loss of eyesight is another obstacle to independence.

- Visual acuity is only one aspect of functional vision that may be affected by eye diseases. Color perception and contrast sensitivity are often affected as well.

- Many elderly people live alone, so a small change in objective acuity may cause a big change in functional ability; for example, changing from 20/30 to 20/40 may seem trivial, but it may make the difference between being able to read the newspaper or the label on a medication container easily and with confidence.

- Having to give up shopping alone, driving, or other independent activities because of declining abilities and eyesight can be a very difficult adjustment, and one that requires sensitivity and compassion on the part of health care providers.

Age-Related Vision Changes

Many changes in vision in elderly patients occur as a result of age-related alteration of the ocular tissues. With age, the lens gradually yellows, resulting in some difficulty with color discrimination. It also becomes increasingly rigid, resulting in a significant loss of accommodative ability. Therefore, the patient has difficulty shifting focus from distance to near. Over time the lens becomes opaque (cataractous), creating difficulty in reading clearly at near, intermediate areas, and for long distances with or without corrective lenses.

When ophthalmic medical assistants appreciate and understand the problems that elderly patients face daily, they can become more sensitive and responsive to their needs. This sensitivity and care will help you achieve more accurate and complete results.

Table 16.1 lists common complaints and ophthalmic entities of seniors. Some elderly patients may have one or more chronic illnesses or limitations on their ability to maneuver easily through their daily activities. Their current visual loss may be just the latest event to occur among other medical concerns.

The special needs of elderly patients can be multisystemic.

Table 16.1 Common Visual Complaints of Seniors

Floaters

Watery, dry, or itchy eyes

Difficulty seeing when going down stairs

Decreased vision at night

Decreased contrast sensitivity

Difficulty with glare

Extra time needed to adjust when entering a darkened room

More light needed to read, yet have problems with glare

Diminished color discrimination, especially blues and greens

Changes in visual ability related to cataract (present to some degree in 95% of people over age 65), glaucoma, or diabetes

Some elderly patients also have loss of hearing, which can compound their sense of isolation. Speak slowly and distinctly to patients who have difficulty in hearing, but do not assume that an elderly patient will have difficulty hearing based on his or her age alone. If you determine that the patient is having trouble hearing you, face your patient squarely and allow the patient to see your lips so he or she can obtain extra clues to what you are saying. It is rarely necessary to raise your voice excessively and never necessary to shout.

Many elderly people who are "partially sighted" do not get around as well as younger individuals who may have their own visual impairment but who may be in better general health, be more optimistic and have a broader support system. However, no one can predict a patient's reaction based on age. A sudden loss of vision for one patient may be far more devastating than a slowly progressive one for another.

Some older persons mistakenly believe they should "preserve" their eyes by not "using them up." Tell them it is not possible to "use up" their eyesight, even if a visual abnormality exists. Encourage them not to sit in the dark, not to give up hobbies, and to continue reading or doing other near work. By participating in living as fully as possible, they will have a better quality of life.

Visual Acuity Testing

As with most adult patients, visual acuity in elderly persons is tested using a standard Snellen chart and procedure (see Chapter 8). When distance acuity is less than 20/200, you usually would have the patient walk toward the chart. As an example, if a patient reads the 200 line at 10 feet, record the vision as 10/200. With elderly patients, however, consider their ability to get in and out of the examining chair; instead, move the chart toward the patient if possible.

Check the near acuity of elderly patients even if distance acuity is poor. The importance of near vision in this age group cannot be overestimated. Reading, needlework, or arts and crafts may be the person's major, if not only, independent activity and source of enjoyment. It is particularly important to adjust the near vision test appropriately to avoid glare, which can be a problem for patients in the initial stages of cataract formation. Glare presents a paradox for the elderly person, who may benefit from additional lighting for reading but at the same time may be bothered by the glare it creates. Maintain the standard distance required for a particular test but allow the patient to adjust the tilt of the near card. The ideal situation is to have the highest contrast with the least amount of glare. Good contrast can often be an easier

and better solution to comfortable reading than high magnification.

When checking both distance and near visual acuity, remember that the elderly patient may require extra time to search for and locate the letters, especially the patient with macular degeneration. Give these patients coaching and extra prompting as needed. Elderly patients may have a slower reaction time than younger patients, so it is important also to give them some additional time to respond.

If an elderly patient is unable to read a distance or near acuity chart at all, proceed with low vision testing as described earlier in this chapter. Elderly patients may also require additional tests of visual abilities, such as contrast-sensitivity and glare testing. (Chapter 10 discusses these and other specialized vision tests.)

Patients Who May Be Suffering from Abuse

Patients who are difficult to examine may be suffering from physical, emotional, or other abuse. Children and the elderly are especially vulnerable because they are more often dependent on others for care. They may be afraid to report any abuse for fear of reprisal, rejection from the abuser, and possibly due to feelings of low self-esteem. Symptoms of abuse can be similar to many of the symptoms discussed in regard to difficult patients throughout this chapter. They may include withdrawal, irritability, anxiety, physical symptoms, and vague complaints.

All 50 states have laws regarding the reporting by medical professionals of suspected child or elder abuse. If you suspect any domestic abuse, immediately discuss your concerns in private with your ophthalmologist.

Patients With Physical Disabilities

Ophthalmic medical assistants may expect to help physically disabled patients in wheelchairs during the course of the office visit (Figure 16.4). Sometimes, moving a patient into and out of a wheelchair can be difficult. This occurs especially with patients who have disabling multiple sclerosis or rheumatoid arthritis or who have experienced a stroke. Some of these patients may need to be belted into the wheelchair for safety. An increasing number of children with cerebral palsy use wheelchairs

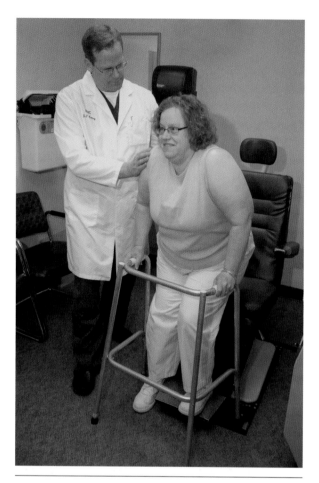

Figure 16.4 Helping a physically disabled individual during an office visit. *(Image courtesy of Brice Critser, CRA, Department of Ophthalmology and Visual Sciences, University of Iowa.)*

equipped with straps that hold them upright. Communication boards allow them to "speak" with others.

Always ask patients in wheelchairs (or their caregiver if the patient is unable to respond) if the patients can be moved from the chair, if they need assistance, or if they can walk to an examination chair. Remember to lock the wheels and to support the chair from behind while the patient is getting in or out or being moved to the examination chair; otherwise, the wheelchair may accidentally roll backward.

If possible, it is advisable to have at least one examination area in the office that can accommodate patients in wheelchairs. Having to move a patient into and out of a wheelchair can cause a patient undue stress or embarrassment. Under certain circumstances, the ophthalmic medical assistant may be asked to accompany a patient in a wheelchair to the restroom. If you have never helped anyone in and out of a wheelchair in a restroom, you should ask for assistance.

Patients With Diabetes

Diabetes mellitus is a chronic disease that inhibits the proper processing of carbohydrate (sugar) in the body. Diabetes can affect many body systems, including the eye (the retina, specifically). The effect of diabetes on the retina is known as *diabetic retinopathy*. Because diabetic retinopathy can lead to visual impairment that requires treatment or may even result in blindness, the ophthalmic medical assistant is likely to encounter patients with diabetes in the ophthalmologist's practice. Patients with diabetes also may have cataracts or glaucoma. Understanding the condition of, and daily problems faced by, patients with diabetes can help the ophthalmic medical assistant appreciate their special needs and thereby provide the appropriate care for these patients.

People with diabetes monitor the level of sugar in their blood, which for some means pricking their finger several times a day to draw blood and using special meters to perform this test (Figure 16.5). Some patients control their blood sugar level by frequent self-administered insulin injections, while others manage to control their blood sugar by a combination of diet, exercise, and stress reduction. The diabetic patient's daily health management can be a source of personal stress.

Diabetes-related eye symptoms, such as double vision, visual fluctuations, or sudden loss of vision, coupled with frequent eye examinations or treatments also create stress. Patients may have high blood pressure, kidney problems, nerve disease, and other conditions related to the diabetes in addition to their visual difficulties. They may be undergoing treatments for these various problems, all of which can add stress and anxiety to their lives.

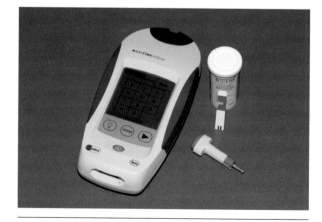

Figure 16.5 Supplies for monitoring the level of glucose in the blood of people with diabetes. *(Image courtesy of Brice Critser, CRA, Department of Ophthalmology and Visual Sciences, University of Iowa.)*

Medical providers need to be sensitive to these issues when performing any examination.

Special Help for Patients With Diabetes

The doctor who treats a patient for diabetes often refers the patient to the ophthalmologist for diagnosis and treatment of related eye conditions. The referring doctor usually forwards the patient's medical history, but the ophthalmologist will also wish to have a baseline ophthalmic and medical history. During this procedure, the ophthalmic medical assistant may expect to record some of the general complaints associated with diabetes. These are listed in Table 16.2.

The medical history should also include a comprehensive list of all medications the patient is taking. This is especially important for patients with systemic disease (such as diabetes), and for those whose disease or medication(s) can affect the health of the eye. It is appropriate and important for the ophthalmic assistant to inform the doctor of any confusion by the patient about medication dosage(s) and frequency. Also confirm that the patient is taking all medications as prescribed.

Patients with confirmed or suspected diabetes may have to undergo lengthy ophthalmologic office procedures, such as fluorescein angiography, ultrasonography, electrophysiologic testing, ophthalmic photography, and laser surgery. Many of these procedures, especially laser surgery, can cause discomfort or pain. Ophthalmic medical assistants often are called upon to inform the patient about what will happen before, during, and after the procedure or test. Therefore, they should understand their office policy and their role in assisting patients who are scheduled for any of these procedures.

TREATMENT OF A HYPOGLYCEMIC REACTION Ophthalmic medical assistants should be alert to the possibility of a diabetic patient having a hypoglycemic reaction while in the office. **Hypoglycemia** results from low blood sugar levels, which can be affected by the amount of food consumed that day, degree of exercise and exertion, medications, or stress. Patients having a hypoglycemic reaction may become weak, sweaty, shaky, or dizzy at first. This initial phase may be followed by numbness of the lips, changes in vision or mood, disorientation, or irritability. Finally, the patient may suffer a seizure or go into a coma.

Ophthalmic medical assistants should be familiar with the office policy for treating a hypoglycemic reaction of a patient in the office. Ask the ophthalmologist or senior staff member to clearly define your role in assisting these patients. Which should you do first: notify the doctor or apply first aid measures? Many patients are prepared to care for themselves if a sudden hypoglycemic episode occurs. Even so, many ophthalmology offices store a quick-acting sugar—such as fruit juice, sugar cubes, or candy—to give the patient immediately or on the patient's request. Then the ophthalmic assistant would notify the doctor of the patient's state.

When scheduling an appointment for a patient with diabetes (especially a patient dependent on insulin), try to choose a time that does not interfere with mealtimes, because many patients must eat at very specific times to ensure an acceptable blood sugar level. If an unexpected test or wait becomes necessary during the office visit, keep in mind that the waiting patient may need a snack or glass of juice.

Table 16.2 General Complaints Associated With Diabetes

Increased hunger or thirst

Increased urination

Sudden weight loss

Fatigue

Blurred eyesight

Numbness or tingling of the hands or feet

Frequent infections

Slow healing of cuts and sores

Impotence

SELF-ASSESSMENT TEST

1. The doctor is with a patient who requires unexpected additional examination time. You have apologized to the waiting patients and explained that the doctor will be delayed another 15 minutes, but Mrs. Wright now tells you she is concerned about getting home later than she had planned. Which of the following would be the best action for you to take? (Check all that apply.)

    a. Explain the nature of the test the doctor is conducting on the patient presently being seen so that Mrs. Wright can appreciate its importance.

    b. Suggest that Mrs. Wright take a walk and return in 15 minutes.

    c. Ask Mrs. Wright to step into a private part of the office with you and explain that you understand how important her time is to her.

    d. Offer to reschedule Mrs. Wright's appointment or allow her to telephone home to say she will be delayed.

    e. Tell Mrs. Wright that an emergency has occurred but that she should have to wait only a few more minutes.

2. List 4 areas of common deficits of visual impairment.

3. Describe how you might handle being called away while guiding a visually impaired patient to a room.

4. Write the visual acuity recording for patients who require the Snellen chart to be 8 feet away before they can see the 200 optotype.

5. Name the 3 principal procedures for determining visual acuity in an older child or adult patients who cannot read the Snellen chart at 3 feet.

6. A papoose board is principally used for which of the following tasks?

    a. Carry an infant from the waiting room to the examination room.

    b. Allow an adult to hold an infant in the lap.

    c. Immobilize an infant during an ophthalmologic examination.

    d. Give an infant a sense of security during an ophthalmologic examination.

    e. Calm a crying infant.

7. Visual acuity in elderly patients is first tested using which of the following?

    a. an Allen chart

    b. the finger-counting procedure

    c. a standard Snellen chart

    d. a near vision card

    e. a letter-matching test

8. In a patient with diabetes, a low blood sugar level can cause a reaction known as _____.

SUGGESTED ACTIVITIES

1. With an ophthalmologist or senior staff member in your office, review the office protocol for assisting patients with the special concerns discussed in this chapter. If your office deals with patients who have special concerns other than those mentioned in this chapter, ask for practical tips to help you give these patients any needed special assistance as well.

2. Determine your office's protocol for summoning assistance when you find yourself in a situation with a patient that you cannot or do not know how to handle.

3. Ask an experienced assistant on your office staff to role-play the part of an irate, visually impaired, elderly, or other type of patient so you can practice performing appropriately. Have the experienced assistant critique your verbal and physical behavior in a discussion afterward.

4. To understand the kind of guidance a visually impaired patient might need, ask another assistant to guide you from the office waiting room to an examining room with your eyes shut or blindfolded. Then switch roles and guide your colleague. Afterward, discuss the exercise with the other assistant and with senior staff members.

5. Ask permission to observe specialized visual acuity testing procedures when they are performed with children, patients who are visually impaired, and elderly patients. Take notes and ask questions in a meeting with the ophthalmologist or other examiner later.

6. If your ophthalmology office treats many children, you may wish to watch television programs such as "Sesame Street" to gain pointers on how to work with youngsters 2 to 6 years old. Stopping by a local store to learn what toys are popular with children of specific ages may help you relate to the young patient.

7. If the ophthalmology practice you work for has a large proportion of elderly patients, consider attending an orientation program at a local senior center to gain an understanding of some aspects of their lives.

SUGGESTED RESOURCES

Centers for Medicare and Medicaid Services. HIPAA general information. http://www.cms.gov/HIPAAGenInfo/. Accessed August 15, 2011.

Cheng H, Moorman C, Buckley S, et al. *Emergency Ophthalmology: A Symptom Based Guide to Diagnosis and Early Management*. London: BMJ Publishing Group: 1997.

DuBois LG. Assisting patients, patient services, pediatric exam. In: *Fundamentals of Ophthalmic Medical Assisting*. DVD. San Francisco: American Academy of Ophthalmology; 2009.

DuBois LG. *Basic Procedures*. Thorofare, NJ: Slack; 1998.

Freeman PB, Jose RT. *The Art and Practice of Low Vision*. 2nd ed. Boston: Butterworth-Heinemann; 1997.

Low Vision. Brochure. San Francisco: American Academy of Ophthalmology; 2011.

Movaghar M, Lawrence MG. Eye exam: the essentials. In: *The Eye Exam and Basic Ophthalmic Instruments*. DVD. San Francisco: American Academy of Ophthalmology; 2001. Reviewed for currency: 2007.

Stein HA, Stein RM. *The Ophthalmic Assistant: A Text for Allied and Associated Ophthalmic Personnel*. 8th ed. St Louis: Mosby; 2006.

Wright KW, Spiegel PH. *Requisites in Ophthalmology: Pediatric Ophthalmology and Strabismus*. St Louis: CV Mosby; 1999.

17 MINOR SURGICAL ASSISTING IN THE OFFICE

Ophthalmologists do not perform surgery exclusively in an operating room. The ophthalmologist can treat many minor ocular health problems that require some type of surgical procedure in the office. Such procedures are known as *minor surgery*, *office surgery*, or *office procedures*. Ophthalmic medical assistants serve as invaluable team members in the care of patients undergoing minor surgery. They can help to answer patients' questions, provide printed informational materials, and prepare patients for surgery. In addition, the ophthalmic medical assistant may sterilize and prepare surgical instruments and materials for surgery, assist the doctor during the procedure, attend to cleanup after the operation, and instruct the patient in postoperative care.

This chapter presents information about patient preparation, surgical materials and instruments, and practical skills that make the ophthalmic medical assistant an important aide to the ophthalmologist before, during, and after minor surgery. It discusses the different types, principles, and requirements of several common minor surgical procedures.

Patient Preparation Before Surgery

Before performing any surgical procedure, the surgeon must prepare patients, not only physically, but also intellectually and emotionally. The ophthalmic medical assistant plays a vital role in patient preparation.

Informed Consent

Before any patient has a surgical procedure, the surgeon discusses the operation, its risks and benefits, and any possible alternative treatments with the patient. This is necessary for the patient to make an informed decision as to whether or not to have the operation. This process, known as obtaining **informed consent**, protects the surgeon and the patient. It ensures that everyone involved understands the purpose and risks of the planned surgery, and that everyone agrees that it should take place.

255

The process of informed consent usually starts during the office visit when the physician makes a diagnosis, begins to inform the patient about the condition, and discusses the information about the proposed procedure. As the final part of the informed consent process, the ophthalmologist judges whether the patient understands all the pertinent information and records the discussion of informed consent on the patient's chart. The surgeon may also obtain the patient's signature on a written operative permit, which documents the informed consent for the patient record, or he or she may delegate this responsibility to another individual in the office. It is important to understand that informed consent is a process and not simply the patient's signature on a written document. Ophthalmic medical assistants should become familiar with the routine of their ophthalmologist's practice for obtaining and documenting informed consent.

Preoperative Assessment

Even with minor procedures, a brief assessment of the patient's current and past physical health is necessary. In most cases, the doctor, nurse, or assistant will simply ask patients about allergies, current medications, significant health history, and current health status. Depending on the procedure and office policy, the surgeon may also require a preoperative blood pressure and pulse. It is important to determine whether female patients are pregnant or nursing an infant, because some medications used during a surgical procedure may affect the fetus or a nursing baby.

Patient Assistance

Because ophthalmic medical assistants are often the first to greet patients and prepare them for their surgical office visit, they have the opportunity to put patients at ease and make their visit as comfortable as possible. A reassuring, calm, and professional manner helps reduce patient anxiety. Informing patients about what to expect throughout the visit by describing the preparatory steps as you perform them also decreases their anxiety and increases their cooperation. Ophthalmic medical assistants should avoid detailed comments about the nature or extent of the patient's condition or the procedure being performed, because such comments can make a patient anxious or apprehensive. It may reassure patients to tell them the doctor is experienced in treating conditions like theirs.

Patient preparation for most minor surgical procedures is similar. Escort patients to the office surgery room and ask them if they need assistance to lie down on the operating table or to sit in the examining chair. Whether patients will lie down or sit in a reclining examining chair will depend on the procedure, office policy, and surgeon preference. Assure that patients are in a comfortable and appropriate position for the surgeon to perform the procedure (Figure 17.1). Depending on the procedure and office policy, you may need to help patients remove or loosen clothing.

HANDLING PATIENT QUESTIONS   When ophthalmic medical assistants are preparing patients for their surgery, patients may ask questions about the operation. You may answer questions regarding how patients will feel during and after the procedure if you are confident of the appropriate answers. Refer patients' questions about the actual surgical procedure or its outcome to the doctor. Bring up these questions when the surgeon enters the room so patients get satisfactory answers before surgery begins.

Administration of Anesthetics

Most minor surgical procedures require an anesthetic (numbing medicine). The most common methods of anesthetizing the surgical area in the office setting are to place topical medications on the ocular surface or to inject an anesthetic agent into the appropriate area. Ophthalmic medical assistants may instill topical anesthetic agents, but a physician or nurse must perform any necessary injections.

Common topical anesthetic agents include proparacaine, tetracaine, and lidocaine, usually administered as eyedrops. Lidocaine is also available as a topical gel. These agents anesthetize the ocular surface and some

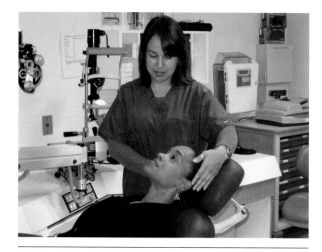

Figure 17.1   Helping position the patient in the operating chair. *(Image courtesy of Mitchell J. Goff, MD.)*

adnexal structures prior to surgery. They are also useful before the surgical prep to alleviate stinging or burning from the antiseptic solution. The surgeon may want a topical agent applied with a soaked **pledget**—a small tuft of cotton, or a cotton-tipped applicator soaked in anesthetic solution. This allows the anesthetic agent to stay in contact with the surgical area for a longer period (Figure 17.2).

The most commonly used injectable anesthetic is lidocaine. It is available in several different strengths and either with or without added epinephrine. The addition of epinephrine helps to prolong the anesthetic effect and reduce bleeding by constricting blood vessels. The initial needle stick can be painful and the medication usually burns as it infiltrates into the tissue. Advise patients of these possible reactions so they will expect the sensations and not react abruptly. The ophthalmic medical assistant can help the surgeon by steadying the patient's head, holding the patient's hand, and asking the patient to gaze in the direction indicated by the doctor. Even though an allergic or sensitivity reaction to injected or topical anesthetics is rare, they do occur. For this reason, do not leave the patient alone for more than a few moments at a time after the patient has any medication administered. Chapter 15 describes appropriate actions to take in case of a drug reaction.

Surgical Materials and Instruments

The ophthalmic surgeon uses a variety of specialized instruments and materials for minor surgery. Commonly

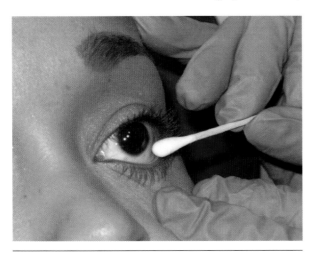

Figure 17.2 Applying an anesthetic-soaked pledget. *(Image courtesy of Mitchell J. Goff, MD.)*

used materials and instruments include sutures and suture needles, forceps, scissors, needle holders, clamps and curettes, blade handles and blades (scalpels), lacrimal instruments, cannulas, and syringes and needles. Every surgeon has individual preferences for supplies and equipment. In addition, surgeons will vary in how they accomplish the specific steps of each surgical procedure. Because the exact procedure and the supplies and equipment needed for each procedure will vary from surgeon to surgeon, it is important to become familiar with the preferences of the ophthalmologist with whom you work.

Ophthalmic medical assistants perform a valuable service by preparing materials and instruments for use and caring for them before and after surgical procedures. In many cases, ophthalmic medical assistants may help during surgery by passing materials and instruments to the doctor as requested. Ophthalmic medical assistants should learn the names and appearances of common instruments and materials used in minor surgery.

Sutures and Suture Needles

Sutures are the thread-like material used to close surgical wounds. They differ in the type of needle attached, the kind of material from which they are made, and in the diameter of the suture (Figure 17.3). Sutures may be either *absorbable*, or *nonabsorbable*.

The body degrades *absorbable sutures* over time so they do not need to be removed. Examples of absorbable natural suture materials include surgical gut and collagen. An example of an absorbable synthetic suture material is polyglactin 910 (brand name: Vicryl).

The body does not degrade *nonabsorbable sutures*. They remain in place until removed. Sometimes this type of suture is intended to be left in place permanently. Nonabsorbable sutures are made of silk, nylon, polypropylene, or polyester fibers, such as Dacron and Mersilene.

Sutures labeled with higher numbers denote smaller diameters. Conversely, those with lower numbers are larger in diameter. For example, a 6-0 (pronounced "six-oh") suture is larger than a 10-0 suture. In general, the largest diameter of suture used in ophthalmic surgery is 4-0 silk. Surgeons often use finer sutures such as a 10-0 nylon to close the eye in intraocular surgery. Eyelid procedures usually require 5-0 to 8-0 sutures.

Suture needles also vary in their characteristics. These characteristics include the curvature and the point of the needles. Needle curvature is measured in degrees of extent: one-quarter of a circle equals 90°E, one-half of a circle equals 180°E, and five-eighths of a circle equals

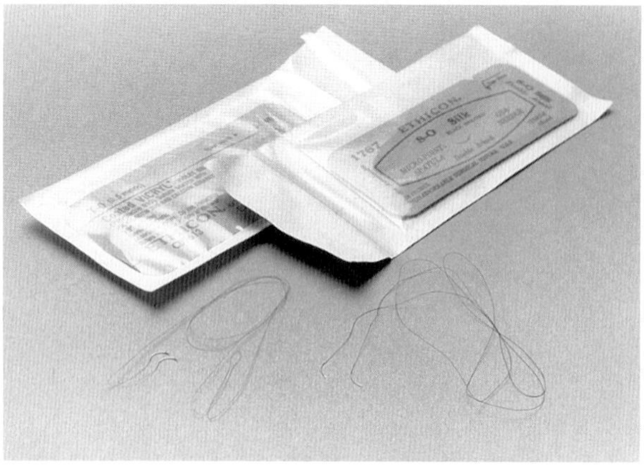

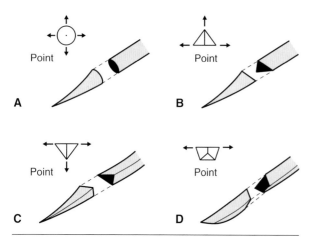

Figure 17.3 Packaged suture materials and unwrapped suture.

225°E. Needle points are available in 4 basic shapes (Figure 17.4):

- Taper point: a cone-shaped single point on a round shaft; it is used for delicate tissues.

- Cutting: a triangular point with 2 side-cutting edges and an upper-cutting edge; the reverse-cutting needle is most commonly used.

- Reverse cutting: a triangular point with 2 side-cutting edges and a lower-cutting edge; it is used for resistant tissue.

- Spatula: a rhomboid-shaped point with 2 side-cutting edges; it is used in the cornea and the sclera where the plane of penetration must be precise.

Suture needles also come in different diameters, usually to match the diameter of the suture material to which they are attached.

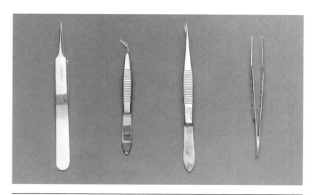

Figure 17.4 Four basic shapes of needle points used in ocular surgery. **A.** Taper point. **B.** Cutting. **C.** Reverse cutting. **D.** Spatula.

Forceps

In general shape and manner of operation, forceps resemble tweezers with very delicate and fine points (Figure 17.5). Forceps are useful for grasping or moving body tissues, sutures, or other materials. Each has a handle and a set of jaws. The inner surface of the jaws may be rounded, flat, serrated, or toothed. The instrument itself may be curved, angled, or straight and may contain a locking device on its handle.

The basic categories of forceps—toothed tissue forceps and nontoothed tying forceps—reflect the different purpose of each. Tissue forceps usually have teeth or serrations that grasp ocular tissues to allow suturing, fixation, or dissection. Tying forceps aid the surgeon in tying sutures and usually have a broad, flat, nontoothed tip to permit grasping suture materials without damaging it. Nontoothed forceps are available for other surgical uses as well.

Scissors

A variety of scissors are available for ocular surgery (Figure 17.6). The type of scissors used during an operation depends on what type of tissue the scissors must cut. Scissors may have blunt or sharp points, may be curved

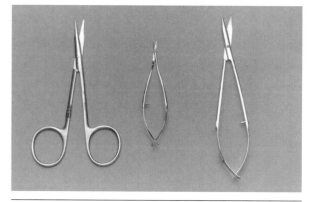

Figure 17.5 Forceps.

Figure 17.6 Ophthalmic surgical scissors.

or straight, and may feature either spring action or direct action.

Needle Holders

Needle holders hold the suture needle, providing more control during suturing (Figure 17.7). In appearance, needle holders resemble a combination of tweezers and scissors. These instruments may be nonlocking or have a locking device. The handle may or may not be spring-loaded, and the tips may be curved or straight, wide or narrow, serrated or nonserrated, or any combination of these features. Some are held like a pencil; others have finger loops like ordinary scissors.

Clamps and Curettes

Clamps (Figure 17.8 left) are used in ophthalmic surgery to hold or fasten onto an area of tissue, either to provide exposure for the procedure or to aid in **hemostasis** (control of bleeding). **Curettes** (Figure 17.8 right) consist of a slim handle with a small bowl-shaped end, which may have either smooth or serrated edges. The surgeon uses curettes in scooping actions (curettage) to remove unwanted tissue.

Blade Handles and Blades (Scalpels)

Minor office surgeries may require a variety of blades (scalpels). The blades are usually disposable and attach to reusable blade handles (Figure 17.9). The specific type of scalpel needed depends on the procedure and the surgeon's preference.

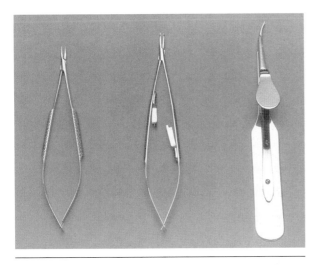

Figure 17.7 Needle holders.

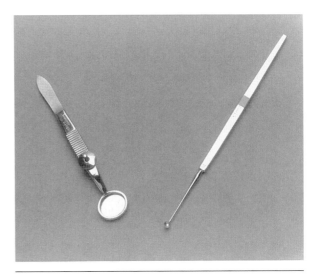

Figure 17.8 Chalazion clamp (left) and curette.

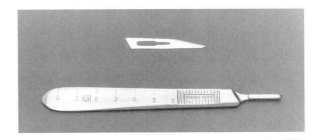

Figure 17.9 Blade and handle.

Lacrimal Instruments

Clearing tear duct obstructions requires special instruments. Sometimes called a **lacrimal set** (Figure 17.10), this group of instruments includes:

- a **punctum dilator** to enlarge the punctum
- a sterile *medicine glass* to hold sterile saline solution or an antibiotic solution, or a *vial* of sterile saline solution from which to draw up irrigating solution using a syringe and needle
- a **syringe** and a **blunt lacrimal cannula** to introduce solution into the duct
- several sizes of **lacrimal probes** to clear the duct

Cannulas

A **cannula** is a hollow, needle-like instrument with a blunt tip used during ophthalmic surgery to inject or extract fluid or air (Figure 17.11).

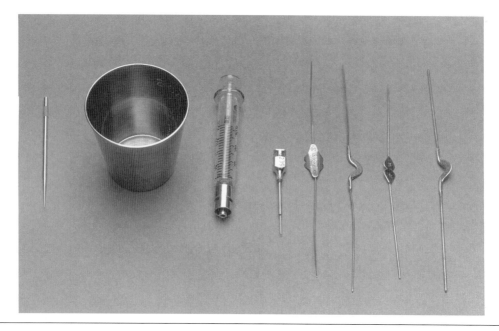

Figure 17.10 Lacrimal set. Left to right: punctum dilator. Holder for sterile saline solution or an antibiotic solution. Syringe. Lacrimal needle. Set of lacrimal probes.

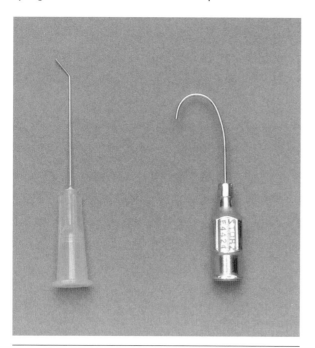

Figure 17.11 Cannulas.

Syringes and Needles

Syringes are used to administer medicines, lubricants, dyes, and gases to the eye during minor surgery. Syringes come in many sizes denoted by the volume they can hold, expressed in milliliters (ml) or cc's. Common sizes used in ophthalmic minor surgery are 5 ml, 3 ml, and 1 ml (also commonly referred to as a TB or tuberculin syringe). Hypodermic needles attach to syringes and come in a variety of sizes or gauges. Similar to suture

material, the larger the gauge number the smaller the diameter of the needle. For example, a 30-gauge needle has a much smaller diameter than an 18-gauge needle. Needles also come in various lengths, usually expressed in inches.

Generally, hypodermic needles used to inject into the eye are short and have a small diameter (large gauge). One of the most common office procedures performed is an intravitreal injection, using a 1 ml syringe and either a 5/8-inch, 30-gauge or a 27-gauge needle (Figure 17.12).

Other Surgical Supplies

All surgeries require at least some appropriate protective attire such as masks, eye protection, head covers, and/or

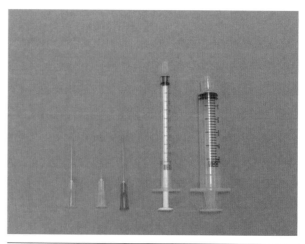

Figure 17.12 Needles and syringes. *(Image courtesy of Mitchell J. Goff, MD.)*

sterile gloves and gowns. These items protect the patient by limiting the risk of infection. In addition, they protect the surgeon and assistant by providing a barrier to avoid exposure to the patient's body fluids. The surgeon or surgical supervisor will determine what protective attire is necessary based on considerations of the principles of universal precautions (see Chapter 7) and aseptic technique (discussed later in this chapter). Ophthalmic medical assistants should be fully knowledgeable about these principles for their own safety as well as for the patient's safety.

In addition to protective attire and the instruments and sutures already discussed, you should become familiar with the appearance and purpose of other supplies commonly used in office surgery (Table 17.1).

Common Minor Surgical Procedures

The range of procedures the ophthalmic surgeon may perform in the office setting is broad and ranges from very minor procedures such as removing small skin lesions to more extensive procedures such as suturing complex eyelid lacerations. In general, the decision whether to do a procedure in the office setting is made by assessing whether the necessary space, equipment, and supplies are available as well as whether personnel have the necessary expertise to assist the surgeon. This chapter covers those procedures most commonly performed in the office setting.

General Considerations

The ophthalmic medical assistant should become familiar with some general responsibilities and concepts applicable to all minor surgeries:

Table 17.1 Supplies Commonly Used in Office Surgery

Surgical scrub brushes containing germicidal solutions

Sterile gauze sponges (various sizes)

Sterile cotton-tipped applicators or cellulose sponges

Cautery devices (various types)

Medications (anesthetic agents, other medications for injection, and eyedrops or ointments)

Germicidal solutions (povidone-iodine or hexachlorophene) for surgical preparation

Dressings, eye patches, shields, and tape

Sterile drapes

- Ensure that surgical areas are clean and uncluttered. Disinfect all surfaces with a germicidal solution to minimize possible sources of contamination.

- Inspect all surgical instruments to ensure they are sterile and in good repair.

- Carefully check any medication needed to make sure it is the right medication in the correct strength and is not expired. Adverse reactions may occur if the patient receives the wrong anesthetic agent or other medication.

- Be sure all supplies and equipment are available and in working order before the procedure begins. It is very inefficient and stressful to be searching for needed equipment or supplies after the surgeon begins the procedure.

Table 17.2 lists the purpose for some of the most common office surgical procedures. Although some of these procedures may not seem like "surgery," they all include some form of tissue invasion or manipulation (for example, *epilation*, or *foreign body removal*). Table 17.2 also lists the type of anesthetic, preparations, the necessary supplies and equipment, and the basic steps for each procedure. Finally, the table includes some common postoperative considerations for each type of surgery.

Postsurgical Medications, Dressings, and Patches

Following some procedures, the surgeon may want certain drops or ointments applied to the operated eye or surgical site. In addition, many procedures require some type of dressing over the surgical area or a patch over the eye. In certain cases, the surgeon may request a pressure patch, which is an eye patch that will provide enough pressure on the eye to prevent lid movement or to limit bleeding. Circumstances may additionally require a protective eye shield. The specific procedure and surgeon preference determine which types of medications, dressings, or patches may be required. In some situations, the patient may not need any ocular dressing. Procedure 17.1 describes the steps in applying a pressure patch and shield.

First Surgical Experience

It is not unusual for ophthalmic medical assistants to feel faint when observing surgery the first few times. If you feel faint, excuse yourself, sit down, and place your head

Table 17.2 Common Office Surgical Procedures

Procedure and Purpose	Anesthesia	Prep	Supplies and Equipment	Procedural Steps	Postoperative Considerations
Epilation To remove abnormally directed eyelashes that rub against the ocular surface	Topical for manual epilation Local injection for cryosurgery, electrosurgery, or laser surgery	Povidone-iodine prep of involved lid	Anesthetic for topical application and/or local injection Syringe and needle Povidone-iodine prep solution Slit lamp or loupes for magnification Nitrous oxide cryotherapy unit or electrolysis unit or laser instruments Smooth forceps	1. Cryosurgery, electrolysis, or laser a. Topical anesthesia applied b. Involved eyelid area prepped with povidone-iodine c. Local anesthetic injected d. Freeze cycles applied, laser or electrolysis to individual misdirected eyelashes e. Lash(es) removed with forceps 2. Manual epilation a. Topical anesthesia applied b. Area of involved eyelid prepped with povidone-iodine c. Lash(es) removed with forceps	Topical antibiotic drops or ointment Usually no dressing required
Anterior chamber tap To obtain sample of aqueous humor for culture To quantify drug penetration in clinical studies To relieve acute elevated intraocular pressure (rare)	Topical Systemic sedation if necessary to assure patient cooperation	Topical 5% povidone-iodine or antibiotic drops	5% povidone-iodine solution or antibiotic drops Topical anesthetic Systemic sedation if indicated Tuberculin syringe and small-gauge needle Toothed forceps Culture media or collection container Slit lamp or loupes for magnification	1. Systemic sedation administered, if indicated 2. Topical anesthesia applied 3. Topical povidone-iodine or antibiotic solution applied to ocular surface (if povidone-iodine used, ocular surface rinsed with sterile saline solution before tap) 4. Area draped as needed 5. Needle inserted through limbus into anterior chamber 6. Aqueous withdrawn 7. Specimen placed in appropriate container for culture or other assessment	Topical antibiotic Usually no dressing required
Foreign body removal To remove a foreign body (FB) from the cornea or conjunctiva	Topical Systemic sedation if necessary to assure patient cooperation	Usually none	Topical anesthetic Systemic sedation if indicated Sterile gauze pad (for wiping spatula or burr, as needed) Corneal burr and/or spatula Slit lamp or loupes	1. Systemic sedation administered, if indicated 2. Topical anesthesia applied 3. FB removed with spatula; rust ring removed with corneal burr or manually removed with spatula	Topical antibiotic solution or ointment Systemic and/or topical medications to control post-procedure pain Patch applied if requested by physician (patching after FB removal is not done universally)

(continued)

Table 17.2 (continued)

Procedure and Purpose	Anesthesia	Prep	Supplies and Equipment	Procedural Steps	Postoperative Considerations
Corneal debridement To remove corneal epithelium in patients with recurring corneal erosion	Topical Systemic sedation if necessary to assure patient cooperation	Usually none	Topical anesthetic Systemic sedation if indicated Sterile gauze pad (for wiping spatula, as needed) Corneal spatula Slit lamp or loupes for magnification	1. Systemic sedation administered, if indicated 2. Topical anesthesia applied 3. Corneal epithelium removed with spatula	Topical antibiotic solution or ointment Patch applied Systemic and/or topical medications to control post-procedure pain Requires periodic follow up during re-epithelialization process
Nasal lacrimal duct (NLD) probing and irrigation[a] To open obstructed NLD	Topical	Usually none	Topical anesthetic Sterile normal saline Fluorescein dye Syringe and needle Sterile gauze pad Appropriate restraining device for infants Suction device and catheter Punctum dilator or large safety pin NLD probes in various sizes NLD cannula May use loupes for better visualization	1. Adequate restraint absolutely imperative for infants 2. Topical anesthetic applied 3. Punctum dilated with dilator 4. Appropriately-sized probe inserted through punctum into NLD to relieve obstruction 5. Normal saline irrigated through punctum with NLD cannula (with or without fluorescein) 6. Post-procedure patency assessed a. Ask adult patients if salt taste perceived (or to blow nose gently to assess for presence of fluorescein) b. Suction nasal passageways of infants to assess for presence of fluorescein	Topical antibiotic or antibiotic/steroid solution or ointment Usually no dressing required
Insertion of punctal plugs[b] To occlude 2 or more puncta in patients with symptomatic dry eye	Topical	Usually none	Topical anesthetic Collagen plugs and forceps, or silicone plugs in preloaded applicator Gauge to measure puncta Slit lamp or loupes	1. Topical anesthesia applied 2. Puncta measured to determine appropriate plug size 3. Plug(s) inserted a. Collagen plugs into all 4 puncta, upper and lower, using forceps b. Silicone plugs into 2 lower puncta only or into all 4 puncta using preloaded inserter	Artificial tears Follow up in 1 to 2 weeks

[a] With infants, the ophthalmologist may prefer to do this procedure in a surgery center, but almost all adult patients have the procedure in the office setting.

[b] The ophthalmologist will usually insert dissolvable collagen plugs as a trial to see if occlusion relieves the patient's symptoms; if temporary occlusion is successful in relieving symptoms, the surgeon will then insert silicone plugs that do not dissolve.

(continued)

Table 17.2 (continued)

Procedure and Purpose	Anesthesia	Prep	Supplies and Equipment	Procedural Steps	Postoperative Considerations
Excision of chalazion To remove a chalazion from the eyelid	Topical and local injection	Topical 5% povidone-iodine	Topical anesthetic Local anesthetic Povidone-iodine 5% solution Syringe and needle Sterile gauze pad Disposable blade Blade handle Chalazion clamp Chalazion curette Toothed forceps Cautery device	1. Topical anesthesia applied 2. Topical 5% povidone-iodine applied 3. Local anesthesia injected 4. Chalazion clamp applied and tightened to provide exposure and prevent excessive bleeding 5. Lid everted 6. Incision into tarsal conjunctiva over lesion 7. Inflammatory material, sac removed with curette 8. Clamp slowly released; surgical area cauterized as needed for bleeding	Topical antibiotic or antibiotic/steroid drops or ointment Patch may be applied
Excision of conjunctival or skin lesions To remove neoplasms (new growths) from the skin on or around the eyelids or from the conjunctiva	Conjunctival: topical and/or local injection Skin: local injection	Conjunctival: 5% povidone-iodine solution Skin: 10% povidone-iodine solution	Topical and/or local anesthetic Conjunctival: 5% povidone-iodine solution Skin: 10% povidone-iodine solution Syringe and needle Sterile gauze pad Disposable blade Blade handle Scissors Suture Specimen container with formaldehyde Slit lamp or loupes for magnification Toothed forceps Needle holder Cautery device	1. Topical anesthesia applied and/or local anesthesia injected 2. Conjunctival: 5% povidone-iodine applied 3. Skin: 10% povidone-iodine prep of involved area 4. Area draped as needed 5. Lesion excised with blade and/or scissors 6. Surgical area cauterized as needed 7. Incision sutured if necessary	Topical antibiotic drops or ointment Dressing or patch as needed Follow up in 1 week for suture removal if necessary
Suture removal To remove suture(s) from the eye or skin	Topical for corneal or conjunctival sutures None needed for skin sutures	Sutures in the eye: topical 5% povidone-iodine (rinse ocular surface before suture removed) Sutures in the skin: 10% povidone-iodine	Topical anesthetic for sutures in the eye Topical antibiotic drops Sutures in the eye: 5% povidone-iodine solution Sutures in the skin: 10% povidone-iodine solution Sterile gauze pad Smooth forceps or needle holder Pointed scissors, blade, or needle	1. Topical anesthesia applied for sutures in the eye 2. Sutures in the eye: 5% povidone-iodine applied 3. Sutures in the skin: 10% povidone-iodine prep of suture area 4. Suture secured with forceps or needle holder 5. Suture cut with scissors or blade, gently pulled free with forceps or needle holder	Sutures in the eye: topical antibiotic drops or ointment Sutures in the skin: topical antibiotic ointment Usually no dressing or patch (Some surgeons use topical antibiotics after suture removal.)

(continued)

Table 17.2 (continued)

Procedure and Purpose	Anesthesia	Prep	Supplies and Equipment	Procedural Steps	Postoperative Considerations
Intravitreal injection To place needed medication into the vitreous	Topical	Antibiotic drops Topical 5% povidone-iodine	Topical anesthetic Antibiotic drops Topical 5% povidone-iodine TB syringe and small-gauge needle Eyelid speculum Intraocular medication Microscopic loupes Sterile cotton tip applicators	1. Topical anesthetic applied 2. Lids, lashes, and eye prepped with povidone-iodine 3. Speculum inserted, topical antibiotic applied 4. Injection made at pars plana using needle on syringe with medication 5. Speculum removed	Intraocular pressure monitored Monitoring for endophthalmitis Topical antibiotic
Retinal lasers To seal retinal breaks To treat swelling in the retina	Topical Retrobulbar injection (occasionally) Systemic sedation if necessary to ensure patient cooperation	Usually none	Anesthesia for topical application or retrobulbar injection Syringe and needle if necessary Systemic sedation if indicated Viewing lenses Lubrication/coupling agent for lenses Laser (usually a slit lamp laser or indirect laser worn on surgeon's head) Sclera depressor Eye pads and tape if necessary	1. Topical anesthesia applied 2. Retrobulbar injection of anesthesia if necessary 3. Systemic sedation if indicated 4. Lens placed with lubricant/coupling agent on eye 5. Lasering of retina performed by surgeon 6. Patch applied if necessary	Patch applied if necessary (usually done if retrobulbar anesthesia used)
Iridotomy To lower intraocular pressure by creating a hole in the iris that allows aqueous fluid to drain out of the eye when the normal route of drainage is blocked during angle-closure glaucoma To prevent angle-closure glaucoma in eyes at risk (those with narrow angles)	Topical	Usually none	Anesthetic for topical application Medications to constrict pupil Viewing lenses Lubricant/coupling agent for lenses Laser (slit-lamp mounted, usually a YAG or argon or both) Medications to lower intraocular pressure	1. Topical anesthesia applied 2. Drops to constrict pupil applied 3. Drops to lower intraocular pressure applied 4. Lens placed with lubricant/coupling agent on eye 5. Lasering of iris performed by surgeon 6. Additional drops to lower intraocular pressure applied	Patient monitored for 30 to 60 minutes to re-evaluate intraocular pressure Often postoperative steroid drops are used
Argon laser trabeculoplasty and selective laser trabeculoplasty To lower intraocular pressure by creating small burns in the trabecular meshwork that stretch the drainage holes in the meshwork, allowing aqueous fluid to drain more easily	Topical	Usually none	Anesthetic for topical application Eyedrops to lower intraocular pressure Viewing lenses Lubrication/coupling agent for lenses Laser	1. Topical anesthesia applied 2. Medication to lower intraocular pressure applied 3. Lens placed with lubricating/coupling agent on eye 4. Lasering of trabecular meshwork 5. Additional drops to lower intraocular pressure applied	Patient monitored for 30 to 60 minutes to re-evaluate intraocular pressure Often postoperative steroid drops used

265

Procedure 17.1 Applying Pressure Patches and Shields

1. Set out 2 sterile eye pads and adhesive surgical tape. Tear the tape into 5- to 6-inch lengths to facilitate the patching process.

2. Instruct the patient to close both eyes tightly.

3. Clean the forehead, the area around the cheekbone, and toward the ear with an alcohol pad to remove skin oils. This helps the tape stick to the skin.

4. Fold a pad in half, place it over the closed eye, and hold it in place with one hand.

5. Apply an unfolded eye pad over the folded one.

6. Tape the unfolded pad firmly to the forehead and cheekbone (Figure A). To prevent blinking, further bleeding, or swelling, the patch must exert some pressure on the lids. The patient should not be able to open the eyelid beneath the patch. The tape should not extend to the jawbone because jaw movement could loosen the patch, nor should it extend into the hair.

7. If the patient has any contusion or laceration of the globe or its adnexal structures, do not apply a pressure patch. Instead, apply and tape a fenestrated aluminum (Fox) shield over the globe to protect these tissues from further damage until healing occurs or the surgeon performs a definitive repair. Rest the shield on the bony eyebrow and cheekbone (Figure B). Never patch an open globe tightly.

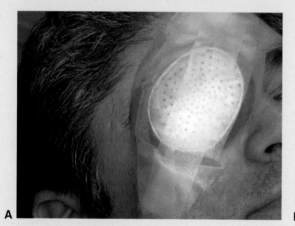
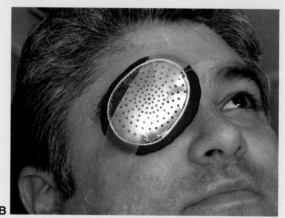

(Images courtesy of Mitchell J. Goff, MD.)

between your knees. It is important to recognize and deal with faintness before you actually collapse, because you could injure yourself and others if you fall.

Some patients may also feel faint during eye surgery. If this happens, ask the patient to stay seated for a few minutes after the procedure until the feeling passes. The ophthalmic medical assistant should be alert to any signs that the patient feels weak or dizzy when asking the patient to sit up after minor surgery. If the patient complains of feeling hot, dizzy, or weak, help the patient lie down again. Do not dismiss any patient until the ophthalmologist thinks the patient is steady enough to leave the office. A drink of water or a snack may help if the patient feels faint. If at any time the patient loses consciousness or falls, do not move the person, and seek immediate emergency help. See Chapter 15 for procedures for helping a patient who feels faint.

Surgical Assisting Skills

When assisting in minor surgery, the ophthalmic medical assistant's main responsibilities are to provide an aseptic (sterile) surgical environment, prepare the instrument tray, assist the doctor during the procedure, and clean and dispose of instruments and materials after surgery.

Aseptic Technique and Minor Surgery

Surgical aseptic technique (also called *sterile technique*) includes all procedures designed to maintain a sterile surgical environment. This limits the risk of infection following the surgery by helping reduce the number of microorganisms that may come into contact with the surgical wound. Although some surgical procedures performed in the office setting require strict observance of aseptic technique, many do not. The ophthalmic assistant should have masks, eye protection, head covers, sterile gowns, gloves, and drapes available to maintain the appropriate level of aseptic technique for each type of procedure as requested by the surgeon.

The main components of aseptic technique applied in the context of minor surgery include the following:

- using sterile instruments and supplies

- preparing the patient's operative site with germicidal (organism-killing) solutions (an activity called *prepping*)

- performing a surgical scrub prior to putting on sterile gloves (some surgeries may also require using head covers, masks, and sterile gowns)

- handling all instruments, solutions, protective drapes, and sterile supplies in such a way that prevents contamination with microorganisms

Aseptic technique is critical during any surgical procedure because it greatly reduces the incidence of postoperative infection. In the formal or hospital operating room, surgeons and other personnel follow strict aseptic technique at all times. In minor surgery performed in the office, the same principles apply but in many cases, strict observance of aseptic technique is not necessary.

The **sterile operating field** (or simply, *sterile field*) is the aseptic area maintained for the sterile instruments and other sterile supplies and equipment. The area designated as the sterile field includes the following:

- tables, trays, and any accessory instruments covered with sterile drapes

- the cleansed (prepped) parts of the patient's body covered with sterile drapes

- portions of the bodies of the surgical personnel (such as the physician, nurse, and ophthalmic assistant) covered with sterile gloves and gowns

Anything lower than the level of the patient's involved body part is not part of the sterile field, even if covered with the sterile drape. Only the front portion of the sterile gown from the chest to the level of the sterile field and the sleeves from 2 inches above the elbow to the tip of the sterile gloves are part of the sterile field.

SURGICAL SCRUB AND PROTECTIVE ATTIRE   When assisting the ophthalmologist during minor surgery and before the procedure begins, ophthalmic medical assistants must scrub their hands and forearms and then put on appropriate protective attire such as sterile gowns and/or gloves. For the majority of office surgery, most surgeons will require their assistants to scrub with warm water and germicidal soap for 3 to 5 minutes, using standard hand-washing technique (described in Chapter 7). Surgical scrubbing usually includes the forearms. Because scrubbing procedures as well as surgeon preference may vary, you should request specific scrubbing instructions from the surgeon or nurse in your office. After scrubbing, put on sterile gloves while maintaining sterility to their outside working surfaces. Your surgeon, nurse, or another trained assistant can show you this simple technique. Put on masks and covers for feet and head, if required, before scrubbing and before gloving. Put on gowns, if required, after scrubbing and before gloving. After gowning and gloving, do not touch anything outside the sterile field. If gloves or gowns become contaminated before surgery begins, remove them and put on new ones. You should practice gowning and gloving with nonsterile supplies while the surgeon or nurse observes and helps you with appropriate techniques.

SURGICAL SITE PREPARATION   For minor office surgery, prepping consists of washing the external area around the operative eye with a sterile cotton ball, swab, or gauze pad soaked with a germicidal solution (such as povidone-iodine or hexachlorophene) while wearing sterile gloves. Prep the area in concentric circles, starting at the center of the surgical site. Never prep back toward the center—always move *outward* from the surgical site in concentric circles. This avoids bringing microorganisms from the outer edges of the prepped area toward the operative site. Repeat this procedure 3 times, using a fresh cotton ball, swab, or gauze pad each time. Although chlorhexidine is acceptable for use as a preoperative hand scrub, it is not recommended for preoperative prepping of the face or head. Take precautions to avoid dropping or splashing any of the prep solution into the patient's eye. If this occurs, rinse the eye well with sterile saline solution to prevent possible irritation. Ophthalmic medical assistants should be aware of the existence of iodine allergy in some patients. Figure 17.13 shows a series of images related to the application of antiseptic agents.

DRAPING   After prepping the surgical area, perform the surgical scrub and put on the appropriate protective attire (caps, masks, gowns, and/or gloves). Then place **sterile drapes** (large, sterilized protective sheets or cloths) around the operative area to provide an aseptic operating field. Draping also provides a sterile area on which the doctor and assistant may rest their hands and instruments during the procedure. It is important to make sure the patient has adequate airflow and is comfortable underneath the sterile drapes.

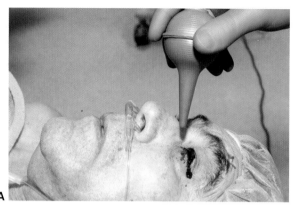

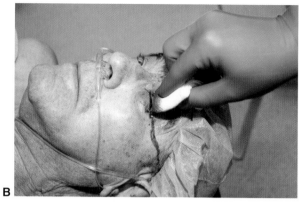

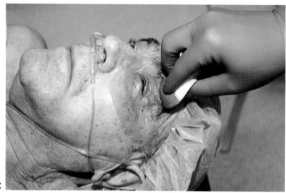

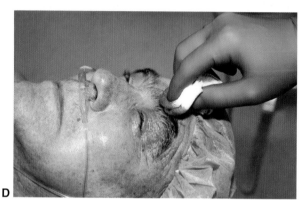

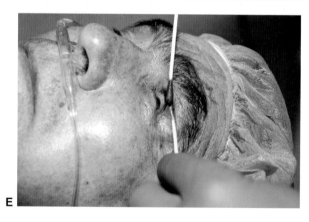

Figure 17.13 Prepping procedure. **A.** For periocular or intraocular surgeries, povidone-iodine 5% solution is placed directly on the conjunctiva. **B–D.** The solution is wiped from central to peripheral in a circular motion. **E.** The lashes are cleaned with a cotton-tipped swab. *(Reprinted, with permission, from Oetting TA,* Basic Principles of Ophthalmic Surgery, *2nd ed, San Francisco: American Academy of Ophthalmology, 2011.)*

Preparing the Instrument Tray

The ophthalmic medical assistant will set up the tray containing the necessary instruments and materials as part of the sterile field. You should prepare the instrument tray after scrubbing and putting on the appropriate protective attire.

Cover the instrument tray with a sterile cloth or paper drape to provide a sterile surface for the sterile instruments and supplies. These drapes are usually impermeable to moisture to prevent contamination from the nonsterile surface below the drape in case any sterile liquids present on the tray soak through the drape. Drapes permeable to moisture are nonsterile if they become wet because microorganisms on the nonsterile surface under

the sterile drape wick through the wet area and contaminate the sterile field. If that occurs, the sterile field must be set up again with fresh drapes and sterile equipment.

You may have commercially prepared surgical packs available with all the needed basic supplies included, or you may be required to prepare packs yourself. Surgical packs have an outer, nonsterile covering and an inner sterile wrapping. Before scrubbing and putting on protective attire, remove the nonsterile packaging and place the pack on the tray or surface you will use for the sterile field. Next, open the inner sterile wrapping, touching only the very edges of the covering to expose the sterile supplies inside. You will need to open any additional instruments or supplies needed and carefully slide them out of the packaging onto the tray to avoid contaminating the sterile field or damaging delicate instrument tips. An experienced assistant or nurse can show you these techniques.

After you have all the needed equipment and supplies on the sterile field, perform a surgical scrub and put on the appropriate protective attire, including sterile gloves so you can handle items on the sterile field. Organize the supplies on the tray, placing the instruments on the sterile tray in the order of use (Figure 17.14). This allows the ophthalmologist and assistant to know where each instrument is for the next step in the procedure.

Count all sharp-pointed instruments (also called *sharps*), such as suture needles, hypodermic needles, and disposable blades, when you prepare the tray. You will recount these sharp instruments after surgery to ensure that you did not leave any near the patient.

In addition to the sterilized instruments on the sterile tray, the surgeon may need sterile cotton-tipped applicators or cellulose sponges (spears) to absorb fluids, hold back certain tissues, and apply solutions or ointments. The surgeon may prefer cellulose sponges or spears to cotton-tipped applicators because they do not shed cotton fibers and tend to be more absorbent (Figure 17.15). Other supplies you may need to place on the sterile tray include suture materials, sterile syringes, needles, or solutions, depending on the procedure and the personal preferences of the surgeon.

Assisting During Surgery

During most minor surgical procedures, the ophthalmic medical assistant can best help the ophthalmic surgeon by anticipating the next step of each procedure. This requires a good understanding of the surgical procedure and a working knowledge of the surgeon's preferences. By anticipating the surgeon's needs, the ophthalmic medical

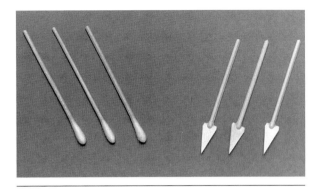

Figure 17.15 Cotton-tipped applicators and cellulose spears.

assistant helps expedite the operation and minimize the chance for complications. Knowing which instrument the surgeon will need next comes with practical experience in assisting over time.

During the actual surgical procedure, the duties of the ophthalmic medical assistant center on providing better operative exposure for the surgeon. In chalazion surgery, for example, this might be accomplished by holding the chalazion clamp during the incision and curettage. In addition, the surgeon may ask the ophthalmic medical assistant to use a cotton-tipped applicator or a cellulose sponge to blot any blood to maintain *hemostasis* so the surgeon can work in an unobstructed field. In many procedures another important function of the assistant is to keep the ocular surface moist, usually by applying lubricating drops or gels to the ocular surface as directed by the surgeon.

The ophthalmic medical assistant can also help the operation go smoothly by passing the surgeon the necessary instruments when requested. It is very important not to pass instruments over the eye or face of the patient, especially sharp instruments such as scalpels or needles. Pass instruments with sharp ends pointed away from the surgeon to avoid an inadvertent injury (Figure 17.16).

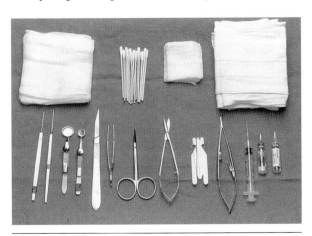

Figure 17.14 Arrangement of instruments and supplies typically used in minor surgery.

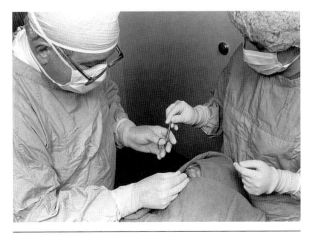

Figure 17.16 Correct technique for passing instruments.

When placing instruments back on to the sterile tray, be very careful. Do not touch the tips of instruments to any hard surface because the delicate tips are easily damaged.

Disposition of Instruments and Materials

At the conclusion of the surgical procedure, the ophthalmic medical assistant removes all instruments and supplies used during the operation. As noted previously, you should recount sharps, such as suture needles, hypodermic needles, and disposable blades, to ensure that you did not leave any sharp objects near the patient. Place disposable sharps in special sharps containers, so they will not injure office personnel or waste collectors. Discard other disposable supplies, including drapes, into appropriate containers. In general, any material that is soaked through or stained with bodily fluid or blood is disposed of in a specially marked biohazard container. Place nondisposable drapes and gowns in the office linen hamper for laundering and resterilization.

Take instruments used during surgery to a sink to be washed, rinsed, and prepared for sterilization. Wear protective gloves while handling and cleaning the instruments. Ophthalmic medical assistants must be careful not to expose their skin or eyes to any of the patient's body fluids. You may need protective eyewear to prevent splashing body fluids or other solutions into your eyes when processing used instruments and supplies.

Separate each instrument from the others and clean them individually, using a commercial instrument cleansing solution. Remove all blood, tissue, and solution from the instruments before re-sterilizing them. Clean jointed instruments thoroughly and carefully. Open scissors to their fullest position and remove all blood, paying special attention to the area around the joints. Remove any blood or tissue from the jaws and tips of all instruments. Cover sharp and delicate instrument tips with an instrument guard after completely cleaning and drying them to protect the points, teeth, or cutting edges as well as to protect office personnel. This step is important because many instruments used in ophthalmic surgery are delicate and easily damaged. Mishandling these instruments can cause the jaws to become misaligned or the points to become bent or dull. After cleaning, rewrap instruments for sterilization.

SELF-ASSESSMENT TEST

1. Name the process by which the physician and patient discuss the risks and benefits of a proposed surgical procedure.

2. A patient asks you a specific question about the outcome of surgery just before the operation. Which is the best action to take?

   a. Answer the question as best you can, based on your experience with similar surgical situations.

   b. Excuse yourself, leave the room to ask the doctor, and report the answer to the patient.

   c. Reassure the patient that there is nothing to worry about.

   d. Suggest that the patient ask the doctor, and bring up the question as soon as the doctor arrives.

3. Name the 2 principal methods used to deliver anesthetizing medication to the eye for minor surgery.

4. Identify from left to right the instruments shown in the photograph.

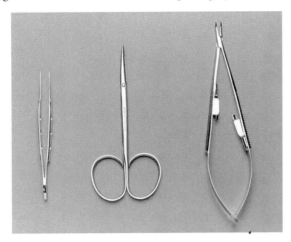

5. What are the 4 types of suture needle points?

6. Name the 2 classifications of suture materials, and identify at least 2 materials used for each kind.

7. List at least 3 minor surgeries commonly performed in the office setting.

8. What are the main purposes of a pressure patch?

9. State the principal purpose for aseptic technique in the office surgical environment.

10. List the 4 components of aseptic technique most applicable to minor office surgery.

11. What does prepping the patient for minor surgery mean?

12. Name the elements of the sterile field.

13. Why is a drape used in ophthalmic minor surgery?

14. Describe the special actions taken with sharps after surgery and explain why they are necessary.

SUGGESTED ACTIVITIES

1. Discuss your responsibilities related to minor surgery with the ophthalmologist for whom you work. Be sure to ask any questions now, rather than during the surgery itself.

2. With the ophthalmologist in your office supervising, role-play with a fellow employee the following minor surgery activities:

   a. Assist the patient onto the operating table, position the patient's head, and give instructions for fixation of gaze to prepare the patient for an anesthetic injection.

   b. Handle some typical patient questions.

   c. Using an inert fluid suggested by the doctor, practice administering anesthetic by the topical drop and the pledget methods.

   d. Prepare (prep) the patient's operative area with germicidal solution, using sterile inert liquid.

3. With the senior technician or ophthalmologist supervising, practice scrubbing, gloving, and postsurgical instrument removal and cleaning.

4. Under supervision, lay out an instrument tray for

   a. chalazion surgery

   b. other lid-lesion removal

   c. lacrimal-system probing

5. Discuss with the ophthalmologist the correct procedure to follow when you or the patient feels faint.

6. With the ophthalmologist's permission, observe several different minor surgical procedures. Take notes and ask questions in a discussion with the surgeon and assistant afterward.

7. Practice applying a pressure patch on either a dummy head or a coworker. Have an experienced person critique your technique.

SUGGESTED RESOURCES

Boess-Lott R, Stecik S. *The Ophthalmic Surgical Assistant.* Thorofare, NJ: Slack; 1999.

Cassin B. *Fundamentals for Ophthalmic Technical Personnel.* Philadelphia: Saunders; 1995: chap 25.

DuBois LG. Patching, patient services, sterile technique. In: *Fundamentals of Ophthalmic Medical Assisting.* DVD. San Francisco: American Academy of Ophthalmology; 2009.

Phillips NF. *Berry & Kohn's Introduction to Operating Room Technique.* 11th ed. St Louis: Mosby; 2007.

Stein HA, Stein RM. *The Ophthalmic Assistant: A Text for Allied and Associated Ophthalmic Personnel.* 8th ed. St Louis: Mosby; 2006.

18 REFRACTIVE SURGERY CONCEPTS AND PROCEDURES

Advances in refractive surgery have reduced the need, in a safe and effective manner, for spectacle lenses required to correct myopia, hyperopia, and astigmatism. This chapter reviews indications and contraindications for refractive surgical procedures and what is involved in evaluating refractive surgical patients. It describes and discusses refractive procedures commonly performed today, the most prevalent of which is laser in situ keratomileusis (LASIK), Several others performed on a regular basis include surface ablation (including photorefractive keratectomy (PRK), LASEK (laser epithelial keratomileusis, and EPI-LASIK), astigmatic keratotomy (AK), conductive keratoplasty (CK), laser thermal keratoplasty (LTK), and use of intrastromal corneal ring segments, and phakic intraocular lenses.

Despite the availability of these procedures, it may not be possible to meet the expectations of potential refractive surgery candidates. Patient selection and counseling are extremely important. A good candidate should have realistic expectations and adequate knowledge of the risks, the benefits, and alternatives to any refractive surgical procedures. This information is also valuable for the ophthalmic medical assistant interacting with refractive surgical patients in the clinic and the operating room.

The reversibility and accuracy of spectacles and contact lenses make them reasonable alternatives to refractive surgical procedures. With modern advancements in technology it is acceptable to operate on a normal eye to reduce the dependence on eyeglasses or contact lenses because most patients are pleased with the ease, safety, and outcomes after successful refractive surgery. However, with newer refractive surgical procedures, less information may be available regarding the long-term safety of the procedure. Validation through controlled and well-designed scientific investigations helps in ensuring high predictability and safety.

History of Refractive Surgery

After the introduction of **radial keratotomy** (**RK**) in Japan in the 1940s, the procedure fell into disfavor because the posterior corneal incisions resulted in endothelial cell injury, irreversible **corneal edema**, and **bullous keratopathy**. Russian investigators used anterior incisions to improve the procedure in the 1970s, followed by continual refinement in the United States during the 1980s, but long-term studies showed significant instability and progressive hyperopic shifts. RK was replaced in the 1990s by procedures using the **excimer laser**, named for the "excited dimer" (a double molecule) of argon and fluoride gas used to generate ultraviolet energy that can precisely vaporize tissue. Trials of PRK by the Food and Drug Administration (FDA) established its efficacy for the correction of myopia, astigmatism, and hyperopia. Subsequent FDA approvals of excimer laser procedures included laser in situ keratomileusis (LASIK), wavefront-optimized and wavefront-guided LASIK.

Indications and Contraindications for Refractive Surgical Procedures

Indications for refractive surgery include occupational goals, cosmetic or recreational desires, contact lens intolerance, or the fear of being unsafe in an emergency without glasses. Patients must understand that refractive surgical procedures usually result in less need for eyewear but, because of the possibility of presbyopia and residual refractive errors after surgery, the ophthalmic assistant should inquire about a patient's motivations for surgery, thereby helping in proper patient selection and evaluation. After refractive surgery, it is not always possible to completely eliminate the need for spectacles or contact lenses to correct for distance, near, or both.

It is essential for the ophthalmologist to ensure that patient expectations match what is realistically offered by surgery, emphasizing that the major motivation for refractive surgery should be the reduction of one's dependence on spectacles or contact lenses. Discussion of the expected outcomes and addressing unrealistic expectations are uniquely the responsibility of the ophthalmologist.

Uncontrolled ocular surface or other eye disease, including blepharitis, dry eye, cataract, or uncontrolled glaucoma, often preclude surgery. Patients who are **immunosuppressed** (lacking the ability to protect against disease), on chronic corticosteroids or **antimetabolites** (agents used for cancer therapy), or suffering from autoimmune connective tissue disease (ie, rheumatoid arthritis, lupus), or other systemic diseases that may have altered wound healing, can compromise the accuracy of intended corrections. Additional contraindications include a refractive condition that is unstable over time. Corneal **ectasias** (thinning with protrusion) such as keratoconus (KC) may yield erratic results postoperatively. Corneal warpage induced by a contact lens should be allowed to resolve before preoperative refractive surgery measurements are performed.

Evaluating Refractive Surgical Patients

In evaluating refractive surgical patients, both preoperative and postoperative tests are necessary. In general, the preoperative visit involves more tests than the postoperative visit. For certain patients with surgical complications, the postoperative visit may be more involved than the preoperative visit.

The ophthalmic medical assistant can play a major role in the preoperative and postoperative evaluation of patients undergoing refractive surgical procedures.

The tests performed most commonly prior to surgery are manifest refraction (Chapter 5) as well as slit-lamp biomicroscopy (Chapter 8) of the anterior segment to identify eye conditions that would be a contraindication for refractive surgery. To avoid overcorrection of myopia or undercorrection of hyperopia, a refraction is repeated after cycloplegia. Near refraction, wavefront analysis, pupillometry, pachymetry, keratometry, and videokeratography are tests that can be conducted in the preoperative and postoperative evaluations.

Refraction in Myopia

In the myopic eye, images are focused in front of the retina. Once the myopic eye is refracted, the minus-powered lens placed in front of the eye corrects the refractive error and allows parallel rays that come from infinity to focus on the retina. Manifest and cycloplegic refractions are performed to determine the degree of nearsightedness. The ophthalmic medical assistant who will be involved in the evaluation of potential refractive surgical candidates needs to master the techniques of refraction reviewed in Chapter 5. The refractive surgeon uses the manifest and cycloplegic results to reduce the refractive power of the cornea (or the crystalline lens) so that parallel rays from infinity focus on the retina.

Refraction in Hyperopia

It is important for the ophthalmic medical assistant to realize that the hyperopic eye focuses parallel rays of light behind the retina. In younger patients with hyperopia, accommodation of the eye may produce enough additional plus power to allow the light rays to focus on the retina, masking the refractive error. Cycloplegic refraction allows for the full disclosure of the hyperopic correction: a plus-powered lens placed in front of the eye will converge parallel rays of light on the retina without the aid of accommodation. In the prepresbyopic age group, hyperopia is less visually significant than myopia for distance, but these patients start experiencing near vision difficulties sooner than their mid-40s by requiring correction for near. Thus, it is important to check uncorrected distance and near vision in these patients prior to cycloplegia. Older patients with hyperopia have insufficient accommodation to compensate for the distance error and require optical correction for clear distance vision. They can benefit from refractive surgical procedures in which the corneal curvature is steepened or the power of the crystalline lens is increased to improve distance and/or near vision.

Refraction in Astigmatism

A skilled ophthalmic medical assistant should be able to use the refraction techniques reviewed in Chapter 5 to determine the magnitude and axis of astigmatism with accuracy. Astigmatism is typically caused by a toric cornea (a cornea whose surface curvature is not uniform) with two principal meridians corresponding to the steepest and flattest curvatures of the cornea. The ophthalmic medical assistant's refraction of the patient with astigmatism will often determine whether the astigmatism is simple or compound, according to whether one or both meridians, respectively, are focused off the surface of the retina. In cases of mixed astigmatism, one meridian focuses in front of the retina (myopic) and the other meridian focuses behind it (hyperopic). In cases of hyperopic astigmatism, it is important to confirm the manifest refraction by performing cycloplegic refraction

to eliminate accommodation during testing. When astigmatism is corrected at the corneal plane, such as with keratorefractive surgery, the full correction of astigmatism is desirable.

Near Refraction in Presbyopic Patients

Presbyopic patients who are considering refractive surgery for myopia must realize that they would be exchanging dependence on distance spectacles for dependence on near-vision spectacles. People with surgically corrected myopia will need reading glasses as they age, whereas before surgery they could remove their spectacles to read. An exception to this is monovision, in which the nondominant eye is left myopic so that reading without glasses can still be performed.

Cycloplegic Refraction

It is important to perform a manifest refraction with fogging (to minimize accommodation during refraction) and near refraction prior to performing the cycloplegic refraction. Cycloplegic refractions are essential for the evaluation of refractive surgery candidates because they ensure complete relaxation of accommodation during testing. One limitation of cycloplegia is that the pupil dilates and therefore other ocular aberrations are produced. The rays of light reaching the periphery of a cornea and lens are bent more than the central rays, causing certain aberrations associated with dilated pupils. Nevertheless, the benefit of relaxing accommodation is very important to avoid over-minusing the patient, especially young patients.

Wavefront Analysis

Wavefront error measurement, or aberrometry, adapted from astronomical optics, is becoming part of the routine evaluation of refractive surgical patients. In a perfect optical system, all the refracted rays are focused on a single plane (wavefront). Optical aberrations induce deformations on this plane and represent the optical performance of the entire visual system, not only the anterior surface of the cornea as measured by most **corneal topography** machines.

In contrast to conventional refraction techniques (determining the sphere and astigmatic correction), wavefront analysis measures higher-order optical aberrations such as spherical aberration, coma configurations, and other forms of irregular astigmatism. These higher-order aberrations cannot be measured by routine refraction techniques, but they can be measured using **aberrometry**. With the use of advanced lasers and wavefront-deformation measuring devices, the correction of these higher-order distortions of the human eye is becoming more common. Aberrometry data is being incorporated into excimer laser nomograms (also known as *customized corneal treatments*). Such data is also taken into account for **phakic IOLs**, which are intraocular lenses surgically implanted without removing the natural crystalline lens, usually to correct high myopia.

Pupil Size Measurements

Keratorefractive procedures are usually centered on the midpoint of the pupil under **mesopic** (vision in dim light levels) or **scotopic** (dark-adapted vision) conditions. Therefore it is important to note during the preoperative evaluation whether the pupil is decentered as well as to measure the pupil size under various lighting conditions. The pupil diameter might reach 6 to 8 mm in dim light, allowing untreated areas of the cornea to leak defocused light onto the retina. Edge glare and halos may ensue with larger pupils, especially at night (or in cases of decentration of the **optical zone**: the area of the central cornea). The role of the ophthalmic medical assistant is important in identifying patients with decentered pupils and/or large pupils to avoid a mismatch between pupil size and optical zone diameter. All patients should be warned by the ophthalmologist prior to surgery about possible postoperative optical distortions after a refractive procedure.

Ultrasound Pachymetry and Keratometry

The techniques of ultrasound pachymetry and keratometry have been described elsewhere in this book. (See Chapters 5 and 10.) There are several methods of obtaining these measurements. Pachymetry readings are important to rule out abnormally thin corneas that would be at greater risk for ectasia after LASIK surgery. Keratometry readings are especially important to identify patients with unusually steep or flat corneas. This information may also be valuable in determining the specific **microkeratome** (a miniature surgical knife) to use during LASIK surgery. Keratometry is additionally helpful in its ability to determine phakic IOL suitability and for implant power calculations, and to uncover early, barely noticeable corneal surface irregularities (seen as distorted mires during testing).

Videokeratography

Computed topography and scanning slit topography, or anterior segment optical coherence tomography (AC-OCT), are essential for appreciating abnormalities of the corneal surface. These techniques provide high-resolution topographic analysis of the cornea. This is especially helpful for discovering subtle abnormal patterns in corneal steepness, often seen in early cases of keratoconus, contact lens corneal warpage, and other cases of irregular astigmatism. The ophthalmic medical assistant should be skilled in using these instruments in order to ensure reproducible and accurate results.

Refractive Surgical Procedures

This section describes refractive procedures commonly performed today.

Laser In Situ Keratomileusis

Laser in situ keratomileusis (LASIK) combines dissection of corneal layers of tissue (lamellae) with the mechanical or laser (femtosecond) microkeratome and a refractive ablation in the stromal bed with the excimer laser. *Ablation* refers to the vaporization of the tissue with laser energy.

In LASIK, an anterior corneal flap is created and lifted. The exposed corneal stroma is treated with the excimer or ultraviolet laser to modify its radius of curvature. During a PRK procedure, the laser is applied directly to Bowman's layer with no corneal flap, whereas in LASIK the laser is applied to the stroma after a flap has been lifted from the cornea. The role of the ophthalmic surgical assistant in LASIK surgery has increased due to the rapid changes in technology of the excimer lasers, microkeratomes, and femtosecond laser keratomes (Intralase, Femto LDV, Visumax). Growth of epithelial cells under the flap may complicate the healing. This complication is sometimes managed by lifting the flap and removing the epithelial ingrowth (Figure 18.1). In some cases sutures may be needed to tightly close the flap margin especially in cases of recurrent ingrowth. Another complication that can occur is flap striae—wrinkles in the flap that may affect vision. An example is shown in Figure 18.2. This is sometimes managed by relifting the flap, irrigating, stretching, and repositioning. Another untoward effect of LASIK is the reduction of corneal biomechanical strength, resulting from a thin residual bed after laser ablation. This instability of the corneal layer under the flap after the laser ablation may rarely result in protrusion and steepening of the central cornea called **ectasia** (Figure 18.3).

Other possible complications of LASIK include flap malpositions and microkeratome malfunction. The latter

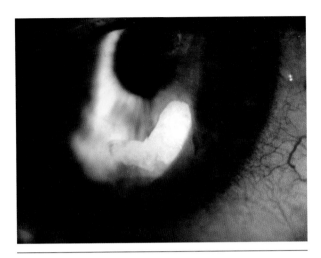

Figure 18.1 Dense ingrowth of epithelial cells in the interface under a LASIK flap.

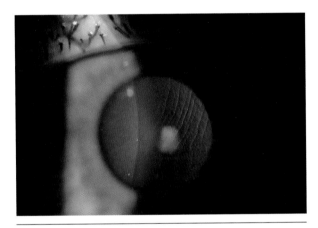

Figure 18.2 Flap striae. *(Image courtesy of David A. Goldman, MD.)*

is less likely to occur if the ophthalmic medical assistants maintain a high level of equipment care and testing prior to surgery. Optical aberrations may also occur after LASIK. They occur more frequently in patients with higher degrees of myopia and hyperopia. While traditional LASIK treatments typically increase the degree of higher-order aberrations, the goal of wavefront-optimized treatment is to create no change in higher-order aberrations, while the goal of wavefront-guided treatments is to decrease higher-order aberrations. It is important to note that larger ablation zone sizes minimize the chance of spherical aberrations; however, the greater depth of an ablation zone may result in irregular astigmatism or instability of the cornea increasing the risk of ectasia.

Photorefractive Keratectomy

In **photorefractive keratectomy** (**PRK**), the corneal epithelium is mechanically removed and the anterior surface

of the stroma is ablated by the excimer laser. Ultraviolet photons break molecular bonds, precisely ablating Bowman's membrane and the anterior corneal stroma while causing minimal residual thermal damage. This central area, or ablation zone, altered by PRK produces corneal flattening over the visual axis, thus reducing myopia. As in LASIK, the surgeon achieves the intended change in dioptric power by varying the diameter and depth of the ablation zone. Treatment of myopia can involve a single ablation, wavefront-guided treatment, or multiple ablations of different diameters. Multizone ablations are often performed for higher degrees of nearsightedness. The fear of deeper ablations in LASIK is ectasia, but in PRK they lead to a greater risk of subepithelial corneal haze (Figure 18.4) caused by growth of scar tissue. Postoperative use of topical corticosteroids is therefore routinely prescribed for 1 to 3 months to limit the haze and its possible refractive regression. The corticosteroid drops work by inhibiting scar-forming cells. Mitomycin C, an antimetabolite (a chemical that inhibits cell growth and, therefore, scar formation) can also be used to reduce postoperative haze. Hyperopia and astigmatism can also be corrected with a LASIK procedure, although in a less predictable fashion than myopia.

Laser Subepithelial Keratomileusis

In **laser subepithelial keratomileusis** (**LASEK**) an epithelial sheet is created and separated with its basement membrane from the stroma with dilute alcohol. The laser is applied as in conventional PRK, and afterward the epithelial sheet is repositioned (Figure 18.5).

EPI-LASIK

In **EPI-LASI**K, an epithelial sheet is created and separated with its basement membrane from the stroma with a device similar to a microkeratome (epi-keratome). The laser is applied as in conventional PRK, and afterward the epithelial sheet is repositioned.

Astigmatic Keratotomy

Several incisional surgical techniques have been described to correct astigmatism. These techniques include transverse and arcuate incisions, and are grouped under the term **astigmatic keratotomy** (**AK**). Very peripheral incisions are sometimes referred to as *limbal relaxing incisions* (LRI). AK involves the placement of transverse or arcuate incisions perpendicular to the steepest corneal meridian of astigmatism. The incised meridian flattens while the meridian 90° away steepens. Incisions are typically placed at or greater than a 7 mm

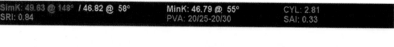

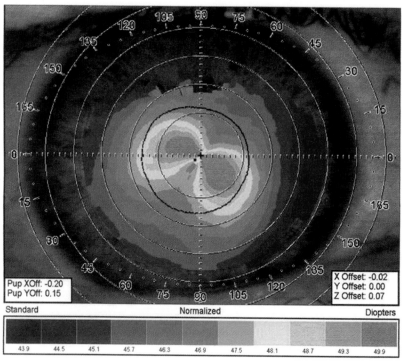

Figure 18.3 Post-LASIK corneal ectasia. Notice irregular central corneal steepening on corneal topography.

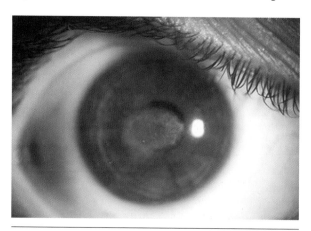

Figure 18.4 Subepithelial haze following PRK procedure.

optical zone diameter. Deeper, longer, and more centrally located AK incisions have greater efficacy in correcting astigmatism, but they also have greater potential side effects, such as irregular astigmatism, overcorrection, and decreased corneal sensation. Irregular astigmatism is not amenable to correction by AK or by conventional lenses. It can be corrected with the application of a rigid contact lens or by surface ablation of the cornea with phototherapeutic keratectomy (PTK). Radial keratotomy (Figure 18.6) is no longer a procedure indicated for low levels of nearsightedness.

Conductive Keratoplasty and Laser Thermokeratoplasty

Conductive keratoplasty, or CK (Figure 18.7), is used to treat low degrees of hyperopia and to induce myopia in the nondominant eye for emmetropic presbyopia (creates monovision). The near vision is created by shrinking the peripheral and paracentral corneal stroma, thereby steepening the central cornea. The solid-state infrared laser, such as the holmium:YAG (Ho:YAG) laser, is used for this procedure. The Ho:YAG laser has been previously employed in a peripheral intrastromal radial pattern (laser thermokeratoplasty) to treat hyperopia of 2.50 D or less. However, the long-term effects and refractive stability of laser thermokeratoplasty have been shown to be inferior to those of CK. Newer generations of CK techniques, such as "light touch CK" (for near vision correction), may have less regression of the effect over time.

Intrastromal Corneal Ring Segments

Intrastromal corneal ring segments (ICRS, or Intacs prescription inserts) were originally used to treat low degrees of myopia, but a more common use is in the treatment of early keratoconus (Figure 18.8) and ectasia after LASIK surgery. The segments are placed in the

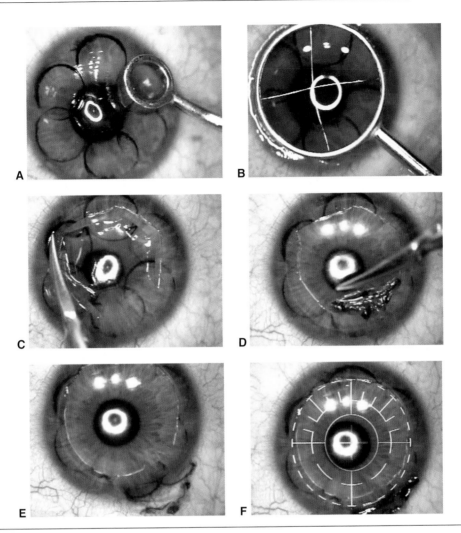

Figure 18.5 Azar's LASEK technique. **A.** Multiple marks are applied in the cornea periphery. **B.** An alcohol dispenser consisting of a customized 9 mm marker attached to a hollow metal handle serves as a reservoir for 18% alcohol. Firm pressure is exerted on the cornea and alcohol is released into the well of the marker for 35 seconds. **C.** A superiorly hinged flap is created with a modified Vannas scissors. **D, E.** The loosened epithelium is peeled as a single sheet, leaving it attached at its superior hinge. **F.** Laser ablation is applied to the exposed Bowman's layer and stroma. After laser ablation, the epithelium is repositioned and aligned. A bandage soft contact lens is applied.

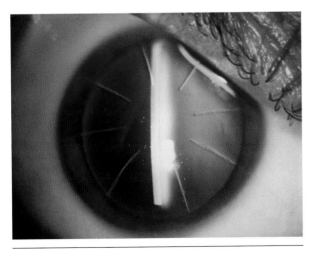

Figure 18.6 Radial keratotomy. Eight corneal incisions are observed radiating from the paracentral area.

midperipheral cornea to flatten the curvature of the central cornea. This technique takes advantage of the fact that the distance from limbus to limbus remains constant at all times, so when the anterior surface is lifted focally over the segments, a compensatory flattening of the central cornea occurs. The segments are threaded into a peripheral midstromal tunnel. The use of the Intra-Lase femtosecond laser has facilitated this surgical step. Despite its limited applications, the main advantage of an ICRS over other corneal refractive surgical techniques is that the segments can be removed.

Phakic Intraocular Lenses

The Verisyse phakic IOL (Abbott Medical Optics, Santa Ana, California), approved by the FDA, is an iris-claw

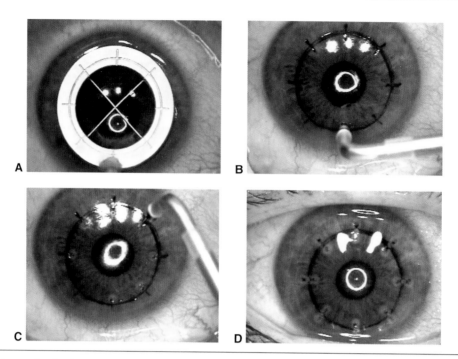

Figure 18.7 In conductive keratoplasty (CK), radiofrequency energy is delivered in a series of spots to the corneal periphery. Higher hyperopic corrections require more circles of spots. **A.** A corneal marker is placed on the cornea to guide the spot placement. **B.** The working tip of the instrument is inserted into the stroma of the cornea at defined spots around the peripheral cornea, oriented perpendicular to the surface, beginning with the 12 o'clock 7.0 mm optical zone spot. **C.** Subsequent spots are applied in a cross-corneal pattern (180° away). The 6.0 and 8.0 mm rings are then sequentially treated, according to the nomogram. **D.** Operative appearance after treatment with 24 spots.

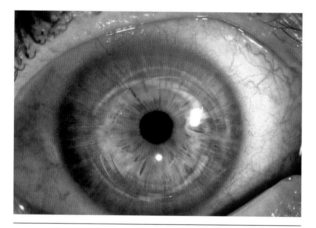

Figure 18.8 Intrastromal ring segments implanted in an eye to treat keratoconus.

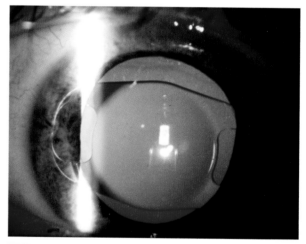

Figure 18.9 Artisan-Worst iris-fixation phakic intraocular lens (Verisyse lens) for myopic correction.

lens originally devised for the correction of aphakia and later modified to correct high myopia in patients whose natural crystalline lenses were intact (phakic). The lens is enclaved (attached) in the midperipheral, less mobile iris and requires a 6.0 mm incision for its insertion (Figure 18.9). Another phakic IOL available for use in the United States is the Visian ICL implantable collamer lens (STAAR Surgical, Monrovia, California). This posterior chamber phakic IOL fits in the space between the posterior iris and the crystalline lens. Several other phakic

IOLs are approved outside the United States including the angle-supported phakic IOL, which was introduced for the correction of myopia and has gone through several modifications. (Figure 18.10 shows an example of an earlier phakic lens.) Long-term follow-up of the original angle-supported lens has shown progressive pupil ovalization. Despite phakic IOL approval in the United States and overseas, longer-term follow-up is ongoing

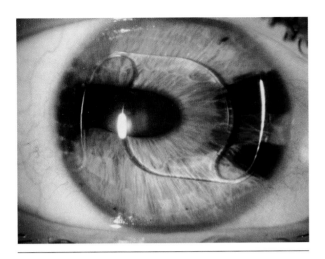

Figure 18.10 An angle-supported phakic IOL causing areas of iris atrophy and pupil ovalization.

for all types of these lenses regarding endothelial cell loss, glaucoma, iris abnormalities, cataract formation, and ease of explantation. It is expected that the role of the ophthalmic medical assistant will undergo substantial modifications as the experience with these lenses increases. In the future, the use of ultra high-frequency ultrasound (UBM) and anterior segment optical coherence tomography (OCT) techniques will increase in the perioperative evaluation of patients undergoing phakic IOL surgery.

In Review

The role of the ophthalmic medical assistant has increased with the advent of refractive surgical techniques, requiring sophisticated and technically demanding perioperative testing and meticulous attention to detail during surgery. In addition, the future of keratorefractive surgery will likely include a wide array of more-complicated surgical procedures with unique indications and technologies. Predictability, stability, and safety will continue to be the goal for all refractive procedures.

Refractive surgeons depend upon skilled ophthalmic technical assistants to help evaluate and treat patients using one or more procedures, among the large number of possible techniques that best fit the needs of the patients. In some patients, a combination of procedures may be used. Postoperative assessments focus on evaluating the surgery of the original procedure or plans for future procedures or glasses or contact lenses. In the short term, LASIK and surface ablation are likely to continue as the procedures of choice for most patients. A monovision approach is commonly employed to treat presbyopic patients with myopic or hyperopic refractive errors. CK is a viable alternative for emmetropic presbyopia. Accommodating and multifocal IOLs, which are gaining greater acceptance for treating cataracts, may become more commonly employed to treat presbyopic patients with relatively high hyperopic errors (even before the onset of visually significant cataracts). This adds to the responsibilities and expectations of the ophthalmic medical assistant.

SELF-ASSESSMENT TEST

1. Name 4 indications for refractive surgery.

2. List at least 4 eye conditions that preclude refractive surgery.

3. Explain why cycloplegic refraction is important in the preoperative evaluation for refractive surgery.

4. What 2 aspects of the pupil examination are important in determining risk of postoperative optical distortions?

5. Describe the procedural differences between LASIK and PRK.

6. Discuss the indications for conductive keratoplasty.

7. What are the main uses of intracorneal ring segments?

8. Why are keratometry readings important in the preoperative evaluation of refractive surgery patients?

9. Why are pachymetry readings important in the preoperative evaluation of refractive surgery patients?

10. Describe some of the problems encountered with placement of a posterior chamber phakic IOL.

SUGGESTED ACTIVITIES

1. Practice measuring a coworker's pupillary diameter and midpoint under scotopic conditions.

2. Demonstrate the steps involved in keratometry to a senior staff member.

3. Tour your clinic's refractive surgery center and observe the preoperative evaluation of a refractive surgery patient.

4. Ask permission to observe a refractive surgery procedure.

5. Talk to several individuals who have had refractive surgery. Ask them about their visual function after surgery.

SUGGESTED RESOURCES

Azar DT. Keratorefractive surgery. In: Pavan-Langston D, ed. *Manual of Ocular Diagnosis and Therapy.* 5th ed. Philadelphia: Lippincott Williams & Wilkins; 2002.

Azar DT, Koch DD, eds. *LASIK: Fundamentals, Surgical Techniques, and Complications.* Refractive Surgery Series; 1. New York: Marcel Dekker; 2002.

Azar DT, Camellin M, Yee R, eds. *LASEK and Stromal Surface Excimer Laser Ablation.* Refractive Surgery Series; 3. New York: Marcel Dekker; 2005.

Boxer Wachler BS, Christie JP, Chandra NS, et al. Intacs for keratoconus. *Ophthalmology.* 2003;110:1031–1040.

Refractive Surgery. Basic and Clinical Science Course, Section 13. San Francisco: American Academy of Ophthalmology; 2011.

Schallhorn SC, Kaupp SE, Tanzer DJ, et al. Pupil size and quality of vision after LASIK. *Ophthalmology.* 2003;110:1606–1614.

19 UNDERSTANDING PRACTICE MANAGEMENT

The goal of an ophthalmologist's office is to provide quality eye care to each patient in an efficient, cost-effective manner that meets or exceeds the patient's expectations. In order for a medical practice to succeed, available resources must be utilized effectively to provide excellent care: claims must be filed and effectively collected in a timely manner, expenses must be paid, and the practice must adhere to all applicable laws and regulations. This does not occur unless someone is managing the operation of the practice effectively. Either a doctor or a practice manager will normally have that overall responsibility.

This chapter highlights the practice management side of the ophthalmologist's office: the responsibilities, accountabilities, and policies and procedures that are vital to the overall success of the practice. In addition, you will be introduced to the basic principles and purposes of coding, the "language" that facilitates the processing of insurance claims.

A superbly managed practice attains satisfied patients and has a strong demand for its services. The practice has low staff turnovers and efficient work processes. Such practices are highly profitable, with a pleasant work environment and minimal work errors. The staff is courteous, dedicated, and involved. The patient's needs are considered primary and the staff works as a team. They are proud to be a part of the organization and understand and are enrolled into the mission and vision of the practice.

The Ophthalmic Practice and You

As an ophthalmic assistant, you are primarily involved in assisting the doctor to render eye care. However, there are other considerations related to your work. These include how you understand management and treat your job responsibilities and how you impact upon the efficiency and operational effectiveness of the practice. In addition your impact on the efficiency and operational environment of the practice will affect your performance reviews and eventually your compensation.

For Whom Do You Work?

Whether this is your first job or you have been working for some time, you may not understand for whom you work. First, you work for yourself. Although you are being paid by an ophthalmology practice, you are managing your own career. By taking this course, you have chosen to improve your skill and knowledge level. By learning what the doctor and practice manager expect of you and by doing your best to meet those expectations, you are managing yourself to improve your opportunities for advancement, greater compensation, and future opportunities.

Second, you work for the practice. You may have an intermediate supervisor, but you are ultimately responsible to the doctor or doctors who own the practice. Every task you undertake should be to meet the goals of the practice and be done within the policies and procedures established by the practice.

You Are Part of a Team

To serve patients effectively, ophthalmology practices employ individuals with different skills. Everyone must coordinate their activities to assure that patients are scheduled, registered, examined, treated, discharged, and billed, and that out-of-pocket expenses are collected. Each staff member has a critical role that links with everyone else. In a small office, employees may be cross-trained for all jobs. In a large office there may be several different departments with unique responsibilities. Even though your primary responsibility may be direct patient care, there may be times that you may need to assist in appointment scheduling (Figure 19.1), medical records,

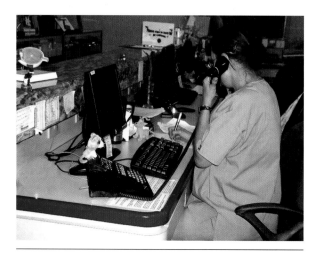

Figure 19.1 Effective team players are flexible, helping out in other areas as needed. Employees may receive cross-training in a variety of skill sets, from direct patient care to appointment scheduling and handling medical records. *(Image courtesy of Emanuel Newmark, MD.)*

or other areas. The best team players are always ready to pitch in where they are needed. This also means you are part of a team, which requires organization and management. In turn, the collected receipts pay office staff salaries and overhead expenses (rent, electric, telephone, insurance, supplies, maintenance, and so on).

Why Management Matters

Without organization, assignment of responsibilities, and accountability, a medical practice would experience inefficiencies and even chaos. Management adds the structure to produce order and efficiencies for a practice. Through this structure, employees are able to complete their jobs in a cost-effective, efficient manner. When management functions at its best, each employee's job is made easier, patients receive the care they expect, and the practice will be successful.

Management and the Patient

Our patients are the fundamental reason we have jobs. The practice must meet the patient's expectations or that patient will not return. A satisfied patient may tell three people about your practice. A patient who is dissatisfied will tell at least 10 people about your practice. At every turn, you are an ambassador for your practice. Courteous service and concerned listening will bring more patients to your practice than any outside marketing program. Your ability to promote good patient relations will be a key factor in reviewing your job performance (Figure 19.2).

Chapter 1 discusses what constitutes professional and ethical behavior by the ophthalmic medical assistant.

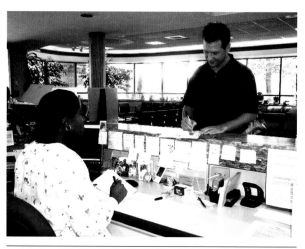

Figure 19.2 Courtesy counts. At every turn, you are an ambassador for your practice. *(Image courtesy of Emanuel Newmark, MD.)*

Chapters 15 and 16 provide additional information about ways to interact with patients as part of a medical process, including patients with special concerns. A key point to remember is that at times, a patient's demands may seem unreasonable or even distasteful in word or deed. Such patients may be undergoing a time of illness and worry that, in turn, affects their behavior. During these situations, patients need your support and understanding. The ophthalmic medical assistant who can communicate with individual patients in a compassionate and courteous manner is more effective and will earn the patients' trust and cooperation.

Although you may mean well by calling patients "dear" or "honey," some patients consider this demeaning. Because a medical practice is a professional organization, most practices insist that you refrain from using these casual terms, and instead call the patient by his or her first name, title, or last name, depending upon the practice and patient preference. In talking to a fellow staff member about a patient, never refer to a patient as "this guy" but instead say "this patient" or mention the person by name.

In order to meet or exceed the patients' expectations for service, a medical practice must have operating policies and procedures to aid in reaching this mission. The objective of the mission is more important than the rule itself. If a rule seems to interfere with the goal of helping the doctor or the patient, then any changes or exceptions to the rules should be discussed with your supervisor. "Management Through Policies and Procedures," a topic discussed later in this chapter, reviews the importance of standardization for decision-making and how tasks are accomplished.

Management and Your Doctor

In a medical practice, the most expensive and productive resource is the physician's professional time. The physician is the individual producing the highest billable services per hour. An efficient and effective staff will enable each physician to spend quality time with each patient and produce his or her optimal billable service per hour. As an ophthalmic assistant, you can assist your doctor by managing your tasks in a manner that optimizes the doctor's time. Everything you do should help the doctor better manage his or her time in treating patients.

Here are some ways to facilitate that:

- Have a pre-clinic meeting with the doctor or other ophthalmic assistants to review the morning or afternoon schedule to plan that half day (Figure 19.3).

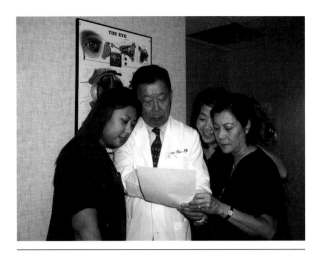

Figure 19.3 A pre-clinic meeting to review the schedule helps everyone manage tasks efficiently. *(Image courtesy of Emanuel Newmark, MD.)*

- Work up patients efficiently prior to their being seen by the physician. A "workup" may consist of a review of systems and the patient's past, family and social history as well as documenting the chief complaint and elements of the history of the present illness. It may also indicate performance of specific elements of the exam and other ancillary testing.

- Gather in the exam room all the ancillary instruments, equipment, and medications anticipated for this visit. Depending on the intended purpose for the appointment, additional supplies may include forceps, lacrimal instruments, dye strips, prisms, trial lens frame, contact lens solution and case, and possibly a suture removal set.

- Be readily available to assist with special-concern patients, such as patients using a walker or wheelchair or having little or no vision.

- Record your notes clearly, simply, and legibly in the medical record in order to meet the needs of the physician as well as the requirement of the payer.

Here are some behaviors to avoid:

- Avoid spending more than minimal time socializing with the patient.

- Do not discuss medical findings with the patients.

- Avoid discussing nonclinic topics with the doctor. This includes discussion of personal problems during working hours. If personal problems arise, consider talking about them with your direct supervisor. When the doctor is your supervisor and is willing to discuss the issues with you, then allow the doctor to set the time and scope of any discussions.

See "Additional Duties" later in this chapter for more information.

The Office Manager's Role

It is not uncommon for employees to wonder what office managers really do. As in watching a talented athlete, when managers are most effective, the job appears easy. In reality, the manager's job is quite complex. The manager must direct all the practice resources: personnel, cash flow, facilities, equipment, and supplies. The manager must ensure that systems are in place for scheduling patients, registering patients, documenting services, filing charges, collecting professional fees, depositing funds, making payroll, paying office overhead expenses (accounts payable), and complying with government laws, rules, and regulations.

The Chain of Command

An essential role of management is to establish and maintain a management chain of command. Everyone in the office needs to know to whom they are accountable and to whom they can go for reliable answers. As you can imagine, it is practically impossible to work for two bosses and please them both. In an ophthalmic practice, unless one of the doctors has assumed the role of practice manager, you will report directly to the practice manager or a mid-level supervisor for all administrative matters. For medical matters you will usually report to your doctor. In some larger practices it is common to have a clinical manager who may be a nurse, a Certified Ophthalmic Technician (COT), or a Certified Ophthalmic Medical Technologist (COMT). In that case that individual may be responsible for managing both administrative matters and medical matters for other ophthalmic assistants and technicians.

Management of Communications

Many problems in the practice stem from inadequate communication. Sometimes this is called "people skills" since communication is the primary way we relate to each other. Good "people skills" include not just how we communicate with others, but also how we listen to others. The best ophthalmic assistants are the best listeners. They really hear what the patients, the doctors, their manager and their coworkers are saying.

Effective communication must be "top down," "bottom up" and "across." "Top down" is when the owners and managers distribute necessary information to all employees to convey the goals, expectations, policies, and procedures of the practice. "Bottom up" communications include suggestions, questions, and feedback from the staff. "Across" communications are communications between coworkers, between departments, with patients, and with outside parties such as insurance companies, regulatory officials, and vendors.

All three types of communication are essential for an effective office. Regarding "top down" communications, you will be expected to thoroughly comprehend the message and if it is unclear ask questions. Regarding "bottom up" communications, you will be expected to offer practical ideas that might contribute to cost savings, operating efficiencies, better quality care, or more satisfied patients. Many practices have a suggestion box or other means to encourage staff ideas. Regarding "across" communications, you will be expected to be fully engaged with patients, coworkers, and outside parties. In all your communications with everyone, you will be expected to be respectful, courteous, and tolerant.

Management by the Numbers

In order to pay staff and doctor salaries as well as other operating expenses, an ophthalmic practice must operate efficiently and profitably. A practice's efficiency can be measured in many ways. Some measures include the number of new and established patient visits per year; number of visits per full-time equivalent (FTE) doctor; number of visits per treatment room per hour; number of patient work ups per FTE assistant; revenue generated per patient visit; annual revenue per FTE staff person; and annual revenue per FTE technician.

As you can see, the productivity of each individual ophthalmic assistant and technician has a significant effect on the overall productivity and financial success of the practice. Measuring productivity should be an important part of your annual performance review.

Many practices will compare their productivity statistics with other similar practices to measure their productivity in comparison to those practices. This is called *benchmarking*. Benchmarking can also be accomplished within your practice by establishing statistics for a base year and then comparing future periods to that base year. Benchmarking is a great way of measuring a practice's success.

Management Through Policies and Procedures

Organizations can achieve operational efficiencies through consistency. Consistency requires that policies and procedures be established to standardize how decisions are made and tasks are accomplished. Policies and procedures are usually established by those individuals or committees governing the practice. In the case of a solo practice that would be the doctor. In a multiple-doctor practice, the practice owners decide who will establish policies. That may be the entire board, an executive committee, or the president of the practice. Clinical procedures will probably be established by your doctor or doctors. Administrative procedures will probably be established by your office manager. Ideally, administrative procedures are documented in procedure manuals, although frequently this is a task in process. Occasionally, a manual may not be available. In that instance, show your doctor this chapter and offer your assistance in establishing an office policies and procedures manual. Even when procedures are written down they should be reviewed annually to be certain they are still appropriate.

You will be expected to understand and comply with the practice's policies and procedures. You will need to know where to find written procedures. You may even be asked to help rewrite or review existing procedures. It is truly everyone's job in a practice to assure that written procedures are designed to accomplish the mission of the practice most efficiently and effectively. If a procedure or a policy seems to be in conflict with the practice's mission statement then it should be reviewed and/or amended.

Commitments and Responsibilities

You have chosen to work in health care and specifically in an ophthalmology practice. Patients trust us to protect and care for two of their most precious assets: their eyes. This is a most serious responsibility, and all our actions and attitudes must convey our respect for the patient and our professionalism in accepting that responsibility. You have obligations and responsibilities toward the practice.

Is It All About Attitude?

Attitude truly affects everything you do and, interestingly, attitude is perhaps the only thing about your job that you have control over. Of course, you can voluntarily give up that control and allow others to manipulate your attitude; when that happens you tend to blame your attitude on other people or on circumstances.

Life is not perfect and neither are you or the people with whom you live and work. In spite of that truth, most people are pleasant and desire to be around cheerful people, not gripers. People who are optimistic, smile, and encourage others are also more successful than those who are negative, fault-finding, and grumpy. The good news is that you get to choose which attitude you will have.

Understanding Your Commitment

What did you agree to when you accepted the job? First, you agreed to show up promptly for work for the days and hours agreed upon. That is a major obligation because the rest of the team is counting on you. It is your responsibility to be prepared for other expected and unexpected events that can impede your fulfilling that commitment. Therefore, you must manage your vacation, sick, or paid time off (PTO) to allow for unexpected circumstances such as sick family members or car and home repairs. Second, you agreed to fulfill the tasks outlined in your job description in a manner that is responsible, efficient, and cost-effective. Assisting in providing quality eye care is only part of your responsibility. Assuring correct coding, proper documentation, office safety, confidentiality, patient relations, cooperation, and harmony in the office are critical parts of your job and no less important than direct patient care.

Optimizing Your Work Time

The best ophthalmic assistants understand that a primary goal of the practice is to see patients efficiently with minimal wait time and with compassion and quality eye care. For example, if you have down time and the doctor is with a patient and has no one assisting him or her during the patient visit, help out rather than taking a break, playing on the Internet, or making personal phone calls. Also if you have down time with no patients to be seen, you may want to check room inventory so that when you are busy later, you have everything you need.

Other impediments to practice efficiency are incomplete patient workups, not signing the chart, or not answering simple questions for the patient prior to the doctor entering the exam room (not medical questions, of course). Leaving telephone messages for patients without leaving your name means that when the patient returns the call, the front desk may spend 15 minutes trying to track down whomever the patient is calling back. Not re-filing medical charts promptly and to their proper location is problematic; it is amazing how much time is spent in the office hunting for "missing" charts.

Your practice should have written personnel policies that discuss how to record your work time and that enumerate what personal activities, if any, are permitted during work time. The use of office equipment such as computers, copy machines, and telephones for personal use is usually permitted with restrictions and significantly limited.

It is your management responsibility to record your work time accurately. The practice wants to pay you accurately for the time you work and are expected to work. Recording time falsely or clocking in or out for another employee may be grounds for dismissal.

Leave any personal problems at the door. This advice is intended not to be callous or insensitive, but practical. The staff is not paid to unload personal problems on the patients or each other. Any discussion of such matters is best avoided with patients and saved for nonworking hours with others.

Understanding Expectations

Most conflicts in the office—as well as in life—stem from conflicts in expectations. Expectations may not have been conveyed, may be misunderstood, or may be reluctantly accepted. Regarding your employment, understanding expectations starts with recruiting and continues throughout employment and even applies to termination.

The practice's expectations of you will be expressed in the policies and procedures manuals and in your job description. If the policies are unclear, ask your manger to clarify. Your practice's personnel manual will not only explain the practice's performance expectations, but it also will explain what benefits are available to you. Read the manual carefully so that you will understand what is expected of you as well as what you can expect from your practice.

Additional Duties

From time to time clinical personnel may be requested to assist in certain administrative duties, some on a regular basis and others occasionally. This section will discuss the most common responsibilities.

Understanding Patient Prescriptions

Almost gone are the days of the handwritten prescription and having the patient take it to the local pharmacy. More frequently now prescriptions are telephoned, faxed, or transmitted electronically (e-prescribed) to a local pharmacy. The objective is to prevent unauthorized use of prescription drugs and to reduce errors in filling patient prescriptions. Many large health care institutions dispense all of their outpatient medications completely electronically. Only the physician has control of the access and process of the e-prescribing program. This process eliminates unauthorized prescriptions. In addition, the programs have "alert pop-ups" indicating incompatibilities (untoward reactions between medications) of the prescribed drug and any recorded allergies to that drug class. The physician can override the alerts based upon his or her medical judgment.

Coordinating Patient Flow

Patient flow is everyone's responsibility, and it starts at the front desk check-in. Failure to alert the clinical staff of the patient's arrival will delay the process and upset the patient when he or she is not taken to the examining room in a timely fashion. A system should be established that conveys the patient's arrival to the clinical care staff. A "no-show" communication to the clinical staff is also important. This opens extra time that may allow for a required diagnostic test for a patient who is already in the office, and thereby reduce medical costs, increase efficiency, and possibly avoid an additional patient visit.

Managing patient flow in a busy ophthalmology office is more complex than in other medical specialties. Eye care patients have an unusual amount of diversions on the way to the doctor's exam: visual field room, computerized imaging, pachymetry test, dilating room, and photography study. Not all visits are the same nor is the time needed for patients to complete each test. Some eyes dilate slower than others, some patients take longer to conclude a visual field test, and there is a great variation in time to complete a manifest refraction. This complexity of visits can create more chaotic and unpredictable patient flow and longer waiting times than anticipated.

While patients are in the clinical area, they should be informed of any delays and asked if they have any subsequent appointments that may conflict with the additional time they will have to spend during this office visit. If a conflict exists, the assistant should notify the doctor so that he or she can expedite the visit.

In a respectful and helpful manner, the assistant should help the doctor to keep on task and negotiate him or her out of a situation that is consuming an inordinate amount of patient care time. Common examples that will delay the doctor are being on the telephone, speaking to pharmaceutical and equipment representatives and "chewing the fat" with a patient who is a friend or relative.

It is your responsibility to do all you can to help keep the doctor running on time. Do the clinical workup and all the special tests before the doctor sees the patient; if it is unclear what special tests are needed ask, the doctor. It is more efficient if you review the charts for the day and know which patients are in for short follow-up visits, and get them in and out quickly.

On any given day, most busy practices have 20% to 30% of the patients that can be seen in a 5- to 10-minute visit. The technician should concentrate on getting them quickly seen by the doctor and happily on their way home or back to work. Delaying a "quick check-up" patient visit for an hour or more reflects poorly on the practice. After a long wait, the patient seems to expect more time from the doctor and that further delays the patient flow. Work with the doctor and appointment personnel to create a schedule that enhances patient flow and fits with the doctor's practice style. Keep the schedule format a work in progress over time, because new technologies, personnel, patient demographics, and allocated office space will change.

A follow-up protocol for missed appointments is essential. Not following up conveys a message to patients that your office does not care about them. It is possible that the patient became gravely ill or was involved in an auto crash just prior to the missed appointment and your timely contact with the patient enhances the "we care about you" type of practice. Some practices charge a minimum fee for missed office visits. Policies may differ from practice to practice or in what circumstances a missed visit fee will be waived.

Elderly patients and patients with disabilities are especially vulnerable to missed appointments because they frequently rely upon others for their transportation, which complicates the visit by involving a third party. For rescheduling they require additional time to arrange for their transportation for their new appointment.

With all that said about patient flow, there is hope on the horizon that computer software programs will become available to greatly assist and enhance the movement of patients through the office visit more efficiently.

Answering the Phone

A superbly managed practice has a strong demand for its services. Timely answering of the telephone is a first step for practices that want to grow by word-of-mouth referrals. Some practices spend a lot of money on advertising but then hinder their efforts by not adequately staffing for incoming telephone calls. In a well-performing practice, the phone should be answered within three rings and hold times should be kept to less than 30 seconds. Always let the patient "see you smile" on the phone.

Sometimes answering the telephone in a timely manner or keeping patients waiting on hold for long periods cannot be avoided. Anyone who is near a phone that has rung three times or notices that a line has been blinking on hold for some time should pick it up and state that the appointment secretaries are busy with other patients and

ask how you can help. Take the name, address, and telephone number of the person calling and ask when it will be a good time for the appointment secretary to call back. Also gather as much information as possible that allows you to determine the urgency of the patient's problem.

Working With Patient Charts

How many times have you heard an office staff member say "We can't find the chart"? Proper storage and retrieval of patient medical records is necessary for quality care and billing for ophthalmic services. Special efforts must be made to file medical records accurately for easy retrieval and rapid access.

The office personnel should be aware that at times medical records may be temporarily filed elsewhere for specific purposes such as pulled for tomorrow's office visit, set aside for accounting, on the doctor's desk, or with the surgical scheduler. When a chart is "pulled" (removed) from the storage area, a "dummy record" should be inserted in its place. A dummy record is a colorful hard cardboard or plastic folder that has a clear pocket to insert a card stating the patient's name or chart number and where the "real" chart may be found.

After personnel have obtained a signed records release, copies may be made of the patient's chart to be forwarded to another physician or facility. Sometimes patients want copies of their medical record for a personal health folder. A signed records release also is necessary as the patient will now be personally responsible to safeguard the privacy of their health record. A dated note should be made in the chart stating to whom copies were sent. Portions of a patient's record (laboratory results, operative reports) are frequently faxed. Each fax should have a disclosure indicating that "this transmission is privileged and confidential and intended only for the addressee and if you have received this communication in error please notify the sender immediately."

An electronic health record (EHR) will help eliminate the need to search for misplaced and misfiled charts. However, concerns over lost patient records still exist if proper steps are not taken to back up computer files and other electronic media. An EHR can be easily printed on the office printer. A hard copy of the EHR also requires a record release.

Scheduling

Inefficient patient scheduling can impede the progress of the day. Scheduling covers appointments for office visits as well as appointments for outside tests.

SCHEDULING APPOINTMENTS Proper staff training is essential to establish and maintain an office appointment schedule. New employees should be mentored by model workers so they understand your practice's appointment schedule. An untrained employee scheduling a new patient appointment will not be able to convey what will actually occur during the office visit. The patient thus arrives at the scheduled time without fully understanding the likely length of the visit and the nature of financial responsibility for the consultation. Such a patient is unlikely to leave the office feeling that the experience rated "5 stars." Return patients may be easier to schedule but when indicated it is important to remind them that they will have their pupils dilated on their next visit and they may want to bring a driver to help take them home. Additional advantages of a well-run schedule are an improved employee environment with less stress and greater satisfaction at work.

SCHEDULING OUTSIDE TESTS Be sure you clearly communicate with the patient the details of an ordered test to be performed at an outside location. Preparatory instructions and directions to the facility should be conveyed to the patient. Knowledge of the patient's insurance coverage and benefits when ordering outside testing is essential to determine whether the test will be a covered service, needs preapproval or must be performed at a specific laboratory, hospital, service company or office.

Spend the extra time with the patient to answer any questions. Ask if there are any questions or concerns and always request the patient to call you if any new questions or concerns arise. Patients who do not understand the importance and purpose of a test are less likely to keep a scheduled appointment. Keep a log of ordered outside studies with the patient's name, medical record number, date, place and name of the ordered test so that you can follow up with the result. Even with your good efforts some patients fail to keep their designated appointment or a test result is improperly forwarded. The lack of followup then becomes a medical legal issue, especially if the test result would have changed the medical treatment of the patient's disease or diagnosis and an adverse outcome occurs.

Scribing

Scribing is the accurate recording of the doctor's findings in legible handwriting. Do not summarize but record the exact words. If records are electronic, the findings are to be transcribed in a similar fashion as the handwritten record. The doctor must sign off that the transcription is accurate. Obviously, the scribe must possess the correct spelling knowledge of the anatomy and diseases of the eye. Documentations in the medical record are permanent and cannot be altered. However, an addendum can be made to the record to correct or amplify any prior notation, and the addition is dated and signed by the author. Again the doctor will co-sign as to the validity of the addendum. In a handwritten note a single line may be drawn through the incorrect item but "white-out" is not to be used. A completed (signed) note in an electronic record cannot be deleted but only amended.

Compliance

Your practice has an obligation to comply with all applicable federal, state, and local laws, rules, and regulations. As an employee you have an obligation to assist the practice in legal compliance. Your practice should have a compliance officer and policies and procedures established to assist the staff in assuring compliance. The compliance officer will probably be either your office manager/administrator or a doctor.

As discussed in "Scribing" above, you will be recording your findings in a legal document—the patient's medical record. Your notes are a part of the documentation that is used to submit a claim to Medicare or insurance companies for payment. The accuracy of your notes is very important in documenting the services the physician has rendered both for insurance and medical legal purposes.

The **Health Insurance Portability and Accountability Act** (HIPAA) has significantly impacted how medical practices secure and transmit medical information. HIPAA regulations prescribe how practices must protect the dissemination of specific information about patients. As an ophthalmic assistant, you will be required to know and comply with these requirements.

The **Occupational Safety and Health Administration** (OSHA) of the U.S. Department of Labor establishes regulations to protect the health and safety of employees. Your practice will have policies and procedures to comply with OSHA regulations. Again, as an ophthalmic assistant, you will be required to know and comply with these requirements.

The **Centers for Medicare and Medicaid Services** (CMS) has established an Internet-based Provider Enrollment, Chain and Ownership System (PECOS). The PECOS program allows physicians, nonphysician practitioners, and provider and supplier organizations to enroll, make a change in their Medicare enrollment, view their Medicare enrollment information on file with Medicare, or check on status of a Medicare enrollment application, all online. Physicians who have not opted out of Medicare need to be enrolled in PECOS if they want to continue seeing or referring Medicare patients for most items and services. In November 2006, CMS approved 10 national accreditation organizations that will accredit suppliers of durable medical equipment, prosthetics, orthotics and supplies (DMEPOS) as meeting new quality standards under Medicare Part B.

In order to enroll or maintain Medicare billing privileges, all DMEPOS suppliers must become accredited. The accreditation requirement applies to suppliers of durable medical equipment, medical supplies, home dialysis supplies and equipment, therapeutic shoes, parenteral/enteral nutrition, transfusion medicine and prosthetic devices, and prosthetics and orthotics.

Other federal and state laws pertain to fraudulent billing practices. If you become aware of any suspicion of fraudulent billing occurring in your practice, you are expected to bring the circumstances to the attention of your practice's compliance officer.

For more information, visit:

- PECOS (www.aao.org/pecos)

- DMEPOS (www.aao.org/dme)

Coding

Coding is a vital process for ophthalmic practices. It is important for all personnel involved in the practice to understand the basic principles and purposes of coding. Coding errors can be costly to the practice when incorrect or no payment is made. Coding errors may also result in third-party payer audits, which often result in the practice refunding significant dollars back to the payer. Ophthalmic medical personnel need to know what the physician requires for documentation, but also the rules and regulations of the payers.

Coding Systems

Coding is the application of selecting appropriate Current Procedural Terminology (CPT) code(s) for exams, testing services, and surgical procedures and linking them to associated International Classification of Diseases Clinical Modification (ICD-9-CM) diagnosis code(s).

CPT   The CPT system is divided into numerous sections. Those sections most commonly used to describe ophthalmic services are Evaluation and Management; Integumentary System; Eye and Ocular Adnexa (Table 19.1 shows examples from this section); Radiology; Special Testing Services; Category II codes, which are designed to report Physician Quality Reporting

Table 19.1 Examples of CPT Codes, Eye and Ocular Adnexa Section

Code	Indication
66984	Extracapsular cataract removal with insertion of intraocular lens prosthesis
67904	Repair of blepharoptosis, levator resection or advancement, external approach
67810	Biopsy of eyelid
67800	Excision of chalazion, single
67820	Correction of trichiasis, epilation, by forceps only
65730	Keratoplasty (corneal transplant); penetrating (except aphakia)

System (PQRS) measures; and Category III codes, which are codes designed to describe new technology. Category II and III codes are numeric-alpha. See Table 19.2 for examples of these codes.

Appropriate coding requires adherence to the rules of CPT. Two extracted rules are described here:

- Although the index may be used to initially locate a code, do not code directly from the index. Always read the complete description in the main body of the manual before selecting a code.

- Do not choose a code that only approximates the service that was performed. CPT specifically indicates that a code should only be selected if it accurately describes the service. There are "unlisted" codes that can be utilized when necessary to describe services for which no specific CPT descriptor applies.

Table 19.2 Examples of Category II and Category III Codes

Category II	
0014F	Cataracts: comprehensive preoperative assessment for cataract surgery with intraocular lens (IOL) placement
2027F	Primary open-angle glaucoma: optic nerve evaluation
2022F	Dilated eye exam in diabetic patient
Category III	
0187T	Scanning computerized ophthalmic diagnostic imaging, anterior segment, with interpretation and report, unilateral
0192T	Insertion of anterior segment aqueous drainage device, without extraocular reservoir; external approach

ICD-9-CM The ICD-9-CM coding system under the auspices of the World Health Organization. ICD-9-CM is a listing of illnesses, symptoms, injuries, and other factors influencing a patient's condition. It consists of 3- to 5-digit codes with narrative descriptors. The examples shown in Table 19.3 are from Section 6, Diseases of the Nervous System and Sense Organs.

V codes are those that describe other factors influencing a patient's condition, but do not specifically describe an illness from which the patient is suffering. V codes also include issues of a family history of a particular condition (Table 19.4).

E codes describe external causes of injury and poisoning. They are of greatest use when submitting claims for which the patient's insurance company may not be responsible for payment, such as for worker's compensation benefits (Table 19.5).

In addition to the tabular list, ICD-9-CM contains an alphabetic index that closely correlates with the tabular list. For example, the alphabetic index contains a section named "glaucoma," with the subtypes of glaucoma indicated under the main heading. The index will help you find the detailed tabular section for the specific code you may be seeking.

It is important to abide by the rules of ICD-9 coding. Three extracted rules are described here:

- Diagnosis selection should never be prepared from the alphabetic index. Any code that appears correct in the alphabetic index should be crosschecked in the tabular list, where a more detailed descriptor can be found.

- The diagnosis code should be finalized to the highest level of specificity. For example, assume the correct diagnosis is "primary open angle glaucoma." It is then appropriate to choose this code (365.11), rather than the code for "open angle glaucoma" (365.1) or, simply, "glaucoma" (365).

- A "suspected" diagnosis should not be coded. A diagnosis of symptoms or signs is instead appropriate when a definite diagnosis has not been made. For example, an elderly patient may present with headaches and transient visual loss. The doctor may suspect a diagnosis of temporal arteritis. The appropriate diagnosis in this example would be "headache" or "transient visual loss," depending on the principal complaint. It would not be appropriate to code "temporal arteritis." If the patient is later found to actually have temporal arteritis, then "temporal arteritis" would be an appropriate diagnosis to use on follow-up visits.

Table 19.3 Examples of ICD-9-CM Codes

Code	Indication
366.16	Cataract, senile, nuclear sclerosis
365.11	Primary open angle glaucoma
373.2	Chalazion
378.05	Alternating esotropia
366.53	After-cataract, obscuring vision
361.32	Horseshoe tear of retina without detachment

Table 19.4 Examples of V Codes

Code	Indication
V43.1	Lens pseudophakia
V45.61	Cataract extraction status
V19.0	Family history blindness or visual loss
V41.0	Problem with sight
V52.2	Fitting and adjusting artificial eye

Table 19.5 Examples of E Codes

Code	Indication
E800	Railway accidents
E810	Motor vehicle traffic accidents
E830	Water transport accidents
E880	Accidental falls
E900	Accidents due to natural and environmental factors

HEALTHCARE COMMON PROCEDURE CODING SYSTEM This is a third system for coding. This system is a group of alpha-numeric codes that cover injectable drugs and optical codes for glasses and contact lenses.

The Benefits of Proper Coding

Specifically, coding facilitates the processing of insurance claims. Payment is more appropriately directed when the proper codes are used. Coding also provides a benefit in the area of research. Imagine that a researcher was interested in studying the characteristics of patients with lesions of the eyelid margin. A search could be conducted on patients on whom CPT code 67840 had been performed. This would provide a quick source of data on patients with this condition.

Perhaps the most important benefit of the coding system is enhanced patient satisfaction. Patients expect, and have a right to, information regarding the care they receive. The coding system is designed to provide straightforward information about what services have been rendered and why they were medically necessary.

Documentation

A key principle of coding is that documentation in the medical record must support code selection. It is commonly stated that "if it isn't documented, it didn't happen." The use of a particular code implies that specific services were rendered. The best, and sometimes the only, way in which these services can be substantiated is through the medical record. Practically speaking, the appropriate code for a service is based upon the recorded events rather than what actually may have transpired face-to-face with the patient.

About ICD-10

In the United States, the ICD-9 system is being replaced by the ICD-10 system, effective October 1, 2013. The ICD-10 diagnosis code set is a 6-digit code with a seventh digit extension that allows for greater specificity. ICD-9 has approximately 17,000 diagnosis codes and ICD-10 has approximately 141,000. Additional ICD-10 benefits include better profiling due to the specificity of data collected, improved clinical information for research, clearer code choices, clearer reimbursement guidelines, and, ultimately, fewer denials of claims. The transition is necessary because ICD-9 was introduced in 1983 and terminology and classification for some conditions are outdated and obsolete. Because many European countries have already converted to ICD-10, comparison with international data is hindered.

Here's a peek into ICD-10:

- There will be specific codes for right and left eyes.
- E codes will become W, X, and Y codes.
- Injuries and surgical complications will become S and T codes.
- Congenital problems are found in the Q codes.

Table 19.6 gives an example of detail found in ICD-10, compared to ICD-9.

Code Linking and Medical Necessity

Successful coding practice requires that an appropriate "linkage" be established between a service (CPT code) and the diagnosis (ICD-9 code) for which the service was rendered. This is largely because the payer will expect that there was a legitimate need for a particular service.

One way in which legitimacy is demonstrated is through the listing of a plausible diagnosis for a particular service.

For example, it is reasonable to see a diagnosis of 365.11, "primary open-angle glaucoma," linked to service 92083, "visual field examination, extended examination." It is less reasonable to see a diagnosis of 374.11, "ectropion, senile" linked to service 92083.

It is very likely that inappropriate linkages will result in a denied claim. In the first example, there is a good chance that the claim will be paid. In the second example, the claim will be denied.

Closely related to code linking is the concept of medical necessity. Medical necessity can be defined as services that are "furnished in accordance with accepted standards of medical practice for the diagnosis or treatment of the patient's condition or to improve the function of a malformed body member." Basically, medical necessity means the service meets, but does not exceed, the patient's medical need.

Medical necessity is required for appropriate code linking to occur. However, just because a diagnosis is listed in a manual as linked to a particular service does not mean that the service is always medically necessary. For example, medically necessary services in a glaucoma patient might include 92020, "gonioscopy" and 92250, "fundus photography with interpretation and report." However, these services would not in general be considered medically necessary if they were repeated within a short time in an otherwise stable glaucoma patient. All Medicare payers have local coverage determination (LCD) coverage policies for many ophthalmic tests and surgical procedures. LCDs detail coverage policies as well as provide a list of covered diagnosis codes. This information can be found on each Medicare payer website. For a list of payer websites, visit www.aao.org/coding.

Table 19.6 Comparison of Chalazion Diagnosis Codes, ICD-9 CM and ICD-10 CM

ICD-9 CM	
373.2	Chalazion

ICD-10 CM	
H00.11	Chalazion right upper eyelid
H00.12	Chalazion right lower eyelid
H00.13	Chalazion right eye, unspecified eyelid
H00.14	Chalazion left upper eyelid
H00.15	Chalazion left lower eyelid
H00.16	Chalazion left eye, unspecified eyelid
H00.19	Chalazion unspecified eye, unspecified eyelid

Coding for Ophthalmology Office Visits

Coding for an office visit in ophthalmology requires some initial thought. One of the biggest issues that ophthalmologists face is whether to use codes from the Evaluation and Management (E&M) section or from the General Ophthalmological Services section of the CPT manual to describe these services.

E&M codes include 99201 through 99205 (new patients) and 99211 through 99215 (established patients). These codes are available to describe office or outpatient services in any field of medical practice. As such, ophthalmologists may use them.

Codes from the General Ophthalmological Services section include 92002 and 92004 (new patients) and 92012 and 92014 (established patients). Eye care is unique in that special codes are available (distinct from E&M management codes) for describing common office visits. These services are generally known as the "Eye codes."

Ophthalmologists and other eye care practitioners may select between E&M and Eye codes for any given encounter. Documentation standards for management E&M services are recognized on a national basis. However, the standards for the Eye codes vary by state and by payer. The CPT manual contains descriptions for both E&M and Eye codes. However, for the Eye codes, payer descriptions (when provided) override the CPT descriptions when it comes to adjudicating a claim.

EVALUATION AND MANAGEMENT SERVICES Specific criteria must be followed if codes from the E&M section of the CPT are used to describe office services. The key components used to determine the appropriate level of code from this section are history, examination, and medical decision making.

The history component includes the chief complaint (CC), history of present illness (HPI), review of systems (ROS), and past medical, family, and social history (PFSH). Of these, the chief complaint is the most important since it "drives" all the other elements of the encounter with the patient.

The CC is the statement that describes the reason for the visit, usually in the patient's own words. The HPI expands upon the chief complaint. According to CPT, the HPI includes these elements: location, quality, severity, duration, context, modifying factors, and associated signs and symptoms.

The ROS is a battery of questions that investigates the status of various body systems. CPT has identified 14 different body systems of potential interest. These 14 systems taken together incorporate the entire spectrum of body functions.

The past history is the history of the patient's past illnesses and surgeries. Also included in the past history are the patient's current medications and allergies.

Family history refers to the medical status of relatives of the patient. Of particular interest here would be the existence of hereditary illness that place the patient at risk. Social history includes information use of alcohol and tobacco. It may also include information about a patient's employment, use of other drugs, marital status, educational level, and sexual history.

The eye exam, from a coding perspective, includes all of the familiar components such as visual acuity, extraocular motility, slit lamp examination, tonometry, and ophthalmoscopy. The examination is broken down in such a way, for purposes of coding, to represent 12 separate elements and a mental assessment of the patient.

Medical decision making refers to the complexity of the patient's number of problems and diagnosis; the type of data, such as ordering and/or reviewing tests, reviewing old records, or receiving history from someone other than the patient; and the amount and/or complexity of data, which includes the level of risk and management options.

Eye Codes

Comprehensive ophthalmological services are defined by CPT as the general evaluation of the complete visual system, including initiation or continuation of diagnostic and treatment programs. In order to qualify, a service must include these elements: chief complaint, history, general medical observation, external examination, gross visual fields, sensorimotor exam, and fundus exam. Often, this service will include slit lamp exam, tonometry, and the use of dilation.

Intermediate ophthalmological services are defined by CPT as the evaluation of a new or existing condition complicated with a new diagnostic or management problem not necessarily relating to the primary diagnosis, including initiation or continuation of a diagnostic and treatment program. This level of service requires chief complaint, history, general medical observation, and external ocular and adnexal examination. Dilation is sometimes performed as a component of this service.

As may be apparent, the Eye codes are less specifically defined than are the E&M codes. Partially in response to this, a number of insurance companies (including Medicare carriers) have created their own definitions for comprehensive and intermediate ophthalmological services. These are generally much more specific than the guidelines in CPT.

An ophthalmology practice must be familiar with the descriptions of the Eye codes for all the various payers with whom they interact. This is the only way in which the practice can intelligently choose between use of the eye codes and the E&M codes for any given encounter.

Coding, although challenging, need not be made overly complex. An appreciation of fundamentals is an excellent first step toward achieving competency in this area.

Ophthalmic Coding Specialist

For many ophthalmic medical personnel, coding is a new skill. Those who acquire this skill bring much greater value to their practices. Educational opportunities in the area of coding are available through several organizations including the American Academy of Ophthalmology and the Joint Commission on Allied Health Personnel in Ophthalmology (JCAHPO).

The American Academy of Ophthalmic Executives in conjunction with JCAHPO offer a coding competency exam. Those who successfully pass the online exam are given the title of Ophthalmic Coding Specialist (OCS). For additional information, visit www.aao.org/ocs.

In Review

Management is the key to your success and the success of the practice. You are taking this course to develop the knowledge and skills necessary to be a valuable member of the eye care team. How successful you become will depend upon the effective management of your attitude, your time, your communications and your clinical skills. You can become extremely valuable to the practice by assisting your office manager and doctor through learning and complying with the management policies and procedures developed by the practice.

SELF-ASSESSMENT TEST

1. How many people will a patient that is dissatisfied tell about your practice?

2. List 6 measures of practice productivity.

3. What is ophthalmic practice benchmarking?

4. List 3 positive ways you can help the doctor to better manage his or her time seeing patients.

5. List 3 behaviors that you should avoid that will help assure clinic efficiency.

6. What one thing do you control at work that always affects patient and staff satisfaction?

7. List 4 impediments to practice efficiency that technicians must avoid.

8. How do the Federal laws known as HIPAA, OSHA, DMEPOS, and PECOS impact your office?

9. Name at least 4 reasons for correct coding for services provided in a doctor's office.

10. What are codes called that describe services and procedures?

11. What are codes called that describe illnesses, symptoms, and injuries?

12. What do E-codes describe?

13. What are 3 rules of ICD-9 coding?

14. What are the 4 components of a history in E&M coding?

15. What are 2 rules of CPT coding?

SUGGESTED ACTIVITIES

1. With the assistance of your coworkers compile a list of at least 5 items that would improve patient satisfaction during their office visit.

2. To impart better team work and establish cross-training ask your practice manager or doctor for an opportunity to learn some of the business office procedures.

3. Use an ICD-9 code book to find the numerical designation for the following diagnoses:

    a. alternating exotropia

    b. acute angle-closure glaucoma

    c. hordeolum externum

    d. blepharitis, unspecified

    e. traumatic cataract

4. Use a CPT book to find the numerical designation for the following procedures:

    a. repair of retinal detachment by scleral buckle

    b. insertion of intraocular lens prosthesis (secondary implant)

    c. repair of brow ptosis, supraciliary

    d. trabeculoplasty by laser surgery

    e. discission of secondary membranous cataract (posterior capsulotomy) by laser surgery

SUGGESTED RESOURCES

American Academy of Ophthalmic Executives. *Ophthalmic Coding Series.* This multi-part series walks ophthalmologists, technicians, and coding staff through the what, why, and how of ophthalmic coding. It's the most comprehensive and up-to-date ophthalmic coding training available. For more information, visit www.aao.org/aaoe.

American Medical Association (AMA). The AMA offers various online and print resources related to coding and compliance. For more information, visit www.ama-assn.org.

Practice Management Information Corporation. This publisher offers a variety of medical coding and compliance resources such as the *ICD-9-CM Code Book* and *ICD-10-CM Code Book.* For more information, visit http://pmiconline.stores.yahoo.net.

20 MEDICAL ETHICS, LEGAL ISSUES, AND REGULATORY ISSUES

Ethical behavior is guided by moral principles and values that dictate standards of conduct that must be met. Guiding principles are inspirational goals that may be difficult to achieve, but should always be something professionals strive to achieve. The importance of ethical behavior on the part of health care providers has long been recognized. Although the principles remain the same, the requirements as set forth in law and regulations affect everyone in health care. It is therefore essential that all ophthalmic technicians know both the principles and the regulations to avoid unethical behavior. In addition to reviewing the history and principles of ethical behavior in ophthalmology, the chapter also provides an overview of your responsibilities as an ophthalmic medical assistant, including your role in the office or clinic.

History

At the completion of medical school, new doctors receive a diploma, but many also recite and adopt a statement of ethical principles often referred to as the Hippocratic Oath. Although it is not binding, this statement of ethical principles has guided doctors for 2500 years. At the very first official meeting of the American Medical Association in 1847, the only items on the agenda were the establishment of minimum standards of education and training for physicians and the establishment of a code of ethics for physicians. Many ethical concepts are now codified by federal and state law, and the field of medical ethics is considered so important and complex that advanced degrees in medical ethics are granted at many universities. Hospitals and large offices have a designated individual or department to be sure they are in compliance with legal regulations and ethical requirements, and a well defined process for resolving any ethical conflicts. Continuing education (CE) requirements for physicians often include a requirement for a minimum number of hours of CE courses in ethics.

Code of Ethics of the Academy

The American Academy of Ophthalmology has developed a Code of Ethics for its members. This code addresses the ophthalmologist's conduct and relates to what behavior is appropriate or inappropriate as determined by the Academy. The principles of ethics contained in the Academy's code are paraphrased in Table 20.1. The ethical guidelines they present are applicable only to ophthalmologists, but ophthalmic medical assistants who work with them will benefit from understanding the ethical goals they represent.

Ethics for Assistants

Because ophthalmic technicians work under the direct supervision of their ophthalmologists, the same principles and rules that guide your doctor should guide you, with some modification to reflect your role as an assistant. In addition, you must be aware of the laws and regulations that govern your actions as an ophthalmic assistant in the state or country in which you work. For

Table 20.1 Guidelines from the American Academy of Ophthalmology Code of Ethics

An issue of ethics in ophthalmology is resolved by the determination that the best interest of the patient is served.

Ophthalmologic services must be provided with compassion, respect for human dignity, honesty, and integrity.

An ophthalmologist must maintain competence by continued study. That competence must be supplemented with the talents of other professionals and with consultation when indicated.

Open communication with the patient is essential. Patient confidences must be safeguarded within the constraints of the law.

Fees for ophthalmologic services must not exploit patients or others who pay for the services.

If a member has a reasonable basis for believing that another person has deviated from professionally accepted standards in a manner that adversely affects patient care or from the Rules of Ethics, the member should attempt to prevent the continuation of this conduct by communicating with the other person or by notifying the appropriate authorities.

It is the responsibility of an ophthalmologist to act in the best interest of the patient.

It is the responsibility of the ophthalmologist to maintain integrity in clinical and basic research.

example, care must be taken to avoid interpreting tests for patients or recommending treatments or medications on your own as this would be considered practicing medicine and could even lead to criminal charges. Other tasks such as refractometry or administration of eyedrops—often considered routine for ophthalmic assistants—may be prohibited in some areas. When in doubt, check with your ophthalmologist to determine what tasks you are permitted to perform.

> Beyond the letter of the law, your professional conduct should always be impeccable and mirror the Academy's Code of Ethics that guides ophthalmologists.

Ethical Behavior

As an ophthalmic technician, you should always keep the best interests of the patient in mind. It is often said we should treat our patients as we would want our family members treated. This guiding principle will go a long way to resolving ethical questions regarding the conduct of ophthalmic technicians when they arise.

All patients should be greeted in a professional, friendly manner that will help set the tone for the visit. It is often best to start with an introduction when you see a new patient and clearly state that you are an ophthalmic assistant working with Dr. Jones and you will gather information to assist the doctor with their visit today. If you are certified, you can mention your credential when you introduce yourself. You should only use the credentials that you have actually attained through the appropriate means and maintained as required. If a patient mistakes you for a doctor, nurse, or other licensed health care provider, you must clarify your status immediately. Some formal training programs have clinical rotations and, if you are participating in patient testing or evaluation during your training period, you should make this fact clear as well and assure the patient that you are working under the guidance of experienced technicians and the ophthalmologist. Some patients may not wish to have a trainee involved in their care, but more often they are glad to interact with a young professional entering the field of eye care. Be sure to thank the patients who make this important contribution to your training.

All patients should have a clear explanation of any test that you perform, including how the test will be done, why the test is being done, and what they should expect during the test. You should, however, refrain from discussing test results, diagnoses, or treatment options until the ophthalmologist asks you to do so. Making diagnoses and prescribing treatment is the practice of medicine and if you do so without the guidance of an ophthalmologist you could be guilty of practicing medicine without a license. You should avoid giving advice to friends, neighbors or family members, even if the situation seems obvious.

Ophthalmic medical assistants should always remember that office supplies, materials, and medications are the property of the office and should never be removed for personal use—or to give to someone else—without permission. It is also important to be diligent in refraining from personal use of office computers and personal cell phones during business hours.

Providing Technical Services

As an ophthalmic technician you will play an integral part in providing compassionate care for the patients who come to your office. It has been said that your integrity is shown by what you do when no one is watching. All evaluations and tests should be performed to the best of your abilities, and you must carefully document the results. It is important to realize that patients are often anxious or frightened when they have a problem, and you must treat them with understanding and compassion.

You must carefully document the results of your evaluation of the patient and never claim to have done exam elements or tests that were not performed. It is important to deal honestly with your doctor, colleagues, and patients. If you make a mistake, you must inform the doctor so any necessary corrective action can be taken.

Competence of Technicians

As a technician, your competency in performing your tasks has a direct impact on the ability of the ophthalmologist to make appropriate diagnoses and decisions. Whether your training was the result of a formal training program or obtained on the job, you must be able to perform all required tasks and tests. However, as an eye care professional, simple competency is not enough. You should strive to enhance your knowledge and skills through continuing education and study.

One way that you can validate your competency is through JCAHPO Certification as discussed in Chapter 1. In review, the Joint Commission on Allied Health Personnel in Ophthalmology was established in 1969 and grants certification to ophthalmic assistants at these core levels:

- Certified Ophthalmic Assistants (COA)—individuals typically new to the field who have met minimum standard of competency for common tasks

- Certified Ophthalmic Technicians (COT)—the intermediate level of certification for those with more experience

- Certified Ophthalmic Medical Technologist (COMT)—the highest level of certification

The certification process is based on a careful analysis of tasks being performed by technicians at the various levels of certification and assures you, the ophthalmologist, and your patients that you have met minimum standards of competency in key areas. For the COA level, only a written test is required. For higher levels of certification, a written test followed by a skills evaluation is required. Candidates must first meet requirements to qualify for the examination.

JCAHPO expects their certificants to adhere to the highest ethical and professional standards and will investigate alleged violations. If it is determined that a certificant has not adhered to the standards, their certification may be suspended or revoked. Table 20.2 lists grounds for JCAHPO to deny, revoke, or otherwise act upon certification or recertification eligibility.

Communication With Patients

All patients have the right to clear and open communication, but it must be remembered that medical information is confidential and under most circumstances, only the patient can give permission for their protected health information to be shared with others, and that permission must be obtained in writing. This principle has been codified in law under the Health Insurance Portability and Accountability Act of 1996—often referred to as "HIPAA regulations." You should be familiar with the requirements of this law as the penalties for violation are severe. There are certain exceptions. You are allowed to share information with other health care professionals for continuity of care, and insurers who are responsible for payment are also permitted to get protected health information without written permission from the patient.

Adherence to the principle of confidentiality requires great care and awareness, and doing so may sometimes seem rude or illogical. Communication with a spouse or relative requires written permission. Well-meaning inquiries regarding a friend or acquaintance who is also a patient in your office must be gently rebuked: "I am sorry; we are not allowed to share any patient information without their permission."

In addition all written patient information must be protected from casual discovery by other patients or visitors to the office, such as salespeople and spouses. This applies to charts, test results, and information on computer

Table 20.2 Grounds for JCAHPO to Deny, Revoke, or Otherwise Act on Certification or Recertification Eligibility

Obtaining or attempting to obtain certification or recertification for oneself or another by fraud or deception of material fact in an application or any other communication to JCAHPO, including but not limited to: (a) misstatement of a material fact, and (b) failure to make statement of a material fact, or (c) failure to provide information requested by JCAHPO.

Providing or attempting to provide ophthalmic services except as specifically delegated by an ophthalmologist.

Misrepresentation of JCAHPO certification or certification status, including but not limited to falsification of documents, use of credential while on non-certified status, and use of credentials without attainment.

Irregularity in connection with any JCAHPO examination, including but not limited to copying answers or permitting another to copy answers for any examination.

Unauthorized distribution of, possession of, use of or access to pertinent materials or information regarding questions or answers relating to any JCAHPO examination or other confidential JCAHPO documents.

Gross or repeated negligence or malpractice in providing ophthalmic care.

Personal use of alcohol or any drug or substance to a degree which impairs professional performance providing ophthalmic care.

Any physical or mental condition which impairs competent professional ophthalmic care performance.

Physical or sexual abuse of a patient.

The conviction of, plea of guilty, or plea of nolo contendere to a crime which is directly related to public health, safety, or professional performance providing ophthalmic care.

Failure to cooperate reasonably with any JCAHPO investigation of a disciplinary matter.

Unauthorized disclosure of confidential information.

(From JCAHPO *Criteria for Certification & Recertification,* ©2008, pages 43–44. Used with permission.)

screens. Care must also be taken to avoid discussions with patients within the earshot of other people, which may take place when patients are checking in or out, or walking from room to room in the examination area.

Informed Consent and Ophthalmic Assistants

The concept of informed consent is based on the principle of individual autonomy and the ultimate right of each patient to weigh information from health care providers and other sources and decide what treatments and interventions they will allow.

Informed consent for a procedure or treatment can only be obtained by the physician. However, ophthalmic assistants often play an important role in preparing the patient with written or verbal educational materials. Patients often have questions they will ask you before they see the doctor, and you should be able to answer simple questions about the procedure. In addition, many offices utilize videotapes or DVDs to educate patients on common procedures. If you are asked questions that you are not comfortable answering, tell the patient to be sure to ask the doctor during his or her visit, and make a note for the doctor as the patient may not remember to ask the question after the doctor begins to talk.

Many individuals of all ages now approach a surgical procedure or intervention with considerable information they have gleaned from the Internet and other sources. It is important to assess the knowledge that the patient already has and correct any misconceptions. Written materials for the patient to take home and review at leisure are often part of the informed consent process.

An informed consent must include the following elements:

- The planned procedure or intervention, expected benefit of the procedure, and any reasonable alternatives should be discussed.

- Possible adverse events should be discussed in detail.

- Patients must understand what they need to do to prepare for the surgery, test, or treatment.

- Patients must know what to expect after the surgery, test, or treatment.

- Patients must have the opportunity to ask any questions before signing the consent form. Many patients will ask questions about insurance or financial information as well.

Some individuals still prefer that the doctor simply take charge and tell them what they should do. This may be based on a deep sense of trust that has developed over a long professional relationship, but sometimes it is simply the recognition on the part of patients that additional knowledge of possible complications will only make them more anxious. Even if a patient communicates to you that he or she does not wish to hear all the details, it does not relieve the doctor of the responsibility of explaining the potential complications and alternatives. It is important, however, to inform the doctor if the patient seems anxious, as the doctor may elect to provide the information in broad terms rather than great detail.

Rarely, individuals may be unable to adequately understand the information given to them in the informed consent process and do not have the capacity to give informed consent. Hopefully, a family member or a legal representative will have already obtained medical power of attorney and will be able to assist the patient in the decision. Often, you will spend a fair amount of time with a patient making surgical arrangements, performing biometry, and providing educational materials. If you believe a patient does not have the capacity to make an informed decision, you should report your concerns to the surgeon, who must then make a judgment regarding the competency of the patient to give informed consent.

In the area of refractive surgery and other elective procedures, it is known that certain types of patients are more likely to be unhappy with the outcome. For instance, demanding, precise people, sometimes referred to as "Type A," are sometimes not satisfied with their results, even if their acuity is quite good. If you feel that a patient you are seeing for evaluation of such a procedure may have unrealistic expectations, it is important to alert the ophthalmologist so he or she can assess that person's appropriateness as a candidate for the proposed surgery.

Ethics and Pharmaceutical Company Representatives

The relationship between physicians and the pharmaceutical industry has come under increased scrutiny in recent years, and there are now regulations that prohibit many practices that were common in the past. In 2002 the Pharmaceutical Research and Manufacturers of America (PhRMA) adopted voluntary policies for dealing with health care professionals, and revised the guidelines in 2008. The rules that went into effect in January of 2009 include the provisions highlighted in Table 20.3.

Although these rules apply primarily to physicians, you will have to abide by them as well, and remember that some offices and institutions (especially academic institutions) have adopted even stricter policies than those outlined above and refuse all materials including educational materials and patient samples. Be sure you understand and adhere to the policies adopted by your office.

Professional Conduct

It is important to remember that you represent the practice in which you work. Your appearance and conduct will often have a tremendous impact on a patient's impression of the practice. You will often see the patient before the ophthalmologist and may spend more time with the patient than the doctor. Patients will assume that your conduct has been approved by the doctor as appropriate for a professional office.

> Your appearance should be professional and conform to the standards of your office.

Appearance

Clothing should be neat and clean and appropriate for a professional office. For example, sandals, jeans, revealing clothing and elaborate jewelry are inappropriate. Some

Table 20.3 Selected Examples, PhRMA Code on Interactions With Health Care Professionals

Category	Interaction
Practice-related items	These items are explicitly prohibited including items of minimal value, such as pens, notepads, mugs or similar "reminder" items that are branded with the company's name or logo. The revised Code permits practice-related items that relate to a patient's disease or are intended to educate the patient.
Meals	Sales representatives may continue to host meals only if accompanied by a legitimate educational presentation.
Entertainment and recreation	Entertainment or recreational items including tickets to theatrical or sporting events, sporting equipment, or leisure or vacation trips, are prohibited—even if they are associated with a heath care provider's engagement as a speaker or consultant.
Consultants and speakers	All compensation and reimbursement of expenses should be based on fair market value.
Continuing medical education (CME)	All companies must separate grants for CME events from sales and marketing functions and follow the standards for commercial support of CME established by the Accreditation Council for Continuing Medical Education or other accrediting bodies.

offices have specific dress codes or require a uniform to avoid some of these issues, and you should be sure to conform with the office policy and have neat, clean uniforms available at all times.

Careful attention to personal hygiene is a must for ophthalmic medical assistants who work in close contact with patients daily. Personal cleanliness and daily use of a deodorant is important, along with careful attention to oral hygiene. Strong perfumes, colognes, and aftershaves should be avoided as they can irritate sensitive individuals. Fingernails should be clean and trimmed, as long nails could cause discomfort for patients.

Respect and Sensitivity

Patients who come to the office with serious problems are often frightened, anxious, or uncomfortable. It is important to deal with them in a compassionate, comforting manner. Most offices are very busy, but if patients feel you are rushing through their exam, or that you appear disinterested, they may believe you and the doctor do not care about their problem. It is important to remember that everyone's time is valuable and if patients are kept waiting you should explain the reason for the delay and apologize. Many offices have a policy for handling patients who are kept waiting and you should be familiar with your office's protocol.

In addition to ocular problems that are more common as we get older, many older patients also have other conditions that impair their hearing or mobility; be ready to assist them and put them at ease. It is important to remember that you can be professional and friendly at the same time. However, your friendliness should always respect the dignity and boundaries of the patient. Many individuals, especially older patients, do not wish to be addressed by their first name, but rather as Mr., Mrs., or Ms. You should only address an individual by his or her first name if they request you do so and it is in accordance with office policy.

It is also important to remember that in most parts of the country we find increasing diversity in the population. Dealing with a multicultural population requires some sensitivity and awareness of cultural norms for various groups, and insofar as is possible, their preferences and expectations should be respected. In addition, you will sometimes have patients with disabilities who require special accommodations, such as wheelchair accessibility or an interpreter who is able to sign for a hearing impaired patient. Federal law requires that accommodations be made for these special needs, but you must also be especially sensitive to treating these patients with dignity and respect.

The same respect and sensitivity you show patients should govern your interactions with others in your office. Doctors and other ophthalmic assistants should be treated with respect, and all interactions within the office should be professional, cordial, and appropriate. Casual conversations should not take place in the presence of patients, and any conflicts with co-workers should be addressed in a civil and professional manner. Many offices have defined processes for dealing with such conflicts, and you must know who mediates such issues in your office.

When one chooses to enter a health care profession, it is a commitment that goes beyond a simple job. You have chosen to become a professional who cares for patients and always keeps their best interests at heart. Standards of ethical conduct are mostly common sense and common courtesy, but legal and regulatory requirements can be complex. You must know the law in the state, province or country in which you work and you must always strive for the highest standards of professionalism. The experience can be demanding, but it can also be very satisfying. The opportunity to make a difference in the lives of your patients will be extremely rewarding to you.

Supplementary Topics

Many of the topics related to ethics and medical legal issues in this chapter are expanded in other sections of this study guide. Refer to the following chapters and topics for additional information:

- Chapter 6: Basics of Ophthalmic Pharmacology. Administration of eyedrops and the patient prescription.
- Chapter 7: Microorganisms and Infection Control. OSHA regulations and Universal Precautions.
- Chapter 15: Patient Interaction, Screening, and Emergencies. Patient greeting, triage procedures, appointment scheduling and emergencies.
- Chapter 16: Patients With Special Concerns. Relationship to families, confidentiality of health information, office waiting time, disruptive patient, responsibilities of treating children and the elderly, domestic violence (abuse), physically disabled patient and patient greeting.
- Chapter 17: Minor Surgical Assisting in the Office. Informed consent.
- Chapter 19: Understanding Practice Management. Office relationships, the medical record, practice policies and procedures, scribing, compliance issues, missed appointments, patient prescription, scheduling appointments, scheduling outside tests and copying medical records for a third party.

SELF-ASSESSMENT TEST

1. Informed consent must contain which group of the following elements?

    a. reason for procedure, alternatives, expected benefits, expected risks

    b. reason for procedure, doctor's qualifications, expected benefits, expected risks

    c. reason for procedure, alternatives, expected benefits, disclosure of any history of malpractice

    d. reason for procedure, alternatives, number of times the doctor has performed the procedure, expected risks

2. The doctor has asked you to explain to a patient what to expect after cataract surgery, including activity limitations. As you begin, the patient tells you she does not want to know any details. What should you do?

    a. Discontinue your discussion.

    b. Continue gently to explain that for the best result after surgery she will need to know this information.

    c. Inform the doctor and allow him or her to decide how to proceed.

    d. Continue as planned without any change to your discussion as this is required for informed consent.

3. A pharmaceutical sales representative is in your office providing information and medication samples. He goes to the chart staging area. To comply with HIPAA regulations, what should you do?

    a. Remove all charts from the area before he enters.

    b. Cover all patient identifiers—names on charts, patient lists, and so on.

    c. Do not allow the representative to enter the area under any circumstance.

    d. Do nothing; he is leaving materials and supplies to benefit the patients so no precautions are needed.

4. A pharmaceutical sales representative offers to take you and several other assistants to lunch. To comply with PhRMA guidelines, how should you proceed?

    a. It is acceptable to go to lunch as you are on your own time at lunch.

    b. You may never accept lunch from a pharmaceutical representative.

    c. You may accept lunch only if there will be educational activities associated with the lunch.

    d. You may accept lunch but it must be reported to the doctor or office manager.

5. You are seeing a patient with impaired hearing who uses sign language to communicate. He has requested an interpreter for the examination. What should you do?

    a. Explain that he must arrange for an interpreter to be present for all exams.

    b. Determine if anyone is available in the office to act as interpreter.

    c. Offer a note pad and pen as an option for completing the visit.

    d. Be certain an interpreter is available as required by federal law.

6. On the first hot summer day in a new office, you choose to wear sandals to work as you did in your last office, but the office manager informs you that they are not acceptable. What is the best way to proceed?

    a. Continue to wear what you wish; your personal choice of footwear should be of no concern to the office.

    b. Respect the standards for your new office; professional standards for dress may differ from office to office.

    c. File a complaint against the office with the State Medical Society.

    d. Check OSHA regulations to see if this is within the office manager's rights.

7. A new patient is in the waiting room for an urgent visit. After you take the patient to the exam room, you note that she looks anxious. What is the best way to begin?

    a. Help calm the patient by calling her by her first name to create a friendly atmosphere.

    b. Proceed with the history; an urgent visit requires the history taking begin without delay.

    c. Introduce yourself and explain that you will be gathering information and performing tests to help the doctor.

    d. Get the doctor immediately.

8. You have performed corneal pachymetry on a glaucoma suspect and you later realize you have reversed the right and left eye readings. What is the correct action to take?

    a. Disregard if the readings were similar within 5 micrometers of each other.

    b. Correct the mistake with a notation in the chart.

    c. Follow the office protocol or ask your supervisor on how to proceed.

    d. Do nothing; if the patient is stable and does not progress to glaucoma no correction is needed.

9. You are seeing a patient for a 2-week follow-up visit and there have been no changes in her problem list or medications for several visits. What is the best way to proceed?

    a. Transcribe the information from prior visits as the patient is stable.

    b. Ask the patient "Is everything the same?"

    c. Ask the patient how she is using her medications and if there are any new problems or symptoms.

    d. Ask the patient if she has any new symptoms.

10. You have been certified as a Certified Ophthalmic Technician (COT) by JCAHPO, but your certification expired. You intend to get the necessary continuing medical education credits and reinstate your certification, but you are not certain how long it will take. What is the best course of action to take?

    a. Discontinue use of "COT" after your name until the reinstatement is complete.

    b. Continue to use the credential, but explain renewal is in progress.

    c. Continue to use the credential because you still have the knowledge and skills required for certification.

    d. Continue to use the credential with existing patients who know you to be certified, but not with new patients.

SUGGESTED ACTIVITIES

1. To help in understanding the best ways to communicate with patients, comply with HIPAA regulations and deal effectively with difficult or unusual patients, try a role-playing session with some assistants acting as patients and others playing the role of ophthalmic medical assistant. Specific situations can be written on slips of paper and drawn randomly for performance. All participants should observe and exchange feedback and ideas.

2. Play medical ethics "Jeopardy." A quiz format game can be utilized as a fun way of exploring legal and ethical issues in the office or as part of a state society meeting.

3. Play HIPAA compliance "Scavenger Hunt." With your supervisor's permission challenge yourself and others in the office to look throughout your office for any places or situations where HIPAA violations may potentially occur.

4. Certification reflects your commitment to the profession of ophthalmic medical assisting and ensures that your training meets minimum professional standards for competence and conduct. Make a commitment to become certified after fulfilling the qualifications.

5. Join a national or state society for ophthalmic medical assistants. Association with other professionals from your area and around the country helps ensure high professional standards and gives you access to continuing education in all areas including ethics and regulatory matters. In addition, it provides a forum for discussion of professional concerns in all areas.

SUGGESTED RESOURCES

The following websites have specific information about ethics, legal and regulatory matters:

American Academy of Ophthalmology. *Code of Ethics.* Revised 2009. www.aao.org/about/ethics/code_ethics.cfm. Accessed August 3, 2011.

American Medical Association. *AMA Medical Assistant Code of Ethics and Medical Assistants Creed.* www.aama-ntl.org/about/code_creed.aspx. Accessed August 15, 2011.

In addition, most states have a Departments of Public Health and a Consumer Protection Agency with websites, and for the truly adventurous, most federal and state statutes are available online.

These organizations often have resources available online or at educational events that may assist you with questions regarding legal or ethical questions:

- American Medical Association (www.ama-assn.org)
- American Academy of Ophthalmology (www.aao.org)
- Joint Commission on Allied Health Personnel in Ophthalmology (www.jcahpo.org)
- Association of Technical Personnel in Ophthalmology (www.atpo.org)
- State medical societies
- State eye societies
- State societies for ophthalmic medical assistants (not all states have active societies)

21 COMMUNITY HEALTH EYE CARE

The term *community health* refers to the health status of a defined group of people or community, such as a country's or state's population, and the actions and conditions that protect and improve their health. Thus, community health eye care involves identifying and treating vision problems of a population. This includes attention to sociocultural aspects of patient care and the community's resources.

This chapter introduces you to the concepts, issues, and difficulties in delivering effective community eye care. It describes definitions of vision impairment and blindness; identifies the major global and local causes of reversible and irreversible blindness and vision loss; and describes VISION 2020 principles and strategies for implementation at a global and local level. In addition, it describes a team approach to eye care, basic features of community eye care programs and methods to develop and deliver health education information within the local community.

As ophthalmic assistants assume larger and more important roles in the delivery of eye care throughout the world, it is important to gain a broader perspective on ophthalmic care issues in the local and international arenas. Although the practice of ophthalmology varies by geographic region, socioeconomic strata and city vs rural settings, certain unifying principles are constant.

An *International Core Curriculum for Ophthalmic Assistants* was published in March 2009 in conjunction with the International Council of Ophthalmology and the International Joint Commission on Allied Health Personnel in Ophthalmology. This chapter was created to fulfill one of the outlined requirements for the international student; however, by reading this chapter, students in the United States will gain an understanding of the "bigger picture" of eye health care and the methods being applied to combat worldwide blindness.

Definitions of Vision Impairment and Blindness

Definitions of the severity of visual loss help to identify vision disorders affecting a population and the kind of treatment needed. However, these definitions may vary from country to country when used for determining visual impairment.

The World Health Organization's International Classification of Diseases, 10th edition, Clinical Modification (ICD-10-CM), defines 5 levels of visual impairment (Table 21.1). These levels are based on best-corrected vision. In the United States, the 1935 Aid to the Blind program in the Social Security Act defines legal blindness as either central visual acuity of 20/200 or less in the better eye with corrective glasses or central visual acuity of more than 20/200 if there is a visual field defect wherein the widest angle of the visual field is no greater than 20° in the better eye. This would correspond to the ICD-10-CM level category of visual impairment level 2. In the United States if your vision with eyeglasses or corrective lenses is 20/60 or worse, you are considered visually impaired (ICD-10-CM level 1). Limitation of side vision, abnormal color vision, or presence of double vision in a single eye may also determine visual impairment. (Chapter 17 introduces systems and concepts of coding.)

In 2002, the International Council of Ophthalmology (ICO) drafted a resolution regarding suggested changes to the ICD-10-CM. The most important change was to base visual impairment on "presenting" visual acuity not "best-corrected" acuity. The reason for this change was that the inability to obtain glasses results in visual impairment in many parts of the world. Indeed, this change in definition increases the worldwide incidence of visual impairment from 150 million to about 300 million. The visual impairment categories (1 to 5) were also assigned text descriptors.

Based on these criteria, the World Health Organization estimates that globally about 314 million people are visually impaired. Forty-five million of these people are blind. It has been estimated that over 80% of global visual impairment is preventable or treatable. Almost 90% of blind and visually impaired people live in low- and middle-income countries where access to eye care is often unavailable.

Governmental Definitions of Visual Impairment and Blindness

It is beyond the scope of this chapter to describe all governments' definitions of visual impairment. This information and statistics about individual nation demographics should be available through an Internet search.

Based on demographics from the 2000 United States Census, an estimated 937,000 (0.78%) Americans older than 40 years were blind (United States definition). An additional 2.4 million Americans (1.98%) had low vision. The study reports that low vision and blindness increase significantly with age, particularly in people over age 65. People 80 years of age and older currently make up 8% of the population, but account for 69% of blindness.

According to a 2008 report by Prevent Blindness America (see "Suggested Resources"), there are more than 3.6 million visually impaired and more than 1 million cases of blindness in the group of Americans 40 years and older. Data indicates that the prevalence of blindness and vision impairment increases rapidly in the later years, particularly after age 75. In addition, blindness affects African Americans more frequently than Caucasians and Hispanics.

Table 21.1 World Health Organization's ICD-10-CM Levels of Visual Impairment

Category of visual impairment	Visual acuity with best possible correction	
	Maximum less than:	Minimum equal to or better than:
1	6/18 3/10 (0.3), 20/70 6/60	6/60 1/10 (0.1), 20/200 3/60
2	1/10 (0.1), 20/200 3/60	1/20 (0.05), 20/400 1/60 (finger-counting at 1 meter)
3	1/20 (0.05), 20/400 1/60 (finger-counting at 1 meter), 1/50	1/50 (0.02), 5/300 (20/1200) Light perception
4	(0.02), 5/300	
5	No light perception	
9	Undetermined or unspecified	

Depending upon the demographics of the practice or clinic and the aging population, ophthalmic assistants will find increasing numbers of senior patients with visual impairment seeking care at ophthalmic offices.

Major Causes of Reversible and Irreversible Blindness

Based on 2004 data (Figure 21.1), globally, the major causes of blindness are cataract (39%), uncorrected refractive errors (18%), glaucoma (10%), age-related macular degeneration (AMD) (7%), corneal opacity (4.3%), diabetic retinopathy (4%), trachoma (3%), eye conditions in children (3%), and onchocerciasis (0.7%). Of these conditions, only glaucoma, AMD and diabetic retinopathy are considered irreversible but they are treatable. See Chapter 7 for additional information about trachoma (3%) and onchocerciasis (0.7%). Although these conditions are unlikely to be encountered in most ophthalmology offices and clinics in the United States, they are problematic in the developing world.

In the United States, the leading causes of blindness among the Caucasian population are AMD (54.4%), cataract (8.7%), glaucoma (6.4%) and diabetic retinopathy (DR) (5.4%). While among African Americans, cataract (36.8%), glaucoma (26%), and DR (5.4%) were most common. Cataract was the leading cause of low vision in America, responsible for approximately 50% of bilateral vision worse than 6/12 (20/40) among Caucasian, African American, and Hispanic persons.

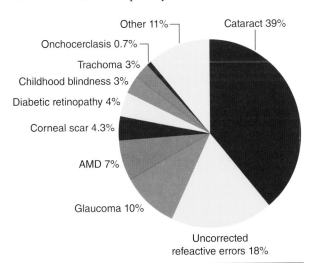

Figure 21.1 Global causes of blindness due to eye diseases and uncorrected refractive errors. *(Reprinted, with permission, from "VISION 2020, The Right to Sight, Global Initiative for the Elimination of Avoidable Blindness, Action Plan 2006–2011," page 4, © 2007. www.who.int/blindness/ Vision2020_report.pdf.)*

VISION 2020: The Right to Sight

In 1999 the World Health Organization and the International Agency for the Prevention of Blindness, in collaboration with international nongovernmental organizations, launched a program called "VISION 2020: the Right to Sight." The strategy of VISION 2020 is built upon a foundation of community participation, with 3 essential components or elements: cost-effective disease control interventions; human resource development (training and motivation); and infrastructure development (facilities, appropriate technology, consumables, funds).

Its mission is to develop the infrastructure, personnel, and economic strategy to address the problems of visual impairment worldwide. VISION 2020 seeks to eliminate the main causes of avoidable blindness in order to give all people in the world, particularly the millions of needlessly blind, the right to sight. Over two decades, it is hoped that VISION 2020 will prevent 100 million people from becoming blind. The goal is to eliminate avoidable blindness by the year 2020. This goal should be achieved through the establishment of a comprehensive eye care system as part of every national health system.

In 2009, the World Health Organization announced an action plan for continued progress on VISION 2020, which included the following objectives:

- Strengthen advocacy to increase Member States' political, financial and technical commitment in order to eliminate avoidable blindness and visual impairment. (The United States has many representatives in this effort, along with the American Academy of Ophthalmology.)

- Develop and strengthen national policies, plans, and programs for eye health and prevention of blindness and visual impairment.

- Increase and expand research for the prevention of blindness and visual impairment.

- Improve coordination between partnerships and stakeholders at national and international levels for the prevention of blindness and visual impairment.

- Monitor progress in elimination of avoidable blindness at national, regional and global levels.

VISION 2020's focus is on planning eye care needs for populations of about one million people has led to a shift in how the planners think about human resources for eye care; the days of just training a clinician or nurse and "parachuting" him or her into a clinic or hospital without technical support are waning. Planning now entails consideration of the entire support team needed to provide eye care: ophthalmologist, ophthalmic nurse, optometrist or refractionist, and surgical and ophthalmic technician. One measure of success of VISION 2020 is that the most recent World Health Organization estimates indicate that visual impairment has been reduced worldwide from 314 million people in 2004, to 285.3 million in 2010.

Strategies for Improving Utilization of Eye Care

Tragically, an estimated 80% of the world's blindness could be treated or altogether avoided with access to quality eye care. Almost 90% of these individuals live in the developing world. Estimates from 1995 suggest that more than 80% of cataract-blinded individuals would die before they had an opportunity for surgery and many of those in the developing world were dissatisfied or even blinded in the operative eye due to low-quality outcomes. Thus, despite the tremendous backlog for eye care services, the quality of that care must be sufficient to meet this need.

Critical barriers to worldwide quality eye care and successful approaches to overcoming them are outlined below:

- physical and geographical barriers worsened by the disproportionate distribution of adequately skilled health care providers to major cities or private practice clinics

- language, educational, and cultural barriers

- financial limitations, especially to expenditure on the elderly

- fear of surgery, lack of knowledge, poor quality services, and mistrust of the medical community

Community mobilization is a process through which action is stimulated by a community itself, or by others, that is planned, carried out, and evaluated by a community's individuals, groups, and organizations on a participatory and sustained basis to improve the health, hygiene and education levels so as to enhance the overall standard of living in the community. A critical component to any successful blindness prevention program is to reach those of greatest need living in remote or lower-resource conditions with limited education and/or social support. Community engagement and managed resources are critical to overcoming the barriers described above and maintaining an ongoing network to locate and assist patients suffering from blindness.

Without a social network and community empowerment, the individual patient often lacks the adequate support to initiate the process toward sight restoration. The key points and objectives to recognize and incorporate into such community-based strategies in global blindness include:

- attitudes and resources within the community

- creating public awareness and appropriate education programs about blindness

- managing participation in the community

- self-management of programs, ownership, and sustainability of community mobilization

- the rights of and decisions of the individual

In summary, successful community-based eye care programs that have overcome such barriers have commonly raised public awareness with an educational program and used high-quality patient screening programs and surgical interventions.

In the United States, medical societies, hospitals and other community health groups have organized health fairs inviting the public to be screened for various medical conditions including eye problems. Ophthalmic assistants frequently volunteer to screen patients for glaucoma and macular degeneration.

Local Delivery of Health Education Information

While the focus of many efforts in international ophthalmology is often on surgical care and "curable" blindness, many commonly encountered causes of blindness (especially infectious and nutritious) could be best addressed by nonsurgical, public health strategies that avoid the initial cause of blinding conditions altogether. Such etiologies of "preventable blindness" include trauma, vitamin A deficiency, and infectious causes (including trachoma, infectious keratitis, river blindness, rubella, cataract, and HIV).

Screening Programs

The impact of early intervention can be profound in the life of a blinded patient. The importance of school screening programs for children cannot be overlooked. For example, childhood cataract is the most common treatable cause of childhood blindness, being responsible for 10% to 30% of all childhood blindness. Preventing blindness from childhood cataract requires not only high-quality pediatric surgery, but also an awareness of the parents' ability to understand and comply with treatment. Childhood blindness has huge socioeconomic costs, and restoring the sight of a single child blind from cataract is considered equivalent to restoring the sight of 10 elderly adults. It is important to recognize that such screening and prevention programs are not only important in diseases like pediatric cataract but also in amblyopia, glaucoma, and diabetic retinopathy.

Surgical Programs

While many surgical programs that address international blindness focus on the numbers of eyes treated, the need to monitor impact or skill transfer to local eye care professionals should not be ignored. This builds capacity (through human resource development) within the local community. Additionally, at no time should the rights of the patient, the quality of surgery, or patient safety be compromised to achieve higher numbers of patients treated. The quality of overall patient care, the relationship with the local community, and the standards and systems employed are critical to the long-term viability of any eye care system.

Worldwide, it is important to adhere to World Health Organization initiatives such as safe site surgery,

informed consent, and hand hygiene campaigns, which all have significant impact on nonsurgical aspects of care. Organizations such as the American Academy of Ophthalmology, the American Society of Anesthesiology, and the Association of periOperative Registered Nurses all provide practice statements for the implementation of such standards. (See Appendix B for additional resources.)

SAFE SITE SURGERY GUIDELINES   The World Health Organization's Safe Site Surgery Guidelines were developed by an international health care team. These guidelines are designed to provide a starting point for safe surgery and ensure that the correct patient receives the correct treatment and surgery on the correct part of the body, with the correct methods at the correct time. The guidelines include a checklist that is to be completed by all members of the medical team, including the surgeon and anesthetist. The safe site surgery checklist (Figure 21.2) has been used in hospitals around the world with demonstrated reduction in medical errors. It notes whether the following criteria have been met:

- Correct patient and surgical site have been identified.

- Consent form is signed and correct.

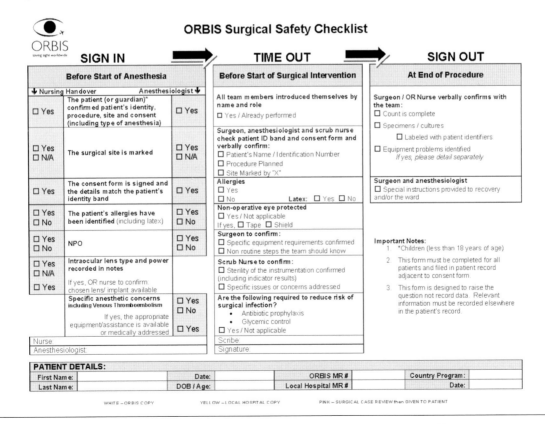

Figure 21.2   Example of a surgical checklist. *(Reprinted, with permission, from ORBIS International.)*

- All required fasting, medications and doses, anesthetic options, and skin preparations correspond with standing orders and/or the doctor's documented request.

- Prior to commencing surgery, all members of the team, within a particular clinical area, have checked that the patient's details in the chart correspond with the patient before them and that they have all the required equipment, stock, medications, and instruments required before commencing the procedure. The medication and stock must also be in-date. No expired medications are to be used.

The operating room surgical nursing team will also complete an additional surgical count at these intervals during the procedure: before the surgery commences, before the surgeon starts to close the wound, and at the end of surgery when the wound is closed. A surgical count also takes place to ensure those items used during surgery are accounted for prior to wound closure. This process is designed to prevent instruments and/or items such as suture needles being retained inside the patient.

Through the use of the safe site surgery checklist, the entire medical team becomes involved in improving patient outcomes and works toward a collaborative patient management team with open communication. Without such a process, patient error and mismanagement increases. Therefore, all such clinical and surgical eye care programs should consider a component of their work for training local workers in eye care and blindness prevention not only in individual clinical/surgical skills but systems transfer that prioritize efficient and safe clinical practice and protocols.

Community Eye Care Programs and the Team Approach

Many types of clinical and surgical program models have been employed to address the blindness issues facing communities. Whatever the program model, these key components have been found fundamental:

- careful planning of the program or what needs to be done before going beyond the clinic

- community involvement and ownership

- government involvement and leadership

- a good monitoring and evaluation system

- a structure and clear mechanisms for dialogue, problem-solving and co-ordination among all stakeholders

The Aravind Eye Hospital in Madurai, India, demonstrates many of the principles discussed in this chapter. It provides an excellent model hospital system in blindness prevention and treatment as well as an internationally recognized research and training facility. This hospital respects local customs, maximizing available resources (including human resources) to deliver an extremely efficient system to provide high-quality, high-volume, cost-effective cataract surgery. Aravind's focus on quality outcomes has created tremendous community demand, which has allowed the hospital to develop standardized systems for cost-recovery, local ownership, financial self-sufficiency, social marketing, and supply chain management.

Local Resources Available to Assist Visually Impaired Patients

Availability of resources varies greatly from country to country and even within countries. Part of an effective community health plan is being able to identify local health resources, mechanisms for patient education and rehabilitation for visually impaired patients. In the United States and many parts of the world, the Internet serves as a searchable tool for local resources. The Internet also can be utilized to contact philanthropic international nongovernmental organizations who in turn may provide resources and information regarding your country, region, or population of interest. In North America and English-speaking countries, many Internet resources are available. It is beyond the scope of this book to feature an exhaustive list.

In summary, the issue of international blindness is incredibly complex involving such social issues as poverty, gender, and culture. A community-based approach that engages and empowers the patient and community has demonstrated significant success and developed new models of health care delivery.

SELF-ASSESSMENT TEST

1. Describe the government and World Health Organization's definition of vision impairment and blindness.

2. Name the major global and local causes of reversible and irreversible blindness and vision loss.

3. Describe the VISION 2020 goal and strategies for implementation at a global and local level.

4. Describe a team approach to eye care.

5. Describe basic features of community eye care programs (eg, cataract, surgical).

6. Describe methods to develop and deliver health education information within the local community.

7. Identify the criteria of the safe-site surgery checklist.

SUGGESTED ACTIVITIES

1. Identify local resources (health, education and rehabilitation) available in your community to assist visually impaired patients.

2. Visit the website of ORBIS International (www.orbis.org). Browse the E-Resources link where you will find valuable information about international ophthalmology, online books and manuals, and videos of ophthalmic surgery.

3. Does your office or health care system participate in community health screening activities? If so, volunteer to be part of the vision screening activities.

SUGGESTED RESOURCES

Arivind Eye Hospitals. "Community Outreach Initiatives for High Quality, Large Volume, Sustainable Cataract Surgery Programmes." http://laico.org/v2020resource/files/Communioutreachmodule.pdf. Accessed August 15, 2011.

Buzzard S, Pfohl J, Yudelman Y. *Participatory Approaches for Community Health Worker Training in Primary Eye Care.* New York: Project Orbis International; 2003.

Cains S, Sophal S. Creating demand for cataract services: a Cambodian case study. *Community Eye Health.* 2006;19:65–66.

Congdon N, O'Colmain B, Klaver CC, et al. Causes and prevalence of visual impairment among adults in the United States. *Arch Ophthalmol.* 2004;122:477–485.

Courtright P, Kanjaloti S, Lewalen S. Barriers to acceptance of cataract surgery among patients presenting to district hospitals in rural Malawi. *Trop Geogr Med.* 1995;47:15–18.

Delgado-Gaitán C. *The Power of Community: Mobilizing for Family and Schooling.* New York: Rowman & Littlefield Publishing; 2001:200–207.

Dyer G. *A Manual for Vision 2020 Workshops.* International Centre for Eye Health. www.cehjournal.org/files/workshopmanual/V2020_Manual_2005.pdf. Accessed August 15, 2011.

Etya'ale D. Beyond the clinic: approaches to outreach. *Community Eye Health.* 2006;19:19–21.

Faal H. Preventing corneal blindness: working with communities. *Community Eye Health.* 2009;22:36–37.

Fletcher AE, et al. Low uptake of eye services in rural India: a challenge for programs of blindness prevention. *Arch Ophthalmol.* 1999;117:1393–1399.

Foster A, Gilbert C, Rahi J. Epidemiology of cataract in childhood: a global perspective. *J Cataract Refract Surg.* 1997;23:601–4.

Francis V. Cataract services: increasing utilization and creating demand. *Community Eye Health.* 2006;19:57–59.

Hannan Z. Case finding in the community: experience of Jatiya Andha Kallyan Somiti in Comilla, Bangladesh. *Community Eye Health.* 2002;15:40–42.

Haynes AB, Weiser TG, Berry WR, et al. A surgical safety checklist to reduce morbidity and mortality in a global population. *N Engl J Med*. 2009;360:491–499.

International Centre for Eye Health. "Community Eye Health Update 5." www.iceh.org.uk/display/WEB/Community+Eye+Health+Update+5+C. Accessed August 15, 2011.

Johnson JG, Goode Sen V, Faal H. Barriers to the uptake of cataract surgery. *Trop Doct*. 1998;28:218–220.

Krishnatray P, Bisht S, Rao GV, Guha K. The social construction of paediatric cataract: how parents make sense of their child's condition. *Community Eye Health*. 2006;19:48–49.

Michon J, Michon L. Popularising eye health services in southern Mexico: community workers meet a felt need. *Community Eye Health*. 2006;19:64–65.

Natchiar G, Robin AL, Thulasiraj RD, et al. Attacking the backlog of India's curable blind. The Aravind Eye Hospital model. *Arch Ophthalmol*. 1994;112:987–993.

Prevent Blindness America. "Vision Problems in U.S., 2008 Update to the Fourth Edition." www.preventblindness.net/site/DocServer/VPUS_2008_update.pdf?docID=1561. Accessed August 15, 2011.

Resnikoff S, et al. Global data on visual impairment in the year 2002. *Bull World Health Organ*. 2004;82:844–851.

Resnikoff S, Pascolini D, Mariotti SP, Pokharel GP. Global magnitude of visual impairment caused by uncorrected refractive errors in 2004. *Bull World Health Organ*. 2008;86:63–70.

Schwab L. *Eye Care in Developing Nations*. London: Manson Publishing; 2007.

Singh AJ, Garner P, Floyd K. Cost-effectiveness of public-funded options of cataract surgery in Mysore, India. *Lancet*. 2000;355:180–184.

Solomon, AW, Zondervan M, Kuper H, Buchan J, Mabey D, Foster A. *Trachoma Control: A Guide for Programme Managers*. www.who.int/blindness/publications/tcm%20who_pbd_get_06_1.pdf. Accessed August 15, 2011.

SOS Children's Villages. "Vietnan Shows That Blindness From Trachoma Can be Eradicated." Press release, January 7, 2011. www.soschildrensvillages.org.uk/charity-news/vietnam-shows-that-blindness-from-trachoma-can-be-eradicated. Accessed August 15, 2011.

Vaidyanathan K, Limburg H, FosterA, Pandey RM. Changing trends in barriers to cataract surgery in India. *Bull World Health Organ*. 1999;77:104–109.

Vaneeste G. "Breaking Down Barriers: A Practical Guide For Eye Units in Developing Countries." www.ccbrt.or.tz/uploads/media/Breaking_Down_Barriers.pdf. Accessed August 15, 2011.

VISION 2020 e-Resource for Eyecare Management Worldwide. "Outreach Camp Protocol." http://laico.org/v2020resource/files/OutreachProt.pdf. Accessed August 15, 2011.

VISION 2020 E-Resource Library. An online collection of comprehensive resources for eye care programs around the world. www.v2020eresource.org. Accessed August 15, 2011.

VISION 2020. "Blindness and Visual Impairment: Global Facts." www.vision2020.org/main.cfm?type=FACTS. Accessed August 15, 2011.

World Alliance for Patient Safety. *WHO Surgical Safety Checklist and Implementation Manual*. www.who.int/patientsafety/safesurgery/ss_checklist/en/index.html. Accessed August 15, 2011.

World Health Organization. "Prevention of Blindness and Visual Impairment." www.who.int/blindness/data_maps/en/. Accessed August 15, 2011.

Yeung I, Wiafe B. An outreach eye care programme, Zambia. *Community Eye Health*. 2002;15:13–14.

22 CARE OF OPHTHALMIC LENSES AND INSTRUMENTS

Ophthalmic medical practices today employ a large variety of instruments and equipment to diagnose and treat patients with eye disorders; these instruments may be hand-held, freestanding, or mounted on a wall, stand, or console. Whether ophthalmic medical assistants use such equipment themselves or not, they often have the responsibility of caring for, maintaining, and performing minor servicing of ophthalmic equipment in the office. These duties may include cleaning lenses and equipment; protecting instruments from dust and damage; replacing light bulbs, batteries, and fuses; and performing minor adjustments and selective calibration.

Many of the lenses and instruments used in today's ophthalmology practice are delicate and costly. These items must remain clean and in good condition to best perform their diagnostic or other medical function; they should be kept covered when not in use. It is important to observe certain precautions in keeping them clean and in proper working order, not only to protect the instruments themselves but also to protect patients from infection caused by microorganisms left on unclean surfaces. Office efficiency may depend on the accessibility of equipment manuals and maintenance records. This chapter presents general guidelines for the care of lenses and selected instruments, including special cautions to observe and techniques to employ for their handling, cleaning, and maintenance.

Care of Lenses

Lenses, whether hand-held or incorporated into instruments, or whether contact or noncontact, compose a significant portion of the diagnostic equipment in an ophthalmology office. All optical lenses used in the ophthalmic practice must be free of dust, dirt, fingerprints, and oils to perform correctly. However, careless cleaning can mar the antireflective coating on ocular instrument lenses or even ruin a precision optical lens. In addition, not all lenses and mirrored optical surfaces can be cleaned safely. The standard care guidelines below apply to the care of all types of diagnostic lenses in the ophthalmology office.

Standard Guidelines for Care of Lenses

Never rub a dry lens; dragging abrasive dust or dirt across a lens surface can scratch it. Always use wet friction or, if liquid cleaners cannot be used, remove the dust by blowing or brushing it off. Use only those cleaning fluids that are approved by the lens manufacturer or by your office policy. Inappropriate cleaning fluids can scratch and permanently damage a lens. Use only special lens-cleaning paper, cotton balls, or soft lint-free ophthalmic cloths. Avoid using ordinary tissue papers, paper towels, cloths with high lint content, nylon, and handkerchiefs, which can be abrasive enough to scratch the lens surface; plastic lenses are particularly easy to scratch in this way.

To ensure that a given lens can be cleaned safely, always consult the lens manufacturer's instructions or your office policy before attempting a cleaning procedure.

Lenses That Do Not Contact the Eye

Examples of lenses that do not contact the eye are the Hruby lens, condensing lenses, and handheld fundus lenses used in conjunction with a slit lamp or an indirect ophthalmoscope.

The **Hruby lens** is a −55 diopter lens attached to the slit lamp (Figure 22.1). It allows high-magnification binocular examination of the vitreous and central fundus. To avoid accidental damage, always return the Hruby lens to its storage position on the slit lamp after use.

Condensing lenses, also known as aspheric or panretinal viewing lenses, are handheld, noncontact biconvex lenses available in powers of +14 to +40 diopters (Figure 22.2). Condensing lenses are used to view the ocular fundus as a real, inverted image in conjunction with the indirect ophthalmoscope.

Handheld, noncontact **funduscopic lenses** of +60, +78, and +90 diopters are used in conjunction with the slit lamp for stereoscopic observation of the fundus within various fields of vision and under magnification.

Although individual types of lenses require specialized care, the standard care guidelines presented above may be applied to most handheld and instrument lenses, optical filters, and other highly polished glass surfaces (including coated lenses) that do not come into contact

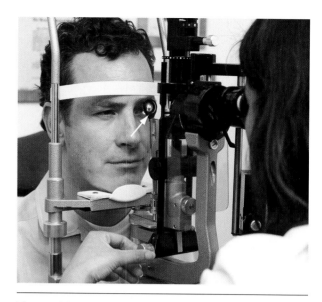

Figure 22.1 Hruby lens in use (arrow). *(Reprinted, with permission, from Wilson FM II, Blomquist PH,* Practical Ophthalmology, *6th ed, San Francisco: American Academy of Ophthalmology, 2009.)*

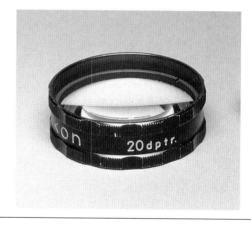

Figure 22.2 Condensing lens used with the indirect ophthalmoscope to examine the fundus.

with the patient's eye. Procedure 22.1 provides instructions for cleaning lenses that do not make contact with the eye.

Lenses That Contact the Eye

Examples of lenses that contact the eye include diagnostic contact lenses, such as the fundus lens and goniolenses like the Goldmann 3-mirror and the Koeppe lens (Figure 22.3). They are used to examine the inner aspects of the eye with greater magnification, often in conjunction with the slit lamp or other magnification and illumination source.

Any lenses that come in contact with the patient's eye may become clouded with diagnostic solutions, smeared

Procedure 22.1 Cleaning Lenses That Do Not Make Contact With the Eye

1. Remove dust from lenses or mirrors that cannot be cleaned with a liquid by blowing it off with a dry, empty bulb syringe or with a blast of air from a can of commercial compressed air or by brushing it off gently with a photographic lens brush or a loosely wadded lens-cleaning paper.

2. Remove fingerprints or oils from cleanable glass and polymethylmethacrylate (PMMA) plastic lenses by moistening a cleaning paper, cotton ball, or lint-free cloth with a special photographic liquid lens cleaner and rubbing the lens surface gently, using a circular motion.

3. Be sure that all cleaning agents are completely removed from the lens surface. Leaving a residue on the lens can diminish its clarity and effectiveness.

4. Dry lenses with clean lens paper or a lint-free cloth.

Additional Tips

Clean only the exposed front and back surfaces of a complex lens system. Never disassemble such a lens system; that procedure is reserved only for the instrument specialist or manufacturer's representative.

Generally, thorough cleaning of optical mirrors in ophthalmic instruments is best left to professionals. For routine cleaning, a blast of air from a dry bulb syringe or from a can of commercial compressed air will usually suffice.

Clean the trial lens set lenses, diagnostic lenses, and easily accessible phoropter lenses regularly. Do not wait until the ophthalmologist or other user becomes aware of a dirty lens.

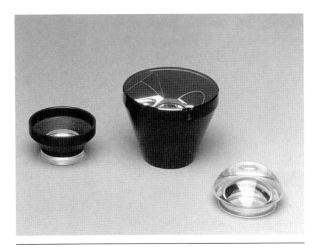

Figure 22.3 Diagnostic contact lenses. Left to right: fundus contact lens, 3-mirror Goldmann lens, Koeppe goniolens.

or on a recently operated eye. Generally, lenses cannot be sterilized in an autoclave, although some made specifically for use in an operating room can be.

Some general guidelines concerning sterilization of these special lenses are as follows. Use ethylene oxide gas and nonheat aeration that does not exceed 125°F. Use the appropriate gas-sterilization container bags with safety markers to ensure complete sterilization according to the operations manual of the sterilizer; be sure to write on the sterilization bag the date of processing. Use the standard unit cycle and aeration time specified in the operations manual of the sterilizer. Finally, do not use wood storage cases in the gas-sterilization process because the gas will not sterilize wood.

GLASS SURGICAL LENS STERILIZATION Before sterilization of glass surgical lenses with stainless-steel components, clean the lenses with soap and water to remove ocular secretions and debris. Sterilize the components with ethylene oxide or autoclave for 5 minutes at 270°F.

Procedure 22.2 Cleaning Lenses That Make Contact With the Eye

1. Using a rotary motion, carefully wash the lens in lukewarm water with a moistened cotton ball that contains a few drops of clear dishwashing liquid.

2. Rinse the lens completely with lukewarm water.

3. Blot the lens dry using a lint-free lens-cleaning paper or a soft lint-free absorbent lens cloth.

4. The lens is now ready for disinfection.

with eye make-up, or contaminated with ocular secretions that could become a source for the spread of infection. These lenses must be cleaned immediately after contact with the eye, generally by rinsing thoroughly with water to remove the contaminants. Lenses that contact the eye may also be either disinfected or sterilized. The appropriate procedure depends on the purpose of the lens (such as diagnostic or surgical), the type of lens, and the materials used in its manufacture. Procedures 22.2 and 22.3 review the steps on cleaning and disinfecting lenses that make contact with the eye.

GENERAL GUIDELINES FOR LENS STERILIZATION Lenses usually do not need sterilization unless they have been grossly contaminated or will be used during surgery

Procedure 22.3 Disinfecting Lenses That Make Contact With the Eye

1. Soak the lens for either

   a. 10 minutes in a disinfecting solution such as 2% aqueous solution of glutaraldehyde, or

   b. 5 minutes in fresh 3% hydrogen peroxide or a 1:10 dilution of household bleach and water, or the length of time indicated on a prepackaged commercial disinfectant solution

      Note: To be sure the solution will not damage the lens, consult the lens and solution manufacturers' directions.

2. Remove the lens from the disinfecting solution and rinse thoroughly with cool running water to remove all residual disinfectant solution.

3. Blot the lens dry, using a lint-free lens-cleaning paper or a soft lint-free absorbent lens cloth.

4. The lens is now ready for disinfection.

Procedure 22.4 Troubleshooting Instrument Failure

If an electrical instrument fails to work, check the following:

1. Is the instrument plugged into an electrical outlet?

2. Are all plugs and connections on the instrument securely in place?

3. Is the bulb burned out or darkened?

4. Is the instrument fuse burned out?

5. Are the central wall outlet and electrical fuse for the circuit functioning?

If a battery-powered instrument fails to work, check the following:

1. Is the battery fresh or recharged?

2. Is the bulb burned out or darkened?

For glass surgical lenses used during fluid–gas exchange procedures (such as intravitreal surgery), first make certain that any oil on the lens surface is removed by careful cleaning with soap and water. Next, fully rinse the lens, blot dry with lint-free lens-cleaning paper, and wipe with alcohol before placing the lens in the receptacle for sterilization.

STERILIZATION OF OTHER LENSES Never autoclave or boil ocular instrument lenses made of polymethylmethacrylate (PMMA). In addition, never use cleaning agents such as acetone, alcohol, or peroxide for PMMA lenses. Consult the manufacturer's information as to which fluid to use.

Care of Instruments

Ophthalmic medical assistants often clean electrical and battery-powered office instruments and perform simple maintenance, such as bulb replacement or minor calibration. The general guidelines below apply to the care and maintenance of all instruments in the ophthalmology office. Procedure 22.4 provides a simple checklist to follow when an ophthalmic instrument fails to operate.

Standard Care Guidelines

Read the operations manuals or user guides for each piece of equipment for which you are responsible. For

easy reference keep the manuals in one place in the office. If any instruction manuals or user guides are missing, request a replacement set from the manufacturer, supplier, or distributor. Check each instrument's user manual for instructions on the proper cleaning solutions and methods and follow the recommended procedures given.

To prevent instrument optics or other delicate components from becoming dusty, dirty, or accidentally damaged, ensure that each instrument is in its storage or carrying case. Alternately, protect the instrument with an individual dust cover when it is not in use.

Always check the instrument user's manual for the correct bulb type, battery type, and replacement procedure. Because oil from fingers can etch an instrument bulb once it heats up, diminishing its effectiveness and life, always handle instrument bulbs with lens tissue paper. If you or someone else has handled an instrument bulb without using tissue paper, remove fingerprints from the bulb with photographic-lens cleaning fluid and lens tissue or a soft lint-free lens cloth.

To avoid burning your fingers when servicing an instrument or replacing a bulb, make certain the instrument is turned off and the housing is cool. A recently burned-out bulb can be very hot; you may need to use a protective cloth to remove it. Maintain an adequate reserve of bulbs, batteries, and fuses for all instruments used in the office by checking the office inventory frequently and reordering as necessary. Keep these supplies handy so that replacement can be immediate. Turn off all instruments when they are not in use to prolong the life of bulbs and batteries. Finally, for rechargeable instruments, check that the recharger is plugged in and turned on as needed.

To avoid electrical shock, always disconnect an instrument from its power source before any servicing, even changing light bulbs or fuses.

Retinoscope

The retinoscope is a handheld instrument used with either trial lens set lenses or the phoropter to define a patient's objective refractive error before beginning subjective tests. The instrument contains a light source at the top of the handle, and a mirrored light-projection and viewing system is in the head of the instrument (Figure 22.4). Most retinoscopes today are powered with batteries or rechargeable power packs.

CARE AND CAUTIONS Clean the front surface of the mirror by blowing off dust with a dry, clean, empty bulb syringe. Always maintain an adequate supply of spare bulbs in the examining room.

Phoropter

The phoropter, or manual refractor, is used in performing refraction/refractometry. A phoropter consists of a unit that holds a series of trial lenses, both spheres and cylinders, mounted on a wheel used to select lenses to place before the patient's eye (Figure 22.5). The instrument includes built-in accessory lenses such as a pinhole, retinoscope lens, Maddox rod, Risley prism, polarizing lens, cross cylinder, and others that aid in measuring the refractive error of the eye.

CARE AND CAUTIONS Never put your finger into the lens aperture because you can get fingerprints on the phoropter's enclosed lenses. To blow dust away from these lenses, use a clean, dry, empty bulb syringe or canned compressed air. A photographic lens cleaner and

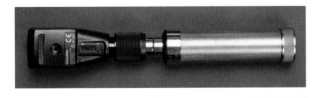

Figure 22.4 Example of retinoscope. *(Image courtesy of Brice Critser, CRA, Department of Ophthalmology and Visual Sciences, University of Iowa.)*

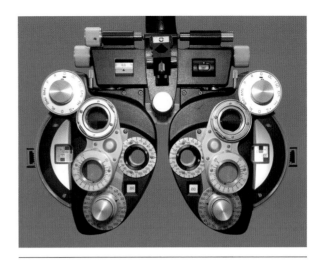

Figure 22.5 Phoropter. *(Image courtesy of Brice Critser, CRA, Department of Ophthalmology and Visual Sciences, University of Iowa.)*

lens tissue can be used for cleaning the accessory lenses located on the outside of the phoropter casing. Schedule authorized maintenance service every 2 years to clean the internal trial lenses and to prevent any major malfunctions. Never use alcohol on any part of a phoropter, except for the plastic face shields. Finally, never use cleaning solutions on the lens power number; instead, use a dry, soft cloth.

MANUFACTURER-SPECIFIC INSTRUCTIONS If your office has a Reichert Technologies Phoroptor®, clean only the lenses located on the back side (that is, the retinoscopic and polarizing lenses) with photographic-lens cleaner and cotton-tipped swabs. Periodically wash the reusable nylon face shields with soap and water and wipe them off between patients with alcohol or antiseptic wipes. The shields also may be disinfected by soaking for a few minutes in alcohol or disinfectant solution or boiling in water, then rinsed and allowed to air-dry. Other brands of manual refractors have disposable shields, which should be discarded after each patient use.

If your office has a Green's manual refractor, clean only the retinoscopic and +0.25-diopter lenses with photographic-lens cleaner and cotton swabs. These lenses become soiled easily because they may come in contact with the patient's eyelashes.

If your office has another brand of manual refractor, review the instruction manual to find out which accessory lenses you should clean.

Lensmeter

The lensmeter is used to determine the prescription of an eyeglass or contact lens. The lensmeter measures the spherical and cylindrical powers in diopters and can define the optical center of a lens, the axis of a cylindrical lens, the presence and direction of a lens prism, and the power of a bifocal or trifocal lens. The lensmeter unit includes a focusing eyepiece, lens holder, light source, and adjustment knobs (Figure 22.6A). Automated lensmeters (Figure 22.6B) have a housing that should be wiped clean and kept covered when not in use.

CARE AND CAUTIONS If dust falls onto the surface of the lenses of the lensmeter, blow it off with a clean, dry rubber bulb syringe, dust brush, or compressed canned air. Wipe the instrument's enamel finish with a soft cloth occasionally to prevent dust collection. Finally, do not attempt to lubricate the instrument. If it feels tight to the operator, call a qualified service technician.

Keratometer

The keratometer, or ophthalmometer, is used to measure corneal curvature objectively and to fit contact lenses (Figure 22.7). It uses the mirror effect of the cornea's surface to measure the curvature of the central 3.3 mm of the anterior corneal surface in its 2 meridians.

CARE AND CAUTIONS Check the lamp bulb for sooty carbon deposits, which can obscure the mirror image. Replace the bulb with a new bulb if these are present. The calibration of the keratometer is checked periodically using metal spheres of known curvature. Refer to the instrument manual for instructions. Do not attempt

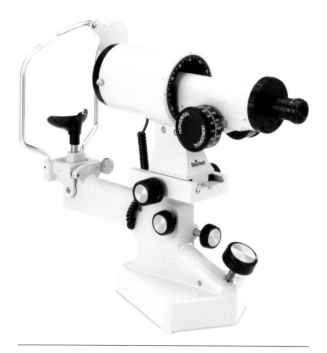

Figure 22.7 Keratometer. *(Image courtesy of Reichert Technologies.)*

to adjust the instrument if it seems out of alignment. Call an optical service technician to repair it.

Slit Lamp

The slit lamp, or biomicroscope, combines a microscope and specialized illumination system that delivers a freely movable slit beam of light (Figure 22.8). It provides a

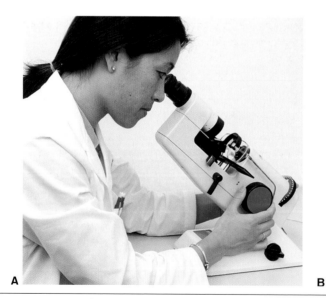
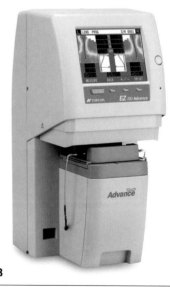

Figure 22.6 Examples of lensmeters. **A.** Manual lensmeter. **B.** Automated lensmeter. *(Part A reprinted, with permission, from Wilson FM II, Blomquist PH, Practical Ophthalmology, 6th ed, San Francisco: American Academy of Ophthalmology, 2009; Part B image courtesy of Topcon Medical Systems, a subsidiary of Topcon Corporation.)*

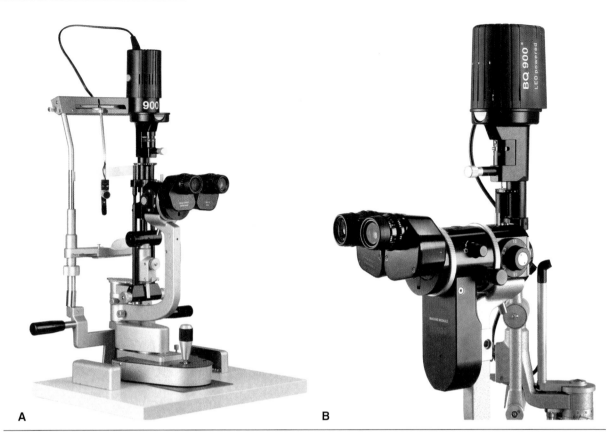

Figure 22.8 Slit lamp, or biomicroscope (**A**) and closeup of oculars (**B**). *(Images courtesy of Haag-Streit USA, Inc.)*

binocular, stereoscopic view of the cornea, sclera, and anterior segment of the eye (lens, iris, anterior chamber, and anterior vitreous) at magnification levels ranging from 10× to 40×. The instrument can also be used with handheld specialty lenses to more closely examine the anterior chamber of the eye, the vitreous, and the central and peripheral fundus. In addition, the slit lamp can function with a special instrument attachment to perform applanation tonometry.

CARE AND CAUTIONS A lens dust brush is usually sufficient for routine maintenance of the mirror on a Haag-Streit type of slit lamp. Always return the brush to its case after use, in order to keep it clean. If that does not work, try dusting and then wiping carefully with a soft lint-free cloth or chamois that will not scratch the mirror surface. If dirt remains, carefully spray the mirror with a photographic-glass cleaner. Wipe the surface dry with cotton balls, using downward strokes only. Be careful not to scratch the mirror surface. Repeat wiping with fresh cotton balls until dry. If the operating handle becomes difficult to move, clean the pad with a standard household cleaning solution. Then apply a thin coat of sewing-machine oil to the pad in the area of the ball joint.

During maintenance, the instrument must be unplugged from its power source. Always check any electrical connections, making sure that all wires are plugged into the transformer after each cleaning and maintenance procedure. If the slit-lamp light does not operate after you have checked all electrical connections, replace the bulb even if it seems to be in good condition, using the standard guidelines for bulb replacement given earlier.

Special instructions for cleaning the tonometer used with the slit lamp appear later in this chapter.

Projector

The projector—with accompanying slides, mirrors, and screens—is used to conduct the Snellen or other visual acuity tests. The projector unit (Figure 22.9A) consists of a housing for the bulb, a tube containing a lens system for focusing, and an opening between the bulb and the lens system for glass target slides (Figure 22.9B). The projector directs images from the glass slides onto a projection screen located 20 feet away or employs multiple mirrors to create the visual effect of 20 feet. Automated projectors (Figure 22.9C) have the different slide images, lenses and bulb housed in a single unit that is run by remote control. Another system is a self-contained automated screen also run by remote control (Figure 22.9D).

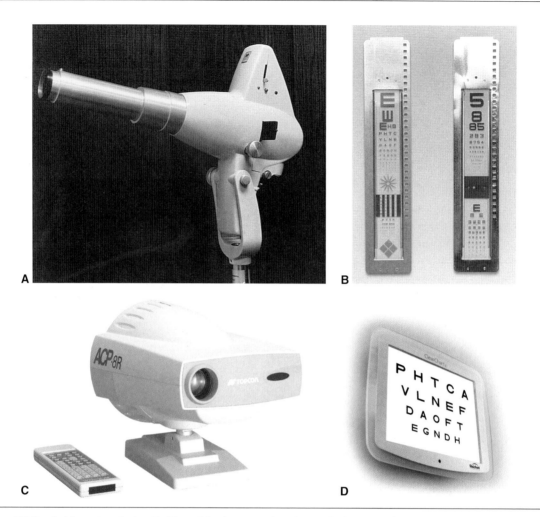

Figure 22.9 **A.** Manual projector. **B.** Glass slides for manual projector. **C.** Automated projector. **D.** Self-contained automated screen also run by remote control. *(Part C courtesy of Topcon Medical Systems, a subsidiary of Topcon Corporation; Part D courtesy of Reichert Technologies.)*

CARE AND CAUTIONS Blow or brush superficial grit off the projector. Automated projector housings and external lenses must be kept free of dust and oil. Do not attempt to remove lenses from the projector barrel. Wipe the glass slides when cooled to room temperature and external lens surfaces of the focusing tubes with a soft clean lint-free cloth or photographic-lens paper at appropriate intervals to prevent dust from accumulating. Clean the projector slides only with a dry photographic- or optical-lens tissue. Do not use water or other cleaning agents. Automated projectors are run by remote control and do not have removable slides.

Clean the patient viewing mirrors (plate glass with silvering on the back surface) and projecting mirrors (silvering on the front surface) with a blast of canned air or with a lint-free photographic cloth. To remove stubborn dirt, use a small amount of household glass cleaner and dry with cotton balls, using downward strokes only, not back-and-forth rubbing motions. Repeat with fresh cotton balls until the surface is dry.

Never take apart the lamp reflectors, which are assembled and positioned at the factory. The reflector behind the bulb can be cleaned as above.

Check to determine whether your office's projector screen can be cleaned (some cannot). If it can, clean the projector screen carefully because it is easily scratched or smeared with fingerprints and scratches can never be removed. To remove fingerprints, use a mild household detergent solution and damp cotton balls or a damp lint-free cloth to wipe the screen surface gently.

Never operate the projector with the lamp compartment open. The lamp operates under pressure and at a high temperature and must be protected at all times from abrasion and contact to avoid shattering.

Finally, you may observe that the projected image becomes dim, particularly in one half of the screen, shortly before the bulb fails. You may wish to replace the bulb at this point to ensure that acuity testing remains accurate.

Applanation Tonometer

The Goldmann-type applanation tonometer consists of a biprism in an eyepiece, attached by a rod to a housing that delivers measured pressure by use of an adjustment knob (Figure 22.10). The Goldmann applanation tonometer, usually attached to a slit lamp, measures intraocular pressure by flattening a small area (3.06 mm) of the cornea with the biprism by a known pressure or force. The intraocular pressure is given directly (in 10 mm Hg units) from a calibrated dial on the adjustment knob.

Because the tip of the Goldmann tonometer contacts the patient's eye during use, it must be carefully cleaned after each use to avoid the possibility of spreading infection. Although ophthalmic medical assistants should consult the ophthalmologist for the preferred cleaning method in their office, either of the two methods below is generally acceptable. Disposable tonometer tips are now available but they are not recommended to be used for glaucoma patients.

CARE AND CAUTIONS To clean the tonometer tip, remove the entire plastic tip from the tonometer and soak it for 5 minutes (no longer than 20 to 30 minutes) in 3% hydrogen peroxide or a 1:10 dilution of household bleach and water. Then rinse the tip under running tap water for 5 minutes and allow it to dry before reuse. The bleach solution should be changed at least once a day, and the peroxide solution twice a day. Although not preferable, some practices wipe the entire tonometer tip carefully and thoroughly with an alcohol swab and allow it to air-dry for 1 to 2 minutes before reuse. Be sure to rinse off the disinfectant and allow for thorough air-drying; if the patient's eye comes in contact with a disinfectant solution, corneal damage, pain, and discomfort could result.

Check the calibration of the tonometer at the intervals determined by the ophthalmologist, but at least once a month. Use the controlled weight supplied with the instrument by the manufacturer.

Indentation Tonometer

Although seldom used in most offices, the indentation, or Schiøtz, tonometer consists of a plunger in a barrel, attached to a footplate assembly that includes a pressure scale (Figure 22.11). The plunger is fitted with one of several available weights, and intraocular pressure is measured by indenting the cornea with the plunger. The intraocular pressure reading shown on the pressure scale is interpreted by using a printed conversion table.

CARE AND CAUTIONS Like the Goldmann applanation tonometer, the Schiøtz indentation tonometer contacts the patient's eye directly. Therefore, to prevent contamination and the spread of infectious diseases, the tonometer must be disassembled and its barrel, plunger, and footplate must be cleaned and disinfected after use with each patient. Use acetone or a disinfectant solution recommended by the manufacturer. Alcohol should

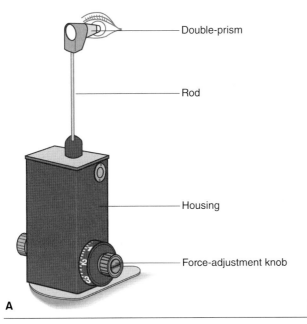

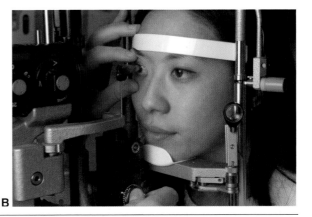

A   B

Figure 22.10 Goldmann applanation tonometer. **A.** Parts. **B.** Slit-lamp–mounted Goldmann applanation tonometer in use. (Note: The examiner's fingers are on the bony orbit, thereby avoiding pressure on the globe.) *(Part B courtesy of Brice Critser, CRA, Department of Ophthalmology and Visual Sciences, University of Iowa.)*

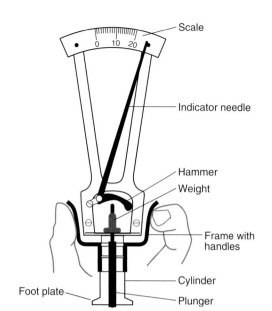

Figure 22.11 Parts of the Schiøtz tonometer. *(Reprinted, with permission, from Wilson FM II, Blomquist PH,* Practical Ophthalmology, *6th ed, San Francisco: American Academy of Ophthalmology, 2009.)*

never be used to clean the Schiøtz tonometer as it can stay in the crevices of the cylinder and cause corneal abrasions.

Do not touch the plunger directly with your fingers after cleaning. Allow all tonometer surfaces to dry before reassembling.

Check that the calibration is at zero between each use, using the zero test block. Be careful not to damage the delicate indicator needle. Never bend it if the calibration is not at zero; this adjustment must be made at the factory. Finally, do not interchange weights between 2 or more separate tonometers because the weights are calibrated specifically for each individual tonometer.

Tono-Pen

The Tono-Pen is a combination indentation and applanation instrument that is handheld and measures IOP electronically (Figure 22.12). It has an internal calibration system and a digital display on the handle that shows the IOP and a reliability factor.

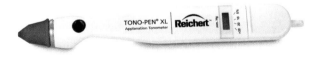

Figure 22.12 Tono-Pen applanation tonometer. *(Image courtesy of Reichert Technologies.)*

CARE AND CAUTIONS The tonometer tip is covered by a thin latex cap that is discarded after use on each patient. The metal tip should be cleared of debris periodically with compressed canned air. To calibrate the Tono-Pen, press the activation button until "CAL" appears in the window. Hold the Tono-Pen with the tip straight down toward the floor. When the instrument beeps and "UP" appears in the window, rotate the instrument so the tip is straight up. If "GOOD" appears in the window, press the button again until a double line = = = = appears. When performing the calibration, if the word in the window consistently reads "BAD", it may help to press the RESET button on the handle or it may indicate that the batteries need to be replaced (refer to the manual). The instrument should be handled with care and stored with a cover over the tip in order to prevent dust and debris from entering the tip.

Direct Ophthalmoscope

The direct ophthalmoscope is a handheld instrument, either battery-powered or electrical, that consists of a light source, built-in dial-up lenses and filters, and a reflecting device to aim light into the patient's eye (Figure 22.13). The ophthalmologist uses this instrument to examine the fundus directly. The direct ophthalmoscope is capable of larger magnification (15×) than is the indirect ophthalmoscope, but provides a more restricted view of the fundus. In addition, because only a single eye can be used for viewing at a time, the direct ophthalmoscope does not provide a stereoscopic view.

CARE AND CAUTIONS Portable scopes require periodic attention to recharging and replacing batteries. The light source will require replacement when the bulb burns out. The hard-wired scopes need bulb replacement and periodic inspection of the cord to detect fraying.

Indirect Ophthalmoscope

The indirect ophthalmoscope is used to examine the complete fundus in stereopsis. The instrument consists

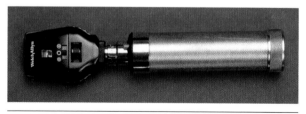

Figure 22.13 Example of direct ophthalmoscope. *(Image courtesy of Brice Critser, CRA, Department of Ophthalmology and Visual Sciences, University of Iowa.)*

of a transformer power source and a headset that fits on the ophthalmologist's head, with a bulb light source and binocular magnifying lenses attached for viewing (Figure 22.14). The ophthalmologist uses a handheld condensing lens (usually +20 diopters) to magnify the image of the fundus. Magnification is usually 2× to 4×, and the image appears as a real, 3-dimensional, inverted image of the retina at the focal point of the handheld lens.

CARE AND CAUTIONS Bulb replacement and cord maintenance is needed on a periodic basis, and a battery-powered instrument will require periodic recharging and replacing of the batteries.

Potential Acuity Meter

The potential acuity meter (PAM) is used to determine potential visual acuities in patients with cataracts. The device consists of a pinpoint light source, a transilluminated Snellen visual acuity chart, and a lens that projects the highly illuminated acuity chart through an opening about 0.1 mm in diameter (Figure 22.15).

CARE AND CAUTIONS To clean the exterior of the instrument, use a clean, damp cloth. Keep optical surfaces clean with a lens brush and always have a spare light bulb on hand.

Perimeters

These instruments provide a formal estimate of the boundaries and abnormalities of the visual field. They typically employ a bowl-shaped light-standardized background onto or from which small, round lights

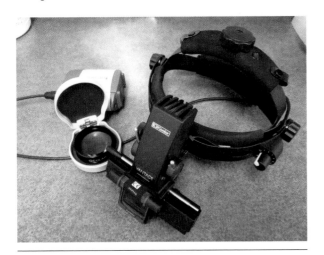

Figure 22.14 Indirect ophthalmoscope with a portable transformer and handheld condensing lens and carrying case (left), ophthalmoscope (right). *(Image courtesy of JoAnn A. Giaconi, MD.)*

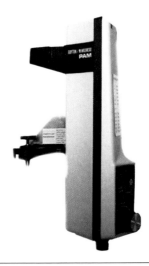

Figure 22.15 Potential acuity meter. *(Image courtesy of Neal H. Atebara, MD.)*

are projected. Perimeters are usually computer automated, but some practices still use manual instruments (Figure 22.16).

CARE AND CAUTIONS The outside of the instruments may be dusted with a soft, lint-free cloth. The inside of the bowls must be kept dust-free with compressed air and/or a soft brush. Be careful not to touch the inside of the bowl as oil and dirt from fingers can change the reflective properties of the surface.

The movable projector arm of the manual perimeter should be lubricated two or three times a year with a very small amount of a thin oil. The data screen of the automated instrument should be cleaned with static- and lint-free wipes. The response button that is held by the patient should be cleaned with a sanitizing wipe between each use.

Lasers

The word laser is an acronym for "light amplification by stimulated emission of radiation." Lasers are a source of an extremely intense form of monochromatic light organized in a concentrated beam that can cut, burn, disrupt, destroy, alter, or vaporize tissue (Figure 22.17). Common types of ophthalmic lasers include the argon, krypton, excimer, diode, and neodymium:yttrium-aluminum-garnet (Nd:YAG). The ophthalmologist uses lasers in a variety of treatments.

- Creating multiple burns in the retina of a diabetic patient to decrease the adverse effects of diabetic retinopathy

- Sealing burns around potential holes or tears associated with retinal detachment

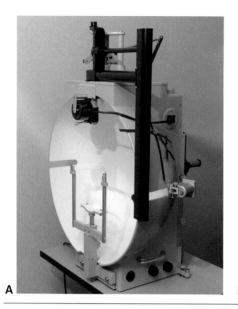
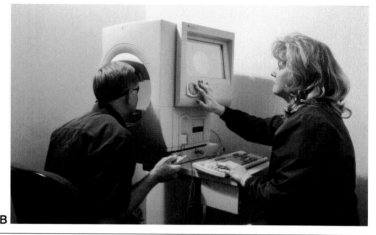

A   **B**

Figure 22.16 Examples of perimeters. **A.** Goldmann manual perimeter. **B.** Humphrey automated field analyzer. *(Part A courtesy of Brice Critser, CRA, Department of Ophthalmology and Visual Sciences, University of Iowa.)*

- Cutting a hole in the periphery of the iris to make an outflow channel for aqueous in patients with acute narrow-angle glaucoma

- Cutting the posterior capsule of the lens if it becomes opaque after cataract surgery

- Treating chronic open-angle glaucoma by applying laser treatment to the trabecular meshwork through a gonioprism lens

- Performing blepharoplasty (cosmetic eyelid surgery) and skin resurfacing

- Correcting refractive errors and removing superficial corneal opacities

- Treating with nonthermal laser to close abnormal blood vessels in the macula previously treated with an injected agent (photodynamic treatment)

CARE AND CAUTIONS Because lasers are powerful instruments that can cause damage if improperly focused on the eye (a patient's or your own), review the instruction manuals for specific safeguards before you begin to assist the ophthalmologist in the laser work area. Always wear the approved protective eye goggles when assisting the ophthalmologist in the laser work area. Never attempt to demonstrate how the laser works without the correct and appropriate knowledge, permission, and supervision. Maintenance should be performed only by a qualified service technician.

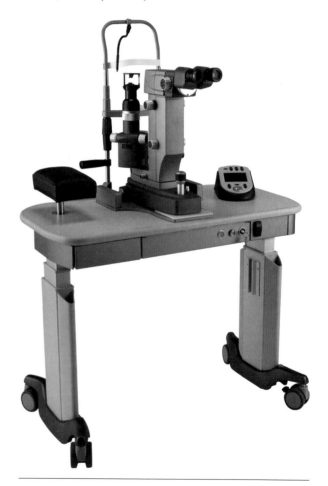

Figure 22.17 Nd:YAG laser. *(Image courtesy of Lumenis Vision.)*

SELF-ASSESSMENT TEST

1. Name 3 diagnostic lenses that do not make contact with the eye.

2. Outline the steps involved in cleaning the retinoscope.

3. What equipment is used to calibrate the keratometer?

4. Describe the 2 preferred methods used to clean the Goldman tonometer.

5. Is the Tono-Pen an indentation or an applanation instrument?

6. Name 4 types of ophthalmic lasers.

7. Outline the steps involved in cleaning lenses that do not make contact with the eye.

8. Outline the steps involved in cleaning lenses that make contact with the eye.

9. What 5 things should you check if an electrical instrument fails to work?

10. What 2 things should you check if a battery-operated instrument fails to work?

SUGGESTED ACTIVITIES

1. Ask your ophthalmologist or senior technician if he or she could supervise you in cleaning noncontact lenses.

2. Observe the senior technicians as they prepare lenses for sterilization.

3. Obtain the user's manuals for the 3 most commonly used instruments in your clinic and review the instructions on proper cleaning techniques.

SUGGESTED RESOURCE

DuBois LG. Instrument maintenance. In: *Fundamentals of Ophthalmic Medical Assisting.* DVD. San Francisco: American Academy of Ophthalmology; 2009.

23 ANSWERS TO CHAPTER SELF-ASSESSMENT TESTS

Chapter 1

1. a, e, d, b, f, c

2. certified ophthalmic assistant (COA), certified ophthalmic technician (COT), certified ophthalmic medical technologist (COMT)

3. d

4. b

5. b

Chapter 2

1. Light rays reflected from an object are focused by the cornea and the lens to produce an upside-down image of the object on the light-sensitive retina. The retina converts the image to electric impulses, which are carried by the optic nerve to the brain's visual cortex, where they produce the sensation of sight.

2. orbit, extraocular muscles, eyelids, lacrimal apparatus

3. the bony cavity in the skull that houses the globe, extraocular muscles, blood vessels, and nerves; protects the globe from major injury by a rim of bone

4. d, a, b, c, f, e

5. to protect the eye from injury, to exclude light, to aid in lubricating the ocular surface

6. outer layer of skin, middle layer of fibrous tissue and muscle, inner layer of tissue (conjunctiva)

7. to produce and drain tears

8. ocular comfort, clear vision, provide moisture, nourish eye

9. Tears are produced by the lacrimal gland; tears are collected in the lacrimal sac; tears drain into the nasal cavity by means of the nasolacrimal duct.

10. The outer, oily layer helps prevent evaporation of moisture from the middle, aqueous layer; the middle layer provides moisture, oxygen, and nutrients to the cornea; the inner mucinous layer promotes even spread of the tear film.

11.

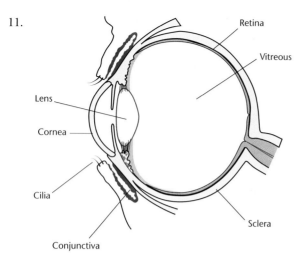

12. to focus light rays reflected to the eye, contributing about two-thirds of the focusing power of the eye

13. d, a, c, b, b

14. to protect intraocular contents

15. to maintain intraocular pressure

16. Aqueous humor enters the eye from behind the iris, flows across the back of the iris, through the pupil, and into the anterior chamber; it leaves the anterior chamber at the filtration angle and passes through the trabecular meshwork, the canal of Schlemm, aqueous veins, and into the blood vessels.

17. iris, ciliary body, choroid

18. Fibers of the dilator muscle that extend from the pupil to the boundary of the iris contract to dilate the pupil; contraction of the sphincter muscle that encircles the pupil makes the pupil smaller.

19. to secrete aqueous humor

20. to supply blood (nourishment) to the outer layers of the retina

21. lens

22. The curvature of the lens can change, becoming rounder, to focus images of objects that are closer to the eye.

23. zonules

24. to act as a shock absorber for the eye and help maintain the spherical shape of the globe

25. rods, cones

26. Rods are largely responsible for vision in dim light ("night vision") and for peripheral vision; cones provide sharp central vision and color perception.

27. The retinal rods and cones receive light rays and, in turn, generate electric (nerve) impulses. These impulses are transmitted to the brain, where the visual messages they carry are converted to the sensation of sight.

28. cone

29. The optic nerves from each eye merge at the optic chiasm. Axon fibers from the nasal retina of each eye cross to the opposite side of the chiasm, while axons from the temporal retina of each eye continue on the same side. The realigned axons emerge from the chiasm as the left and right optic tracts, ending in the left and right lateral geniculate bodies. There the axons synapse (connect) to the optic radiations, which travel to the right and left halves of the visual cortex of the brain.

Chapter 3

1. infectious, inflammatory, allergic, ischemic, metabolic, congential, developmental, degenerative, neoplastic, traumatic

2. *Sign*: a change that can be observed by a physician. *Symptom*: a change experienced by a patient (a sign is usually more objective; a symptom, more subjective). *Syndrome*: a group of signs or symptoms characteristic of a particular condition.

3. proptosis, exophthalmos

4. grossly swollen lids, red eyes

5. misalignment of the eyes; greater than normal tissue bulk in orbit, loss of muscle elasticity from scarring, muscle paralysis due to nerve damage, congential weakness of one or more extraocular muscles

6. a, c, d, g, b, h, i, e, f

7. dry eyes; artificial tears in the form of eyedrops

8. dacryocystitis

9. *Bacterial*: mucopurulent discharge. *Viral*: watery discharge, palpebral conjunctiva is covered with small bumps. *Allergic*: tearing, itching, redness, swelling.

10. rupture of a conjunctival blood vessel, allowing blood to flow under the conjunctival tissue; may occur after violent sneezing or coughing

11. *Pinguecula*: small, benign yellow-white mass of degenerated tissue beneath bulbar conjunctiva that does not cross onto the cornea and that can cause minor eye irritation. *Pterygium*: wedge-shaped growth of abnormal tissue on bulbar conjunctiva that can cross onto the cornea and can cause irritation, redness, foreign-body sensation, sensitivity to light

12. pain, sensitivity to light, tearing; treat with antibiotics

13. symptoms not as severe; dense corneal opacity, branch-shaped figure on cornea

14. center of cornea thins and acquires a cone shape, which affects vision

15. abnormal rise in intraocular pressure, with eventual damage to the optic nerve and sign loss; glaucoma

16. c, d, b, a

17. a, b, c, d, e, f, g

18. opacification, or loss of transparency

19. aging, injury, disease, congenital

20. small particles of dead cells and other debris in vitreous and collagen fibers from vitreous degeneration; experienced by patient as spots or cobwebs

21. endophthalmitis

22. separation of sensory and pigment layers of retina

23. The patient notices stars or flashes of light at the corner of the eye, followed some hours later by sensation of a curtain moving across the eye and by painless loss of vision.

24. Sensory cells of macula deteriorate, causing loss of central vision.

25. swelling of optic disc with engorged blood vessels, causing enlargement of the normal physiologic blind spot

26. tumor, stroke, trauma, inflammation

Chapter 4

1. insulin, thyroid hormone, estrogen, testosterone

2. inflammatory and autoimmune, metabolic, vascular, infectious, malignant

3. photophobia, burning sensation, grittiness, foreign body sensation

4. blood vessel leakage of fluid and exudation of protein substances into the retina, very poor retinal circulation, retinal ischemia, retinal neovascularization

5. less than 7%

6. a clot of cholesterol, blood cells, or calcium

7. cytomegalovirus, herpes zoster

8. breast, lungs

9. visual field defects, pupillary abnormalities

10. examination of spinal fluid, MRI scans, assessment of the patient's long-term pattern of symptoms

Chapter 5

1. *Refractive index*: the ratio of the speed of light in a vacuum to its speed in a specific substance. *Focal point*: the point somewhere along the principal axis of a lens at which the paraxial rays converge or diverge. *Focal length*: the distance between the focal point and the lens. *Diopter*: the unit of measure of the power of a lens.

2. A convex lens converges light rays; a concave lens diverges light rays.

3. *Emmetropia*: the normal refractive state of an eye, in which light rays from distant objects are focused clearly on the retina by the relaxed lens without any accommodative effort. *Ametropia*: the abnormal refractive state of the eye, in which light rays from distant objects cannot be focused clearly on the retina due to a refractive error.

4. *Myopia*: nearsightedness; the cornea and lens have too much plus power for the length of the nonaccommodating eye, so that the light rays from distant objects are focused in front of the retina. *Hyperopia*: farsightedness; the cornea and lens have too little plus power for the length of the nonaccommodating eye, so that light rays from distant objects are focused theoretically behind the retina. *Astigmatism*: blurred vision of both distant and near objects due to a toric cornea or one whose surface is irregular, so that light rays are not brought to a single focal point.

5. progressive loss of accommodative ability of the crystalline lens due to a natural process of aging

6. eyeglasses, contact lenses, intraocular lens implants, refractive surgery

7. lower segment(s) of a multifocal lens; used to provide near vision to patients with presbyopia

8. lens that has different curvatures in each of two perpendicular meridians (like a football), each of which possesses refractive power

9. refracts light rays towards its base

10. to correct diplopia caused by visual misalignments

11. prism diopters

12. 2

13. *Myopia*: concave, or minus, sphere. *Hyperopia*: convex, or plus, sphere. *Astigmatism*: spherocylinder, or cylinder.

14. process of measuring a person's refractive error and determining the optical correction required to provide clear vision

15. refractometry and clinical judgment

16. retinoscopy (objective refractometry), refinement (subjective refractometry), binocular balancing

17. *Cycloplegic refraction*: uses cycloplegic drops to temporarily paralyze the ciliary muscle and block accommodation. *Manifest refraction*: is obtained without cycloplegia.

18. *Objective refractometry* is retinoscopy, which does not require responses from the patient. *Subjective refractometry* is refinement, which requires the patient to participate by choosing the lens (usually presented by means of a phoropter or trial frame and lenses) that provides the better clarity.

19. retinoscope, refractor (or phoropter), trial lens set and trial frame, cross cylinder

20. *With motion*: the retinoscopic reflex of the eye that moves in the same direction as the retinoscope streak of light. *Against motion*: the retinoscopic reflex of the eye that moves in the opposite direction from the retinoscope streak of light.

21. a. Sign and power of sphere. b. Sign and power of cylinder. c. Axis of cylinder.

22. +5.75 –1.50 × 45

23. measurement of the prescription of eyeglass lenses or the power of contact lenses

24. power in diopters, axes of cylinder component, presence and direction of prism, optical centers

25. sphere

26. +1.75

27. measurement of a patient's corneal curvature; provides an objective, quantitative measurement of corneal astigmatism

28. (1) The reticule is in the center of the bottom-right circle. (2) The instrument is focused with fusion of the bottom-right circles. (3) The pluses between the circles are in the same plane and are fused. (4) The minuses between the circles are in the same plane and are fused.

Chapter 6

1. topical, injectable, oral

2. solutions, suspension, ointments and gels, inserts

3. redness, tearing, pain

4. drug remains in contact with eye or lid longer

5. registered nurse or doctor

6. c, a, d, b, e

7. b

8. d

9. a

10. b

11. d

12. c

13. b

14. a

Chapter 7

1. bacteria, viruses, fungi, protozoa

2. airborne droplets and particles, direct contact with an infected person, indirect contact with a contaminated person or object, common vehicles, vector-borne spread

3. to prevent the spread of infectious microbes to or from patients and medical office personnel

4. (1) Wash hands between contacts with patients. (2) Wear disposable gloves to avoid contact with body fluids or contaminated objects. (3) Use special receptacles ("sharp containers") for disposal of contaminated needles, blades, and other sharp objects. (4) Properly dispose of, disinfect, or sterilize contaminated objects between uses with patients. (5) Wear a fluid-impermeable gown and mask when there is potential for splash of bloody or contaminated body fluids. (6) Dispose of eye patches, gauze, and the like that are saturated with blood (blood that can be wrung or squeezed out) in a special red impermeable isolation bag.

5. (1) Assistants with a fever blister should be excused from hands-on contact with patients until recovery. (2) If the patient has a fever blister, assistants should avoid touching the patient near the mouth with fingers or instruments. Assistants should wash their hands after completing any tests and be certain instruments used with the patient are properly disinfected or sterilized.

6. (1) Turn on the faucets and adjust the water to the warmest comfortable temperature. (2) Wet your hands, wrists, and about 4 inches of the forearms. (3) Apply antiseptic soap from a dispenser, and wash your hands with circular strokes for at least 15 seconds. (4) Rinse your hands and forearms. (5) Hold dry paper towels to close the faucets, discarding the paper towels when finished. (6) Dry your hands with clean paper towels.

7. *Disinfection* inactivates or eliminates most disease-causing microorganisms. *Sterilization* destroys all microorganisms.

8. moist heat, ethylene oxide gas

9. Handle the sterile item only by a nonfunctional part (a part that does not come in contact with the patient or other sterile materials).

10. Avoid finger contact with the lip, tip, or inner lid of the bottle. Never permit the tip of the dropper bottle to touch the patient's eyelashes, lid, or eye. Check the liquid in the bottle for cloudiness or particulate matter and discard if present. Discard single-dose containers after one use.

11. Contaminated sharp objects are placed in a rigid, puncture-proof biohazard container (a "sharps container"). When the container is full, it is disposed of according to standard procedures.

Chapter 8

1. to reveal both existing and potential eye problems, even in the absence of specific symptoms

2. Certain eye diseases cause no symptoms until they are too advanced for effective treatment. Eye health is an important indicator of general health. Individuals who are at high risk for developing certain eye diseases can be monitored.

3. chief complaint and present illness; ocular history; general medical and social history; family ocular and medical history; allergies, medications, vitamins and supplements

4. Refer the patient to the ophthalmologist for a diagnosis or medical advice, even if you think you know the answer.

5. the ability to discern fine visual detail

6. The first number represents the distance in feet at which the test was performed (distance of patient from chart). The second number indicates that the patient can read at 20 feet what a normal eye can read at 40 feet.

7. $\bigvee \begin{array}{l} \text{OD } 20/60 \\ \text{OS } 20/40 \end{array} \overline{sc}$

8. The pinhole acuity test can reveal whether a patient's below-normal visual acuity is the result of a refractive error or is due to some other cause.

9. The patient complains that reading or other close work is difficult. There is reason to believe that the patient's ability to accommodate is insufficient or impaired.

10. eye movement (motility), eye alignment, fusional ability

11. right and up, right, right and down, left and up, left, left and down

12. to measure the extent of a misaligned eye's deviation

13. to determine whether the eyes are perfectly aligned and, if so, whether the brain acknowledges the visual information from both eyes or suppresses the information from one eye; the test will also reveal diplopia

14. to determine whether the patient has fine depth perception and to qualify it in terms of binocular cooperation

15. A manifest deviation (tropia) is an ocular misalignment that is clearly evident on inspection. A latent deviation (phoria) is an ocular misalignment that reveals itself with special testing because ordinarily it is prevented from becoming apparent by the patient's normal fusional ability.

16. afferent pupillary defect

17. to measure the expanse and sensitivity of vision surrounding the direct line of sight (peripheral vision)

18. on each other's uncovered eye

19. the presence and location of defects in the central portion of the visual field

20. for early detection of abnormal intraocular pressure and glaucoma, which may be present long before patients notice any symptoms such as visual loss

21. applanation and indentation

22. c

23. Accurate measurement of the corneal thickness is necessary for diagnosis of many corneal diseases and aberrations such as corneal edema, keratoconus, and irregular astigmatism. Pachymetry has been found to be an important parameter in the diagnostic evaluation of glaucoma.

24. to assess the ocular adnexa, external globe, and anterior chamber

25. to estimate the depth of the anterior chamber and the chamber angle; to alert the physician to avoid dilating the pupil as it may precipitate an attack of acute angle-closure glaucoma

26. to obtain a magnified view of the patient's ocular adnexa and anterior segment structures; to perform applanation tonometry with the Goldmann tonometer; to examine the fundus; to perform gonioscopy

27. noncontact lenses used with a slit lamp that examine the optic nerve head and small areas of the posterior retina, macula, and vitreous

28. a special viewing method for examination of the anterior chamber angle; employs a mirrored or high-plus contact lens

29. (1) The direct ophthalmoscope is a handheld instrument with a light-and-mirror system that affords an upright, monocular survey of a narrow

field of the ocular fundus magnified 15-fold. (2) The indirect ophthalmoscope is worn on the physician's head and consists of a binocular viewing device and an adjustable lighting system wired to a transformer power source; the binocular system allows for a stereoscopic view of the fundus.

30. pseudoisochromatic color plates, 15-hue (Farnsworth-Munsell D-15) test

31. to measure the patient's tear output

32. The purpose is to test the structural integrity of the corneal epithelium. Defects seen with corneal abrasions or punctate staining in dry eye disease are common examples of staining.

33. The examiner touches the central portion of the cornea with a sterile wisp of cotton to determine whether the patient has normal corneal sensation.

34. to measure the position of the eyeball in relation to the bony orbital rim surrounding it and record the existence and extent of proptosis

Chapter 9

1. Medial rectus: in-turning (adduction). Lateral rectus: out-turning (abduction). Superior rectus: up-turning (supraduction). Inferior rectus: down-turning (infraduction). Superior oblique: in-twisting (incyclotorsion). Inferior oblique: out-twisting (excyclotorsion).

2. (1) up and in; (2) up and out; (3) down and in; (4) down and out; (5) straight in; (6) straight out

3. Versions are tested by observing the eye movements of the patient with both their eyes open. One observes ductions by occluding one eye and observing eye movements of the uncovered eye and then occluding the other eye and observing that eye's movements.

4. Suppression is the brain's mechanism that can develop in young children to avoid double vision (diplopia). When the eyes are not aligned, the brain will ignore or "suppress" the image of one eye to prevent diplopia. The not aligned eye is usually the eye that is suppressed. The brain loses this ability after childhood.

5. Amblyopia is decreased vision in one or both eyes due to vision deprivation during early childhood.

In conditions like strabismus, congenital cataract, or large refractive states, the young child's brain does not receive adequate stimulation to develop normal vision and as an adult is uncorrectable by spectacles or contact lenses.

6. The corneal light reflex test can be confounded by deformed pupils or abnormal retinal architecture.

7. The cover-uncover test is performed first because it tests for tropias. The cross cover test cannot distinguish between tropias and phorias. Therefore, once a tropia is ruled out by the cover-uncover test, the cross cover test is used to detect a phoria.

8. prism and cover test

9. fusion, suppression, diplopia

10. depth perception (stereopsis)

Chapter 10

1. to determine the potential visual status of a patient with a media opacity and the extent to which surgery or other types of therapy may improve vision

2. potential acuity meter, super pinhole, interferometer, retinal acuity meter

3. when basic assessment reveals a deficiency or ophthalmic condition

4. vision testing in patients with media opacities, tests for corneal structure and disease, photography of the external eye and fundus, ultrasonography

5. to determine whether a patient's visual complaints are due to cataract and whether the patient requires surgery for cataract

6. to determine whether sensitivity to glare is contributing to a patient's visual symptoms

7. corneal thickness, that is, the distance between the epithelium (front layer of cells) and the endothelium (back layer of cells) of the cornea

8. to diagnose the cause and determine the extent of corneal swelling and the thickening and to help estimate the cornea's ability to withstand the stress of an operation

9. to photograph the cornea's endothelial cells at great magnification for cell counting to assess the health

of the cornea and its ability to withstand certain intraocular surgical procedures

10. b

11. d

12. Fluorescein, a fluorescent dye, is injected into a vein in the patient's arm; the dye is delivered to the retinal blood vessels by the vascular system; the fundus camera photographs the appearance of the vessels in rapid sequence.

13. temporary nausea, a severe allergic reaction

14. The reflection (echo) of high-frequency sound waves defines the outlines of ocular and orbital structures, measures the distance between these structures, and determines the size, composition, and position of intraocular abnormalities.

15. a

16. e

17. b

Chapter 11

1. testing procedures for measuring the expanse and sensitivity of a patient's peripheral vision and visual field and for pinpointing possible defects

2. because of the high concentration of cone cells in this area and the "one-to-one" wiring of the cones to the retinal nerve fibers

3. The physiologic blind spot corresponds to the point at which the optic nerve exits the eye; sight is not possible there because of the absence of rods and cones at the head of the optic nerve.

4. to create a meaningful representation of the patient's visual field for the purpose of diagnosing and monitoring diseases of the eye and visual pathways

5. fovea

6. circles off center; radial meridians

7. about 15° off center on the 0° or 180° (horizontal) meridian in the temporal field

8. about 90° temporally; 60° nasally, superiorly, and inferiorly

9. inferior nasal

10. to detect abnormalities in the visual field; to monitor diseases of the eye and visual pathways

11. *Kinetic perimetry*: uses a moving test object (target) of predetermined size and brightness. *Static perimetry*: employs a stationary target of fixed size that can be changed in brightness, and position within the visual field but is not displayed until it has stopped moving.

12. a contour of the visual field obtained with a single target of a particular size and brightness, representing a line of equal or better sensitivity to the stimulus

13. A scotoma is an area of reduced sensitivity in the visual field. A shallow scotoma is a mild visual defect; a deep scotoma, a serious defect. An absolute scotoma is an area that could not elicit a response to the largest, brightest test object available on a particular machine.

14. The main tests are the confrontation field test, tangent screen test, Goldmann perimetry. Simplicity of the confrontation field test makes it useful for screening patients with major defects, particularly children, the very old, and the mentally impaired. The tangent screen test is more sensitive than the confrontation test, but still relatively simple to perform. Goldmann perimetry is more sensitive and reproducible than the other two procedures; it is also able to measure the entire visual field.

15. simple to understand for both the patient and the examiner; produces a pictorial result that is easy to interpret

16. The patient is slow to respond, either because of a long reaction time or because of a poor understanding of the test. The examiner moves the target too fast or too slow.

17. suprathreshold perimetry, threshold perimetry

18. more sensitive at detecting small or shallow defects in the visual field; can eliminate the burden on the technician for actually performing the test

19. takes longer to perform; is more tedious; is more difficult for patients to understand; is less reliable for use with patients with limited mobility, attention span, or knowledge of the examiner's spoken language

20. generalized defects, focal defects

21. glaucoma, retinal ischemia, optic nerve atrophy, media opacity (cataract or corneal scarring)

22. In kinetic perimetry, too rapid movement of the test object, poor understanding of the test by the patient, and patient slowness in signaling that the target has been seen; also, small pupils, interference with vision by eyeglass rims, aphakia, or a target that seems to be out of focus due to refractive error

23. location, size, shape, depth, slope of margins

24. *Hemianopia*: the right or left half or entire lower or upper portion of the visual field is defective or missing. *Homonymous hemianopia*: the right or left half of the visual field is defective or missing in both eyes.

25. Bjerrum scotoma, paracentral scotoma, nasal step

26. loss of the entire upper or lower visual field

27. environment-, device-, patient-, and examiner-related factors

28. *Environment*: room too hot or cold; room lights too bright or fluctuate; intrusion, movement, noise, and other distractions. *Device*: perimeter, illumination not calibrated; paper, pencils, and other markers are unavailable; if computer-controlled, incorrect disk or door of disk drive not closed. *Patient*: misunderstanding the test, slow reaction time, poor physical condition, distractibility, boredom, anxiety, discomfort, abnormal pupil size, visual acuity, refractive error. *Examiner*: failure to calibrate perimeter illumination or to ensure that environmental conditions are suitable for testing, failure to properly cover eye not being tested, failure to instruct the patient properly in the test, procedure, moving or presenting test targets too rapidly or too slowly.

Chapter 12

1. b, c, d, a

2. b, a, e, d

3. c

4. plastic

5. b

6. the front curve of the lens surface

7. black

8. The angle by which the frame front deviates from the vertical plane when worn. The bottom of the eyeglass frame is closer to the face than the top.

9.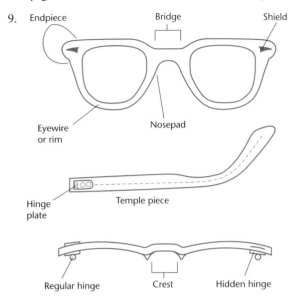

10. Cover the tips of the temple pieces of the frames with your fingers until you have moved them past the patient's eyes.

11. lower eyelid margin

12. c, d, e, b, a

Chapter 13

1. The World Health Organization definition of low vision is a visual acuity of less than 6/18 (20/60) and equal to or better than 3/60 (20/400) in the better eye.

2. cataract, ocular trauma, high refractive error, corneal scarring, macular degeneration, glaucoma, onchocerciasis, diabetic retinopathy, congenital causes, retinopathy of prematurity

3. 1.25×

4. c

5. handheld magnifying lenses, high plus reading spectacles with prismatic correction, telescopes fitted on spectacle lenses

Chapter 14

1. A layer of tears lies between the contact lens and the cornea, filling out corneal irregularities and converting the interface between the contact lens and the cornea into a smooth, spherical surface; the contact lens provides a radius of curvature different from that of the cornea, allowing light to focus on the retina.

2. allow adequate oxygen to reach all of the cornea, promote flushing of metabolic waste from underneath the lens, sustain the integrity of the corneal epithelium, sustain normal corneal temperature

3. spherical power, keratometry readings, lens diameter, base curve, lens thickness, lens material, water content (soft lens), specific brand or type of lens, edge blends or peripheral curves, tint, desired wearing schedule

4. b, c, f, a, e

5. Soft lenses diffuse oxygen and carbon dioxide through the lens material, with a minimal tear pump; PMMA lenses deliver oxygen only by pumping oxygenated tears under the lens; RGP lenses provide oxygen and carbon dioxide diffusion through the lens material and a tear pump.

6. Cleaning removes protein, deposits, and other debris that can blur vision or irritate the eye and act as a reservoir for microorganisms; disinfection prevents the growth of bacteria, viruses, and fungi on the lens.

7. chemical, heat

8. to keep the lens surface hydrophilic; to provide a lubricating cushion between the contact lens and the cornea and between the contact lens and the eyelid

9. Wash hands and dry them with a lint-free towel; be sure all traces of soap are rinsed off.

10. irritation, fogging, redness, tearing, decreased wearing time, blurry vison

11. Warping is a semipermanent change in the corneal curvature; it is caused by an improperly fit contact lens, usually due to rigid contact lenses.

12. edema, vascularization, ulcer, abrasion, keratitis, infection

13. The conjunctiva, which lines both the globe and the inner lid, prevents the lens from disappearing behind the eye.

14. pathologic conditions such as allergies, chronic blepharoconjunctivitis, pterygium, seventh-nerve paresis, anesthetic cornea; inappropriate nervous and emotional temperament; poor or no blink reflexes; dry eyes; disabilities such as parkinsonism or arthritis; ongoing exposure to dust, dirt, particles, or caustic chemicals

Chapter 15

1. a preliminary interview with a patient to determine the urgency of the situation and to schedule a visit with the doctor accordingly

2. What is the basic medical complaint or symptom? How did the complaint or symptom originate? When did the complaint or symptom start?

3. The triage process typically begins when the ophthalmic medical assistant performs a preliminary interview with a patient by phone to determine the urgency of the patient's situation and to schedule his or her visit with the ophthalmologist appropriately.

4. b, c, d

5. a, b, c, d

6. acid, alkali, organic solvents

7. Irrigate the affected eye immediately by holding it open either under a continuous flow of running tap water or a basin filled with water for at least 15 to 20 minutes before proceeding to the office or emergency facility.

8. a, b, d

9. c, d

10. If possible, get the patient's head below the heart.

11. c

12. d

13. a, b, c, d, e

14. a, b, c

Patient Screening Exercises

1. b, c, e, f, h *Discussion*: Any screening evaluation requires you to obtain the most important information in the shortest time. The principal questions to ask in assessing the urgency of a complaint of visual disturbance are how long the symptom has been present (b), how rapidly it has occurred (c), how severe it is (f), and whether one or both eyes are affected (e). For any complaint, it is useful to document any noticeable associated symptoms (h). The other questions might be useful in a more detailed history, but they do not help to establish the urgency of the patient's complaint.

2. a, c, d, e, i *Discussion*: A chemical injury should always be considered an emergency, and the screening evaluation should seek only the most crucial pieces of information. For injuries that have just occurred, immediate irrigation should always supersede all other instructions or inquiries (a). Timing of the accident (c) is relevant because the more recent the occurrence, the greater the benefit of immediate irrigation and prompt medical attention. This information tells the doctor how far, if at all, damage has progressed and helps in patient evaluation. Impaired vision (d) may suggest a more serious injury, and knowing the chemical involved (e) can provide information about the potential for serious eye damage. Both of these facts help the ophthalmologist make the most informed treatment decisions. It can help to know whether a patient can see well enough with at least one eye to get to the water faucet or drive to the doctor's office, although it may not ordinarily matter which eye was involved (h). Always ask patients with potential emergencies if they have transportation to the office or a medical facility (i); if not, an ambulance or a taxicab may have to be summoned. The presence or absence of glasses (b) is usually critical only if there was an explosion that may have caused fragments from the glasses to penetrate the eye. History of glaucoma (f) and presence of tearing (g) are not considered crucial information in this case.

3. b, c, e, f, h *Discussion*: All patients should be questioned about the duration of their symptoms (b). Mild symptoms of long duration, such as burning eyes over a 3-month period, typically do not represent an emergency. However, a patient with sudden, unexplained burning and/or redness (e) of previously normal eyes may be experiencing an acute reaction to an environmental irritant and

should be handled expeditiously. Knowing whether and when symptoms seem most noticeable (c), whether and what other symptoms are present (f), and what activities relieve the patient's symptoms (h) can better indicate the nature of the problem and may allow the doctor to recommend relief measures until the patient can be seen. Questions a, d, and g are not necessarily inappropriate but may be better left for a more detailed history at the time of the visit.

4. a, b, d, e *Discussion*: Whenever a patient reports visual impairment, such as this one and the patient reporting blurred vision in exercise 1, it is important to define the nature of the visual loss precisely. This includes the time of onset (a) and whether one or both eyes are affected (b). If the patient had not volunteered that the episodes were transient, it would be appropriate to ask if the visual loss was intermittent or persistent. This information, as well as the length of time of each episode (d), gives the doctor important diagnostic clues that would bear on the urgency. For patients such as this one with repeated episodes, identifying associated symptoms can be important (e). Specifically asking about discharge and tearing (c) or headaches (g) is not usually useful in determining the nature of the visual loss itself. These questions and questions about family history (f) may be asked during a more detailed history-taking at the office.

Chapter 16

1. a, d

2. no peripheral vision but good central vision, no central vision, less than 20/200 visual acuity, only portions of the visual field perceived, light perception only, no light perception, fluctuations in vision

3. Either proceed to a room with the patient or have another office staff member take over guiding the patient for you.

4. 8/200

5. see and count fingers, detect hand movements, perceive light

6. c

7. c

8. hypoglycemia

Chapter 17

1. informed consent

2. d

3. topical eyedrops, infiltrative injection

4. forceps, scissors, needle holder

5. taper point, cutting, reverse-cutting, spatula

6. *Absorbable*: surgical gut, collagen, polyglactin 910. *Nonabsorbable*: silk, nylon, polypropylene, polyester.

7. epilation, anterior chamber tap, suture removal, foreign body removal, punctal plug insertion, excision of conjunctival and lid lesions

8. to minimize postsurgical bleeding and immobilize the eyelid

9. to reduce the number of microorganisms that come in contact with the surgical wound, thus minimizing the chance of infection

10. instrument sterilization, germicidal prepping of the operative site, scrubbing and gloving (also gowning and masking if required), handling materials in a way that prevents contamination

11. cleansing the patient's operative site with germicidal solution

12. sterile table and trays containing instruments, portions of the patient that have been prepped and draped, portions of the surgical personnel that have been cleansed and gloved

13. to provide a clean operating field and a sterile area on which personnel may rest their hands and instruments during surgery

14. Sharps must be re-counted to ensure that none remains near the patient; disposable sharps are placed in safety containers so that they will not injure office personnel or waste collectors.

Chapter 18

1. occupational requirements, cosmetic or recreational needs, contact lens intolerance, fear of being unsafe in an emergency without glasses

2. uncontrolled ocular surface or other eye disease, immunosuppression, autoimmune diseases that

alter wound healing, corneal ectasias, contact lens–induced warpage

3. Cycloplegic refraction allows the exact determination of the preoperative refraction in that it eliminates accommodation as a source of refractive variability. By completely relaxing accommodation, the refractionist can avoid over-minusing myopic patients and under-plusing hyperopic patients.

4. pupil centration, pupil size under various lighting conditions

5. In LASIK, an anterior corneal flap is created and lifted. The exposed corneal stroma is then treated with the laser. In PRK, the corneal epithelium is mechanically removed and the anterior stroma is then ablated with the laser.

6. low degrees of hyperopia, the induction of myopia in the nondominant eye of a person with emmetropic presbyopia (monovision)

7. low degrees of myopia, early keratoconus, and ectasia post-LASIK surgery

8. to identify patients with abnormally steep or flat corneas and thereby help determine the most appropriate microkeratome to use in LASIK surgery, to determine suitability for phakic IOL, for implant power calculations, to uncover early, barely noticeable corneal surface irregularities.

9. to rule out abnormally thin corneas that would be at greater risk for ectasia after LASIK surgery

10. pigment dispersion, pupillary block, cataract

Chapter 19

1. 10

2. number of new and established patient visits, number of visits per hour per doctor, number of visits per treatment room per hour, number of patient workups per hour per assistant, revenue generated per patient visit, annual revenue per full-time equivalent staff person, annual revenue per full-time equivalent technician

3. the comparison of productivity statistics from one practice with other similar practices to measure their productivity in comparison to those practices

4. (1) Have a preclinic meeting with the doctor or other ophthalmic assistants to review the morning or afternoon schedule to plan that half day. (2) Work up patients efficiently. (3) Determine precisely why the patients is visiting the office. (4) Record your notes clearly, simply, and legibly in the medical record. (5) Be present to assist with special concern patients. (6) Gather ancillary supplies needed for the office visit.

5. (1) Avoid spending more than minimal time socializing with the patient. (2) Do not discuss medical findings with the patient. (3) Do not discuss nonclinical topics with the doctor during clinic time.

6. your attitude

7. performing incomplete patient workups, not signing the chart, not answering simple nonmedical questions for the patient prior to the doctor entering the exam room, leaving telephone messages for patients without leaving your name

8. *HIPAA*: patient records and information must be protected from improper dissemination or transmittal. *OSHA*: personnel must practice certain procedures to protect the health and safety of you, other employees, and patients. *DMEPOS*: suppliers must become accredited in order to enroll or maintain Medicare billing privileges. *PECOS*: physicians who have not opted out of Medicare need to be enrolled in PECOS if they want to continue seeing or referring Medicare patients for most items and services.

9. simplification of insurance claims, standardization of services among physicians, facilitation of appropriate reimbursement by insurance companies, avoidance of payment penalties in the event of an audit, research benefits, patient satisfaction

10. CPT codes

11. ICD codes

12. external injuries and poisonings

13. (1) Coding should never be prepared from an alphabetical list. (2) Coding should be finalized to the highest degree of specificity. (3) Do not code "suspected" or "rule out" diseases.

14. chief complaint; history of present illness; review of systems; past, family, and social history

15. (1) Although the index may be used to initially locate a code, do not code directly from the index. Always read the complete description in the main body of the manual before selecting a code. (2) Do not choose a code that only approximates the service that was performed. CPT specifically indicates that a code should only be selected if it accurately describes the service. There are "unlisted" codes that can be utilized when necessary to describe services for which no specific CPT descriptor applies.

Suggested Activities

3. ICD codes:

378.15	Exotropic
365.22	Acute glaucoma
373.11	Hordeolum
373.0	Blepharitis
366.20	Traumatic cataract

4. CPT codes:

67112	Retinal detachment repair
66985	2° IOL
67900	Repair brow ptosis
65855	Trabeculoplasty
66821	Posterior capsulotomy

Chapter 20

1. a
2. b
3. b
4. c
5. d
6. b
7. c
8. c
9. c
10. a

Chapter 21

1. The World Health Organization defines 5 levels of visual impairment. Its definition is based on best-corrected vision in the better-sighted eye. The mildest category encompasses visual acuities from 20/70 to 20/200. The intermediate categories are 20/200 to 20/400, 20/400 to 20/1200, and 20/1200 to bare light perception. The last category is no light perception. Individual government definitions for vision impairment may vary. In the United States, if your vision with eyeglasses or corrective lenses is 20/60 or worse, you are considered visually impaired (ICD-10-CM level 1). The 1935 Aid to the Blind program in the Social Security Act defined legal blindness as either central visual acuity of 20/200 or less in the better eye with corrective glasses or central visual acuity of more than 20/200 if there is a visual field defect wherein the widest angle of the visual field is no greater than 20° in the better eye. This would correspond to the ICD-10-CM level category of visual impairment level 2.

2. cataract, uncorrected refractive errors, glaucoma, age-related macular degeneration, corneal opacity, diabetic retinopathy, trachoma, eye conditions in children, onchocerciasis

3. The goal of the VISION 2020 initiative is to eliminate avoidable blindness in the world by the year 2020. Its strategy is built on a foundation of community participation, with 3 essential components or elements: cost-effective disease control interventions, human resource development (training and motivation), and infrastructure development (facilities, appropriate technology, consumables, funds).

4. The team approach to eye care recognizes that multiple individuals and resources are needed to support the individual eye care patient. Key components of the team approach are careful planning prior to the beginning of a project, community involvement, government involvement, a monitoring and evaluation system for outcomes, and clear mechanisms for dialogue, problem-solving, and coordination between all members of the team.

5. Key features of successful community eye care programs include careful planning of the project, community involvement and ownership, government involvement and leadership, a good

monitoring and evaluation system for outcomes, and a structure and clear mechanisms for dialogue, problem-solving, and coordination among all stakeholders.

6. Raising public awareness with an educational program and providing high-quality patient screening programs are very effective methods to provide health education information within the local community. In the United States, medical societies, hospitals, and other community health groups have organized health fairs inviting the public to be screened for various medical conditions, including eye problems.

7. Criteria include the following: correct patient and surgical site have been identified; consent form is signed and correct; all required fasting, medications and doses, anesthetic options, and skin preparations correspond with standing orders and/or the doctor's documented request. Prior to commencement of surgery, all members of the team, within a particular clinical area, have checked that the patient's details in the chart correspond with the patient before them and that they have all the required equipment, stock, medications, and instruments required before commencing the procedure. The medication and stock must be in-date. No expired medications are to be used.

Chapter 22

1. Hruby lens, condensing lenses, funduscopic lenses

2. Clean the front surface of the mirror by blowing off dust with a dry, clean, empty bulb syringe.

3. metal spheres of known curvature

4. To clean the tonometer, wipe the entire tonometer tip carefully and thoroughly with an alcohol sponge and allow it to air-dry for 1 to 2 minutes before reuse. Alternatively, remove the entire prism from the tonometer and soak it for 5 minutes in 3% hydrogen peroxide or a 1:10 dilution of household bleach and water. Then rinse the tip

under running tap water and allow it to dry before reuse. The bleach solution should be changed at least once a day, and the peroxide solution twice a day. Be sure to rinse off the disinfectant and allow for thorough air-drying; if the patient's eye comes in contact with a disinfectant solution, corneal damage, pain, and discomfort could result.

5. It is a combination indentation and applanation device.

6. argon, krypton, Nd:YAG, excimer, diode

7. (1) Remove dust from lenses or mirrors that *cannot* be cleaned with a liquid by blowing it off with a dry, empty bulb syringe or with a blast of air from a can of commercial compressed air or by brushing it off gently with a photographic lens brush or a loosely wadded lens-cleaning paper. (2) Remove fingerprints or oils from cleanable glass and polymethylmethacrylate (PMMA) plastic lenses by moistening a cleaning paper, cotton ball, or lint-free cloth with a special photographic liquid lens cleaner and rubbing the lens surface gently, using a circular motion. (3) Be sure that all cleaning agents are completely removed from the lens surface. Leaving a residue on the lens can diminish its clarity and effectiveness. (4) Dry lenses with clean lens paper or a lint-free cloth.

8. (1) Using a rotary motion, carefully wash the lens in lukewarm water with a moistened cotton ball that contains a few drops of clear dishwashing liquid. (2) Rinse the lens completely with lukewarm water. (3) Blot the lens dry using a lint-free lens-cleaning paper or a soft lint-free absorbent lens cloth. (4) The lens is now ready for disinfection.

9. Is the instrument plugged into an electrical outlet? Are all plugs and connections on the instrument securely in place? Is the bulb burned-out or darkened? Is the instrument fuse burned-out? Are the central wall outlet and electrical fuse for the circuit functioning?

10. Is the battery fresh or recharged? Is the bulb burned-out or darkened?

Appendix A   GLOSSARY

This glossary includes pronunciations for many ophthalmic technical terms. Accented syllables are indicated by CAPITAL LETTERS. Vowel sounds are indicated and pronounced as shown in the table below. Pronunciations are approximate, and alternative pronunciations are often acceptable.

Vowel	Written	Pronounced as in
A	ay	may
	a + consonant	tap
	ah	father
	uh	about
	ae	pair
E	ee	bee
	e + consonant or eh	bet
	ur	term
I	iy	eye
	consonant + y	dye
	i + consonant + e	bite
	i, ih	bit
O	oh	oh
	uh	mother
	o + consonant	hot
	ah	fog
	oo	do
U	yoo	cute
	u + consonant, or uh	hut
Y	ee	happy
	ih	myth
	y	my

abduction (ab-DUK-shun)   The movement of the eye outward toward the temple.

aberrometry (ab-er-ROM-uh-tree)   The measurement of optical aberrations of the visual system using a device called a wavefront analyzer or an aberrometer. *See also* **wavefront analysis**.

abrasion   A scratch.

abscess (AB-sehs)   A localized collection of pus surrounded by inflamed tissue.

absolute scotoma (skoh-TOH-muh)   A severe visual field defect in which the largest and brightest stimulus cannot be seen; blindness at that specific location.

accommodation   The change in the curvature of the crystalline lens that helps to focus images of objects close to the eye.

acidic burns   A chemical injury to tissue, caused by an agent of low pH.

acquired immunodeficiency syndrome (AIDS)   An infection with human immunodeficiency virus (HIV) that causes a compromised immune system.

acute   Refers to a condition that flares up suddenly and persists for only a short time.

add   The portion of the multifocal lens (usually the lower part) that provides correction for near vision. Also called *segment* or *near add*.

adduction (ad-DUK-shun)   The movement of the eye inward toward the nose.

adenovirus (ad-een-oh-VY-rus)   A family of viruses involved primarily in respiratory infections; can cause highly contagious forms of conjunctivitis.

adnexa (ad-NEK-suh)   The tissues and structures surrounding the eye; includes the orbit, extraocular muscles, eyelids, and lacrimal apparatus.

afferent pupillary defect (APD)   A pupil with normal iris function that fails to constrict normally with direct light stimulation but reacts strongly consensually, or when the fellow eye is stimulated. Usually secondary to optic nerve disease.

"against motion"   The retinoscopic reflex movement that is in the opposite direction from the movement of the streak of light from the retinoscope; typical of the myopic eye.

age-related macular degeneration (MAK-yoo-lahr)   A disease in which sensory cells of the macula degenerate, resulting in a loss of central vision; usually affects older people.

AIDS   *See* **Acquired immunodeficiency syndrome**.

alkali burn   A chemical injury to tissue, caused by an agent of high pH.

allergic reaction   A condition in which the body produces antibodies to foreign materials such as food, plant pollens, or medications.

alternate cover test   A test performed by placing an occluder over one eye and then moving it slowly over to the other eye to detect a tendency for the eyes to deviate while under the occluder (such an ocular misalignment is known as a phoria). Also called *cross-cover test*.

altitudinal scotoma (skoh-TOH-muh)   The joining and enlargement of a nasal step visual field defect and an arcuate scotoma to cause loss of the entire upper or lower visual field.

amblyopia   Decreased vision present without apparent abnormalities in the ocular anatomy and uncorrectable by spectacles or contact lenses; results from visual deprivation in early childhood.

ametropia (am-eh-TROH-pee-uh)   The refractive state of an eye that is unable to focus correctly due to a refractive error.

A-mode ultrasonography   *See* **A-scan ultrasonography**.

Amsler grid test (AHM-zler)   A test for determining the presence and location of defects in the central portion of the visual field.

anatomy   The structure of an organism.

anesthetic   A drug that causes a temporary deadening of a nerve, resulting in loss of feeling in the surrounding tissue.

angiogenesis   The formation of new blood vessels.

angiography   A method of examining and recording size, structure, and location of blood vessels in organ systems, using fluorescent dyes.

anisocoria (an-ih-so-KOH-ree-uh)   A condition in which the pupils are of unequal size.

anterior   The front part of a structure

anterior chamber angle   The junction of the cornea and the iris, from which aqueous humor leaves the eye. Also called *filtration angle*.

anterior chamber   The small compartment between the cornea and the iris that is filled with a clear, transparent fluid called aqueous humor.

anterior ischemic optic neuropathy (AION)   Insufficient blood flow to the optic nerve head resulting in a lack of oxygen and subsequent infarction of (loss of) the nerve fibers and loss of vision.

anterior limiting membrane   *See* **Bowman's membrane**.

anterior segment   The front of the eye; includes the structures between the front surface of the cornea and the vitreous.

anti-angiogenesis   A process or agent that prevents new blood vessel growth

antibiotic   A drug that combats a bacterial infection.

antibody   A chemical substance that the body manufactures to neutralize an infecting microorganism, toxin, or foreign agent.

antifungal   A drug that combats a fungal infection.

antimetabolite   A substance that interferes with a metabolite necessary for normal metabolic functions; often used to disrupt proliferation of cancerous or other abnormal cells, antimetabolites may also be used to prevent normal re-growth in circumstances where it is not desirable.

antireflective (AR)   A treatment that reduces or eliminates reflections from the surface of a lens.

antivascular endothelium growth factor (anti-VEGF)   A therapeutic drug used in intravitreal injections that targets vascular endothelial growth factor (VEGF). It acts by diminishing the stimulus for abnormal new vessel growth (angiogenesis), a known cause of wet age-related macular degeneration.

antiviral   A drug that combats a viral infection.

apex   The top, as of a prism.

aphakia (ah-FAY-kee-uh)   The absence of the crystalline lens, usually because of cataract extraction.

aphakic correction (ah-FAY-kik)   The use of a contact lens, eyeglasses, or an intraocular lens to improve visual acuity in aphakic patients.

applanation (ap-lah-NAY-shun)   A form of tonometry in which the force required to flatten a small area of the central cornea is measured and extrapolated into intraocular pressure.

aqueous humor (AY-kwee-us)   The clear, transparent fluid that fills the anterior chamber.

AR   *See* **antireflective**.

arc perimeter   An instrument used to test peripheral vision using bands of half circles placed at various meridians.

arcuate scotoma (AHR-kyu-at skoh-TOH-muh)   An arc-shaped area of reduced sensitivity, or blindness, in the visual field. Also known as *Bjerrum scotoma* or *comet scotoma*.

arcus   *See* **arcus senilis**.

arcus senilis (AR-kus sih-NIL-us)   A common degenerative change in which the outer edge of the cornea gradually becomes opaque, generally in both eyes; usually affects people over the age of 50.

A-scan ultrasonography (ul-trah-son-OG-ruh-fee)   A diagnostic procedure in which sound waves traveling in a straight line are used to reveal the position of, and distances between, structures within the eye and orbit. This technology helps to determine the power selection of an intraocular lens. Also called *A-mode ultrasonography*.

aseptic technique (ay-SEP-tik) A range of procedures used in medical environments to prevent the spread of infectious microbes.

astigmatic keratotomy (AK) A surgical technique to correct astigmatism that employs transverse or arcuate incisions perpendicular to the steepest meridian of the cornea.

astigmatism (uh-STIG-muh-tizm) The refractive error of an eye whose corneal surface curvature is greater in one meridian than another; both distant and near objects appear blurred and distorted.

asymptomatic Without symptoms of disease.

atrophic Loss of tissue or cellular density.

autoclave A metal chamber equipped to use steam or gas under high pressure and temperature to destroy microorganisms.

autoimmune diseases Diseases in which normal immune function is altered, causing the body to produce antibodies against its own cells; examples include Sjögren syndrome, systemic lupus erythematosus, and ulcerative colitis.

Autoplot Brand name for a refined version of the tangent screen (older kinetic perimetric device) for measuring the central 30° of vision.

axial *See* **axial ray**.

axial length of the globe The length of the eyeball from front (cornea) to back (retina), measured through the optical center.

axial ray (AK-see-al) A light ray that strikes the center of a lens of any shape and passes undeviated through the lens material. Also called *principal ray*.

axis The meridian perpendicular to the meridian with curvature in a cylindrical lens.

axon The long fiber-like portion of a ganglion cell that courses over the surface of the retina and converges at the optic disc.

bacteria (singular: bacterium) Single-celled microorganisms, widely dispersed in nature; some bacteria are capable of causing disease in humans.

balancing A procedure performed on both eyes at once to ensure that the optical correction determined by refractometry for distance vision does not include an uneven overcorrection or undercorrection. Also called *binocular balancing*.

basal cell carcinoma (kar-sih-NOH-muh) The most common malignant lid tumor; has a characteristic appearance of a pit surrounded by raised "pearly" edges.

base The bottom, as of a prism.

base curve The curve of the lens surface, usually the outer or front side of the lens, from which the other curves necessary for sight correction are calculated.

benign (beh-NINE) Refers to any tumor that is not dangerous to the well-being of the individual. Also known as *nonmalignant*.

Berlin's edema *See* **retinal edema**.

bifocal lens One that has two powers: usually one for correcting distance vision and one for correcting near vision.

bifocals A lens with two visual purposes; commonly the correction of both distance and near vision.

binary fission The form of cellular reproduction by a bacterium, by splitting in two.

binocular balancing *See* **balancing**.

binocular vision The blending of the separate images seen by each eye into one image; occurs when both eyes are directed toward a single target and perfectly aligned.

biometry *See* **ultrasonography** and **A-scan ultrasonography**.

biomicroscope *See* **slit lamp**.

bipolar cell A type of retinal cell that accepts electric (nerve) impulses from the photo-receptors and passes them to the ganglion cells.

bitemporal hemianopia (hem-ee-uh-NOH-pee-uh) A visual field defect affecting the temporal half of the field of both eyes.

Bjerrum scotoma (BYER-oom skoh-TOH-muh) *See* **arcuate scotoma**.

blended bifocal *See* **invisible bifocal**.

blepharitis (blef-ah-RY-tis) A common inflammation of the eyelid margin.

blowout fracture An injury caused by blunt force applied to the eye, creating pressure that fractures the orbital bones.

blunt lacrimal cannula An unsharpened needle used to pass into the tear system puncta and canaliculus.

blunt trauma Tissue damage caused by a nonpenetrating force.

B-mode ultrasonography *See* **B-scan ultrasonography**.

Bowman's membrane The second corneal layer that lies under the outermost epithelium and above the stroma; also known as the *anterior limiting membrane*.

branch retinal artery occlusion (BRAO) Obstruction of blood flow in a tributary vessel of the central retinal artery.

brightness acuity tester (BAT) A handheld instrument used to assess the disability that occurs when glare interferes with a patient's visual acuity or quality of vision. *See also* **glare testing**.

bruise *See* **ecchymosis**.

B-scan ultrasonography (ul-trah-son-OG-ruh-fee)   A diagnostic procedure that provides two-dimensional reconstruction of ocular and orbital tissues, using radiating sound waves. Also called *B-mode ultrasonography*.

bulbar conjunctiva (kon-junk-TY-vuh)   The portion of the conjunctiva that covers the globe to the edge of the cornea

bullous keratopathy *See* **corneal bullous edema**.

calibration   The testing of any device against a known standard; for example, the illumination of a perimetric device.

canal of Schlemm (SHLEM)   A structure that drains the aqueous humor from the anterior chamber after it has flowed through the trabecular meshwork.

canaliculus (kan-ah-LIK-yu-lus; plural: canaliculi)   *See* **lacrimal canaliculus**.

cannula   A blunt-tipped tube used during surgery for injecting or extracting fluid or air.

canthus (KAN-thus; plural: canthi)   The point where the upper and lower eyelids meet on the nasal (inner) side (medial canthus) and the temporal (outer) side (lateral canthus).

cardinal positions of gaze   The 6 points to which a patient's eyes are directed, to test the major function of each extraocular muscle; the positions are right and up, right, right and down, left and up, left, and left and down.

cardiovascular system   The body system consisting of the heart and blood vessels (arteries and veins).

cataract (KAT-ah-rakt)   An opacified or clouded lens.

cautery (KAW-ter-ee)   The application of heat by electric current by means of a specialized instrument; used to destroy a lesion or to stem bleeding.

cells   The primary building blocks of biologic tissue.

central retinal artery occlusion (CRAO)   Obstruction of blood flow in the main feeder vessel of the retina (central retinal artery).

central scotoma (skoh-TOH-muh)   A visual field defect in the center of the field.

chalazion (kah-LAY-zee-on)   A chronic inflammation resulting from an obstructed meibomian gland in the eyelid; associated with infection. The acute condition is called an internal hordeolum. *See also* **external hordeolum**.

chemical trauma (TRAW-muh)   Refers to injury caused by a chemical, such as an acid or an alkali.

chief complaint   That part of the health history in which the patient describes the primary reason for seeking health care; it should be recorded in the patient's own words as nearly as possible (eg, "patient states he has a red eye" not, "patient has conjunctivitis"). *See also* **history of present illness**.

Chlamydiae (klah-MID-ee-ee; singular: *Chlamydia*)   A type of bacteria.

choroid (KOR-oyd)   A layer of tissue largely made up of blood vessels that nourishes the retina; it lies between the sclera and the retina in the uveal tract.

choroidal neovascularization (CNV)   An abnormal collection of fragile new blood vessels growing in the choroid under the retina, responsible for hemorrhages and fluid leakage, which can lead to loss of central vision when present in or near the macula.

chronic   Refers to a condition that has persisted for some time.

cilia (SIL-ee-ah; singular: cilium)   The eyelashes.

ciliary body (SIL-ee-ehr-ee)   A band-like structure of muscle and secretory tissue that extends from the edge of the iris and encircles the inside of the sclera.

ciliary muscle (SIL-ee-ehr-ee)   The muscle fibers in the ciliary body of the uveal tract that are involved in accommodation.

ciliary process (SIL-ee-ehr-ee)   A finger-like extension of the ciliary body that produces aqueous humor.

ciliary spasm   A painful contraction of the ciliary muscle commonly caused by inflammation of the cornea or iris.

cilium   *See* **cilia**.

circles of eccentricity   A series of concentric circles at intervals of 10° from the point of central visual fixation, providing coordinates for mapping the visual field.

clamp   A surgical instrument used to compress or crush tissue, or temporarily hold surgical sutures or drapes.

CLPU   *See* **contact lens peripheral ulcers**.

CNV   *See* **choroidal neovascularization**.

codes for diagnoses   A numerical designation applied to all known medical conditions; eg, 373.2 in ICD-9 terminology indicates a diagnosis of chalazion. Used for billing and tracking purposes. *See also* **ICD codes**.

codes for procedures and services   A numerical designation applied to medical procedures and services; eg, 67800 in CPT terminology indicates a procedure for excision of chalazion, single. *See also* **CPT codes**.

collagen vascular disease   *See* **connective tissue disease**.

comet scotoma (skoh-TOH-muh)   *See* **arcuate scotoma**.

comitant   A strabismus that is the same in all fields of gaze.

common-vehicle transmission   The form of infection transmission involving the transfer of infectious microbes from one reservoir to many people.

complication   A problem that occurs during or after medical or surgical treatment.

computed tomography   An x-ray technique that produces a very detailed image of a cross section of tissue. The image created is often called *CT scan*.

concave lens   A piece of glass or plastic in which one or both surfaces are curved inward. Also called *negative lens* or *minus lens*.

concave mirror effect   The lighting effect of a retinoscope that produces convergent rays.

condensing lenses   High plus (+14 to +40) handheld, noncontact biconvex lenses used by the physician to view the ocular fundus with the slit lamp or indirect ophthalmoscope.

conductive keratoplasty (CK)   A solid-state infrared laser refractive surgical procedure employed to create heat shrinkage of the peripheral corneal stroma thereby steepening the central cornea and reducing hyperopia.

cone   The retinal photoreceptor largely responsible for sharp central vision and for color perception.

confrontation field test   A test comparing the gross boundaries of the patient's field of vision with that of the examiner, who is presumed to have a normal field.

congenital glaucoma (glaw-KOH-muh)   A rare disease that occurs in infants; due to a malformation of the anterior chamber angle.

congenital   Refers to any disease process or effect that is present from birth.

conjunctiva (kon-junk-TY-vuh)   A thin, translucent mucous membrane extending from the outer corneal border over the globe and the inner surface of the eyelids.

conjunctivitis (kon-junk-tih-VY-tis)   An inflammation of the conjunctiva that causes swelling of the small conjunctival vessels, making the eye appear red; it may be caused by bacterial or viral infection, allergy, or exposure to environmental agents such as chlorinated swimming pool water; also called *pink eye*.

connective tissue disease   Disorders characterized by immunologic and inflammatory changes in the connective tissues, Also called *collagen vascular disease*.

consensual pupillary reaction   Reflexive reaction occurring when a light is directed into one pupil and the pupil of the opposite eye simultaneously and equally reacts. *See also* **direct pupillary reaction**.

contact lens-induced acute red eye (CLARE)   Dilation of blood vessels in the conjunctiva caused by contact lens irritation.

contact lens peripheral ulcers (CLPU)   Contact lens-induced noninfectious corneal ulcers outside the visual axis.

contraindication   Any condition that renders a particular treatment, medication, or medical device inadvisable for a particular patient.

contrast-sensitivity test   A procedure for determining the ability to distinguish between light and dark areas; useful in the diagnosis of cataract.

converge   To come together.

convex lens   A piece of glass or plastic in which one or both surfaces are curved outward. Also called *positive lens* or *plus lens*.

cornea (KOR-nee-uh)   The clear membrane at the front of the globe that begins the process of focusing light the eye receives.

corneal abrasion (KOR-nee-uhl)   A scratch or other defect in the superficial cornea (epithelium) caused by trauma.

corneal bullous edema   Swelling of the corneal tissue severe enough to create blisters on the surface of the cornea and decreased vision. Also known as *bullous keratopathy*.

corneal edema   Swelling of the corneal tissue.

corneal endothelium (KOR-nee-uhl en-doh-THEE-lee-um)   The fifth, innermost corneal layer that lies under Descemet's membrane; it is composed of a single layer of cells that maintains proper fluid balance within the cornea.

corneal epithelium (KOR-nee-uhl ep-ih-THEE-lee-um)   The outermost corneal layer, which lies above Bowman's membrane and provides defense against infection and injury.

corneal infiltrates   A discrete collection of inflammatory cells in the cornea.

corneal stroma (KOR-nee-uhl STROH-muh)   The third, or middle, corneal layer, which lies under Bowman's membrane and above Descemet's membrane; it contributes to corneal rigidity.

corneal topography (KOR-nee-uhl top-OG-rah-fee)   A device that records the surface terrain of the cornea, used to detect aberrations of the contour, as well as regular and irregular astigmatism.

corneal ulcer (KOR-nee-uhl) Pathologic condition involving a defect in the corneal surface and associated with inflammation; infectious ulcers are caused by a pathogenic microorganism.

corneal vascularization Abnormal condition characterized by blood vessel growth in the cornea.

cortex A clear paste-like protein that surrounds the nucleus of the crystalline lens.

corticosteroid A drug, either a natural or a synthetic hormone, that combats an allergic or inflammatory condition. Also called *steroid*.

cover–uncover test A test performed by alternately covering and uncovering each eye to determine if a patient's eyes are misaligned (this misalignment is called a tropia).

CPT codes Codes referring to current procedural terminology published by the American Medical Association, which assigns a number to each procedure or test; updated regularly, the current version is CPT-5.

CR-39 Common plastic lens material with an index of refraction of 1.49.

cranial arteritis *See* **temporal arteritis.**

Creutzfeldt-Jakob disease A rare, progressive encephalopathy associated with aberrant prion protein particles. May be transmitted via organ transplantation (including corneal transplants). "Mad cow" is the prion disease in cattle that when transmitted to humans causes a variant form of Creutzfeldt-Jakob disease.

cross cover test *See* **alternate cover test.**

cross cylinder A special lens consisting of two cylinders of equal power, one minus and one plus, with their axes set at right angles to each other; used for determining the axis and power of an astigmatic correction.

cryopexy (kry-oh-PEKS-ee) Freezing by surgical means.

crystalline lens *See* **lens.**

CT scan *See* **computed tomography.**

cul-de-sac (KUL-deh-sahk) *See* **fornix.**

curette A scoop-shaped surgical tool used to scrape or remove unwanted tissue.

Cushing disease The disease complex caused by excessive secretion of the adrenal hormone cortisol. Predominantly found in women. Also known as *hypercortisolism* or *Cushing syndrome.*

cycloplegia (sy-kloh-PLEE-jee-uh) Temporary paralysis of the ciliary muscle (preventing accommodation) and of the iris sphincter muscle (preventing constriction of the pupil).

cycloplegic refraction (sy-kloh-PLEE-jik) Refractometry performed with the use of a drug that temporarily paralyzes the ciliary muscle, thus blocking accommodation.

cylinder *See* **spherocylinder.**

cylindrical lens A lens that has curvature in only one meridian.

cytomegalovirus (CMV) (sy-toh-Meg-ah-loh-VY-rus) A member of the herpes virus family; causes CMV retinitis.

D segment A portion of a bifocal or trifocal lens; so called because it is shaped like the capital letter D lying on its side.

dacryocystitis (dak-ree-oh-sis-TY-tis) Inflammation of the lacrimal sac; usually caused by blockage or obstruction of the nasolacrimal duct.

daily-wear lenses Rigid and soft contact lenses intended to be worn for fewer than 24 consecutive hours while awake.

DBC *See* **distance between optical centers.**

DCRP *See* **digital corneal reflex pupillometer.**

decibel The unit (one tenth of a log) of measure of the brightness of a test object.

decongestant A substance that reduces congestion or swelling; decongestant eyedrops constrict the superficial conjunctival blood vessels to reduce ocular redness

deep scotoma (skoh-TOH-muh) A visual field defect more serious than a shallow scotoma; appears as a "pit" or "well" in the island of vision.

degenerative Refers to any process in which the structure or function of body tissues gradually deteriorates.

dendritic (den-DRIT-ik) Branch-shaped, such as the corneal ulcers seen after infection with the herpes simplex virus.

density Compactness, with reference to the structure of a particular substance.

depression The type of visual field defect that is like an indentation in the surface of the island of vision.

Descemet's membrane (des-eh-MAYZ) The fourth corneal layer that lies above the innermost endothelium and below the stroma; it contributes to corneal rigidity.

developmental Refers to any disease process or effect that results from faulty development of a structure or system.

diabetes mellitus (dy-uh-BEE-tis MEL-it-us) A disorder of metabolism resulting from insufficient or absent insulin production from the pancreas; may also be due to insulin resistance.

diabetic retinopathy (dy-uh-BET-ik Reh-tin-OP-uh-thee) Pathologic changes in the retina; usually occurs in patients with long-standing, poorly controlled diabetes.

diagnosis (dy-ag-NOH-sis) Determination of a medical condition.

diffuse To spread widely through a tissue. *See* **infection**.

digital corneal reflex pupillometer (DCRP) An instrument that monocularly measures interpupillary distance (PD).

dilator muscle The iris muscle that dilates the pupil in reduced light conditions; fibers from this muscle stretch from the pupil to the outer boundaries of the iris.

diopter (dy-OP-tur) The unit of measure of the power of a lens.

diplopia (dih-PLOH-pee-uh) Double vision.

direct and consensual pupillary reaction (PYU-pih-lehr-ee) The response of the pupils when light is shone in one eye: that eye constricts (direct reaction) and the other eye also constricts, even when light does not reach it (consensual reaction).

direct-contact transmission The form of infection transmission between people usually requiring body contact, or contact with blood and body fluids.

direct ophthalmoscope (ahf-THAL-muh-skohp) A handheld instrument with a light and mirror system that provides a 15-fold magnified, monocular view of a narrow field of the ocular fundus. *See also* **indirect ophthalmoscope**.

direct pupillary reaction A reflexive reaction occurring when a light is directed into one pupil; the normal response is pupillary constriction. *See also* **consensual pupillary reaction**.

disease Abnormal function of a body part or system due to hereditary, infectious, dietary, environmental, or other causes and characterized by a certain set of signs and symptoms.

disinfection The process of inactivating or eliminating pathogenic microorganisms.

disposable lenses Soft contact lenses designed for both daily and extended wear, and then discarded after 1 to 4 weeks.

distance between optical centers (DBC) The distance between the optical center of the right eyeglass lens and that of the left; corresponds to the patient's interpupillary distance.

distometer (dis-TOM-eh-ter) An instrument for measuring vertex distance. *See also* **vertometer**.

diverge To spread apart.

Dk A measurement of the amount of oxygen transmission through a contact lens; high Dk values indicate high oxygen permeability. *See* **oxygen permeable**.

double-D segment A multifocal lens with the distance correction in the middle, a traditional near-power D segment at the bottom, and an intermediate-power inverted D segment at the top.

drusen Light-yellow deposits beneath the retinal pigment epithelium, visible on examination of the ocular fundus.

eccentricity, circles of *See* **circles of eccentricity**.

ecchymosis A visible collection of blood that has leaked from a vessel into the surrounding tissue, usually due to trauma; also called a *bruise*.

ectasia In the eye, refers to a thin, stretched sclera or cornea. A corneal ectasia is thinning with protrusion.

ectropion (ek-TROH-pee-on) A condition in which the eyelid margin is everted (turned) outward from the globe; may be degeneration of or damage to the eyelid tissues.

edema (eh-DEE-mah) Swelling caused by the abnormal presence of fluid in tissues.

electromagnetic radiation Radiation produced through the combination of electrical and magnetic forces; includes rays from the shortest to longest wavelengths, both visible and invisible.

emergency A medical situation that requires immediate attention.

emmetropia (em-eh-TROH-pee-uh) The refractive state of an eye that is able to focus correctly without the need for optical lenses.

emphysema Air trapped in an organ or tissue.

empiric treatment The institution of medical treatment based on probable cause, before test results or other time-consuming procedures confirm a diagnosis.

endocrine system The body system consisting of multiple glands that produce chemicals called hormones, which regulate various bodily functions.

endophthalmitis (en-dahf-thal-MY-tis) A serious inflammation of the intraocular tissues including the vitreous; may be due to bacterial or fungal infection, allergy, or chemical toxicity.

endothelium, corneal *See* **corneal endothelium**.

entropion (en-TROH-pee-on) A condition in which the upper or lower lid margin is turned inward.

enzyme cleaner A specially designed detergent for removing protein deposits from contact lenses.

enzymes Substances produced by cells to accelerate or promote a biochemical reaction.

epiphora (eh-PIF-oh-ruh) Excessive tearing.

episcleral blood vessels Fine blood vessels on the surface of the sclera and under the conjunctiva.

episcleritis (ep-ih-skleh-RY-tis) Inflammation of the surface layer of the sclera.

epithelium, corneal *See* **corneal epithelium**.

eso deviation The inward deviation of the eye.

esophoria (ees-oh-FOR-ee-uh) The inward deviation of the eye that is present only when one eye is covered.

esotropia (ees-oh-TROH-pee-uh) The inward deviation of the eye in which the eyes are misaligned even when uncovered.

etiology (ee-tee-OL-oh-jee) Literally, the study of the causes of a disease; informally, the causes themselves.

excimer laser An ultraviolet laser instrument that vaporizes or ablates tissue.

executive Refers to a bifocal lens consisting of a top distance band and a bottom near band that divide the entire width of the lens into two parts.

exo deviation The outward deviation of the eye.

exophoria (ek-soh-FOR-ee-uh) The outward deviation of the eye that is present only when one eye is covered.

exophthalmometer (ek-sahf-thal-MOM-uh-tur) An instrument that measures the prominence of the eyeball in relation to the bony orbital rim surrounding it.

exophthalmometry (ek-sahf-thal-MOM-uh-tree) The measurement of the prominence of the eyeball in relation to the bony orbital rim surrounding it.

exophthalmos (ek-sahf-THAL-mohs) *See* **proptosis**.

exotropia (ek-soh-TROH-pee-uh) The outward deviation of the eye in which the eyes are misaligned even when uncovered.

exposure keratopathy The pathologic change that occurs to the cornea when it is partially or completely unprotected by the eyelids for extended periods of time.

extended-wear lenses Soft contact lenses that are approved for overnight wear for up to 7 days.

external hordeolum An infection or inflammation of a Zeis gland located on the eyelid margin in a lash follicle. *See* **internal hordeolum**.

extraocular muscles The 6 muscles that attach to the outside of the globe and control its movements.

exudative retinal detachment *See* **retinal detachment**.

eyeball *See* **globe**.

eyelid The complex movable cover of the outer portion of the eyeball. The eyelids consist of an upper and lower component of skin, tarsus, delicate muscles, eyelashes, glands, and conjunctiva.

15-hue test A test that can identify color vision deficits by asking the patient to arrange 15 pastel-colored chips of similar brightness but subtly different hues in a related color sequence. Also called *Farnsworth-Munsell D-15 test*.

Farnsworth-Munsell D-15 test Color vision test. *See* **15-hue test**.

filtration angle *See* **anterior chamber angle**.

fixate To gaze steadily at something.

flashlight test A simple test for estimating the depth of the anterior chamber and the chamber angle.

floaters Small particles of dead cells or other debris that become suspended in the vitreous, or particles of the vitreous itself that degenerate in the normal aging process; they cast shadows on the retina and appear as spots or cobwebs.

fluorescein (FLOOR-uh-seen) A dye solution that is used in applanation tonometry; also used intravenously in fluorescein angiography.

fluorescein angiography (FLOOR-uh-seen an-jee-OG-ruh-fee) Diagnostic photography of retinal vessels that utilizes an intravenous injection of fluorescein dye.

focal defect The type of visual field defect in which a local "pit" or "well" in the field of vision occurs.

focal length The distance between the focal point and the lens.

focal point The point somewhere along the principal axis at which the paraxial rays from a distant source are refracted by a lens and converge in the case of a convex lens and diverge in the case of a concave lens.

foreign-body sensation A feeling of eye irritation or grittiness.

fornix (FOR-niks) The loose pocket of conjunctival tissue where the palpebral and bulbar portions of the conjunctiva meet in the recess of the upper and lower lids. Also called *cul-de-sac*.

fovea (FOH-vee-uh) The center of the macula.

frequency doubling technology (FDT) A perimetry examination using alternating flickers of black and white striated stimuli into the eye at a very high temporal frequency. This test uses an illusion created by the stimuli to detect visual field defects.

functional vision An individual's subjective perception of his or vision during activities of daily living.

fundus (FUN-dus) A collective term for the retina, optic disc, and macula.

funduscopic examination (fun-du-SKOP-ik) Examination of the vitreous and fundus by ophthalmoscope. Also called *posterior segment examination*.

funduscopic lenses   High plus (+60, +78, and +90), noncontact lenses used in conjunction with the slit lamp for stereoscopic observation of the fundus.

fungus (plural: fungi)   A multicelled microorganism that differs from a bacterium in that it has a more complex structure; includes yeasts and molds. Some can live inside the body and cause infection.

fusion   The blending by the brain of the separate images received by the two eyes so that a single view is perceived even when the eyes move.

ganglion cell (GANG-glee-on)   The type of retinal cell that accepts electric (nerve) impulses from the bipolar cells and sends the impulses via axons through the optic disc to the brain.

gel   Thick (viscous) liquid used as a vehicle to deliver a drug topically. *See also* **ointment**.

generalized defect   The type of visual field defect in which the field of vision shrinks symmetrically or is depressed evenly across the entire retina.

genetic   Refers to a trait that is inherited from either or both parents.

Geneva lens clock   An instrument for measuring the base curve of an eyeglass lens.

genus (plural: genera)   A category of biologic classification ranking immediately higher than the species; the general name for a type of organism.

geometric optics   The area of optics that deals with the transmission of light as rays and is concerned with the effect of lenses on light and the production of images.

germicide   A chemical that kills germs.

giant cell arteritis   *See* **temporal arteritis**.

giant papillary conjunctivitis (GPC) (PAP-ih-lehr-ee Kon-junk-tih-VY-tis)   Inflammation of the palpebral conjunctiva, characterized by large raised bumps.

gimbal (GIM-buhl)   The ring-like frame in the lensmeter.

glare   A scattering of a single bright light source across the visual field that interferes with one's sight and markedly reduces the quality of the image received by the retina.

glare testing   A procedure for assessing a patient's vision in the presence of a bright light source to determine whether sensitivity to glare is contributing to visual symptoms. *See also* **brightness acuity tester**.

glaucoma (glaw-KOH-muh)   An eye disease in which the intraocular pressure is high enough to cause damage to the optic nerve, resulting in visual loss; caused by impaired drainage of the aqueous fluid out of the eye.

globe   The eye, without its surrounding structures. Also called *eyeball*.

goblet cell   The type of cell in the conjunctiva that produces the sticky fluid (mucin) that comprises the innermost tear-film layer.

Goldmann applanation tonometer   A tonometer that is attached to a biomicroscope (slit lamp) that measures intraocular pressure by determining how much force is needed to flatten the central cornea.

Goldmann goniolens (GOH-nee-oh-lenz)   A mirrored contact lens used in gonioscopy; reflects an image of the anterior chamber angle, viewed with the aid of a slit lamp.

Goldmann perimeter   A bowl-like instrument for testing visual fields in which targets (lights) of different sizes and intensities are projected onto a standardized background illumination.

gonioscopy (goh-nee-OS-koh-pee)   A method of viewing the chamber angle through a special contact lens placed on the anesthetized eye.

GPC   *See* **giant papillary conjunctivitis**.

Gram staining   The procedure for identifying bacteria and certain other microbes according to their reaction to a dye—either gram-positive or gram-negative.

granuloma (gran-yu-LOH-mah)   A firm collection of a specific kind of inflammatory cell.

granulomatous   A term used to describe a mass lesion resembling a granuloma.

Graves disease   A condition of unknown origin that involves the thyroid gland and causes the soft tissues surrounding the globe to swell.

Health Insurance Portability and Accountability Act (HIPAA)   A federal regulation that mandates how medical practices secure and transmit a patient's medical information.

Heidelberg retinal tomograph (HRT)   An instrument used for analysis of the optic nerve head and other posterior structures by producing a topographic image of the optic nerve head, vitreoretinal interface, and macula.

hemianopia (hem-ee-uh-NOH-pee-uh)   The type of visual field defect in which the right or left half of the field in one eye is missing.

hemorrhage (HEM-or-ij)   Rapid loss of a large amount of blood from a damaged blood vessel.

hemostasis (hee-moh-STAY-sis)   The control of bleeding.

herpes simplex virus (HER-peez SIM-pleks)   In ophthalmology, a type of virus that infects the cornea, producing branch-like ulcers (dendritic keratitis).

herpes simplex virus type 1 (HSV-1) (HER-peez SIM-pleks)   A herpesvirus that causes recurrent fever blisters on the lips and mouth and, if introduced to the eye, causes keratitis.

herpes simplex virus type 2 (HSV-2) (HER-peez SIM-pleks)   Similar to HSV-1, except that it more commonly infects the genital region and is spread by sexual contact.

herpesvirus (her-peez-VY-rus)   A family of viruses.

HIPAA *See* **Health Insurance Portability and Accountability Act.**

history of present illness   The expansion of a patient's chief complaint; includes information about the onset, duration, characteristics, and aggravating or alleviating factors related to the present illness. *See also* **chief complaint.**

HIV *See* **human immunodeficiency virus.**

homonymous hemianopia (hoh-MON-ih-mus Hem-ee-uh-NOH-pee-uh)   The type of visual field defect in which the right or left half of the field in both eyes is missing.

hordeolum (hor-DEE-oh-lum)   *See* **internal hordeolum; stye.**

horizontal and vertical meridians   The radial meridians that divide the visual field into quarters.

hormones   Regulating substances produced by various endocrine glands (such as the thyroid, pituitary, and adrenal), and transported by the blood to targeted organs to initiate a specific reaction or effect.

host   The animal or plant from which a microbe gains nutrients and the conditions necessary for its survival and reproduction.

HRT *See* **Heidelberg retinal tomograph.**

Hruby lens (HRU-bee)   A noncontact lens attached to the slit lamp; useful for examining the optic nerve head and small areas of the posterior retina and vitreous.

HSV-1 *See* **herpes simplex virus type 1.**

HSV-2 *See* **herpes simplex virus type 2.**

human immunodeficiency virus (HIV)   A retrovirus that causes acquired immunodeficiency syndrome (AIDS), a disorder of the immune system that increases the patient's susceptibility to infections such as cytomegalovirus (CMV) retinitis.

hydrophilic (hy-droh-FIL-ik)   Refers to the property of combining with or attracting water.

hydrophobic (hy-droh-FOH-bik)   Refers to the property of resisting or repelling water.

hypercortisolism *See* **Cushing disease.**

hyperopia (hy-per-OH-pee-uh)   Farsightedness. If the eye is too short for its optical system the condition is called axial hyperopia. If the refractive power is insufficient for the length of the eye the condition is called refractive hyperopia.

hyperthyroidism   The disease complex caused by excessive secretion of thyroid hormone.

hyphema (hy-FEE-muh)   The pooling of blood in the anterior chamber as a result of trauma or certain diseases.

hypoglycemia (hy-poh-gly-SEE-mee-uh)   Low blood sugar level, common among patients with diabetes.

hypopyon (hy-POH-pee-on)   The accumulation of pus (white blood cells) in the anterior chamber.

hypoxia (hy-POK-see-uh)   A loss of oxygen.

ICD codes   Code of the *International Classification of Diseases* published by the American Medical Association, a system that assigns a number to each disease or diagnosis; updated regularly, the current version is *ICD-9.*

ICRS *See* **intracorneal ring segment.**

idiopathic   Of unknown cause.

immune reaction   The body's response to infection, in which antibodies are manufactured to neutralize the infecting microorganism and perhaps prevent recurrence of the infection.

immunosuppressed   Lacking the ability to produce a normal immune response to fight infection by bacteria, fungi, or viruses. Also called *immunocompromised.*

incise   To make a deliberate and controlled cut into body tissue.

incision   A cut produced by a sharp instrument.

incomitant *See* **noncomitant.**

indentation   A form of tonometry in which the amount of corneal indentation produced by a fixed weight is measured.

indirect ophthalmoscope (ahf-THAL-muh-skohp)   An instrument with a light and mirror system that provides a binocular and wide view of the ocular fundus. *See* **direct ophthalmoscope.**

indirect-contact transmission   The form of infection transmission involving an intermediate, inanimate object.

indocyanine green   A dye solution that is used intravenously in indocyanine angiography to study choroidal circulation and in situations where an overlying hemorrhage or exudate obscures the visibility of the choroidal vessels.

infection   The invasion and multiplication of harmful microorganisms in the body tissues: a local bacterial or fungal infection begins in the tissues immediately surrounding the microorganism's point of entry; if unchecked, the infection may spread to surrounding tissues, thereby becoming diffuse.

infectious corneal ulcer   An open lesion on the corneal surface caused by a pathogenic microorganism.

inferior oblique muscle   Extraocular muscle attached to the lower, outer side of the globe; 3 functions are to move the eye upward and outward and to rotate the eye outward.

inferior rectus muscle   Extraocular muscle attached to the underside of the globe; 3 functions are to move the eye downward and inward toward the nose (adduction) and rotate the eye outward.

inflammation   A local protective tissue response to infection, injury, or irritation in which specialized cells move to the affected area; characterized by redness, swelling, warmth, and pain in the inflamed area.

informed consent   The process by which a patient receives information from the physician about the risks, benefits, and alternatives of a proposed procedure in order to decide whether or not to have the procedure or treatment.

injection   (1) The delivery system by which a drug is injected into the body with a hypodermic needle. (2) Tissue redness and swelling caused by dilated blood vessels usually as a result of inflammation or infection.

injury   Damage to or destruction of cells that compose a tissue, organ, or system.

insert   The delivery system by which a drug-containing wafer is placed on the conjunctiva under the upper or lower eyelid; releases the drug slowly and steadily over a period of time.

insulin (IN-suh-lin)   A hormone of the body that regulates sugar metabolism.

interferometer (in-ter-feer-OM-uh-ter)   A laser instrument for determining visual acuity in the presence of an opacity, such as a cataract.

internal hordeolum (hor-DEE-oh-lum)   An acute infection of a meibomian gland in the eyelid; when chronic, the condition is called a *chalazion. See also* **external hordeolum**.

interpupillary distance (IPD or PD) (in-ter-PYU-pih-lehr-ee)   The distance from the center of the pupil of one eye to the center of the pupil of the other eye.

intracorneal ring segment (ICRS)   A surgical technique of placing thin plastic half-circle ring segments in the mid-peripheral cornea to flatten the curvature of the central cornea and reduce myopia. Also known as *intrastromal corneal ring segment*.

intracranial   The cavity in the skull that houses the brain.

intrastromal corneal ring segment   *See* **intracorneal ring segment**.

intraocular pressure (in-trah-OK-yu-lur)   Fluid pressure within the eye.

invisible bifocal   A bifocal lens with a softened or blended transitional zone between the segment and the distance portion. Also called *seamless bifocal* or *blended bifocal*.

IPD   *See* **interpupillary distance**.

iridotomy (ihr-ih-DOT-oh-mee)   A type of laser glaucoma surgery in which an opening is made in the iris to allow fluid to drain from the posterior chamber into the anterior chamber.

iris   The colored circle of tissue that controls the amount of light entering the eye by enlarging or reducing the size of its aperture, the pupil.

iritis (iy-RY-tis)   Inflammation of the iris.

irregular astigmatism (uh-STIG-muh-tizm)   The less common form of astigmatism, in which the corneal surface loses its uniformity secondary to scarring or other pathology.

ischemia (is-KEE-mee-uh)   A condition in which the supply of blood to a part of the body is severely reduced.

isopter (iy-SOP-ter)   In visual field tests, a line connecting the points denoting areas of equal sensitivity to a stimulus; similar to contour lines denoting equal elevations of a topographic map.

keratitis (kehr-ah-TY-tis)   Inflammation of the cornea.

keratoconjunctivitis sicca (kehr-ah-toh-kon-junk-tih-VY-tis SIHK-uh)   Inflammation of the cornea and conjunctiva caused by dry eyes.

keratoconus (kehr-ah-toh-KOH-nus)   A rare degenerative corneal disease in which the center of the cornea thins and assumes the shape of a cone, seriously affecting vision.

keratometer (kehr-ah-TOM-eh-tur)   An instrument used to measure corneal curvature. Also called *ophthalmometer*.

keratometry (kehr-ah-TOM-eh-tree)   The measurement of corneal curvature.

kinetic perimetry (kih-NET-ik peh-RIM-eh-tree)   The type of perimetry that uses a moving test object of a predetermined size and brightness.

Koeppe lens (KEP-ee)   A high-plus contact lens used in gonioscopy to examine the angle structures directly with a handheld light source and microscope.

laceration   A traumatic cut.

lacrimal apparatus (LAK-ri-mul)   The structures for tear production and drainage. *See* **lacrimal gland, punctum, lacrimal canaliculus, lacrimal sac, and nasolacrimal duct**.

lacrimal canaliculus (kan-ah-LIK-yu-lus; plural: canaliculi)   One of 2 small channels (plural *canaliculi*) that starts at the punctum in the upper or lower eyelid and drains tears from the surface of the eye to the lacrimal sac.

lacrimal gland   The gland that produces the watery substance making up the middle layer of the tear film; located in the lateral part of the upper lid.

lacrimal needle   *See* **cannula**.

lacrimal probe   An instrument for exploring and clearing an obstruction of the tear duct.

lacrimal sac   The sac that holds tears after they pass through the canaliculi, which empty through the nasolacrimal duct into the nasal cavity.

lacrimal set   A group of instruments for identifying and clearing an obstruction of the tear duct.

lagophthalmos (lag-ahf-THAL-mos)   A condition in which the globe is not completely covered when the eyelids are closed; may be caused by facial-nerve paralysis or by an enlarged or protruding eye.

LASEK   *See* **laser subepithelial keratomileusis**.

laser assisted in situ keratomileusis (LASIK)   A refractive laser procedure using a microkeratome or femtosecond laser keratome to raise a corneal flap followed by ablation of the stromal bed with an excimer laser.

laser photocoagulation   *See* **photocoagulation**.

laser subepithelial keratomileusis (LASEK)   A refractive laser procedure performed after temporary removal of the surface epithelium and basement membrane from the corneal stroma and replacing it after the laser ablation.

LASIK   *See* **laser assisted in situ keratomileusis**.

lateral canthus   *See* **canthus**.

lateral geniculate body (jeh-NIK-yu-let)   The part of the brain along the visual pathway where optic fibers synapse to the optic radiations and transmit visual impulses.

lateral rectus muscle   Extraocular muscle attached to the outer (temporal) side of the globe; moves the eye outward toward the ear (abduction).

legal blindness   A best-corrected visual acuity of 20/200 or less or a visual field reduced to 20° or less in the better-seeing eye.

lens   Part of the optical focusing system of the eye, immediately behind the iris. Also called *crystalline lens*.

lensmeter (LENZ-mee-tur)   An instrument for measuring the prescription of eyeglass lenses or the power of rigid contact lenses. Also called *lensometer*.

lensometry (lenz-OM-eh-tree)   The measurement of certain qualities of lenses by the use of a lensmeter.

lesion   An abnormal tissue or a break in a normal tissue.

levator palpebrae (leh-VAY-tor PAL-peh-bree)   The muscle attached to the tarsal plate in the middle layer of the upper eyelids that raises the eyelid when it contracts.

limbus   The junction between the sclera and the cornea.

lissamine green   A dye solution that is used topically on the cornea for diagnostic purposes to detect dry eye disease.

local   *See* **infection**.

lower canaliculus   *See* **lacrimal canaliculus**.

lower punctum   *See* **punctum**.

LTK   *See* **laser thermal keratoplasty**.

lubricant   *See* **ocular lubricant**.

MacKay-Marg tonometer   An electronic tonometer that measures intraocular pressure.

macula (MAK-yoo-luh)   The specialized area of the retina close to the center of the back of the eye that provides detailed central vision.

magnetic resonance imaging (MRI)   A multisliced imaging technique utilizing a powerful magnetic field.

malignant (mah-LIG-nant)   Term used to describe a condition that tends to become worse and to cause severe problems or death; *malignant myopia* refers to an unusually severe myopia that causes other progressive problems; a *malignant skin lesion* is one that is cancerous with the potential to spread.

manifest refraction   Refractometry performed without the use of cycloplegic drugs. *See also* **refinement**.

media opacities (oh-PASS-ih-teez)   The general term used to describe a variety of conditions that cloud, obscure, or otherwise affect the ocular media and, ultimately, may disrupt vision.

medial canthus   *See* **canthus**.

medial rectus muscle   Extraocular muscle attached to the inner (nasal) side of the globe; function is to move the eye inward toward the nose (adduction).

meibomian gland (my-BOH-mee-an)   Multiple specialized glands in the upper and lower eyelids that secrete the oily part of the tear film.

meridian (meh-RID-ee-an) Geometric plane; used to indicate maximum and minimum corneal curvature.

mesopic vision Referring to the eyesight under dim lighting conditions. *See also* **photopic vision and scotopic vision.**

metabolism (meh-TAB-uh-lizm) The physical and chemical processes by which the body converts food into energy and new body tissues.

metastasis (meh-TAS-tuh-sis) The process by which cancerous tumor cells move from the site of the original growth to other, distant areas of the body, forming new tumors; the verb form is *metastasize.*

metastasize The transfer of disease from one organ or part to another not directly connected, forming a new distant location of that disease.

microbe *See* **microorganism.**

microkeratome A miniature surgical mechanical knife that can cut a thin corneal flap; used in conjunction with laser refractive surgery such as LASIK.

microorganism An extremely small life form invisible to the unaided eye. Also called *microbe.*

minus lens *See* **concave lens.**

miotic (my-OT-ik) A drug that causes the iris sphincter muscle to contract, producing miosis (pupillary constriction), which reduces the amount of light entering the eye.

mires (MY-erz) The perpendicular crossed lines in a lensmeter or the semicircular lines in a tonometer—targets that, when aligned, aid in the acquisition of accurate measurements.

mirror effect Reflection of an image from a clear, smooth, or polished surface.

mold A form of fungus that produces a woolly, fluffy, or powdery growth.

monovision An artificially produced system creating visual clarity for near in one eye and for distance in the other eye. Can be achieved through surgical procedure or external lenses.

mucinous (MYU-sih-nus) Sticky.

mucopurulent discharge (myu-koh-PYUR-yu-lent) A thick fluid containing mucus and pus; symptomatic of bacterial infection.

multifocal lens *See* **bifocal lens; trifocal lens.**

muscle balance The term that describes the alignment of the extraocular muscles; assessing ocular alignment involves several procedures including the cover test, the alternate cover test, and others.

mydriasis (mih-DRY-ah-sis) Increase in pupil size (dilation) that occurs artificially with application of certain drugs or naturally in dim light.

mydriatic (mid-ree-AT-ik) A drug that dilates the pupil by causing the iris dilator muscle to contract and/or by paralyzing the iris sphincter muscle.

myopia (my-OH-pee-uh) Nearsightedness. If the eye is too long for its optical system, the condition is called *axial myopia.* If the refractive power is excessive for the length of the eye, the condition is called *refractive myopia.*

nasal step The type of visual defect that, when plotted, appears as a step-like loss of vision at the outer limit of the nasal field.

nasolacrimal duct (nay-zoh-LAK-rih-mal) The duct through which tears pass from the lacrimal sac into the nasal cavity.

near add *See* **add.**

near visual acuity (uh-KYU-ih-tee) The measurement of the ability to see clearly at a normal reading distance.

negative lens *See* **concave lens.**

neoplasm (NEE-oh-plazm) A new growth of different or abnormal tissue, such as a tumor or wart.

neovascular net *See* **choroidal neovascularization.**

neovascularization (nee-oh-vas-kyu-lar-ih-ZAY-shun) The abnormal growth of new blood vessels.

nervous system The body system consisting of the brain, spinal cord, and peripheral nerves.

neutralization *See* **lensometry.**

neutralization point The lens power that is the approximate correction for a refractive error.

nevi (NEE-vy; singular: nevus) Literally, freckles; common tumors involving the retina, bulbar conjunctiva, and skin, and appearing as yellowish pink or brown areas.

noncomitant A strabismus that has a different deviation in various gaze directions typically caused by either restriction or paralysis of extraocular muscle(s).

nystagmus (nis-TAG-mus) A condition in which the eyes continually shift in a rhythmic, side-to-side, up-and-down, or rotary motion and then snap back to the normal position.

objective refractometry *See* **retinoscopy.**

occluded Totally obstructed or blocked.

occlusion Blockage.

Occupational Safety and Health Administration (OSHA) A federal agency mandated to protect the health and safety of individuals in the workplace.

ocular histoplasmosis Retinal changes presumed to be caused by the microorganism *Histoplasma* with some lesions affecting the macula, resulting in loss of central vision.

ocular lubricant A medication that helps maintain an adequate tear-film balance or keeps the external eye moist.

ocular media The transparent optical structures that transmit light: cornea, aqueous, lens, and vitreous.

ocularist (ok-yu-LEHR-ist) A professional who measures and fits patients with an artificial eye (prosthesis) to replace an absent eye or cover an unsightly one.

oculomotor nerve (Ok-yu-loh-MOH-ter) The third cranial nerve, which supplies the impulses that activate the superior, medial, and inferior rectus muscles, the inferior oblique muscle, and the levator palpebrae.

OD (oculus dexter) Latin for right eye.

ointment or gel The form of a drug in which the drug is dissolved or suspended in a greasy vehicle or a thickened water-soluble matrix.

opacification (oh-pass-ih-fih-KAY-shun) Clouding of a structure, as in the normally clear ocular media, most often seen in the cornea or lens; lenticular opacification (cataract) occurs in many people over age 65.

opaque Refers to a substance that completely blocks light.

ophthalmia neonatorum (ahf-THAL-mee-uh Nee-oh-nay-TOH-rum) Conjunctivitis in the newborn.

ophthalmic medical assistant (ahf-THAL-mik) A professional who assists the ophthalmologist in a variety of diagnostic and administrative tasks, including performing certain tests, administering certain topical medications or diagnostic drugs, and helping with office surgical procedures.

ophthalmic photographer A professional who photographs eye structures for diagnosis and documentation.

ophthalmic registered nurse A registered nurse with additional experience, education, and/or training in caring for patients with ophthalmic problems.

ophthalmologist (ahf-thal-MOL-uh-jist) A medical doctor (MD or DO) who specializes in the prevention, diagnosis, and medical as well as surgical treatment of vision problems and diseases of the eye.

ophthalmology (ahf-thal-MOL-uh-jee) The medical and surgical specialty concerned with the eye and its surrounding structures, their proper function, disorders, and all aspects of vision.

ophthalmometer (ahf-thal-MOM-uh-ter) *See* **keratometer**.

ophthalmoscope (ahf-THAL-muh-skohp) An instrument for examining directly or indirectly the vitreous and fundus.

optical center The point of optimal vision; the single point of a lens through which light may pass without being bent or changed (ie, refracted).

optical centers, distance between *See* **distance between optical centers**.

optical coherence tomography (OCT) A system used for analysis of the optic nerve head and retinal nerve fiber layer as well as the macular tissue layers by producing topographic images.

optical density A lens property that increases the effectiveness to bend light.

optical pachymeter (pah-KIM-eh-ter) A device for measuring corneal thickness using an optical system.

optical zone The major or central focusing area of the cornea or any lens.

optic chiasm (KY-azm) The point behind the eyes in the brain where the 2 optic nerves merge and the axon fibers from the nasal retina of each eye cross to the opposite side.

optic disc The location where the central retinal artery enters and the central retinal vein, as well as the nerve fibers, exit. Also called *optic nerve head*.

optic nerve The nerve that carries electric impulses to the brain's visual cortex, where they are integrated to produce the sensation of sight.

optic nerve head *See* **optic disc**.

optic neuritis (noo-RY-tis) Inflammation of the optic nerve; can produce a sudden, but reversible, loss of sight.

optic radiation The nerve fibers that transmit visual information from the lateral geniculate body to the visual cortex.

optic tract The part of the brain between the optic chiasm and the lateral geniculate body.

optician An independent professional licensed to dispense eyeglasses and contact lenses from the prescription of an ophthalmologist or optometrist.

optics The branch of physical science that deals with the properties of light and vision.

optometrist An independent practitioner trained in the prescription of eyeglasses and contact lenses as well as in the detection of eye disease.

optotypes, Snellen *See* **Snellen chart**.

oral drug delivery The delivery system by which a drug is taken by mouth.

oral Medications taken by mouth.

orbicularis oculi (or-bik-yu-LEHR-is OK-yu-liy) The circular muscle, located in the middle layer of the eyelids, that closes the eye when it contracts, as in winking.

orbit The bony cavity in the skull that houses the globe, extraocular muscles, blood vessels, and nerves. Also called *socket*.

orbital cellulitis A diffuse infection of tissues in the orbit, causing grossly swollen eyelids and red eye, sometimes without proptosis.

organic solvents Liquid substances that are derived from raw petroleum and from other volatile liquid agents.

orthophoric (or-thoh-FOR-ik) Refers to the absence of strabismic deviation; normal.

orthoptist (or-THOP-tist) A professional who works under the direction of an ophthalmologist to help with the diagnosis, management, and nonsurgical treatment of eye muscle imbalance and related visual impairments.

OS (oculus sinister) Latin for left eye.

oscilloscope An instrument box with a TV-type screen that displays the shape of an electric current or ultrasonic wave as seen with ultrasonography.

OSHA *See* **Occupational Safety and Health Administration**.

OU (oculus uterque) Latin for each eye.

oxygen permeable (Dk) The ability of a contact lens to transmit oxygen through its material.

pachymeter (pah-KIM-eh-ter) An instrument that measures the distance between the corneal epithelium and the corneal endothelium (corneal thickness). Sometimes spelled *pachometer*. *See also* **optical pachymeter**.

pachymetry (pah-KIM-eh-tree) The measurement of corneal thickness by the use of a pachymeter. Sometimes spelled *pachometry*.

palpation Medical examination by touch.

palpebral conjunctiva (PAL-peh-bruhl kon-junk-TY-vuh) The portion of the conjunctiva that lines the inner eyelids.

palpebral fissure (PAL-peh-bruhl) The almond-shaped opening between the upper and lower eyelids.

palsy (PAWL-zee) Paralysis or weakness of muscle function, usually due to nerve damage.

pantoscopic angle (pan-toh-SKOP-ik) The angle of an eyeglass frame by which the frame front deviates from the vertical plane when the glasses are worn.

papilledema (pap-il-eh-DEE-muh) A swelling of the optic disc with engorged blood vessels; caused by increased fluid pressure within the skull.

papoose board A padded board with Velcro straps; used for immobilizing an infant during an ophthalmologic examination.

paracentral scotoma (skoh-TOH-muh) A relatively blind area in the visual field, smaller than a Bjerrum scotoma, near the fixation point above or below the horizontal axis.

parallax (PAER-ah-laks) An optical distortion that occurs when the measurer's line of sight is not parallel to that of the patient.

parallel Refers to rays that travel side by side in the same direction, neither diverging nor converging.

paralytic strabismus A misalignment of the eyes when one or more extraocular muscles lose their nerve function (paralysis).

paraxial rays (paer-AK-see-ahl) Light rays that enter a lens system away from the center.

pathologic Abnormal or diseased.

PD *See* **interpupillary distance**.

PDT *See* **photodynamic therapy**.

perimetry (peh-RIM-eh-tree) The measurement of the expanse and sensitivity of peripheral vision and the visual field to pinpoint possible defects.

peripheral vision The visual perception of objects and space that surround the direct line of sight.

Perkins tonometer A handheld applanation tonometer.

phakic An eye with an intact natural crystalline lens.

phakic IOL An intraocular lens surgically implanted in the anterior or posterior chamber of the eye without removing the natural crystalline lens; usually performed to correct high myopia.

pharmacology (fahr-mah-KOL-uh-jee) The study of the medicinal use and actions of drugs (medications).

phenol red thread tear test A test that aids in the diagnosis of dry eyes and uses cotton threads treated with a pH indicator to measure the patient's tear production.

phoria (FOH-ree-uh) A tendency toward ocular misalignment that is held in check by the fusional effort of the extraocular muscles. *See* **esophoria, exophoria,** and **tropia**.

phoropter (foh-ROP-ter) *See* **refractor**.

photochromic (foh-toh-KROH-mik) Refers to a lens specially manufactured to be sensitive to ultraviolet light, so that it darkens in sunlight and lightens when not in sunlight.

photocoagulation (foh-toh-koh-ag-yu-LAY-shun) Use of a xenon or laser light beam to destroy tissue; among other uses, it is often used to treat abnormal leaking blood vessels (neovascularization) or to "weld" a retinal tear.

photodynamic therapy (PDT)   A treatment intended to reduce further vision loss from the "wet" form of age-related macular degeneration (AMD); the patient receives an intravenous injection (injection into a vein) of a light-sensitive substance, verteporfin (*Visudyne*), followed by "cold" laser stimulation of the verteporfin in the area of choroidal neovascularization, causing selective damage to the abnormal tissue.

photopic vision   Referring to the eyesight under daylight lighting conditions. *See also* **mesopic vision** and **scotopic vision**.

photoreceptor   A light-sensitive cell.

photorefractive keratectomy (PRK) (kehr-uh-TEK-tuh-mee)   A refractive surgical procedure that employs the excimer laser to reshape the corneal curvature after removing the epithelium.

phototherapeutic keratectomy (PTK)   An excimer laser is employed to ablate the anterior corneal surface to correct irregular astigmatism, scarring, or other superficial abnormalities.

physical optics   The study of optics that describes the nature of light in terms of its wave properties.

physiologic blind spot   The sightless "hole" in the normal visual field corresponding to the optic disc where there are no photoreceptors.

physiology   Literally, the study of the functions of the human body; refers to the processes by which an organism, cell, or anatomic structure functions.

pigment epithelium (ep-ih-THEE-lee-um)   The outer layer of the retina; lies against the choroid.

pinguecula (ping-GWEK-yu-luh; plural: pingueculae)   A thickened, benign, yellowish area of the bulbar conjunctiva on the temporal or nasal side of the cornea in the exposed portion of the eyeball. May precede pterygium.

pinhole occluder   The handheld device that completely covers one eye and allows the other to view a chart through a tiny central opening; often used to confirm a diagnosis of refractive error.

pink eye   *See* **conjunctivitis**.

placido disk (plah-SEE-doh)   A flat disk with alternating black and white rings encircling a small central aperture, used in evaluating the regularity of the anterior curvature of the cornea. With a normal corneal curvature, the rings are reflected without distortion.

plane   Flat.

planned-replacement lenses   Contact lenses that are designed to be replaced on a regular schedule determined by the ophthalmologist according to patient wearing characteristics and other factors.

plano lens   A lens without any ability to bend light rays; a zero power lens.

plano mirror effect (PLAY-noh)   The flat lighting effect of a retinoscope that produces slightly divergent rays.

pledget (PLEJ-eht)   A small tuft of cotton or other absorbent material that may be soaked with a liquid medication for a more prolonged application time to the surface of the eye; often used with topical anesthetic agents to achieve optimal anesthesia prior to minor surgical procedures.

plus lens   *See* **convex lens**.

PMMA   *See* **polymethylmethacrylate lenses**.

pneumatonometer (noo-mah-toh-NOM-uh-ter)   An instrument that uses compressed air and a piston-like wand to applanate the surface of the eyeball and measure the intraocular pressure.

pneumatoretinopexy (noo-mah-toh-reh-tih-NOP-pek-see)   A surgical procedure for correcting retinal detachment by injecting gas into the eye.

polarized   A specialized lens that reduces glare from a horizontal reflecting surfaces and protects against UV rays.

polycarbonate   A common plastic safety lens material that is resistant to shattering.

polymethylmethacrylate (PMMA) **lenses** (pol-ee-meth-il-meh-THAK-ril-ayt)   Contact lenses that provide oxygen by means of a tear pump only; no oxygen or carbon dioxide diffuses through the lens.

positive lens   *See* **convex lens**.

posterior   Toward the back.

posterior chamber   The space between the back of the iris and the front of the vitreous; the crystalline lens is suspended in this chamber, which is filled with aqueous fluid.

posterior segment   The rear portion of the eye; includes the vitreous and the retina.

posterior segment examination   *See* **funduscopic examination**.

posterior vitrectomy   *See* **vitrectomy**.

posterior vitreous detachment (PVD)   A separation of the posterior vitreous surface from the underlying retina that often occurs when the vitreous liquefies during aging, but may also be caused by certain diseases or trauma; symptoms may include increased floaters and/or photopsia (light flashes).

potential acuity meter   A device for determining visual acuity in the presence of media opacities.

power   *See* **vergence power**.

prepping   Short for preparing; the routines for cleansing a patient's surgical site prior to surgery.

presbyopia (prez-bee-OH-pee-uh) The progressive loss of the accommodative ability of the lens, due to natural processes of aging.

primary angle-closure glaucoma A form of glaucoma associated with a structural abnormality of the eye resulting in a shallow anterior chamber angle; also as the lens increases in size with aging, it blocks the flow of aqueous through the pupil, gradually causing the iris to bow forward until its outer edge blocks the aqueous outflow channels (pupillary block).

primary open-angle glaucoma A form of glaucoma in which the pressure inside the eye is elevated because of increased resistance to aqueous drainage in the outflow channels; accounts for 60% to 90% of all adult glaucoma.

principal axis The pathway of a light ray that strikes the center of a lens of any shape and passes undeviated through the lens material.

principal meridians The meridians of maximum and minimum corneal curvature.

principal ray *See* **axial ray**.

prions Extremely small pathologic protein elements responsible for brain disorders that occur in certain animals (eg, bovine spongiform encephalitis, or "mad cow disease") and humans (eg, variant Creutzfeldt-Jakob disease).

prism A triangular piece of glass or plastic with flat sides, an apex, and a base.

prism and alternative cover test A test to measure the quantity of ocular misalignment using prisms and an occluder.

prism diopter (dy-OP-tur) The unit of measure of the refractive power of a prism.

prismatic effect (priz-MAT-ik) An optical distortion in which images are displaced from their normal position; can occur if the distance between optical centers (DBC) does not correspond to the interpupillary distance (IPD).

PRK *See* **photorefractive keratectomy**.

prognosis (prog-NOH-sis) Prediction of the outcome of a medical condition.

progressive addition multifocals A spectacle lens with multiple areas of different focal points with no discrete visible lines dividing the various segments; rather, the optical power is added progressively in a transitional manner. Also called *progressive add multifocals*.

proliferative diabetic retinopathy Abnormal changes in the retina due to poorly controlled diabetes mellitus, manifested by the presence of hemorrhages, exudates, microaneurysms, and neovascularization. This is a more advanced stage of diabetic retinopathy.

proptosis (prop-TOH-sis) A condition characterized by a protruding eyeball; caused by an increase in volume of the orbital contents. Also called *exophthalmos*.

proteolytic Capable of dissolving protein.

protozoan (proh-toh-ZOH-an; plural: protozoa) A large, single-celled microbe found in fresh and salt water, soil, plants, insects, and animals.

pseudoisochromatic color plates (soo-doh-Iy-soh-kroh-MAT-ik) A book of plates that display patterns of colored and gray dots; used for evaluating color vision.

pseudophakia (soo-doh-FAY-kee-uh) The use of an intraocular lens to correct the vision of an aphakic patient.

pterygium (teh-RIJ-ee-um; plural: pterygia) A lesion of hypertrophied tissue that extends from the medial canthus onto the cornea.

PTK *See* **phototherapeutic keratectomy**.

ptosis (TOH-sis) Drooping of the upper eyelid most commonly caused by the levator muscle's inability to lift the eyelid to its full extent. May be congenital or acquired.

punctum (PUNK-tum; plural: puncta) The tiny opening on the upper eyelid margin (upper punctum) and lower eyelid margin (lower punctum) near the nose, through which tears pass.

punctum dilator Part of the lacrimal set; the instrument used for enlarging the punctum.

pupil The opening in the center of the iris that enlarges or dilates (admitting more light) and reduces or constricts (admitting less light).

pupillometry The measurement of pupillary diameters.

PVD *See* **posterior vitreous detachment**.

quadrant One of 4 quarters of the visual field: upper left, upper right, lower left, and lower right.

radial keratotomy (RK) (kehr-uh-TOT-uh-mee) A refractive surgical procedure that employs anterior radial incisions in the cornea to flatten its curvature and reduce myopia.

radial meridians Dividing sections radiating from the point of central fixation on a visual field chart.

reagent (ree-AY-jent) A special solution designed to react with a specific type of microorganism or chemical; used in microbiologic testing.

refinement   The subjective step of refractometry, requiring patient participation and responses, which confirms the information produced by retinoscopy. Also called *subjective refractometry* or *manifest refractometry*.

refracted   Refers to the change in directions of a light ray when it passes from one medium to another.

refraction   (1) In physics, the bending of a light ray as it passes through substances of different densities. (2) In eye care, the process of measuring a patient's refractive error and the clinical judgment to determine the optical correction needed.

refractive error   A nonpathologic deficiency in the eye's optical system.

refractive index   The ratio of the speed of light in a vacuum to its speed through a specific substance.

refractive state   The relative ability of the refractive components of the eye to bring objects into focus on the retina.

refractive surgery   A type of corneal surgery that modifies the shape of the cornea to correct some types of myopia, hyperopia, and astigmatism. *See also* **phakic IOL**.

refractometry (ree-frak-TOM-eh-tree)   The measurement of refractive error with a variety of instruments and techniques.

refractor   An instrument for determining a corrective lens prescription; stores a range of trial lenses that can be dialed into position. Also called phoropter or *Phoroptor* (brand name).

regular astigmatism (uh-STIG-muh-tizm)   The most common form of astigmatism, in which the cornea resembles a football standing on one end or on its side.

reservoir   An animate or inanimate object that provides a microorganism the means for survival and opportunity for transmission.

respiratory system   The structures primarily involved in exchanging oxygen and carbon dioxide; includes the nasal passages, trachea, bronchi, and lungs.

restrictive strabismus   An ocular misalignment caused by an extraocular muscle that is hindered or physically prevented from moving the eye.

retina (RET-in-uh)   The inner lining of the posterior segment of the eyeball; consists of a layer of light-sensitive cells that convert images from the optical system into electric impulses sent along the optic nerve for transmission to the brain.

retinal detachment   The separation of the sensory layer from the pigment layer of the retina; may be abbreviated RD. There are 3 causes: rhegmatogenous (tear or hole), traction (pulling off by scar tissue) and exudative (fluid accumulation).

retinal edema (Berlin's edema)   Swelling of the retina caused by blunt trauma to the retinal structures that results in release of fluid into the tissues.

retinal tear   A break in the retina. It can develop into a detachment.

retinitis pigmentosa (ret-ih-NY-tis pig-men-TOH-suh)   A hereditary, progressive retinal degeneration that may lead to blindness.

retinoscope (ret-ti-nuh-skohp)   A handheld instrument for measuring refractive error; consists of a light source and a viewing component. It is used with a phoropter or trial lenses.

retinoscopy (ret-tih-NAHS-kuh-pee)   The use of a retinoscope to determine a refractive error; the first step in refractometry. Also called *objective refractometry*.

retrobulbar (ret-roh-BUL-bar)   Behind the eye.

retrobulbar hemorrhage   Hemorrhage behind the eye.

retrobulbar visual pathway   *See* **visual pathway**.

retroscopic tilt   The tilt of an eyeglass frame adjusted so that the lower rim tilts away from the face.

RGP   *See* **rigid gas-permeable lenses**.

rhegmatogenous retinal detachment   *See* **retinal detachment**.

rigid gas-permeable (RGP) lenses   Contact lenses that permit oxygen and carbon dioxide diffusion through both the lens material and a tear pump.

RK   *See* **radial keratotomy**.

rod   The retinal photoreceptor largely responsible for vision in dim light (scotopic or "night vision") and for peripheral vision.

round-top segment   A portion of a circle fused or ground into a distance lens for near vision; may be used in bifocals and trifocals.

routine situation   A medical situation that usually can be scheduled for the next available routine office appointment time, within a few days or weeks.

rubeosis iridis (ru-bee-OH-sis IY-rid-is)   A condition in which the iris develops a reddish color due to neovascularization.

scanning laser polarimeter with variable corneal compensation (model GDx VCC)   A device that measures retinal nerve fiber layer (RNFL) thickness. The VCC (variable corneal compensation) model improves test results for detecting glaucoma.

Schiøtz tonometer (SHEE-ots)   An indentation contact tonometer that uses weights and a table of measurements based on the weight used to determine intraocular pressure.

Schirmer tear test (SHIR-mer)   A test that uses a strip of filter paper to measure the patient's tear output and helps to confirm the diagnosis of dry-eye conditions.

Schlemm's canal   *See* **canal of Schlemm**.

sclera (SKLEH-rah)   The outer fibrous tissue of the globe, which surrounds the cornea and forms the wall of the eye; protects intraocular contents.

scleral buckle (SKLEH-ral)   A surgical procedure for correcting retinal detachment that involves placing a block of silicone or other material on the sclera to indent the wall of the eye.

scleral rigidity   The resistance to stretching of the white fibrous outer layer of the eye.

scleritis (skleh-RY-tis)   Inflammation of the sclera.

scotoma (skoh-TOH-muh)   An area within the contours of the visual field where vision is reduced.

scotopic vision   Referring to the eyesight under dark-adapted conditions. *See also* **photopic vision** and **mesopic vision**.

seamless bifocal   *See* **invisible bifocal**.

secondary glaucoma (glaw-KOH-muh)   Glaucoma that occurs secondary to another, primary disease.

segment height   The distance between the lowest part of an eyeglass rim and the top of the multifocal lens segment.

segment   *See* **add**.

shallow scotoma (skoh-TOH-muh)   A mild visual field defect that appears as a depression in the island of vision.

short-wavelength automated perimetry (SWAP)   A perimetry examination using blue light stimuli on a yellow background. SWAP is considered a more sensitive visual field test than the standard achromatic perimetry (SAP) in identifying early glaucomatous visual field defects.

sign   An abnormal change observed objectively by the physician on examination of the patient.

sinus   A bony cavern of the skull that contains air and connects with the nasal passages.

slit lamp   An instrument used for close examination of the lids and lashes, cornea, lens, membranes, and clear fluids within the eye; consists of a microscope of low magnifying power and a light source that projects a rectangular beam that changes in size and focus. Also called *biomicroscope*.

Snellen acuity test   A measurement of visual acuity by testing the ability to read characters at a standard distance on a special target called the Snellen chart.

Snellen chart   A printed visual acuity chart consisting of Snellen optotypes—specially formed letters of the alphabet arranged in rows of decreasing letter size.

socket   *See* **orbit**.

soft lenses   Flexible contact lenses that permit oxygen and carbon dioxide diffusion through the lens material itself, with a minimal tear pump.

solution   The form of a drug in which the drug is completely dissolved in an inert liquid.

species (plural: species)   A category of biologic classification ranking immediately below the genus; the specific name for a type of organism.

spectacle blur   Temporary blurred vision upon switching from contact lenses to eyeglasses.

specular microscopy/photography   A method of microscopically photographing the cornea's endothelial cells at great magnification and producing photographs on which the cells can be counted.

sphere   *See* **spherical lens**.

spherical cornea (KOR-nee-uh)   A cornea (of the normal eye and most myopic and hyperopic eyes) whose curvature is uniform.

spherical lens   Also simply *sphere*. A concave or convex lens whose curvature is uniform, allowing it to focus light rays to a single point.

spherocylinder (sfee-roh-SIL-in-der)   Also simply *cylinder*. A combination of a spherical lens and a cylindrical lens. Sometimes called *toric lens*.

sphincter muscle (SFINGK-ter)   The muscle that encircles the pupil and makes the pupil smaller in response to bright light.

spore   A resting state of bacterium, protected by a heavy cell wall that permits the bacterium to survive for a long period of time until suitable conditions for growth occur.

standard precautions   A program of sanitation and microbial control in the medical office, intended to reduce the opportunity for harmful microbes to flourish and threaten patients and medical personnel. Includes the provisions of universal precautions and body substance isolation precautions. *See also* **universal precautions**.

static perimetry (peh-RIM-eh-tree)   The type of perimetry that uses a target that can be varied in size, brightness, and position within the visual field but is only displayed when stationary.

stereopsis (stehr-ee-OP-sis)   Three-dimensional visual perception.

sterile drapes   A large, sterile protective barrier sheet made of plastic, synthetic fiber, or cloth, placed around the part of the body that is to undergo surgery.

sterile operating field   The surgical area and the materials within that area that have undergone sterilization. Also called simply *sterile field*.

sterilization A process that utilizes heat or chemicals to destroy all living or dormant microorganisms.

steroid *See* **corticosteroid**.

strabismic amblyopia (struh-BIZ-mik am-blee-OH-pee-uh) The tendency of a child's brain to suppress the image from the deviating eye.

strabismus (struh-BIZ-mus) A misalignment of the eyes that may cause vision to be disturbed; occurs when the extraocular muscles do not work in a coordinated manner.

stroma, corneal *See* **corneal stroma**.

stye *See* **external hordeolum**.

subjective refractometry *See* **refinement**.

subconjunctival hemorrhage (sub-kon-junk-TY-vul HEM-or-ij) A rupture of a conjunctival blood vessel that allows blood to flow under the tissue and produces a bright-red flat area on the conjunctiva.

subjective refractometry *See* **refinement**.

super pinhole A pinhole occluder that helps to determine macular function in a patient with an opacity, such as a cataract.

superior oblique muscle Extraocular muscle attached to the upper, outer side of the globe; 3 functions are to rotate the eye downward and outward and to rotate inward.

superior rectus muscle Extraocular muscle attached to the upper side of the globe; 3 functions are to elevate the eye, turn the eye inward, and rotate the eye inward.

suppression The brain's mechanism to avoid double vision by ignoring the image from one eye. This can lead to amblyopia if not treated. The brain loses this ability after childhood.

suprathreshold static perimetry (soo-prah-THRESH-hold peh-RIM-eh-tree) A type of perimetry in which a light or target of a specific size, brightness, or intensity is chosen so that the patient should be able to see it when it is placed at a particular site in the visual field.

surfactant cleaner (sur-FAK-tant) A specialized contact lens cleaning solution and wetting agent.

suspension The form of a medication in which particles of the drug are suspended in a liquid vehicle.

suture (SOO-chur) To stitch a wound closed; the pattern of the stitch; or the thread-like material used to make the stitch.

SWAP *See* **short-wavelength automated perimetry**.

swinging-light test A test used to define normal binocular pupillary response to a light stimulus; the direct and consensual pupillary reaction. Also called *swinging-flashlight test*.

symptom A subjective abnormality that cannot be directly observed by another person but only perceived by the patient; examples include pain, blurred vision, or itching.

synapse (SIN-aps) The connection between nerves, where electric (nerve) impulses are transmitted.

syndrome A set of signs or symptoms that is characteristic of a specific condition or disease.

syringe (sih-RINJ) An instrument for injecting liquid into or withdrawing liquid from a blood vessel or cavity.

systemic drug delivery Intravenous, intramuscular, or subcutaneous injection or oral administration for absorption into the circulatory system.

tangent screen test A type of manual perimetry used for identifying visual field defects within 30° of a fixation point.

tarsal plate (TAHR-sal) *See* **tarsus**.

tarsus (TAHR-sus) The dense, plate-like framework within the middle layer of each eyelid that gives the eyelids their firmness and shape. Also called *tarsal plate*.

tear film The moist coating, composed of 3 layers, that covers the anterior surface of the globe.

temporal arteritis A systemic autoimmune disease with invasion of large inflammatory cells into arteries that can cause obstruction of the central retinal artery leading to blindness.

thermal trauma (TRAW-muh) Refers to injury that results in the burning or freezing of tissues.

threshold static perimetry The type of static perimetry in which the threshold is that level of brightness at which the patient can just detect a test object about half the time.

Titmus stereopsis test (stehr-ee-OP-sis) A test for determining whether the patient has fine depth perception in terms of binocular cooperation.

tomography A detailed mapping of the contours of a tissue or organ.

tonometer (toh-NOM-eh-ter) An instrument for measuring intraocular pressure.

tonometry (toh-NOM-eh-tree) The measurement of intraocular pressure by means of a tonometer; useful in the diagnosis of glaucoma.

Tono-Pen A portable electronic tonometer used to measure intraocular pressure.

topical application A route of drug administration in which the medication is applied to the surface of the eye or another body part; topically applied medications may be in the form of liquids, gels, or ointments.

toric cornea   A cornea whose surface curvature is not uniform. *See* **astigmatism**.

toric lens   *See* **spherocylinder**.

toxin (TOK-sin)   A poison.

toxoplasmosis   A protozoan organism that can infect the retina and the brain causing specific local lesions. If the lesion is on the macula, it can lead to loss of central vision.

trabecular meshwork (trah-BEK-yu-lar)   The sponge-like structure that filters the aqueous humor from the anterior chamber and controls its rate of flow out of the eye.

transilluminator   A small-tipped flashlight.

translucent   Refers to a substance that transmits light but significantly interferes with its passage.

transparent   Refers to a substance that permits the passage of light without significant disruption.

transposition   The conversion of a lens prescription from plus-cylinder form to minus-cylinder form or vice versa.

trauma (TRAW-muh)   Physical injury to body tissue from various causes, including force, toxins, or temperature extremes.

traumatic hyphema   Bleeding into the anterior chamber as a result of trauma.

traumatic iritis   A blunt injury to the iris causing inflammation; manifested by light sensitivity, conjunctival injection, and pupillary abnormality (miosis or mydriasis). *See also* **injection**.

traumatic optic neuropathy   Edema and vision loss resulting from a noninflammatory abnormality of the optic nerve caused by trauma.

triage (tree-AHZH)   The process of placing patients (screened in person or on the telephone) into a classification system according to need, with those having more serious problems in a different category than those with minor problems; the purpose is to ensure that patients are seen in a timely fashion, based on the severity of their problem.

trial frame   The frame into which various optical lenses are placed; used during refractometry.

trial lens set   A set of various hand-held lenses introduced before a patient's eye to select the appropriate corrective lens.

trichiasis (trih-KY-ah-sis)   An abnormality of the eyelid that causes eyelashes to turn in the wrong direction and rub against the surface of the eye.

trifocal lens   One that has 3 powers: one for correcting distance vision, one for correcting intermediate range of sight, and one for correcting near vision.

triphasic enzyme   A specialized cleaning agent that dissolves adhered substances on contact lenses.

tropia (TROH-pee-uh)   An obvious (manifest) misalignment of the eyes.

ultrasonic pachymeter (pah-KIM-eh-ter)   An instrument that measures corneal thickness, the distance between the corneal epithelium and endothelium by an ultrasonic probe.

ultrasonography (ul-trah-son-OG-ruh-fee)   A method of examination that uses the reflection (echo) of high-frequency sound waves to define the outline of ocular and orbital structures, measure the distance between structures, and identify abnormal tissues inside the eye or orbit.

unilateral proptosis   The forward protrusion of one eyeball from the eye socket.

universal precautions   An approach to infection control in which all human blood and certain human body fluids are treated as if known to be infectious for human immunodeficiency virus (HIV), hepatitis B virus (HBV), or other bloodborne pathogens; this approach is based on the concept that a medical history and examination cannot reliably identify all patients infected (or potentially infected) with a bloodborne pathogen, so the care of all patients should include these precautions.

upper lacrimal canaliculus   *See* **canaliculus**.

upper punctum   *See* **punctum**.

urgent situation   A medical situation, as defined by the American Academy of Ophthalmology, that requires attention within 24 to 48 hours.

uvea   *See* **uveal tract**.

uveal tract (YU-vee-al)   The pigmented layers of the eye (iris, ciliary body, and choroid) that contain the majority of the blood vessel supply. Also called *uvea*.

varicella-zoster virus (VZV) (vahr-ih-SEL-uh ZOS-ter)   A herpesvirus that produces chicken pox and the skin disease zoster, or shingles.

vascular endothelial growth factor (VEGF)   A protein substance that stimulates the formation of new blood vessels.

vascular occlusion   The obstruction of blood flow in a blood vessel.

VEGF   *See* **vascular endothelial growth factor**.

vehicle   The nonmedicinal portion of medication.

vergence power (VER-jens)   Also simply *power*. The measure of a lens's ability to converge or diverge light rays.

vertex distance (VER-teks)   The distance from the back surface of an eyeglass lens to the front surface of the cornea.

vertical meridians *See* **horizontal and vertical meridians**.

vertometer A device for measuring the distance between the posterior surface of an eyeglass lens and the anterior surface of the eyeball (ie, vertex distance), under a closed eyelid. This distance is especially important for high minus or plus eyeglass lens prescriptions. Also called distometer.

videokeratography A computerized technique to provide high-resolution, 3-dimensional topographic analysis of the corneal surface. *See* **corneal topography**.

virtual image The image formed by a concave lens when the paraxial rays from a distant source are refracted and diverge.

virus (plural: viruses) A microorganism smaller than the smallest bacterium that has no cellular structure and can cause infectious disease.

visual acuity (uh-KYU-ih-tee) The ability to discern fine detail.

visual acuity tests Distance and near tests to discern a patient's ability to see fine detail using letters or other symbols and determining the smallest identifiable object at a set distance.

visual cortex The area of the brain responsible for the initial conscious registration of visual information; the designation of electric (nerve) impulses from the retina.

visual field The full view seen by an eye that is fixating straight ahead. *See* **peripheral vision**.

visual field examination A test of the patient's full ability to see central and peripheral objects when the patient's gaze is fixated straight ahead.

visual pathway The route that is taken by light-generated nerve impulses after they leave the eye. Also called *retrobulbar visual pathway*.

vitrectomy The surgical removal of some or most of the vitreous. This can be accomplished by an *anterior* or *posterior* surgical approach.

vitreous (VIH-tree-us) The clear, jelly-like substance that fills the space behind the lens. Also called *vitreous body*.

VZV *See* **varicella-zoster virus**.

wavefront analysis The determination of higher order optical aberrations. The procedure measures optical errors other than those that can be detected with routine refraction. *See also* **aberrometry**.

"with motion" The retinoscopic reflex movement that is in the same direction as the movement of the streak of light from a retinoscope; typical of the hyperopic eye.

Worth 4-dot test A test for determining whether the eyes are perfectly aligned and whether the brain suppresses information from one eye.

yeast A form of fungus that produces creamy or pasty colonies.

zonule (ZOHN-yul) A transparent fiber that supports the lens by attaching to the ciliary body. Assists in the accommodative process. *See* **accommodation**.

Appendix B   RESOURCES

This section highlights some of the many organizations that mobilize efforts to combat blindness and promote eye care in developing countries, where medical resources may be scarce.

American Academy of Ophthalmology

www.aao.org

The American Academy of Ophthalmology provides a wide variety of programs, products, and services to Eye M.D.s and the patients they serve. For example, Smart-Sight™ is an initiative to assist patients who have visual acuities of 20/40 or scotomas, field loss, or contrast loss. The program has downloadable information for patients and physicians concerning visual rehabilitation. The EyeSmart® public awareness campaign aims to help people know their risk factors for eye diseases, infections, and injuries, and to understand how ophthalmologists can help prevent, diagnose, and treat eye conditions. Among the programs of the Foundation of the American Academy of Ophthalmology, the Foundation's International Assistance program contributes to the education of ophthalmologists in developing nations and facilitates international volunteerism. Each year the Academy provides hundreds of boxes of educational materials to ophthalmology residency programs in developing countries. The EyeCare Volunteer Registry connects eye care professionals who are interested in becoming international volunteers with organizations and institutions seeking ophthalmic volunteers.

American Foundation for the Blind

www.afb.org

The American Foundation for the Blind is committed to expanding possibilities for people with vision loss. The organization's website has links regarding support groups and employment for the visually impaired in addition to information for health care workers. There is also a searchable "Directory of Services" database that contains information on more than 1,500 organizations and agencies that serve people who are blind or visually impaired. It compiles listings of schools, agencies, organizations, and programs in the governmental and private nonprofit sectors that provide direct and indirect services, information, and other assistance to blind and visually impaired children and adults, their families, and professionals who work with them.

Aravind Eye Care System

www.aravind.org

The mission of the Aravind Eye Care System (AECS) is to eliminate needless blindness by providing compassionate and high-quality eye care for all. AECS comprises a network of eye hospitals, a comprehensive outreach network, an education and training facility (LAICO) exclusively to teach and train eye care workers, a manufacturing facility (Aurolab) that provides high-quality ophthalmic supplies at costs affordable to developing economies, and an eye bank. In the year ending March 2010, more than 2.5 million outpatients were treated and more than 300,000 eye surgeries were performed.

The Carter Center

www.cartercenter.org

The Carter Center's international health programs focused on visual health include the River Blindness Program and the Trachoma Program. Through the River Blindness Program, The Carter Center has assisted in the delivery of more than 70 million treatments of Mectizan in Africa and Latin America as of January 2006. The Trachoma Control Program has 7 programs in 6 African countries that work with Ministries of Health to fight blinding trachoma.

Christian Blind Mission

www.cbm.org

Christian Blind Mission (CBM) is an international Christian organization that is committed to improving the quality of life of people with visual, hearing, physical, or intellectual disabilities in the poorest countries of the world. CBM supports more than 1,000 projects in more than 100 countries, working in 4 major ways: prevention, treatment, education/rehabilitation, and economic empowerment. CBM works closely with organizations like the World Health Organization (WHO) to understand where the greatest needs are and develop initiatives like VISION 2020, with the goal of eliminating world blindness by the year 2020. The international headquarters is in Bensheim, Germany, with affiliate offices in 10 countries, including the United States.

Dana Center for Preventive Ophthalmology

www.hopkinsmedicine.org/wilmer/ danacenter

The Dana Center for Preventive Ophthalmology, part of the Wilmer Eye Institute, is a joint collaboration of The Johns Hopkins University School of Medicine and The Bloomberg School of Public Health. The Center is dedicated to improving knowledge of risk factors for ocular disease and public health approaches to the prevention of these diseases. It is a collaborating center for WHO, providing consultation and expertise in blindness and vision care programs in every part of the world. The Public Health Ophthalmology program is designed to help eye care professionals to develop skills in applying public health principles to blindness prevention.

Fred Hollows Foundation

www.hollows.org

The Fred Hollows Foundation is inspired by the work of the late professor Fred Hollows, an ophthalmologist who became known for his work helping to restore the eyesight of countless thousands of people in developing countries around the world. Today the Foundation facilitates international eye health programs in Africa, Asia, Australia, and the Pacific. It works to achieve 4 key goals: ending avoidable blindness in the communities and countries where the Foundation works; improving the life chances and choices of Indigenous Australians through improving their health; working through strong partnerships and cross-sector collaborations at local, national and global levels; and building a strong and dynamic organization.

Helen Keller International

www.hki.org

The mission of Helen Keller International (HCI) is to save the sight and lives of the most vulnerable and disadvantaged people. HCI combats the causes and consequences of blindness and malnutrition by establishing programs based on evidence and research in vision, health, and nutrition. HCI operates in Africa, Asia, and the Americas, encompassing 25 nations and directly benefiting millions of people each year. The major areas of focus are eye health and health and nutrition. In addition, HCI promotes timely detection of eye problems, with an emphasis on childhood and adult cataract, in order to provide efficient delivery of intervention. They train surgeons, nurses, and community health workers, and develop basic eye health education programs with government counterparts and local nongovernmental organizations, also providing the equipment and technology necessary for program implementation.

Himalayan Cataract Project

www.cureblindness.org

The Himalayan Cataract Project (HCP) works to eradicate preventable and curable blindness through high-quality ophthalmic care, education, and the establishment of a world-class eye care infrastructure. Today HCP reaches the most unreachable patients wherever its services are needed through a combination of teaching ophthalmic care at all levels; furthering specialized care through training and skills transfer, country by country; establishing self-sustaining eye care centers; and performing sutureless cataract operations in 6 to 7 minutes, at a low cost, with excellent outcomes. Since 1994, more than 100 doctors have been trained in modern cataract surgery and more than 100 ophthalmic assistants and nurses have been trained. On a yearly basis, more than 200,000 patients are screened, and between 12,000 and 15,000 cataract surgeries are performed.

International Agency for the Prevention of Blindness

www.vision2020.org

The International Agency for the Prevention of Blindness (IAPB) is a coordinating, umbrella organization established to lead international efforts in blindness prevention activities. Its first major achievement was to promote the establishment of the World Health Organization program for the prevention of blindness, with which it has remained strongly linked, and which is now embodied in the global initiative, VISION 2020: The Right to Sight. The launch of VISION 2020 has led to concerted international effort in advocacy, resource mobilization, joint planning, strengthening national capacities through human resource development, and the transfer of appropriate technologies to developing countries.

International Centre for Eye Health

www.iceh.org.uk

The International Centre for Eye Health (ICEH) is a Research and Education group based at the London School of Hygiene & Tropical Medicine. The organization works to improve eye health and eliminate avoidable visual impairment and blindness, with a focus on low income populations. ICEH research aims to provide information of value for the cost effective implementation of VISION 2020: The Right to Sight. Research studies encompasses epidemiological studies, operational research, health economics, and qualitative research.

International Council of Ophthalmology

www.icoph.org

The International Council of Ophthalmology (ICO) works with ophthalmologic societies and others to enhance ophthalmic education and improve access to the highest-quality eye care in order to preserve and restore vision for the people of the world. Programs include the World Ophthalmology Congress; international basic science assessment and clinical sciences assessment for ophthalmologists; international fellowships; international clinical guidelines; international standards for

vision, eye care, and ophthalmology; research agenda for global blindness prevention; Vision for the Future, the international ophthalmology strategic plan to preserve and restore vision; advocacy for preservation of vision; and various ophthalmic education initiatives.

International Eye Foundation

www.iefusa.org

The International Eye Foundation (IEF), founded in 1961, is dedicated to the prevention of blindness in developing countries seeking to eliminate the causes of avoidable blindness: cataract, trachoma, onchocerciasis, and childhood blindness; reduce the cost of eye care in developing countries; and create a network of highly efficient, productive, and self-sustaining eye hospitals that treat all persons. Its sight-saving programs have benefited more than 60 developing nations—where 90% of the world's blindness exists. Visit the website for more information about IEF successes and programs.

Kilimanjaro Centre for Community Ophthalmology

www.KCCO.net

The Kilimanjaro Centre for Community Ophthalmology (KCCO) is dedicated to the elimination of avoidable blindness through programs, training, and research, focusing on the delivery of sustainable and replicable community ophthalmology services. KCCO aims to build the capacity of eastern Africans to provide high-quality eye services to meet the needs of the population; develop internationally recognized educational programs; and develop a teaching and research environment that promotes health care measures beneficial to Tanzania and surrounding countries. The KCCO is part of Tumaini University and is associated with the Department of Ophthalmology at the Kilimanjaro Christian Medical College (KCMC) in Moshi, Tanzania.

Korat Institute of Public Health Ophthalmology

www.mnrh.go.th

The Korat Institute of Public Health Ophthalmology was established in 1984 by the Ministry of Public Health of

Thailand. It is attached to Maharat Nakhon Ratchasima Regional Hospital, about 175 miles northeast of Bangkok. The Korat Institute serves as the headquarters for the national program for prevention of blindness and serves as a regional training center for Southeast Asia and the western Pacific World Health Organization region. The Korat Institute is a model center for technical cooperation in developing countries in the areas of eye care, personnel training, and training in management.

Lighthouse International

www.lighthouse.org

Lighthouse International is dedicated to fighting vision loss through prevention, treatment, and empowerment. The organization's programs and services include a low vision center, specialized services, early intervention program, youth services, career and academic services, vision rehabilitation services, occupational therapy, orientation and mobility instruction, social services, assistive technology services, diabetes services, geriatric services, and a print access center. Its 3 schools offer diverse educational opportunities. In addition, the Arlene R. Gordon Research Institute engages in research that benefits low-vision populations; develops methodologies and training programs that maximize sight among low vision populations; and partners with government agencies, businesses, and nonprofits on initiatives and technologies to enhance low vision function.

Lions Club International Foundation

www.lcif.org/EN

Lions Clubs International Foundation (LCIF) is the grant-making arm of Lions Clubs International. Many LCIF grants help the visually impaired or deal with blindness prevention. Begun in 1989, LCIF's SightFirst program is the Lions' main blindness prevention initiative. SightFirst projects typically focus on strengthening eye care infrastructures and eye health delivery systems, training eye care workers, and intervening against the major blinding diseases. SightFirst assists in restoring sight to the cataract blind, provides support for onchocerciasis programs, supports capital construction and renovation of eye clinics and hospitals, and works with local and national organizations to provide training for eye health care workers. SightFirst works in collaboration with the WHO to expand the effort to reduce the prevalence and incidence of blindness in children.

LV Prasad Eye Institute

www.lvpei.org

LV Prasad Eye Institute (LVPEI), Hyderbrand, India, is a center of excellence in eye care services and basic and clinical research into vision-threatening conditions. The institute also focuses on modes of management, training, product development and rehabilitation for those with incurable visual disability. The main focus of all areas of work at LVPEI is to extend equitable and efficient eye care to all in need of care, especially disadvantaged populations in the developing world. LVPEI is a WHO Collaborating Center in the area of blindness prevention, and houses the IAPB Central Office.

Mercy Ships

www.mercyships.org

Mercy Ships is a global charity that has operated hospital ships in developing nations since 1978. As specialists on board, Mercy Ships ophthalmic surgeons perform free, critical eye surgeries providing patients renewed sight and improved quality of life. Community-based eye clinics provide basic eye care to treat acute problems and prevent blindness. Short-term crew can volunteer from 2 weeks to 2 years depending on the position and typically fill service roles or very specialized medical or technical positions. The ability to utilize professional volunteers as crew allows Mercy Ships to maximize donor support and serve those who need help the most.

Nadi Al Bassar

www.nadialbassar.planet.tn

Nadi Al Bassar, Tunisia, was conceived in 1981. It began as a small Center for Ophthalmology and Visual Science mainly for residents and ophthalmology students. Prevention of blindness soon became the main objective. The discovery, in 1982, that 33% of the pupils at the School of the Blind were partially sighted led to the foundation of the low vision clinic, which offers free consultations. Nadi Al Bassar developed rapidly as a national nongovernmental organization dedicated to the prevention of blindness and restoration of sight, one of the first to be thus established in a developing nation.

ORBIS International

www.orbis.org

ORBIS International is a nonprofit organization fighting blindness in developing countries, where it works with its local partners to establish comprehensive, affordable and sustainable eye care. The ORBIS Flying Eye Hospital is literally a hospital with wings, where local doctors, nurses and technicians work alongside ORBIS's international medical team to exchange knowledge and improve skills. In 2011, FedEx donated an MD-10 cargo aircraft to ORBIS to be the third-generation Flying Eye Hospital. ORBIS also conducts training in adult and pediatric ophthalmology at local hospitals and through the awarding of fellowships. Another ORBIS International initiative is Cyber-Sight, a telemedicine program providing ophthalmologists in developing countries the opportunity to connect with expert mentors through online consultation and education.

Francis I. Proctor Foundation for Research in Ophthalmology

www.proctor.ucsf.edu

Established in 1947, the Francis I. Proctor Foundation for Research in Ophthalmology is an internationally renowned, privately endowed Organized Research Unit at the University of California, San Francisco Medical Center. The Foundation is dedicated to research and training in infectious and inflammatory ocular diseases, and the application of this research to the prevention of blindness worldwide. Ninety percent of blind and visually disabled individuals are in developing countries where health care resources and research facilities are most limited. This is a primary area of the Foundation's research activity. The overall mission of the Proctor Foundation is three-fold: education, patient care, and research.

Seva Foundation

www.seva.org

Seva Foundation was founded in 1978 by a group of former WHO smallpox campaign workers and their friends. They came together to prevent and relieve suffering through compassionate and effective action. The Sight Programs, which are among the most enduring of Seva's activities, focus on direct eye care services, sustainable eye care programs, and the Center for Innovation in Eye Care. Seva supports local hospitals and clinics in many developing countries, helping them to provide basic eye care, surgeries, eye exams and glasses at little or no cost. Seva also trains local people to provide care to their own communities. Seva is an active member of the VISION 2020 initiative.

Sight Savers International

www.sightsavers.org

Since 1950, Sight Savers International (SSI), previously known as the Royal Commonwealth Society for the Blind, has been working with local partners to combat blindness in developing countries. Working with partners in 2010, SSI helped to protect more than 23 million people against river blindness, perform more than 270,000 sight-restoring cataract operations, and treat more than a million people with antibiotics for trachoma. Sight Savers International is a founding member of VISION 2020. SSI works with local partners in 30 of the poorest countries in the world to ensure that services are developed that are appropriate to local needs.

Surgical Eye Expeditions International

www.seeintl.org

Surgical Eye Expeditions (SEE) International, founded in 1974, is a nonprofit, humanitarian organization that provides medical, surgical, and educational services by volunteer ophthalmic surgeons. Its primary objective is restoring sight to disadvantaged blind individuals worldwide. At the invitation of eye surgeons in developing countries, and with the approval of local health and civic authorities, SEE International recruits, organizes, and deploys numerous small surgical teams worldwide. In addition to surgeons, teams include registered nurses with ophthalmic experience, certified ophthalmic technicians, surgical technicians, and equipment technicians. Since 1974, SEE International's eye surgeons have examined more than 3 million patients and performed over 384,000 sight-restoring operations.

Unite For Sight

www.uniteforsight.org

Unite For Sight was founded in 2000 by Jennifer Staple-Clark in her dorm room when she was a sophomore at Yale University. As of 2011, Unite For Sight's programs in Ghana, Honduras, and India have provided high-quality care to more than 1,200,000 of the world's poorest people, including more than 44,000 sight-restoring surgeries. The eye care is provided by local eye doctors. Since 2003, Unite For Sight has trained more than 7,900 fellows to eliminate preventable blindness in their local communities and abroad. The organization's ongoing research programs are designed to continually enhance global health delivery, both with eye clinic partners and on a broad scale.

Vision Health International

www.visionhealth.org

Even the most basic vision care is out of reach for most in rural Latin America, where there is perhaps one ophthalmologist for every 350,000 people, and where unemployment, lack of insurance, malnutrition, and the burden of poverty compound an already serious medical problem. Ophthalmologist Rodney E. Abernathy, MD, recognized the need for accessible and affordable vision health services in the developing countries of Latin America. As a tribute to his memory and his pioneering work, Vision Health International (VHI) was founded in 1985. VHI volunteer medical teams have provided more than 15,000 eye exams, dispensed more than 13,000 pairs of eyeglasses, and performed more than 3,000 sight-restoring surgical procedures in Costa Rica, The Dominican Republic, Ecuador, Guatemala, Honduras, Nicaragua, Peru, and Poland.

World Health Organization

www.who.int/en

Established in 1948, the World Health Organization (WHO) is the directing and coordinating authority for health within the United Nations system. It is responsible for providing leadership on global health matters, shaping the health research agenda, setting norms and standards, articulating evidence-based policy options, providing technical support to countries and monitoring and assessing health trends. Recently, the WHO website featured detailed information on more than 200 WHO programs, partnerships, and other projects.

The WHO Program for the Prevention of Blindness was created in 1978 following a resolution adopted by the World Health Assembly in 1975. Examples of key partnerships in this program include VISON 2020, a global partnership between WHO and the International Agency for the Prevention of Blindness (IAPB) aiming to eliminate avoidable blindness by the year 2020. GET 2020, which aims to eliminate blinding trachoma by 2020, is a partnership WHO, U.N. member states, nongovernmental organizations, foundations, and industry engaged in the control and elimination of blinding trachoma. The project on Prevention of Avoidable Childhood Blindness is financially supported by the Lions Clubs International Foundation's SightFirst Initiative. The NGDO Coordination Group for onchocerciasis control coordinates the activities of the main international and national nongovernmental developmental organizations involved in the control of onchocerciasis, mainly in Africa but also in Latin America. Visit the website for more information on the broad range of WHO activities.

INDEX

Murocel, 86
Muscle balance, 120
My Eye Career for Ophthalmic Medical
  Technicians, 6t
Myasthenia gravis, 40, 40f
Mycobacteria, 95
Mycobacterium tuberculosis, 99
Mydfrin. *See* Phenylephrine
Mydriacyl. *See* Tropicamide
Mydriatics
  cycloplegics vs, 80
  description of, 78
  reversal drops for, 80
Myopia
  concave lens correction of, 180f
  description of, 54, 54f, 274–275
  prescription for, 63
  refraction in, 274–275
Myopic astigmatism, 55f

N
Nasal lacrimal duct probing and irrigation,
  263t
Nasolacrimal duct, 14
Natamycin. *See* Natacyn
Natacyn, 84
Nd:YAG laser, 325–326
Near acuity test, 116–117, 119f, 119p
Near refraction, 275
Near visual acuity
  definition of, 200
  test of, 116–117, 119f, 119p
Nearsightedness. *See* Myopia
Nedocromil, 86
Needle(s), 257–258, 258f, 260, 260f
Needle holders, 259, 259f
Needlesticks, 105
Neisseria gonorrhoeae, 95
Neomycin-polymyxin B-bacitracin, 84
Neomycin-polymyxin B-dexamethasone, 84
Neomycin-polymyxin B-gramicidin, 84
Neomycin-polymyxin B-hydrocortisone, 84
Neomycin-polymyxin B-prednisone, 84
Neonatal conjunctivitis, 95, 95f
Neoplasm
  benign, 25
  definition of, 25
  malignant, 25
Neoplastic diseases, 45–46
Neosporin ointment. *See* Neomycin-
  polymyxin B-bacitracin
Neosporin ophthalmic solution. *See*
  Neomycin-polymyxin B-gramicidin
Neo-Synephrine. *See* Phenylephrine
Neovascular net, 34
Neovascularization, 33, 154
Nepafanc, 85
Neptazane. *See* Methazolamide
Nervous system, 39
Neutralization
  definition of, 64
  of progressive addition lenses, 182
Neutralization point, 60
Nevanac. *See* Nepafanc
Nevi, 30

Nizoral. *See* Ketoconazole
Nonabsorbable sutures, 257
Nonsteroidal anti-inflammatory drugs, 85
Nystagmus, 27

O
Objective refractometry, 59
Objective refractors, 64
Objective/subjective refractor, 64
Occluded, 24
Occupational Exposure to Bloodborne
  Pathogens, 100, 101p
Occupational Safety and Health
  Administration, 290
Ocufen. *See* Flurbiprofen
Ocuflox. *See* Ofloxacin
Ocular histoplasmosis, 45
Ocular media, 149
Ocular motility. *See* Motility
Ocularist, 3
Oculomotor nerve
  description of, 139
  paralysis of, 27
Oculus dexter, 63
Oculus sinister, 63
Ocupress. *See* Carteolol
OD. *See* Oculus dexter
Office waiting periods, 242–243
Officer manager, 286
Ofloxacin, 84
Oil, 318
Ointments
  application of, 79p
  definition of, 77
Older adults. *See* Elderly
Olopatadine, 86
Onchocerca volvulus, 100
Onchocerciasis, 100, 309
Opacification, 16
Opacities
  definition of, 149
  vision tests for patients with, 150–151
Opaque, 50
Open-angle glaucoma
  description of, 32, 32f
  low vision caused by, 200
  miotics for, 82
Ophthaine. *See* Proparacaine
Ophthalmia neonatorum, 29
Ophthalmic history
  areas of, 113t
  chief complaint, 111–112, 113t, 294
  family, 113t, 114, 294
  form for, 111, 112f
  guidelines for, 114, 243–244
  history of present illness, 111–112, 113t,
    294
  overview of, 111
  past ocular history, 113, 113t, 294
  purpose of, 111
Ophthalmic medical assistant
  attitude of, 287
  certification as, 4–5
  commitment by, 287–288
  communication by, 241–242

continuing education for, 5
definition of, 4
ethics for, 298–301
expectations, 288
greeting by, 227–228, 243–244
hygiene by, 105
informed consent, 300–301
patient interactions with, 227, 245
professional development of, 5–6
responsibilities of, 4, 283
teamwork by, 284
time management by, 287–288
Ophthalmic photographer, 3–4
Ophthalmic Photographers Society, 5, 6t
Ophthalmic photography
  external, 153
  purpose of, 153
  slit-lamp photography, 153, 154f
Ophthalmologic subspecialists, 3
Ophthalmological services, 294–295
Ophthalmologist
  description of, 2
  pediatric, 3
  referral to, 114
  responsibilities of, 2–3
  subspecialists, 3
  time management, 285–286
  training of, 2
Ophthalmology, 1
Ophthalmometer, 68, 320. *See also*
  Keratometer
Ophthalmoscope
  description of, 1, 2f
  direct, 130, 131f, 324, 324f
  indirect, 130, 131f, 324–325, 325f
Ophthalmoscopy
  definition of, 111, 130
  direct, 130, 131f
  indirect, 130, 131f
Ophthetic. *See* Proparacaine
Opportunistic infections, 44, 95
Optic atrophy, 18
Optic chiasm, 19, 19f, 160
Optic disc, 18, 18f
Optic nerve
  abnormalities of, 34–35
  anatomy of, 10, 10f
  central scotoma caused by damage to,
    172, 175f
  imaging of, 155–156, 156f
Optic nerve head, 18
Optic neuritis, 35
Optic neuropathy, traumatic, 234
Optic radiations, 19, 19f
Optic tracts, 19, 19f
Optical center, 68
  checking of, 194, 195p
  definition of, 186, 194
  distance between, 187, 188, 194
Optical coherence tomography, 154, 155f
Optical density, 50
Optical pachymeters, 128, 152, 152f
Optical prescriptions
  contact lens specification vs, 209
  for hyperopia, 63